Springer Series on Epidemiology and Public Health

Series Editors

Wolfgang Ahrens, BIPS, Leibniz Institute, Bremen, Germany

Iris Pigeot, Bremen, Germany

The series has two main aims. First, it publishes textbooks and monographs addressing recent advances in specific research areas. Second, it provides comprehensive overviews of the methods and results of key epidemiological studies marking cornerstones of epidemiological practice, which are otherwise scattered across numerous narrow-focused publications. Thus the series offers in-depth knowledge on a variety of topics, in particular, on epidemiological concepts and methods, statistical tools, applications, epidemiological practice and public health. It also covers innovative areas such as molecular and genetic epidemiology, statistical principles in epidemiology, modern study designs, data management, quality assurance and other recent methodological developments. Written by the key experts and leaders in corresponding fields, the books in the series offer both broad overviews and insights into specific areas and topics. The series serves as an in-depth reference source that can be used complementarily to the "The Handbook of Epidemiology," which provides a starting point of orientation for interested readers (2nd edition published in 2014 http://www.springer.com/public+health/book/978-0-387-09835-7). The series is intended for researchers and professionals involved in health research, health reporting, health promotion, health system administration and related aspects. It is also of interest for public health specialists and researchers, epidemiologists, physicians, biostatisticians, health educators, and students worldwide.

Hajo Zeeb • Laura Maaß
Tanja Schultz • Ulrike Haug
Iris Pigeot • Benjamin Schüz
Editors

Digital Public Health

Interdisciplinary Perspectives

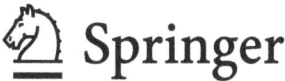

Editors
Hajo Zeeb
Leibniz Institute for Prevention Research
and Epidemiology - BIPS
Bremen, Germany

Tanja Schultz
Cognitive Systems Lab
University of Bremen
Bremen, Germany

Iris Pigeot
Leibniz Institute for Prevention Research
and Epidemiology - BIPS
Bremen, Germany

Laura Maaß
SOCIUM - Research Center on Inequality
and Social Policy
University of Bremen
Bremen, Germany

Ulrike Haug
Leibniz Institute for Prevention Research
and Epidemiology - BIPS
Bremen, Germany

Benjamin Schüz
Institute of Public Health and Nursing
Research
University of Bremen
Bremen, Germany

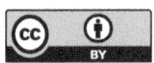

ISSN 1869-7933   ISSN 1869-7941   (electronic)
Springer Series on Epidemiology and Public Health
ISBN 978-3-031-90153-9   ISBN 978-3-031-90154-6   (eBook)
https://doi.org/10.1007/978-3-031-90154-6

The work was supported by the Leibniz ScienceCampus Digital Public Health Bremen (www.digital-public-health.de), which is jointly funded by the Leibniz Association (W4/2018), the Federal State of Bremen and the Leibniz Institute for Prevention Research and Epidemiology – BIPS. This publication was partly funded by the Publication fund of the Leibniz Association.

© The Editor(s) (if applicable) and The Author(s) 2025. This book is an open access publication.
Open Access This book is licensed under the terms of the Creative Commons Attribution 4.0 International License (http://creativecommons.org/licenses/by/4.0/), which permits use, sharing, adaptation, distribution and reproduction in any medium or format, as long as you give appropriate credit to the original author(s) and the source, provide a link to the Creative Commons license and indicate if changes were made.
The images or other third party material in this book are included in the book's Creative Commons license, unless indicated otherwise in a credit line to the material. If material is not included in the book's Creative Commons license and your intended use is not permitted by statutory regulation or exceeds the permitted use, you will need to obtain permission directly from the copyright holder.
The use of general descriptive names, registered names, trademarks, service marks, etc. in this publication does not imply, even in the absence of a specific statement, that such names are exempt from the relevant protective laws and regulations and therefore free for general use.
The publisher, the authors and the editors are safe to assume that the advice and information in this book are believed to be true and accurate at the date of publication. Neither the publisher nor the authors or the editors give a warranty, expressed or implied, with respect to the material contained herein or for any errors or omissions that may have been made. The publisher remains neutral with regard to jurisdictional claims in published maps and institutional affiliations.

This Springer imprint is published by the registered company Springer Nature Switzerland AG
The registered company address is: Gewerbestrasse 11, 6330 Cham, Switzerland

If disposing of this product, please recycle the paper.

Foreword

Digital public health is changing the practice and policy of public health. Digital innovations and applications such as electronic health records, mobile health apps, wearable devices, social media monitoring, personalized medicine, and social data analytics have become hot topics. The opportunities to improve the health and welfare of many—particularly vulnerable populations that are typically ill-served—are impressive. In the wake of the COVID-19 pandemic, some might be most grateful for digital tools' power and effectiveness to survey diseases and predict population outbreaks. Others are most interested in their potential to manage chronic diseases better and growing non-communicable lifestyle challenges, such as obesity. People interested in reducing health inequality and inequity praise the digital tools' potential for increased and simplified access to healthcare services, especially in underserved areas in the Global South and for vulnerable groups worldwide. Those focused on the cost–benefit of health interventions pin their hopes on highly effective personalized interventions designed and tailored to individual needs. Researchers, healthcare professionals, and policymakers have recognized the potential offered by large amounts of high-quality health data. This data is a welcome source of information for health policy and provides the necessary evidence base for interventions. And not very long ago, most of us witnessed, for the first time, the enormous power of artificial intelligence, such as ChatGPT, watching with awe and realizing that the possibilities of digital tools and methods for public health are only in their infancy. Much is still to come in ever-shorter innovation cycles.

Despite these bright looming promises, there is also widespread skepticism around the—largely non-intended, yet hardly avoidable—side effects and social costs that digital public health might bring. The most debated risks of digital health technologies are privacy and security concerns around collecting and sharing sensitive personal data and the fear of biases in data collection and analyses that potentially lead to (or fortify) healthcare access and therapies inequalities. Some voices deplore the field's systemic lack of adequate regulatory oversight, which seems almost impossible to overcome in the notorious "hare and hedgehog race" between fast-paced digitalization and notoriously slow policy processes. Digital sovereignty and autonomy are at stake in public health as in other sectors of society. Moreover, many fear some estrangement from medical care as a human-centered and human-delivered service, the fear of robots, and uncontrollable algorithms taking control of the individual without nuance and empathy. Or even making momentous mistakes that humans allegedly would not have made. Linked to this fear is the risk that healthcare providers may become overly reliant on technology and miss out on learning and developing critical thinking and judgment, for instance, in diagnosis. Pointing to the high cost and needed skill level of digital medical applications, some people also regard digital public health as a threat, rather than a solution, to health inequality worldwide where digital literacy is less pronounced.

This is the backdrop against which this volume on *Digital Public Health* has been developed. This book results from a multi-year interdisciplinary engagement of dozens of public health experts from various social science and science disciplines within a unique research initiative, the Leibniz ScienceCampus Digital Public Health Bremen. The book skillfully compiles over 30 chapters covering many of the abovementioned issues. The first chapters provide novel theoretical approaches to key aspects of digital public health, such as Open Data Science, participation in digital health interventions, and the big questions of evaluation of the latter. The second part compiles papers discussing cross-cutting issues, such as European and global perspectives on regulation and policies, digital health inequality, and literacy. Practical case studies and discussions of concrete digital applications and core themes follow these more conceptual chapters. The authors carefully carve out the specific opportunities and limits, discuss what politics needs to do to create a welfare-creating balance, and develop suggestions on how to unleash the potential of digital tools without harming digital sovereignty. The next part collects chapters on technologies and software engineering in public health, again sharing innovative approaches and weighing costs and benefits.

This work shows that digital public health interventions are highly promising yet still in their infancy. Therefore, we understand that they must be carefully designed, ideally in a participative way, to reduce fears and improve effectiveness and acceptance. And that they have to be permanently evaluated to ensure learning and improvement, to hold unintended consequences at bay, and avoid mistrust and backlash in society.

Overall, this volume mirrors the Leibniz Science Campus's successful and impactful interdisciplinary work, which I was lucky enough to accompany for the past years. I thank the editors and all authors for the immense work pulling all the learnings together for a comprehensive and precious resource.

El-Erian Professor for Behavioural Economics and Policy,   Lucia A. Reisch
University of Cambridge
Cambridge, UK
Leibniz-Institute for Prevention
Research and Epidemiology—BIPS
Bremen, Germany

Preface

We are rehashing a commonplace idea from the last decade by pointing out that digital technology can potentially transform public health. In many instances, digitalization has already changed many aspects and working modes of public health by improving access to healthcare, strengthening disease surveillance, and enhancing health education and promotion.

However, often this development has been driven by new information and communication technology, more processing power, or general technology advances rather than targeted developments that fulfill public health needs—the rapid creep of digital technology into public health at times seems like a solution looking for a problem.

We argue that to harness the full potential of digital technology for public health, it needs to serve public health functions, such as those outlined in the World Health Organization's (WHO) 10 Essential Public Health Operations (EPHOs). Additionally, the development of future technology should be driven by evidence-based public health demands and follow systematic steps to ensure its effectiveness and safety.

This book provides an overview of core concepts, requirements, and frameworks, as well as state-of-the-art research in applying digital technology for public health functions. This book also covers a multitude of relevant interdisciplinary topics related to digital public health, since interdisciplinarity, in our view, is a hallmark of the field. We have invited authors from the Leibniz ScienceCampus Digital Public Health Bremen (www.digital-public-health.de), our interdisciplinary research consortium in Bremen, Germany, as well as other active researchers in the field of digital public health, to provide impulses, theoretical advances, and the state of the art on how digital technology impacts public health in four thematic parts.

Part I: Overarching Issues

In the first part (Chapters "Public Health in the Digital Era: Digital Entry Points for Population Health", "A Framework to Develop and Evaluate Digital Public Health Interventions", "Participatory Approaches for Digital Public Health: Giving Voice to Values", "Open Data for DiPH Research Versus Data Protection", "Evidence-Based Approaches in Digital Public Health", "Digital Interventions for Public Health: A Systematic Planning Approach" and "Evaluation of Digital Public Health Interventions"), this book discusses legal, ethical, conceptual, and theoretical approaches to digital public health. This includes a framework and suggestions for systematically accounting for scientific evidence in developing digital public health applications. Accordingly, suggestions on how to systematically generate evidence on the application of digital technology in public health are provided in a distinct section. The vital importance of interdisciplinarity is underlined in the introductory chapter.

The rapid development of digital technology in health promotion, prevention, and other public health fields has also led to a plethora of concepts and definitions. Here, we build on a definition provided by Wienert et al. (2022), who suggest that digital public interventions are those that operate on a population level and serve public health functions (more below) across a continuum of care, from health promotion and general prevention to improvements in health care and management. The focus on entire populations differentiates this field from more targeted application fields and, at the same time, emphasizes the need to account for key aspects of health interventions provided for populations such as those outlined in the Ottawa Charta (WHO 1986)—focusing on health inequalities, empowering individuals and communities, and reforming health services (Fig. 1).

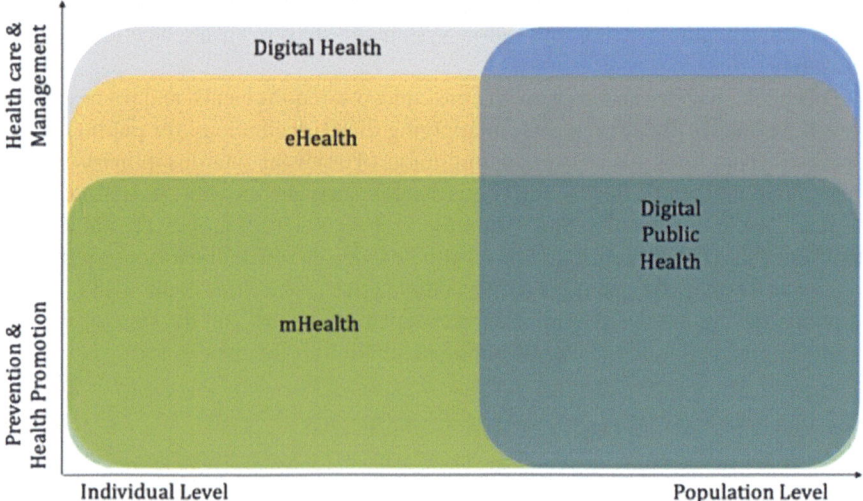

Fig. 1 Digital public health and related fields. (Source: ©Wienert J et al. Originally published in the *Journal of Medical Internet Research* (https://www.jmir.org), 28.06.2022)

Part II: Challenges for Digital Public Health

The second part (Chapters "Cyberspaces: Modifying the Digital Environment for Health Promotion and Prevention", "Digital Public Health in Europe: Was the COVID-19 Pandemic an Enabler for Healthcare Digitalization?", "Global Perspectives on Digital Public Health: A Framework", "Digital Health Inequality", "Digital Health Literacy", "Public Health Goes Digital—Or Not? Ethical Considerations Concerning Limits and Necessary Alternatives" and "Social Media in Digital Public Health") examines cross-cutting challenges for digital public health. These include the potential increase in social and digital inequalities and inequity. In order to realize the potential to transform public health systems positively, digital technology needs to achieve broad reach. Currently, this reach is mainly realized through applications that could be classified as risk exposures rather than health-promoting, namely through health-related misinformation in social media, aggressive and thorough commercialization of personal data (including health data), and concentration of reach within a small number of increasingly powerful corporate IT conglomerates. The second part also contains discussions by international experts regarding the issues of globalizing digital public health applications and modifying digital environments for health promotion. Chapters on approaches to mitigating the effects of individual and societal deprivation and the extent and role of poor digital literacy for public health conclude the section.

Part III: Digital Technology to Serve Key Public Health Functions

The book's third part concentrates on the potential of digital technologies to serve key public health functions organized around the WHO's Essential Public Health Operations (EPHOs; Fig. 2) that include "intelligence" (1–2), "delivery" (3–5), and "enabler" (6–10) functions. Digital technology can support these by providing real-time data on outbreaks, tracking diseases, empowering individuals with health education, and connecting people with needed health services. For instance, mobile health (mHealth) applications can help individuals to manage chronic conditions, access health education materials, and receive alerts on disease outbreaks. Beyond their role in improving communication flows between healthcare providers, electronic health records (EHRs) can facilitate the identification of health trends and outbreaks. Additionally, telehealth services can provide access to healthcare providers remotely, particularly in remote areas or during emergencies. Social media can be used to mobilize communities, and online forums and support groups can help connect people with similar health concerns.

At the same time, the development, implementation, evaluation, and refinement must be driven by the extent to which digital technology can meet these demands. In this part, we critically evaluate the potential of various digital technologies to serve these EPHOs and have asked expert contributors to provide overviews, case studies, and critical perspectives on digital technologies serving EPHOs.

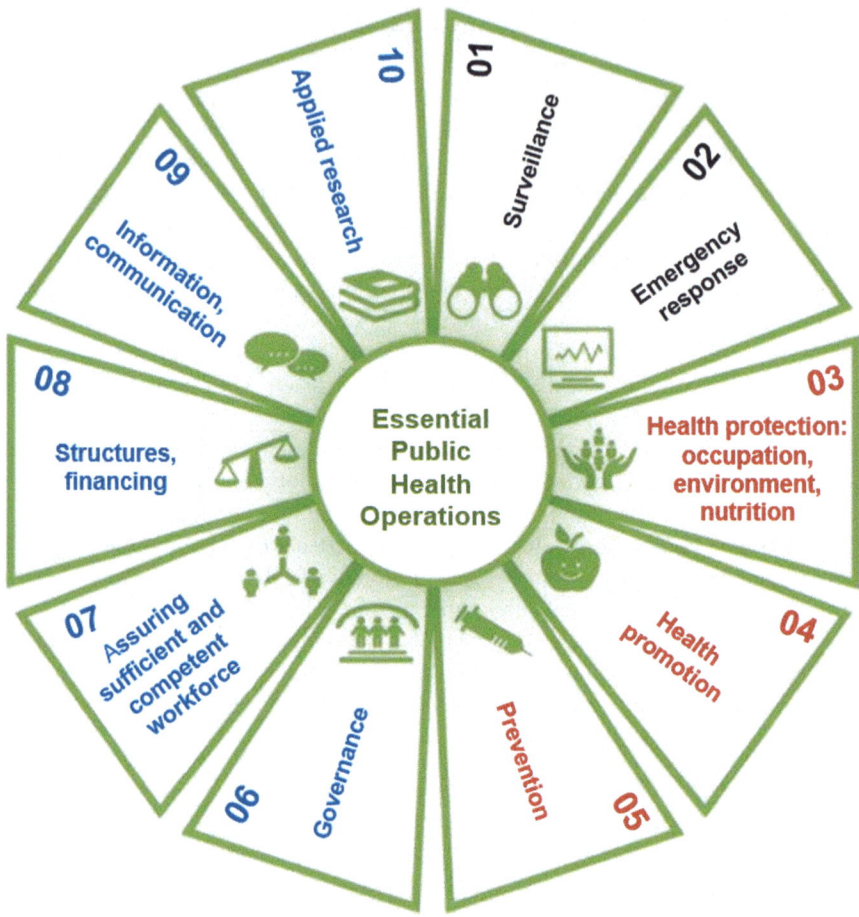

Fig. 2 Essential public health operations. (Own figure, adapted from www.zukunftsforum-public-health.de)

Part IV: Engineering Digital Public Health

The fourth part (Chapters "From Smartwatches to Research Tools: Unlocking the Potential of Modern Health Monitoring Technology", "AI Meets Digital Public Health", "Use of Secondary and Registry Data for Digital Public Health", "Ethical Implications of User Autonomy in Digital Public Health" and "Health Data Pipelines: Moving Away from Excel to Scalable, Sustainable, Insightful, and Future-Proof Infostructure") provides a critical perspective on development and engineering to support development fit for purpose. While we have argued that technology development for digital public health should be guided by serving public health functions rather than technology looking for applications, applying digital technology in public health has led to further developments and new developmental challenges. Further, the fact that advanced technology is being used in the health domain requires retrofitting public health considerations around technological advances. Take the example of artificial intelligence: AI has the potential to revolutionize public health by improving disease diagnosis, predicting disease outbreaks, and identifying at-risk populations. Further, AI can analyze large secondary and registry data sets to identify patterns and trends, enabling early disease detection and personalized treatment. AI-powered systems can, therefore, help predict the spread of infectious diseases and track epidemics, facilitating timely responses to outbreaks. At the same time, the use of AI in public health also poses substantial challenges, particularly concerning the spread of misinformation and algorithmic discrimination if trained on biased data, leading to disparities in health outcomes.

Outlook

Digital technology can potentially transform public health by enhancing disease surveillance, improving access to healthcare, and providing health education and promotion. However, to harness its full potential, digital technology must serve public health functions like those outlined in the WHO's EPHOs. Future technology development must be driven by evidence-based public health demands and follow rigorous systematic steps to ensure its effectiveness and safety and to fulfill the promise of universal access and, consequently, broad reach. Ultimately, integrating digital technology for public health needs to prioritize public health by ensuring transparency, equity, and the ethical use of data. This book aims to support this integration, and it does so through an open-access approach to avoid cost barriers.

Bremen, Germany	Hajo Zeeb
Bremen, Germany	Laura Maaß
Bremen, Germany	Tanja Schultz
Bremen, Germany	Ulrike Haug
Bremen, Germany	Iris Pigeot
Bremen, Germany	Benjamin Schüz

References

Wienert J, Jahnel T, Maaß L (2022) What are digital public health interventions? First steps toward a definition and an intervention classification framework. J Med Internet Res 24(6):e31921

World Health Organization (1986) Ottawa Charter for Health Promotion: First International Conference on Health Promotion, Ottawa. https://www.healthpromotion.org.au/images/ottawa_charter_hp.pdf. Accessed Jul 2023

Contents

Why Is It Essential to Address Digital Public Health in an Interdisciplinary Way? 1
Laura Maaß, Hans-Henrik Dassow, Daniel Diethei, Merle Freye, Jasmin Niess, and Stefanie Do

Overarching Issues

Public Health in the Digital Era: Digital Entry Points for Population Health 29
Tina Jahnel, Benjamin Schüz, and Hajo Zeeb

A Framework to Develop and Evaluate Digital Public Health Interventions 43
Chen-Chia Pan, Núria Pedrós Barnils, Saskia Muellmann, Tina Jahnel, Dorothee Jürgens, Merle Freye, Hans-Henrik Dassow, Wolf Rogowski, and Ansgar Gerhardus

Participatory Approaches for Digital Public Health: Giving Voice to Values 59
Rehana Shrestha, Anke V. Reinschluessel, and Jasmin Niess

Open Data for DiPH Research Versus Data Protection 79
Merle Freye and Benedikt Buchner

Evidence-Based Approaches in Digital Public Health 95
Joanna Albrecht, Pinar Tokgöz, and Christoph Dockweiler

Digital Interventions for Public Health: A Systematic Planning Approach 115
J. Bruinsma and R. Crutzen

Evaluation of Digital Public Health Interventions 135
Oliver Lange, Paula Boskamp, Werner Brannath, Karina Karolina De Santis, Saskia Muellmann, Wolf Rogowski, and Heinz Rothgang

Challenges for Digital Public Health

Cyberspaces: Modifying the Digital Environment for Health Promotion and Prevention 159
A. L. Stark-Blomeier, J. Albrecht, and C. Dockweiler

Digital Public Health in Europe: Was the COVID-19 Pandemic an Enabler for Healthcare Digitalization? 179
Laura Maaß, Brian Li Han Wong, Rok Hrzic, Ave Põld, Juan José Rachadell, Marine Delgrange, Robin van Kessel, and Stefan Buttigieg

Global Perspectives on Digital Public Health: A Framework 211
Luís Velez Lapão

Digital Health Inequality 229
T. Brand, P. S. Herrera-Espejel, and H. Busse

Digital Health Literacy 249
Hajo Zeeb and Julia Dratva

Public Health Goes Digital—Or Not? Ethical Considerations Concerning Limits and Necessary Alternatives 267
Dagmar Borchers and Regina Müller

Social Media in Digital Public Health 281
Elida Sina, Merle Freye, Thomas Eßmeyer, Lara Reich, and Daniel Diethei

Digital Technology to Serve Key Public Health Functions

Surveillance of Population Health and Well-being (EPHO 1) 309
Wolfgang Ahrens and Iris Pigeot

Monitoring and Response to Health Hazards and Emergencies (EPHO2) 329
Göran Kirchner, Robin Houben, Justus Benzler, Tobias R. K. Heller, Tim Einbeck, Katrin Werth, and Patrick Schmich

Health Protection, Including Environmental and Food Safety (EPHO 3) 345
Anna Förster, Gibson Kimutai, Myat Su Yin, Peter Haddawy, and Urte Klink

Health Promotion, Including Action to Address Social Determinants and Health Inequity (EPHO 4) 357
Laura M. König

Disease Prevention, Including Early Detection of Illnesses (EPHO5) 381
Ihoghosa Iyamu, Devon Haag, Heather Pedersen, and Mark Gilbert

Assuring Governance for Health and Well-Being (EPHO 6) 405
Sarah Forberger

**Assuring a Sufficient and Competent Public Health
Workforce for Digital Public Health (EPHO 7)** 429
Monica Georgiana Brînzac, Rok Hrzic, Mariam Hachem,
and Fatai Ogunlayi

**Assuring Sustainable Organizational Structures
and Financing for Digital Public Health (EPHO 8)** 447
Oliver Lange and Wolf Rogowski

**Advocacy, Communication, and Social Mobilization
for Health (EPHO 9)** 471
Rasmus Cloes, Christopher Jones, Hajo Zeeb, and Benjamin Schüz

**Advancing Public Health Research to Inform Policy
and Practice (EPHO 10)** 483
H. Zeeb and S. Forberger

Engineering Digital Public Health

**From Smartwatches to Research Tools: Unlocking
the Potential of Modern Health Monitoring Technology**............. 499
Anke V. Reinschluessel, Bastian Dänekas, Thomas Eßmeyer,
Katharina Hasenlust, and Rainer Malaka

AI Meets Digital Public Health 513
Lars Steinert, Daniel Diethei, Viktoria Hoel, Horst K. Hahn,
Karin Wolf-Ostermann, Marvin N. Wright, and Tanja Schultz

Use of Secondary and Registry Data for Digital Public Health 537
Timm Intemann, Ulrike Haug, and Iris Pigeot

Ethical Implications of User Autonomy in Digital Public Health........ 563
Hans-Henrik Dassow and Thomas Eßmeyer

**Health Data Pipelines: Moving Away from Excel to Scalable,
Sustainable, Insightful, and Future-Proof Infostructure** 585
Martina Cilia and Stefan Buttigieg

Digital Public Health: An Outlook 613
Hajo Zeeb, Laura Maaß, Ulrike Haug, Iris Pigeot, Tanja Schultz,
and Benjamin Schüz

Why Is It Essential to Address Digital Public Health in an Interdisciplinary Way?

Laura Maaß, Hans-Henrik Dassow, Daniel Diethei, Merle Freye, Jasmin Niess, and Stefanie Do

Abstract Public health requires collaborations across several disciplines to meet population health needs. Increasing technological advancements have accelerated the transformation of public health to digital public health (DiPH), including new domains to develop, maintain, and improve evidence-based digital technologies.

L. Maaß (✉)
SOCIUM Research Center on Inequality and Social Policy, University of Bremen, Bremen, Germany

Leibniz ScienceCampus Digital Public Health Bremen, Bremen, Germany
e-mail: Laura.maass@uni-bremen.de

H.-H. Dassow
Leibniz ScienceCampus Digital Public Health Bremen, Bremen, Germany

Institute for Philosophy, University of Bremen, Bremen, Germany

Juniorprofessorship for Medical Ethics with a focus on Digitization, Faculty for Health Sciences Brandenburg, University of Potsdam, Potsdam, Germany
e-mail: dassow@uni-potsdam.de

D. Diethei
Leibniz ScienceCampus Digital Public Health Bremen, Bremen, Germany
e-mail: diethei@uni-bremen.de

M. Freye
Leibniz ScienceCampus Digital Public Health Bremen, Bremen, Germany

IGMR Institute for Information, Health and Medical Law, University of Bremen, Bremen, Germany
e-mail: mfreye@uni-bremen.de

J. Niess
Leibniz ScienceCampus Digital Public Health Bremen, Bremen, Germany

University of Oslo, Oslo, Norway
e-mail: jasminni@uio.no

S. Do
Leibniz ScienceCampus Digital Public Health Bremen, Bremen, Germany

Leibniz Institute for Prevention Research and Epidemiology – BIPS, Bremen, Germany
e-mail: dostef@leibniz-bips.de

© The Author(s) 2025
H. Zeeb et al. (eds.), *Digital Public Health*, Springer Series on Epidemiology and Public Health, https://doi.org/10.1007/978-3-031-90154-6_1

However, having various disciplines collaborating can create unique challenges if there is no mutual understanding of DiPH. This chapter aims to illustrate and discuss interdisciplinary approaches and collaborations in DiPH research and practice. First, we will give an overview of the concept of interdisciplinarity and draw on the practical challenges of interdisciplinary research and best practice examples for promoting such competencies. Second, we will describe traditional public health core functions and their relationship with other disciplines in the social, natural, and environmental sciences and humanities. Third, we will highlight how the extension to DiPH influenced the so-called system of sub-disciplines that form public health. Fourth, we will use a case study on mental health and medical apps to highlight essential strengths and limitations of selected sub-disciplines in DiPH (epidemiology, psychology, philosophy, law, computer science, and implementation science). Finally, we provide seven key recommendations that should promote and foster effective interdisciplinary collaborations in DiPH.

Keywords Computer sciences · Epidemiology · Implementation science · Interdisciplinarity · Law · Psychology · Public health

Abbreviations

DiGA	Digital health applications
DiPH	Digital public health
ECRA	Early Career Researcher Academy
EUPHA	European Public Health Association
GPS	Global positioning system
HCI	Human-computer interaction
LSC DiPH	Leibniz ScienceCampus Digital Public Health Bremen
MDR	European medical device regulation
MHMA	Mental health and medical apps
WHO	World Health Organization

1 Background

1.1 Introduction

In their article on developing interdisciplinary collaborations in academia, Madzvamuse and Lubkin (2016) state that "interdisciplinary research requires the integration and blending of single disciplinary knowledge and methods to bear fruit on a common goal, or scientific problem of significant importance, that cannot be otherwise addressed by single disciplines." This chapter will explore why and how various disciplines should and can effectively collaborate to impact population health in public health and digital public health (DiPH).

While individual health already involves various disciplines to be adequately addressed (like medicine, pharmacology, disease prevention, nutrition science, environmental science, sociology, etc.), even more fields gain importance when it comes to health on a population level, also named public health. Since the goal of public health is to improve population health, it needs to collaborate with all disciplines to improve population health. This includes disciplines focusing or (a) diagnosing and treating diseases on the individual level (e.g., medicine, psychology, etc.), (b) measuring health outcomes and relevant exposures on a population level (e.g., epidemiology), (c) setting the framework for health practices (e.g., law, ethics, etc.), (d) designing interventions (e.g., health promotion, health management), or (e) implementing interventions (e.g., implementation science) (Acheson 1988).

The digitalization of public health goals, also named DiPH (Odone et al. 2019; Wong et al. 2022), which we will describe in detail later, brings even more players on stage (e.g., Human-Computer Interaction (HCI), data analytics, engineering). They need to be involved in developing and improving evidence-based digital tools for use and application at a population level. DiPH tools must be collectively developed by different stakeholders, from the vision and goal-setting to actual design and implementation. It is essential to address user needs before the devices are developed, during, and after implementation to meet their needs and improve acceptability. Collaboration instead of consultation is the key to successful DiPH interventions and tools (Weisel et al. 2019).

This chapter will set the base for interdisciplinarity in DiPH and sensitize the reader to the importance of collaborating with researchers and practitioners from other scientific fields for creating DiPH tools with a sustainable impact on population health. We will start by defining public health and DiPH and provide an overview of the disciplines involved in the field. We do not claim that this overview is complete or intends to suggest a hierarchical order of importance for these topics. Instead, it should display the various fields to consider when working in public health and DiPH. Following this, we will explain what *interdisciplinarity* means, how it differs from *multidisciplinarity*, and highlight the drivers of interdisciplinarity in DiPH. After we have set the frame, we will open the floor to some disciplines involved in DiPH: epidemiology, psychology, philosophy and ethics, law, computer science, and implementation science. These disciplines were chosen based on the authors' expertise and should in no way be understood as more critical to DiPH than other fields. Disciplinary experts will discuss how their fields can contribute to DiPH, but also where the limitations are and where support from other disciplines is required. We will show how DiPH projects and interventions can only be efficient if different disciplines work together, thus using synergies to overcome weaknesses in each respective field. After summarizing the findings on the importance of interdisciplinarity, we will propose ways to incorporate interdisciplinary approaches to (digital) public health research projects and practice. Finally, we will close with a proposal for how future DiPH collaborations should look.

The case studies will focus on mental health and medical apps (MHMA) used to treat diseases or improve general mental health (we differentiated between health apps and medical apps in a previous article (Maaß et al. 2022)). On the one hand, mental disorders are one of the leading public health problems, with over one billion people worldwide suffering from mental or addictive disorders (Rehm and Shield 2019). On the other hand, the shortage of mental health professionals is a crucial problem regarding adequate health services. Several countries struggle to find psychiatrists and nurses for mental health care (Chandrashekar 2018; Rehm and Shield 2019; Rudd and Beidas 2020). Smartphones and, therefore, health and medical apps have become increasingly available worldwide and present a possibility to support professionals and help-seeking individuals in treating mental health disorders (Bucci et al. 2019; Domhardt et al. 2021; Kozlov et al. 2020). Some studies indicated that digital solutions such as MHMAs could provide support during psychological therapies or even replace them to a certain extent where no professional is available (Andersson et al. 2014; Olthuis et al. 2016). Further, evidence-based MHMAs can reduce the stigma of seeking help for mental health disorders and improve mental health awareness (Bakker et al. 2016; Friis-Healy et al. 2021; Luxton et al. 2011; World Health Organization 2013a).

1.2 Definition of Public Health and Digital Public Health

The term "public health" can be divided into two parts in which "public" implies a group of people in a specific community or the whole population rather than an individual. The second term, "health," is defined by the World Health Organization (WHO) as "a state of complete physical, mental, and social well-being and not merely the absence of disease or infirmity" (World Health Organization 1946). Extended definitions include other essential aspects such as what public health is and how it can be achieved (Winslow 1920), living conditions (U.S. Institute of Medicine 1988), the efficient use and equitable distribution of resources (Gerlinger et al. 2012), or sustainability (Beaglehole and Bonita 1998). Nowadays, the most commonly used definition, which the WHO also adopted, characterizes public health as "the art and science of preventing disease, prolonging life and promoting health through the organized efforts of society" (Acheson 1988). Common elements in all preceding definitions include the dual nature of public health as science and practice, its focus on the health of entire populations, and its interdisciplinary nature. Critical tasks of public health aim to protect and promote population health and are summarized by the WHO as the ten Essential Public Health Operations in practice (World Health Organization 2013b).

The digital transformation across sectors emphasizes using Big Data, computing power, mobile technology, or Artificial Intelligence (Bucci et al. 2019), which drives the transition from public health to DiPH. DiPH can be described as a reimagination of public health using new ways of working, blending established public health wisdom with new digital concepts and tools, and an asset to achieve existing public health goals (Iyamu et al. 2021; Iyamu et al. 2022). Traditional application fields such as etiological health research, health promotion, and health services and health care are confronted with newly emerging evaluation criteria, including the efficacy and efficiency, equity, and unintended effects of digital health technologies (Darmann-Finck et al. 2020). Their increasing use and integration into public health functions support the transition from cure to prevention, the centering and empowerment of people and patients, and the facilitation of more efficient, safer, and cheaper healthcare management and delivery (Zeeb et al. 2020; Maaß et al. 2024).

However, effective implementation of digital programs for public health purposes requires the development of an overarching regulatory framework for Artificial Intelligence and a more thorough understanding of digital health technologies (Benke and Benke 2018). Applying these technologies in the public health sphere requires professionals with technical backgrounds (i.e., computer scientists and engineers) (Wong et al. 2022) as well as those with advanced data analytic skills (i.e., data scientists) (Kunkle et al. 2016) who can identify possibilities and existing limitations while shaping workable solutions. For instance, computer scientists are central in providing technical means to use the internet and digital devices to enrich data collection or develop software programs and devices to support clinical work (Epstein 2013). Figure 1 summarizes the different disciplines in DiPH and describes the four traditional core disciplines (Egger and Razum 2012; Maaß et al. 2025; Organisation for Economic Co-operation and Development 2007), i.e., social sciences (red), humanities (purple), natural sciences (blue), and environmental sciences (green), and the newly added core discipline engineering (yellow) (Earnest et al. 2006; Ke and Liu 2012; Wong et al. 2022). Each of these core disciplines is accompanied by different sub-disciplines (outer circles) and can be divided into fields that are either predominantly classifiable by one core discipline (i.e., unicolored) or by at least two core disciplines (i.e., multicolored with a differently colored background). This illustration highlights the interdisciplinary character of (digital) public health that requires joint efforts and collaboration of individual disciplines to develop a novel and comprehensive approach to improving population health.

1.3 Key Characteristics and Definition of Interdisciplinarity

Interdisciplinarity is an integral part of contemporary academia (Medina 2021). In the context of successful academic careers or innovative study programs, interdisciplinarity is often demanded, expected, or required (Jordan et al. 2021). Public health scientists also claim to facilitate health-related interdisciplinary research under the umbrella of public health and apply findings from interdisciplinary research in practice (Prowd et al. 2018; Smye and Frangi 2021). These aspects already point to a problem in the use of the term interdisciplinarity: It is not entirely evident whether this is a solely descriptive term or whether normative expectations are additionally associated with it. For our objectives, we must develop an explanatory understanding of interdisciplinarity as a first step (this section). Based on this, the drivers of

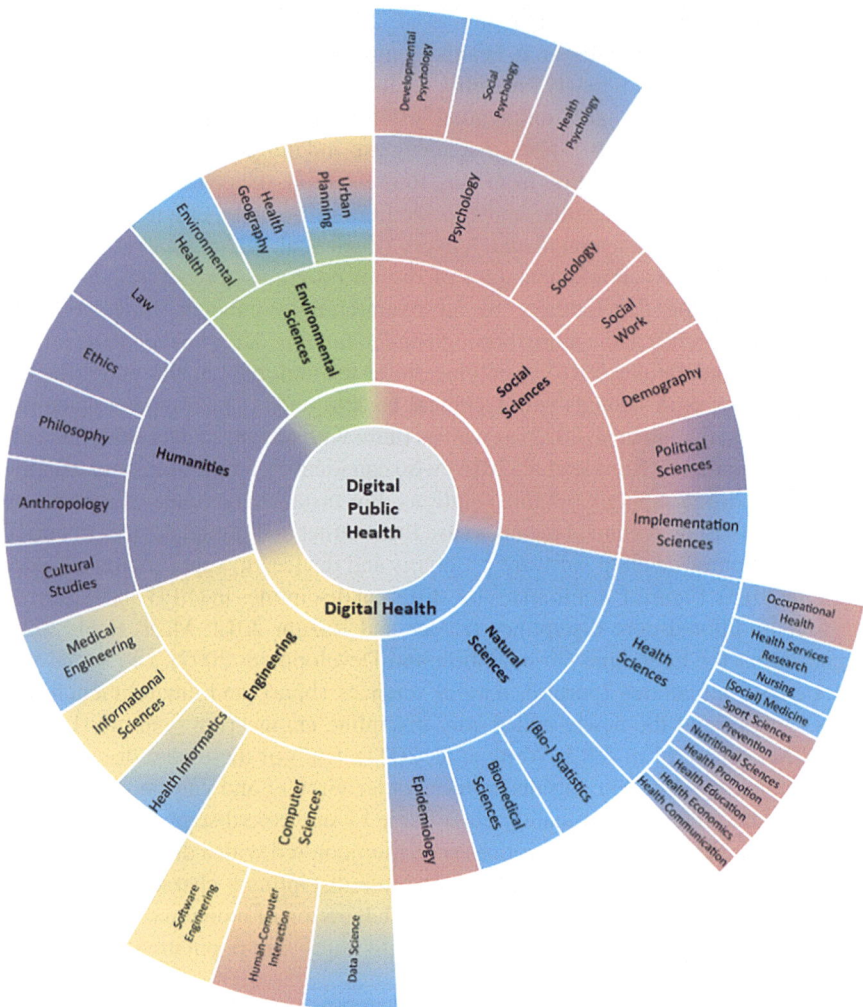

Fig. 1 Disciplines in digital public health. (Source: own figure)

interdisciplinarity in DiPH will be addressed in a normative sense (next section). The interest in better understanding and defining interdisciplinarity is not exclusively theoretical. A shared understanding of interdisciplinarity is essential for successful interdisciplinary research (Morss et al. 2021).

Interdisciplinarity is not a contemporary trend but has been a challenge and requirement for the academic community for a long time (Klein 2018; Morss et al. 2021). The theoretical patterns of justification and historical debates are too broad to be discussed here. At this point, it is reasonable to break down the concept of interdisciplinarity into its essential characteristics. An etymological analysis of the word 'interdisciplinarity' provides indications of two key elements: While the second part of the word (-disciplinarity) refers to scientific disciplines, the prefix "inter" (Latin: between) refers to the relationship among scientific disciplines. Interdisciplinarity thus requires the involvement of at least two scientific disciplines. However, the participation of two or more scientific disciplines is not a unique characteristic of interdisciplinarity: Multidisciplinarity also refers to research in which two or more domains are involved and focus on a shared research object (Serlet et al. 2020). Interdisciplinarity, however, is distinguished from multidisciplinarity by the collaboration of disciplines within research. It constitutes more than just an exchange of results, methods, and theories. The product of multidisciplinary research is no more and no less than the simple sum of its parts. Interdisciplinarity goes beyond the sum of its parts (Wagner et al. 2011), which happens due to its interactive nature between involved disciplines (Kivits et al. 2019).

For this chapter, we will apply the definition by the National Academy of Sciences et al. (2005), which describes interdisciplinarity as "a mode of research by teams or individuals that integrates information, data, techniques, tools, perspectives, concepts, and/or theories from two or more disciplines or bodies of specialized knowledge to advance fundamental understanding or to solve problems whose solutions are beyond the scope of a single discipline or area of research practice".

1.4 Drivers and Rationales of Interdisciplinarity in Digital Public Health

It has always been a critical characteristic in the history of public health to unite different disciplines under its umbrella (Tulchinsky and Varavikova 2014). Indeed, interdisciplinary approaches are a must for successfully addressing global health issues (Medin and Krettek 2008). Yet, despite this, the success of interdisciplinary collaboration in public health does not indicate why interdisciplinarity is essential in DiPH. To that end, four main drivers of interdisciplinarity are of crucial importance (National Academy of Sciences et al. 2005; Klein 2018):

1. DiPH addresses the *complexity of nature and society* in both ways; for example, by monitoring and trying to contain diseases not only at the individual level but also at the population level, a complex interaction between nature and society emerges, which can only be made tangible by several disciplines in interdisciplinary collaboration. This is the case for both public health and DiPH.
2. We assume that *the drive to explore fundamental research problems* is also genuine for DiPH. We will provide evidence for these claims later. The following section will explain the perspectives of individual disciplines on DiPH, their contributions, and their dependencies on the scientific findings of other disciplines. DiPH, by its nature, can only be successful if it transcends the boundaries of individual disciplines instead of remaining within individual disciplines. Therefore, it is both a drive and a necessity for interdisciplinarity in DiPH.

3. Our understanding of public health points to *societal problems* that exist or can newly arise. By combining science and practice, public health aims to solve societal issues in population health. There are no apparent reasons why this should not also apply analogously to DiPH.
4. Finally, *the power of new technologies* can certainly be identified for DiPH. All three of the previously mentioned drivers, which apply equally to public health and DiPH, are reinforced here by the expansion of public health challenges through digital technologies. In addition, digital technologies add a new quality of complexity to public health that can only be understood in its essence through interdisciplinary research.

2 Overview of Disciplines in Digital Public Health

In the following paragraphs, we will introduce selected disciplines in DiPH within the context of MHMAs. These disciplines are chosen due to our expertise and do not necessarily represent traditional core disciplines in DiPH. Each paragraph will briefly introduce the field, highlight what it can contribute to DiPH, and where it needs support from other disciplines.

2.1 The Perspective of Epidemiology

Epidemiology is the science that studies disease occurrence and health states in human populations (Lash et al. 2020). One of its core tasks is to carry out activities within the realm of public health surveillance which is traditionally defined as the "ongoing systematic collection, analysis and interpretation of data, closely integrated with the timely dissemination of the resulting information to those responsible for preventing and controlling disease and injury" (Thacker and Berkelman 1988).

A key strength in epidemiology is the integration of different data sources and their integration of different data sources that can then jointly be used to develop and characterize disease markers. For instance, self-reports are complemented by sensor data which is translated into behavioral markers relevant to mental health and enable surveillance and monitoring of mental health conditions at a population level (Cornet and Holden 2018). In addition, integrating personal sensing data with clinical and genomic databases will offer the opportunity to deepen understanding of the relationship between behavior and its interactions with genes on health and disease (Mohr et al. 2017). Another strength is its systematic collection, analysis, and interpretation of data that contributes to a scientific-driven development and methodologically sound evaluation of MHMAs. Proper evaluation of MHMAs is increasingly needed for measuring efficacy and cost-effectiveness. Previous reviews have indicated that MHMAs are extensively available on commercial markets but very frequently suffer from poor quality regarding the engagement of users, information quality, and privacy features (Bauer et al. 2020; Domhardt et al. 2021).

Despite promising opportunities, it is also essential to acknowledge contemporary challenges that epidemiologists encounter when collecting and using data from digital health technologies. First, potential conflicts may arise regarding data collection when attempting to maximize publicly accessible data, on the one hand, and minimize publicly accessible personal data to protect individual privacy on the other hand (Brockmann 2020; Salathé 2018). Often there is no clear understanding and consensus about the type of person-specific behavioral data which should be protected (Brockmann 2020), resulting in a lack of specific guidelines and subsequent disagreements within the community of researchers (Mohr et al. 2017). One possible solution includes the establishment of data cooperatives with restricted access enabling the extraction of scientific findings while ensuring a high degree of data protection (Salathé 2018).

Further, epidemiologists need to complement their expertise in storing and processing large amounts of data with the expertise of lawyers and data security professionals to handle legal and ethical concerns (e.g., consent, privacy expectations, data protection, and security) for passively collected digital data (Salerno et al. 2017). Possible unintended effects of digitally generated data can lead to a distorted picture of reality. For example, suppose digital approaches captured individual lifestyle risk factors rather than social determinants. In that case, social inequalities may be exacerbated to the extent that the living conditions and access barriers of socioeconomically disadvantaged people are neglected as a result (Darmann-Finck et al. 2020). Lastly, generating and converting large amounts of raw sensor data into meaningful information can fail without deliberate collaboration among disciplines. In this endeavor, epidemiologists need to collaborate with computer scientists to develop and tailor sensors (Søgaard Neilsen and Wilson 2019), and machine learning experts to apply adequate statistical methods to high dimensional data (Morgenstern et al. 2021). Further, they need to work with experts on subject matter and other methods, such as psychologists, clinicians, and implementation scientists, to effectively interpret scientific findings and translate them into practice (Neta et al. 2017).

2.2 The Perspective of Psychology

Psychology is the scientific study of behavior and mental processes (Fernald 2008; Hockenbury and Hockenbury 2010). The discipline encompasses various subdisciplines, such as health psychology, social psychology, developmental psychology, and experimental psychology (American Psychological Association 2013a).

One of the critical aspects that psychologists can contribute to the field of DiPH is in-depth knowledge of human behavior. Some leading public health challenges, such as obesity, smoking, or mental health problems, are closely linked to behavior and habit formation (Gardner 2015). Considering the example of an MHMA, psychologists can contribute evidence-based knowledge on promoting mental health, preventing mental health issues, and improving mental health care solutions. However, psychological principles and theories that relate to interactions between people (e.g., therapy sessions with a psychologist and client) cannot simply be transferred one-to-one to a mobile app (Bucci et al. 2019). Ideally, meaningful design decisions considering the needs of the core stakeholders involved (i.e., psychologists, clients) should be based on a human-centered iterative design process (Thieme et al. 2020) and implemented by someone with programming skills and knowledge of user interface design. Psychologists are not usually trained to design or implement user-centered mobile apps (American Psychological Association 2013b). Consequently, the interdisciplinary collaboration between people with backgrounds in computer science, design, and psychology can lead to the most promising results.

When psychological knowledge has been integrated into the design of a DiPH intervention (e.g., MHMAs), it must be analyzed whether the app is accepted by the users and leads to positive health outcomes (Grossman et al. 2020). Psychology can provide methods for researching acceptance, long-term use of the MHMA, and subjectively perceived health improvements. However, determining an improvement in mental health at the population level (for example, supported by various mental health interventions) requires collaboration with epidemiologists.

Despite the potential that apps offer to improve people's health, it is also vital to consider the risks (Miralles et al. 2020). People potentially interested in an MHMA are potentially vulnerable and looking for health and support (Martinengo et al. 2019). For instance, there may be situations where a person is mentally distressed or ill and urgently needs to see an expert instead of consulting an app. The analysis and mitigation of such risks require close collaboration between law, psychology, ethics, computer science, and psychiatry experts to develop structures and principles which protect all parties involved (e.g., app developers, psychologists, and the app users, amongst others) as much as possible. In summary, psychology plays a central role in the field of DiPH. Still, close collaboration between several disciplines is needed to support society's overall health as effectively as possible.

2.3 The Perspective of Philosophy and Ethics

There is no commonly accepted academic definition of philosophy, as different philosophical schools have always disputed what philosophy can or should accomplish (Williamson 2007). In turn, it is widely accepted that ethics is a central subfield of philosophy. Ethics is a reflective theory of morality. It is devoted to one of the four Kantian questions: "What should I do?" (Bartneck et al. 2021). In addition to normative ethics, which seeks to identify and establish general principles that can systematically guide our actions, applied ethics is devoted to practical ethical challenges of everyday life, politics, or science (Singer 2011).

Within applied ethics, specific public health ethics addresses the ethical challenges of public health as a science and practice. Based on the 'Principles of biomedical ethics' (Beauchamp and Childress 2019), public health ethics commonly applies ethical principles such as respect for autonomy, beneficence, non-maleficence, and justice as ethical criteria for evaluating a public health intervention (Marckmann et al. 2015). Here, philosophy can reflect on the various assumptions and values behind each principle. In this sense, philosophical reflection can develop normative criteria and justify them argumentatively. However, the philosophical method cannot systematically provide empirical findings like epidemiology or psychology. Public health ethics must rely on empirical findings from other participating disciplines to determine whether a particular public health intervention causes harm to specific target groups. Public health ethics is feasible only in an interdisciplinary interaction of empirical science and normative philosophical reflection (Barrett et al. 2016).

There are no apparent arguments for abandoning the application of ethical principles to the evaluation of DiPH interventions: Ethical frameworks for DiPH adopt the basic structure from public health ethics and extend the principles as necessary (Marckmann 2020). Specifying the general DiPH ethics towards mHealth ethics is another reasonable approach (Cvrkel 2018; Williamson 2007). In both cases, privacy and data security aspects were added to the principles.

Our case study of MHMAs addresses the classic principles of public health ethics. It should be ensured that an MHMA does not harm users, and it would be ethically desirable that it does them good. Just as the autonomy of individuals must be protected, it must be ensured that an MHMA in the sense of a DiPH intervention does not lead to inequitable outcomes (Cvrkel 2018; Williamson 2007). A central ethical challenge is to treat users' data appropriately. Yet, the ethics of DiPH follow the same pattern as the ethics of public health: The application of ethical principles depends on other empirical disciplines. A philosopher cannot generate knowledge about mental health, nor can their method succeed in designing infrastructures that adequately respect users' privacy. In this specific case, the ethical evaluation relies, at a minimum, on studies from psychology and computer science to be satisfactorily conducted. The unprecedented capacity of ethics and philosophy to provide normative guidance is thus dependent on empirical science in the case of the ethics of DiPH.

2.4 The Perspective of Law

The law sets binding rules to protect users' and stakeholders' rights for MHMAs. Consequently, the law is a source of knowledge about applicable regulations (Kähler 2018) and a guarantee of rights protection. The applicable rules for MHMAs are diverse and arise from each word in *digital*, *public*, and *health*. Relevant data protection and security laws exist, which constantly develop new standards and norms to keep up with rapid technological progress. Since the potential of apps for health systems and the population is increasingly recognized, applicable laws are also developed in public and social law. In Germany, health insurances reimburse some health apps as digital health applications (DiGA) (§ 33a SGB V 2022), and the German social law contains rules to protect the users and the health system (Kircher 2022). The applicable laws originate from health and medicine. Accordingly, the European medical device regulation (MDR) establishes conditions for entering the market (von Zezschwitz 2020), which may apply to MHMAs depending on the risks posed by the app. Some national laws also include medical confidentiality (Heimhalt and Rehmann 2014) and the conditions for remote treatment (Dochow 2019).

From a more ideological point of view, the law becomes an essential instrument for generating trust in health apps if the regulatory framework is appropriate. Trust is supported by ensuring a high level of user protection (Torous et al. 2021). For example, German social law requires a certain level of evidence for medical benefit, data security, and protection to become a DiGA (Braun 2019; Greiner et al. 2022; § 10 DiGAV 2022). Moreover, by referring to these standards, the law can potentially guarantee that scientific standards from other disciplines are valued in practice. Rules for situations when legal requirements are unmet further enhance trust (e.g., remedies, liability, and penalties) (General Data Protection Regulation 2018).

Although the law can ensure the protection of user rights, trust in apps, and the use of scientific findings in practice, these strengths depend on interactions with other disciplines. A paradigmatic example of this interaction is the term "state-of-the-art data security," which has to be ensured and proved by the manufacturer of a DiGA (§ 139e SGB V 2022). However, this term is a "general technical clause" as the law does not determine the concrete measures for meeting the state-of-the-art, and technological expertise is needed.

Nevertheless, some weaknesses of law cannot be solved by other disciplines either. First, law highly depends on several factors. The applicable law differs from country to country and, therefore, is locational. Additionally, legal statements depend on numerous factors within the legal system: An appropriate protection measure for one specific MHMA does not necessarily apply to another app if the other app has slightly different characteristics. Second, (inter)national legislation is often a slow process conflicting with the rapid development of apps (Torous et al. 2019). The reality of health apps constantly raises questions that the law cannot answer (yet) and needs the flexibility and creativity of legislators and courts. Third, compared to empirical sciences, the law is under-complex in capturing reality (Kähler 2018). This is not a weakness but a logical consequence resulting from the fact that empirical sciences aim at grasping reality, whereas law is not asking what is but what should be (Kähler 2018). Therefore, communicating legal concepts to laypeople from other disciplines should be based on a mutual understanding and acceptance of methodological differences.

2.5 The Perspective of Computer Science

Computer science studies computers and algorithmic processes, including their principles, hardware, and software designs, applications, and their impact on society (Tucker 2003). While it seems evident that computer science is essential for developing DiPH technologies, this section highlights some barriers to current DiPH interventions. Further, we provide some suggestions to advance the field.

Architects, developers, engineers, and designers have traditionally been involved in building systems in computer science. However, following the user-centered design paradigm, end users also need to be incorporated into the design process since the user experience of digital technologies plays a vital role in users accepting and using new technology. HCI addresses the task of involving users in the design process. It is defined as designing, evaluating, and implementing interactive computing systems for human use and studying significant phenomena surrounding them (Hewett et al. 1992).

Digital mental health tools have gained a lot of interest in recent years. They are often delivered through smartphones. Mental health care can benefit from smartphones in multiple ways, including app-based therapeutic interventions, capturing mental health data for diagnosis and monitoring, and analyzing data (Torous et al. 2021). Data collection via smartphones can be active or passive. Active data are usually gathered through smartphone-based surveys, such as active symptom monitoring or momentary ecological assessment. Remotely monitoring symptoms seems feasible even for severe mental illnesses such as schizophrenia. Passive data are collected via smartphone sensors such as the global positioning system (GPS), camera, or audio signals. The main advantages of passive data are the low burden for users and novel digital markers of behavior that can be captured (Torous et al. 2021).

MHMAs have been shown to be beneficial if implemented based on theory, user needs, and interdisciplinary collaboration (Søgaard Neilsen and Wilson 2019). However, while some digital mental health tools are effective, the underlying reasons sometimes remain unclear (Lehtimaki et al. 2021; Philippe et al. 2022). Often, psychological theories are not considered (Torous et al. 2021). This is problematic for the implementation: if we can't explain why such tools work, we can hardly promote their widespread use.

Not all developers adhere to the principles of user-centered design. This leads to products that fail to be effective and sustainable, especially for underserved populations whose needs are not addressed in the design process. To reduce the barriers to access and effectiveness of interventions, researchers and developers should engage in culturally salient recruitment strategies that better capture community mistrust, participant resource constraints, and potential risks (Friis-Healy et al. 2021).

The evidence base for the effectiveness of widely used MHMAs remains poor. A review suggests that only 2% of commercially available MHMAs are supported by original research. Furthermore, the supposedly simple transfer of face-to-face interventions into digital ones remains challenging (Torous et al. 2021). In digital mental health research, there is consensus that interdisciplinary collaboration is essential for effective interventions (Calvo et al. 2018; East and Havard 2015; Friis-Healy et al. 2021). While the potential for advancing and improving mental health through digital tools is immense, their success relies on developing interdisciplinary communities. Developers and mental health experts should work together to ensure that products are theory-based and user-centered.

2.6 The Perspective of Implementation Science

Implementation science has roots in innovation diffusion and technology transfer research (Bauer and Kirchner 2020). Adapted for psychology, medicine, and public health, it supports the implementation of screening programs, hygiene protocols for reduced transmission of infections, or the diffusion of treatment practices in psychotherapy. In addition, implementation science in health provides methods to promote and strengthen the systematic adaptation and integration of evidence-based research findings, procedures, interventions, and policies into routine care to impact population health (Brownson et al. 2017; Eccles and Mittman 2006; National Cancer Institute Division of Cancer Control & Population Sciences 2022).

Unlike epidemiology or medicine, which focus on clinical effectiveness as an outcome parameter, implementation science analyses micro- and macro-level factors that support or hinder the implementation and uptake of interventions (Bauer and Kirchner 2020; Torous et al. 2021). According to Colditz and Emmons (2018), contextual factors are the main elements leading to the wide application of clinical innovations, which is the same for MHMAs. Of course, the clinical efficacy of a mental health or medical app is essential. However, the broader evaluation of aspects that influence its successful implementation is equally crucial for adapting the app. It isn't the most effective app that is most widely used, but the one that targets and responds to its users' needs, skills, and resources best and is the easiest to work with (Connolly et al. 2021). More than applying traditional clinical research methods from epidemiology, psychology, or medicine to assess an intervention's effectiveness, pushing it into the real world is required to achieve a sustainable public health impact. The evaluation should, therefore, also determine factors leading to (non-) adoption. Due to its focus on practical implementation, implementation science bridges the gap between science and practice (Glasgow et al. 2013). It offers methods and strategies to improve trial outcomes and enhance intervention uptake to benefit users (Bauer and Kirchner 2020; Wiltsey Stirman and Beidas 2020). Especially after the actual dissemination, implementation science can develop realistic implementation strategies for digital tools (Connolly et al. 2021).

In interdisciplinary research teams, implementation scientists are advisors based on their expertise in real-world contexts of interventions. They consult topic experts (e.g., experts in programming, financing, or regulating MHMAs) on the dissemination and implementation steps of interventions. In addition, implementation scientists provide information about the dissemination and implementation strategy and its outcomes and develop or test such systems. This makes them the perfect companion for disciplines that program an intervention, assess the app's effectiveness, costs, and regulation, or describe the target population's characteristics to improve the chances of intervention uptake (Tabak et al. 2021).

For implementation science in MHMAs, it is essential to collaborate with psychology, public health, and ethics and to draw from their expertise in equity. Wiltsey Stirman and Beidas (2020) stated that "there is no implementation without equitable implementation." Health equity needs to play a fundamental role in implementation science for health to ensure that evidence-based interventions address the needs of all target groups without excluding vulnerable groups.

3 Summary of Case Studies: What does Interdisciplinarity mean for Digital Public Health?

As described in an editorial article in Nature (2015), "the best interdisciplinary science comes from the realization that there are pressing questions or problems that cannot be adequately addressed by people from just one discipline." DiPH as a field is characterized by many such questions where good collaboration between disciplines is needed for effective and sustainable solutions. The use of mobile technology is one of the drivers that transform public health into DiPH in which traditional disciplines from empirical social and health research (e.g., epidemiology, psychology, philosophy, law, implementation science) are complemented by engineering disciplines (e.g., computer science). MHMAs, for instance, present an evidence-based solution that can complement current mental health care practices.

Developing effective MHMAs requires collaboration across different stages of product development: In the development stage, computer scientists need to collaborate with psychologists, medical practitioners, and epidemiologists to integrate evidence-based knowledge in the design of an MHMA. Due to the ever-changing environment of mobile apps (such as updates in the operating system), IT experts are also required to keep public health apps up to date. Regarding data protection, they also need to collaborate with experts from the fields of law and data security to ensure that MHMAs guarantee data protection for each user. In the implementation stage, implementation scientists (Wienert and Zeeb 2021; Wiltsey Stirman and Beidas 2020) and lawmakers must be consulted to set the frame for MHMAs to operate. Experts in ethics should be considered in the development and implementation stages to ensure accessibility, user-friendliness, equity, and equality within the targeted user group (Friis-Healy et al. 2021). In the final knowledge translation stage, epidemiologists and health economists must work closely with computer and data scientists to evaluate MHMAs. Psychologists, medical practitioners, and implementation scientists translate these findings into mental health practice.

4 Prerequisites for Effective and Sustainable Interdisciplinary Collaborations in Digital Public Health

Throughout this chapter, we have highlighted why different disciplines should closely collaborate on DiPH topics such as MHMAs. In the following section, we will propose seven critical recommendations for interdisciplinary collaborations. These key recommendations are partially informed by the literature and our experiences in the interdisciplinary Early Career Researcher Academy (ECRA), which we established as part of the Leibniz ScienceCampus Digital Public Health Bremen (LSC DiPH) in March 2020. This network comprises early career researchers (Ph.D. candidates and postdocs) from different scientific backgrounds who research a topic related to DiPH (Leibniz ScienceCampus Digital Public Health Bremen 2022a).

1. When collaborating with experts from other fields, one must adapt to a considerable degree of uncertainty outside one's scientific background. As Freeth and Caniglia (2020) wrote, one needs to learn how to "collaborate while collaborating." What we deem most important is to invest in *communication*. When we established the ECRA, we soon realized that the most commonly known construct (may it be a framework, a method, or a study type) for a scholar from one discipline was utterly new to researchers from other fields. While this "problem" of speaking different academic languages might sound superficial, it can potentially harm the fundamental pillars of any interdisciplinary project, as it leads to misunderstandings or the feeling of being excluded (Glänzel and Debackere 2022; Nature 2015). Investing in a community where involved researchers can ask for technical vocabulary or methods is essential when setting up interdisciplinary projects. Some projects even prohibit technical, disciplinary language to facilitate understanding between academic fields from the beginning (Brown et al. 2015). Our approach was different: We created a glossary, which includes all technical terms important for DiPH that come from all the included disciplines. This overview was discussed in two workshops and is now displayed on the website of the LSC DiPH for everyone to access (Leibniz ScienceCampus Digital Public Health Bremen 2022b).
2. Additionally, we see the need to facilitate better *exchange* between members through formal team meetings or spaces for informal exchange. Team meetings can improve the effectiveness and level of innovation if supported by clear goals, objectives, and continuous assessments (Borrill et al. 2000; Xyrichis and Lowton 2008). Further, they reduce professional barriers, support the resolution of conflicts, promote partnerships and collaboration, and improve communication in the network (Wittenberg-Lyles et al. 2009a). During our kick-off workshop, all ECRA participants agreed to meet at least once every month to discuss ideas for shared activities (note that although the ECRA is one research network, most researchers only occasionally collaborate on their main projects, so the ECRA allows them to initiate new interdisciplinary projects). As a result of these meet-

ings, various interdisciplinary papers were published, workshops were organized, and experts from different academic fields were invited for lectures. Elaborating on joint research is crucial for any interdisciplinary project's success (Kivits et al. 2019). Furthermore, the ECRA took advantage of virtual interdisciplinary exchange spaces such as virtual coffee breaks to connect with other peers from the ECRA or a self-organized group of Ph.D. candidates. These "trading zones" (Gorman 2010) are places where the scientific language of each discipline is exchanged as a form of good between researchers to create value. According to the literature, these trading places are vital for interdisciplinary research (Bolger 2021). Ultimately, this approach leads to adopting terminology from another discipline and incorporating these terms into the community's communication style (Bolger 2021; Gorman 2010).

3. Based on the growing interdisciplinary communication, questions arise regarding one's *empathy* towards different scientific approaches. This may relate to a specific method, a framework, or how data are collected. Therefore, it is crucial that the network is an environment where asking questions is not only allowed but also encouraged by all members. Eventually, this will lead to a mutual understanding of how each discipline functions, allowing the network to tackle more complex topics that can only be addressed by researchers from various fields (such as DiPH) (Glänzel and Debackere 2022; Ledford 2015; National Academy of Sciences et al. 2005). Ideally, the interdisciplinary approach is already expressed via phrasing research questions so that the issue under study is not dominated by a discipline but rather in a mutually acceptable way for all participating research fields. Essential for this approach is to receive input from all involved researchers (Glänzel and Debackere 2022; Nature 2015). The question "How do you collect and process data?" is of equal importance to the question "When do you collect data?". While some disciplines prefer to include these steps in their primary research project (which can prolong the time between data collection to data interpretation), others delegate such tasks. For instance, some epidemiologists in our network prefer to delegate questionnaire programming to information technology experts, whereas members from social science prefer to develop this independently. This can lead to conflicting interests and tensions if not discussed before. Therefore, asking the above questions while planning an interdisciplinary project is essential (Kivits et al. 2019).

4. A joint *mission*, a clear vision, and a common goal are crucial for the project's success, particularly in settings where people voluntarily collaborate to strengthen their research (Brown et al. 2015; Nancarrow et al. 2013). While the ECRA, as a sub-section of the LSC DiPH, already had a mission before most members joined, it needed to be more precise. We recognized that many members didn't identify with the mission and did not collaborate. This led to a lack of purpose in their joining the network. In 2021, we opted for a bottom-up approach to redefine our mission and vision together with all ECRA members, which resulted in increased collaboration, participation, and creativity among our members.

5. A person's level of expertise can determine team communication and subsequently set hierarchical structures in a network or project. For instance, groups who had a leader with a medical background focused more on biomedical information rather than on other areas during discussions. The result can lead to tension and dissatisfaction in the team (Wittenberg-Lyles et al. 2009a; Youngwerth and Twaddle 2011). The best way to approach a hierarchical structure is through *mutual trust and respect* toward colleagues in the project (Jünger et al. 2007; Kilgore and Langford 2009; Xyrichis and Lowton 2008; Youngwerth and Twaddle 2011). This can be fostered through an open, friendly, and optimistic environment (Nancarrow et al. 2013; Youngwerth and Twaddle 2011). Eventually, this setting will support open communication and free speech and improve collaboration in interdisciplinary projects (Neumann et al. 2010; Sargeant et al. 2008; Wittenberg-Lyles et al. 2009b; Youngwerth and Twaddle 2011). For the ECRA, we decided to work without a hierarchy (besides two people representing the academy to the outside). This can be different in other interdisciplinary projects or networks. What is more important than the question of leadership is whether or not all people involved in the network can trust that their colleagues (from other fields of research) invest a similar amount of time and attention in the project (Nature 2015).
6. We want to emphasize the importance of *team organization and composition*. If (financially) possible, hiring a facilitator or boundary manager for interdisciplinary research should be considered, as suggested by the literature (von Wehrden et al. 2019). Their job is critical as they guide project managers during team planning and recruitment (Nancarrow et al. 2013). Earlier research identified that team composition and size have an impact on effectiveness. Unsurprisingly, those members with higher occupational diversity had a higher overall effectiveness score (Xyrichis and Lowton 2008; Youngwerth and Twaddle 2011). However, less experienced members also play a valuable role in team composition as they tend to ask more questions, which might raise awareness of different topics and eventually lead to new creative ideas (Neumann et al. 2010; Youngwerth and Twaddle 2011). After they help set up the team structure, facilitators can provide an overview of the required skillset for the project. During the project, they support the team as a mediator for discussions (Bolger 2021; The British Academy 2016). Additionally, the facilitator can serve as an administrative supporter and be in charge of effectively implementing the network (Kilgore and Langford 2009; Wittenberg-Lyles et al. 2009a; Xyrichis and Lowton 2008; Youngwerth and Twaddle 2011). A Ph.D. candidate and a postdoc representative facilitate the ECRA.
7. We are aware that interdisciplinary research requires *patience* as it usually takes longer and is more expensive than single-discipline research. This needs to be acknowledged when planning research projects and applying for funding. The longer duration of such projects comes from the structures mentioned above that

need to be enabled before the project members can start working (such as implementing a shared understanding, overcoming different research approaches and resulting conflicts, or forming joint research questions) (Bolger 2021; Brown et al. 2015).

5 Conclusion

DiPH is a field in which interdisciplinarity is not only possible but essential. To tackle interdisciplinary projects (such as developing MHMAs), one needs to reconsider seven pre-requirements:

1. *Communication*: Aim for an inclusive language between all participating project members.
2. *Exchange*: Invest some time in your project in team meetings to get everyone on board and set up informal interdisciplinary exchange spaces.
3. *Empathy*: Question other research approaches and accept that other fields research differently than your home discipline.
4. *Mission*: Collaboratively develop a mission, vision, and goal that every project member can identify with.
5. *Mutual trust and respect*: Aim for mutual trust in the group, especially between researchers from different disciplines.
6. *Team organization and composition*: Plan project funds for a facilitator and invest in a balanced team composition.
7. *Patience*: Interdisciplinary research takes longer than projects with teams from similar backgrounds.

Finally, the question arises: How can we achieve such requirements and conduct genuinely interdisciplinary research as displayed in this chapter's case study? We emphasize personal training and interdisciplinary education already in the early stages of the training curricula (Kilgore and Langford 2009; Nancarrow et al. 2013; Youngwerth and Twaddle 2011). By teaching students already interdisciplinarity, the future generation of public health researchers and practitioners will adopt the skillset to effectively work in interdisciplinary projects—in digital public health or other fields—to make an impact (Bolger 2021; Buchmüller et al. 2021; Di Giulio and Defila 2017; Downey et al. 2006; The British Academy 2016). To achieve this, universities, faculties, or institutes strive to teach their students through lecturers from different disciplines, by teaching students from various study fields together in one class, and/or through collaborations with stakeholders outside academia that students can actively participate in. Closing this chapter, we would like to highlight that the discussed features are essential for interdisciplinary work in DiPH but also extend to other research areas, with some adaptation.

References

§ 10 (DiGAV) (2022) Studien zum Nachweis positiver Versorgungseffekte (Studies demonstrating positive health care effects). Last changed through article 1 V. from 22.09.2021 BGBl. I p 4355, 2022 BGBl. I p 463, BGBl. I p 768

§ 139e (SGB V) (2022) Verzeichnis für digitale Gesundheitsanwendungen; Verordnungsermächtigung (Digital health application directory; ordinance authorization). Last changed through article 1 G. from 07.11.2022 BGBl. I p 1990, BGBl. I p 1387

§ 33a (SGB V) (2022) Digitale Gesundheitsanwendungen (Digital health applications). Last changed through article 1 G from 7.11.2022, BGBl. I S. 1309

Acheson D (1988) Public health in England. The report of the committee of inquiry into the future development of the public health function. HMSO, London

American Psychological Association (2013a) Psychology subfields. https://www.apa.org/education-career/guide/subfields. Accessed 29 May 2025

American Psychological Association (2013b) APA guidelines for the undergraduate psychology major. https://www.apa.org/about/policy/undergraduate-psychology-major.pdf. Accessed 29 May 2025

Andersson G, Cuijpers P, Carlbring P, Riper H, Hedman E (2014) Guided Internet-based vs. face-to-face cognitive behavior therapy for psychiatric and somatic disorders: a systematic review and meta-analysis. World Psychiatry 13(3):288–295. https://doi.org/10.1002/wps.20151

Bakker D, Kazantzis N, Rickwood D, Rickard N (2016) Mental health smartphone apps: review and evidence-based recommendations for future developments. JMIR Ment Health 3(1):e7. https://doi.org/10.2196/mental.49841 0.2196/mental.4984

Barrett DH, Lortmann LW, Dawson A, Saenz C, Reis A, Bolan G (eds) (2016) Public health ethics: cases spanning the globe. Public health ethics analysis. Springer, Cham. https://doi.org/10.1007/978-3-319-23847-0

Bartneck C, Lütge C, Wagner A, Welsh S (2021) What is ethics? In: Bartneck C, Lütge C, Wagner A, Welsh S (eds) An introduction to ethics in robotics and AI. Springer International Publishing, Cham, pp 17–26. https://doi.org/10.1007/978-3-030-51110-4_3

Bauer MS, Kirchner J (2020) Implementation science: what is it and why should I care? Psychiatry Res 283:112376. https://doi.org/10.1016/j.psychres.2019.04.025

Bauer M, Glenn T, Geddes J, Gitlin M, Grof P, Kessing LV, Monteith S, Faurholt-Jepsen M, Severus E, Whybrow PC (2020) Smartphones in mental health: a critical review of background issues, current status and future concerns. Int J Bipolar Disord 8(1):2. https://doi.org/10.1186/s40345-019-0164-x

Beaglehole R, Bonita R (1998) Public health at the crossroads: which way forward? Lancet 351(9102):590–592. https://doi.org/10.1016/S0140-6736(97)09494-4

Beauchamp T, Childress J (2019) Principles of biomedical ethics: marking its fortieth anniversary. Am J Bioethics 19(11):9–12. https://doi.org/10.1080/15265161.2019.1665402

Benke K, Benke G (2018) Artificial intelligence and big data in public health. Int J Environ Res Public Health 15(12):2796

Bolger P (2021) Delivering on the promise: how are sustainability research institutes enabling interdisciplinary research? Int J Sustain High Educ 22(8):167–189. https://doi.org/10.1108/ijshe-10-2020-0415

Borrill C, West M, Shapiro D, Rees A (2000) Team working and effectiveness in health care. Br J Healthcare Manag 6(8):364–371. https://doi.org/10.12968/bjhc.2000.6.8.19300

Braun J (2019) Die Versorgung mit digitalen Gesundheitsanwendungen nach den Regelungen des Digitale-Versorgung-Gesetzes (The provision of digital health applications in accordance with the regulations of the digital health care act). GesundheitsRecht 18(12):757–771. https://doi.org/10.9785/gesr-2019-181205

Brockmann D (2020) Digitale Epidemiologie (Digital epidemiology). Bundesgesundheitsblatt - Gesundheitsforschung - Gesundheitsschutz 63(2):166–175. https://doi.org/10.1007/s00103-019-03080-z

Brown RR, Deletic A, Wong THF (2015) Interdisciplinarity: how to catalyse collaboration. Nature 525(7569):315–317. https://doi.org/10.1038/525315a

Brownson RC, Colditz GA, Proctor EK (2017) Dissemination and implementation research in health: translating science to practice, 2nd edn. Oxford University Press, Oxford. https://doi.org/10.1093/oso/9780190683214.001.0001

Bucci S, Schwannauer M, Berry N (2019) The digital revolution and its impact on mental health care. Psychol Psychother 92(2):277–297. https://doi.org/10.1111/papt.12222

Buchmüller S, Malhotra S, Bath C (2021) Learning how to engage with another's point of view by intercultural, interdisciplinary and transdisciplinary collaborations. J Univ Teach Learn Pract 18(7):89–111. https://doi.org/10.53761/1.18.7.7

Calvo RA, Dinakar K, Picard R, Christensen H, Torous J (2018) Toward impactful collaborations on computing and mental health. J Med Internet Res 20(2):e49. https://doi.org/10.2196/jmir.9021

Chandrashekar P (2018) Do mental health mobile apps work: evidence and recommendations for designing high-efficacy mental health mobile apps. mHealth 4:6. https://doi.org/10.21037/mhealth.2018.03.02

Colditz GA, Emmons KM (2018) Accelerating the pace of cancer prevention—right now. Cancer Prev Res (Phila) 11(4):171–184. https://doi.org/10.1158/1940-6207.Capr-17-0282

Connolly SL, Hogan TP, Shimada SL, Miller CJ (2021) Leveraging implementation science to understand factors influencing sustained use of mental health apps: a narrative review. J Technol Behav Sci 6(2):184–196. https://doi.org/10.1007/s41347-020-00165-4

Cornet VP, Holden RJ (2018) Systematic review of smartphone-based passive sensing for health and wellbeing. J Biomed Inform 77:120–132. https://doi.org/10.1016/j.jbi.2017.12.008

Cvrkel T (2018) The ethics of mHealth: moving forward. J Dent 74:S15–S20. https://doi.org/10.1016/j.jdent.2018.04.024

Darmann-Finck I, Rothgang H, Zeeb H (2020) Digitalisierung und Gesundheitswissenschaften – White Paper Digital Public Health (Digitalization and health sciences—white paper digital public health). Gesundheitswesen 82(7):620–622. https://doi.org/10.1055/a-1191-4344

Di Giulio A, Defila R (2017) Enabling university educators to equip students with inter- and transdisciplinary competencies. Int J Sustain High Educ 18(5):630–647. https://doi.org/10.1108/Ijshe-02-2016-0030

Dochow C (2019) Telemedizin und Datenschutz (Telemedicine and data protection). Medizinrecht 37(8):636–648. https://doi.org/10.1007/s00350-019-5295-7

Domhardt M, Messner EM, Eder AS, Engler S, Sander LB, Baumeister H, Terhorst Y (2021) Mobile-based interventions for common mental disorders in youth: a systematic evaluation of pediatric health apps. Child Adolesc Psychiatry Ment Health 15(1):49. https://doi.org/10.1186/s13034-021-00401-6

Downey GL, Lucena JC, Moskal BM, Parkhurst R, Bigley T, Hays C, Jesiek BK, Kelly L, Miller J, Ruff S, Lehr JL, Nichols-Belo A (2006) The globally competent engineer: working effectively with people who define problems differently. J Eng Educ 95(2):107–122. https://doi.org/10.1002/j.2168-9830.2006.tb00883.x

Earnest GS, Reed LD, Conover D, Estill C, Gjessing C, Gressel M, Hall R, Hudock S, Hudson H, Kardous C, Sheehy J, Topmiller J, Trout D, Woebkenberg M, Amendola A, Hsiao H, Keane P, Weissman D, Finfinger G, Tadolini S, Thimons E, Cullen E, Jenkins M, McKibbin R, Conway G, Husberg B, Lincoln J, Rodenbeck S, Lantagne D, Cardarelli J (2006) Engineering and public health at CDC. MMWR CDC Surveill Summ 55(Suppl 2):10–13

East ML, Havard BC (2015) Mental health mobile apps: from infusion to diffusion in the mental health social system. JMIR Ment Health 2(1):e10. https://doi.org/10.2196/mental.3954

Eccles MP, Mittman BS (2006) Welcome to implementation science. Implement Sci 1(1):1. https://doi.org/10.1186/1748-5908-1-1

Egger M, Razum O (2012) Public Health: Zentrale Begriffe, Disziplinen und Handlungsfelder (Public health: central terms, disciplines and fields of action). In: Egger M, Razum O (eds) Public health. De Gruyter, Berlin, pp 1–22. https://doi.org/10.1515/9783110255416.1

Epstein JA (2013) Collaborations between public health and computer science: a path worth pursuing. Am J Public Health Res 1(7):166–170. https://doi.org/10.12691/ajphr-1-7-4

Fernald D (2008) Psychology: six perspectives. SAGE Publications, Washington, DC

Freeth R, Caniglia G (2020) Learning to collaborate while collaborating: advancing interdisciplinary sustainability research. Sustain Sci 15(1):247–261. https://doi.org/10.1007/s11625-019-00701-z

Friis-Healy EA, Nagy GA, Kollins SH (2021) It is time to REACT: opportunities for digital mental health apps to reduce mental health disparities in racially and ethnically minoritized groups. JMIR Ment Health 8(1):e25456. https://doi.org/10.2196/25456

Gardner B (2015) A review and analysis of the use of 'habit' in understanding, predicting and influencing health-related behaviour. Health Psychol Rev 9(3):277–295. https://doi.org/10.1080/17437199.2013.876238

General Data Protection Regulation (2018) Regulation on the protection of natural persons with regard to the processing of personal data and on the free movement of such data, and repealing Directive 95/46/EC (Data Protection Directive). Chapter 8 (Art. 77–84). Remedies, liability and penalties. European Parliament, Brussels

Gerlinger T, Babitsch B, Blättner B, Bolte G, Brandes I, Dierks ML, Faller G, Gerhardus A, Gusy B, for the German Public Health Association (2012) Situation und Perspektiven von Public Health in Deutschland – Forschung und Lehre. Positionspapier der Deutschen Gesellschaft für Public Health e. V. (Situation and perspectives of public health in Germany—research and teaching. Position Paper of the German Public Health Association). Gesundheitswesen 74(11):762–766. https://doi.org/10.1055/s-0032-1330011

Glänzel W, Debackere K (2022) Various aspects of interdisciplinarity in research and how to quantify and measure those. Scientometrics 127(9):5551–5569. https://doi.org/10.1007/s11192-021-04133-4

Glasgow RE, Eckstein ET, ElZarrad MK (2013) Implementation science perspectives and opportunities for HIV/AIDS research: integrating science, practice, and policy. J Acquir Immune Defic Syndr 63:S26–S31. https://doi.org/10.1097/QAI.0b013e3182920286

Gorman ME (2010) Trading zones and interactional expertise: creating new kinds of collaboration. The MIT Press, Cambridge

Greiner W, Gensorowsky D, Witte J, Batram M (2022) DiGA-report 2022. Techniker Krankenkasse, Hamburg

Grossman JT, Frumkin MR, Rodebaugh TL, Lenze EJ (2020) mHealth assessment and intervention of depression and anxiety in older adults. Harv Rev Psychiatry 28(3):203–214. https://doi.org/10.1097/Hrp.0000000000000255

Heimhalt D, Rehmann WA (2014) Gesundheits- und Patienteninformationen via Apps (health and patient information via apps). MPR. https://beck-online.beck.de/?vpath=bibdata%2Fzeits%2FMPR%2F2014%2Fcont%2FMPR.2014.197.1.htm. Accessed 29 May 2025

Hewett TT, Baecker R, Card S, Carey T, Gasen J, Mantei M, Perlman G, Strong G, Verplank W (1992) ACM SIGCHI curricula for human-computer interaction. Association for Computing Machinery, New York. https://doi.org/10.1145/2594128

Hockenbury DH, Hockenbury SE (2010) Psychology, vol 5. Worth Publishers, Worcestershire

Iyamu I, Xu AXT, Gómez-Ramírez O, Ablona A, Chang H-J, Mckee G, Gilbert M (2021) Defining digital public health and the role of digitization, digitalization, and digital transformation: scoping review. JMIR Public Health Surveill 7(11):e30399. https://doi.org/10.2196/30399

Iyamu et al. (2022) https://pubmed.ncbi.nlm.nih.gov/35656283/

Jordan EJ, Young SJ, Menachemi N (2021) Expanding the curriculum in a school of public health. Front Public Health 9:700638. https://doi.org/10.3389/fpubh.2021.700638

Jünger S, Pestinger M, Elsner F, Krumm N, Radbruch L (2007) Criteria for successful multiprofessional cooperation in palliative care teams. Palliat Med 21(4):347–354. https://doi.org/10.1177/0269216307078505

Kähler L (2018) Die asymmetrische Interdisziplinarität der Rechtswissenschaft (The asymmetric interdisciplinarity of jurisprudence). In: Rehberg M (ed) Der Erkenntniswert von

Rechtswissenschaft für andere Disziplinen. Springer Fachmedien Wiesbaden, Wiesbaden, pp 105–151. https://doi.org/10.1007/978-3-658-18494-0_5

Ke W, Liu Z (2012) Software engineering in public health: opportunities and challenges. In: 2012 international conference on computer distributed control and intelligent environmental monitoring, 5–6 March 2012, pp 630–637. https://doi.org/10.1109/CDCIEM.2012.155

Kilgore RV, Langford RW (2009) Reducing the failure risk of interdisciplinary healthcare teams. Crit Care Nurs Q 32(2):81–88

Kircher P (2022) Anforderungen an digitale Gesundheitsanwendungen – Wenn Innovationen auf die GKV treffen (Requirements for digital health applications—when innovations meet the SHI system). Medizinrecht 40(4):278–285. https://doi.org/10.1007/s00350-022-6160-7

Kivits J, Ricci L, Minary L (2019) Interdisciplinary research in public health: the 'why' and the 'how'. J Epidemiol Community Health 73(12):1061–1062. https://doi.org/10.1136/jech-2019-212511

Klein JT (2018) Current Drivers of Interdisciplinarity. In: Jennex et al. (Ed.): Promoting Interdisciplinarity in Knowledge Generation, pp 14–28 https://doi.org/10.4018/978-1-5225-3878-3.ch002

Kozlov E, Bantum E, Pagano I, Walser R, Ramsey K, Taylor K, Jaworski B, Owen J (2020) The reach, use, and impact of a free mHealth mindfulness app in the general population: mobile data analysis. JMIR Ment Health 7(11):e23377. https://doi.org/10.2196/23377

Kunkle S, Christie G, Yach D, El-Sayed AM (2016) The importance of computer science for public health training: an opportunity and call to action. JMIR Public Health Surveill 2(1):e10. https://doi.org/10.2196/publichealth.5018

Lash et al. (2020) https://shop.lww.com/Modern-Epidemiology/p/9781451193282?srsltid=AfmBOoqZ15LOVGbtpHj8CpAx_DKkTsXj3YSXwW0rXnypyb_8iYC1c7R2

Ledford H (2015) How to solve the world's biggest problems. Nature 525(7569):308–311. https://doi.org/10.1038/525308a

Lehtimaki S, Martic J, Wahl B, Foster KT, Schwalbe N (2021) Evidence on digital mental health interventions for adolescents and young people: systematic overview. JMIR Ment Health 8(4):e25847. https://doi.org/10.2196/25847

Leibniz ScienceCampus Digital Public Health Bremen (2022a) About ECRA. https://www.digital-public-health.de/ecra.html. Accessed 29 May 2025

Leibniz ScienceCampus Digital Public Health Bremen (2022b) Glossary on core terms for the LeibnizScience Campus Digital Public Health. https://www.lsc-digital-public-health.de/en/research/glossary.html. Accessed 29 May 2025

Luxton DD, McCann RA, Bush NE, Mishkind MC, Reger GM (2011) mHealth for mental health: integrating smartphone technology in behavioral healthcare. Prof Psychol Res Pract 42(6):505–512. https://doi.org/10.1037/a0024485

Maaß L, Freye M, Pan C-C, Dassow H-H, Niess J, Jahnel T (2022) The definitions of health apps and medical apps from the perspective of public health and law: qualitative analysis of an interdisciplinary literature overview. JMIR mHealth uHealth 10(10):e37980. https://doi.org/10.2196/37980

Maaß et al. (2024) https://www.nature.com/articles/s41746-024-01078-9

Maaß et al. (2025) https://link.springer.com/article/10.1007/s00103-024-03989-0

Madzvamuse A, Lubkin SR (2016) A note on how to develop interdisciplinary collaborations between experimentalists and theoreticians. Interface Focus 6(5):20160069. https://doi.org/10.1098/rsfs.2016.0069

Marckmann G (2020) Ethische Fragen von Digital Public Health (Ethical questions of digital public health). Bundesgesundheitsblatt - Gesundheitsforschung - Gesundheitsschutz 63(2):199–205. https://doi.org/10.1007/s00103-019-03091-w

Marckmann G, Schmidt H, Sofaer N, Strech D (2015) Putting public health ethics into practice: a systematic framework. Front Public Health 3:23. https://doi.org/10.3389/fpubh.2015.00023

Martinengo L, Van Galen L, Lum E, Kowalski M, Subramaniam M, Car J (2019) Suicide prevention and depression apps' suicide risk assessment and management: a systematic assessment of adherence to clinical guidelines. BMC Med 17(1):231. https://doi.org/10.1186/s12916-019-1461-z

Medin J, Krettek A (2008) An apple a day keeps the doctor away: interdisciplinary approaches to solving major public health threats. Scand J Public Health 36(8):857–858. https://doi.org/10.1177/1403494808094919

Medina FX (2021) Mediterranean diet: the need for cross-disciplinary perspectives. Int J Environ Res Public Health 18(11):5687

Miralles I, Granell C, Díaz-Sanahuja L, Van Woensel W, Bretón-López J, Mira A, Castilla D, Casteleyn S (2020) Smartphone apps for the treatment of mental disorders: systematic review. JMIR mHealth uHealth 8(4):e14897. https://doi.org/10.2196/14897

Mohr DC, Zhang M, Schueller SM (2017) Personal sensing: understanding mental health using ubiquitous sensors and machine learning. Annu Rev Clin Psychol 13(1):23–47. https://doi.org/10.1146/annurev-clinpsy-032816-044949

Morgenstern JD, Rosella LC, Costa AP, de Souza RJ, Anderson LN (2021) Perspective: big data and machine learning could help advance nutritional epidemiology. Adv Nutr 12(3):621–631. https://doi.org/10.1093/advances/nmaa183

Morss RE, Lazrus H, Demuth JL (2021) The "inter" within interdisciplinary research: strategies for building integration across fields. Risk Anal 41(7):1152–1161. https://doi.org/10.1111/risa.13246

Nancarrow SA, Booth A, Ariss S, Smith T, Enderby P, Roots A (2013) Ten principles of good interdisciplinary team work. Hum Resour Health 11(1):19. https://doi.org/10.1186/1478-4491-11-19

National Academy of Sciences, National Academy of Engineering, Institute of Medicine of the National Academies (2005) Facilitating interdisciplinary research. The National Academies Press, Washington, DC. https://doi.org/10.17226/11153

National Cancer Institute Division of Cancer Control & Population Sciences (2022) About implementation science. https://cancercontrol.cancer.gov/is/about. Accessed 29 May 2025

Nature (2015) Mind meld. Nature 525(7569):289–290. https://doi.org/10.1038/525289b

Neta G, Brownson RC, Chambers DA (2017) Opportunities for epidemiologists in implementation science: a primer. Am J Epidemiol 187(5):899–910. https://doi.org/10.1093/aje/kwx323

Neumann V, Gutenbrunner C, Fialka-Moser V, Christodoulou N, Varela E, Giustini A, Delarque A (2010) Interdisciplinary team working in physical and rehabilitation medicine. J Rehabil Med 42:4–8. https://doi.org/10.2340/16501977-0483

Odone A, Buttigieg S, Ricciardi W, Azzopardi-Muscat N, Staines A (2019) Public health digitalization in Europe: EUPHA vision, action and role in digital public health. Eur J Public Health 29(Suppl 3):28–35. https://doi.org/10.1093/eurpub/ckz161

Olthuis JV, Watt MC, Bailey K, Hayden JA, Stewart SH (2016) Therapist-supported Internet cognitive behavioural therapy for anxiety disorders in adults. Cochrane Database Syst Rev 3(3):CD011565. https://doi.org/10.1002/14651858.CD011565.pub2

Organisation for Economic Co-operation and Development (2007) Revised field of science and technology (FOS) classification in the frascati manual. OECD, Paris

Philippe TJ, Sikder N, Jackson A, Koblanski ME, Liow E, Pilarinos A, Vasarhelyi K (2022) Digital health interventions for delivery of mental health care: systematic and comprehensive meta-review. JMIR Ment Health 9(5):e35159. https://doi.org/10.2196/35159

Prowd L, Leach D, Lynn H, Tao M (2018) An interdisciplinary approach to implementing a best practice guideline in public health. Health Promot Pract 19(5):645–653. https://doi.org/10.1177/1524839917739616

Rehm J, Shield KD (2019) Global burden of disease and the impact of mental and addictive disorders. Curr Psychiatry Rep 21(2):10. https://doi.org/10.1007/s11920-019-0997-0

Rudd BN, Beidas RS (2020) Digital mental health: the answer to the global mental health crisis? JMIR Ment Health 7(6):e18472. https://doi.org/10.2196/18472

Salathé M (2018) Digital epidemiology: what is it, and where is it going? Life Sci Soc Policy 14(1):1. https://doi.org/10.1186/s40504-017-0065-7

Salerno J, Knoppers BM, Lee LM, Hlaing WM, Goodman KW (2017) Ethics, big data and computing in epidemiology and public health. Ann Epidemiol 27(5):297–301. https://doi.org/10.1016/j.annepidem.2017.05.002

Sargeant J, Loney E, Murphy G (2008) Effective interprofessional teams: "contact is not enough" to build a team. J Contin Educ Health Prof 28(4):228–234. https://doi.org/10.1002/chp.189

Serlet et al. (2020) https://www.frontiersin.org/journals/environmental-science/articles/10.3389/fenvs.2020.00063/full

Singer P (2011) Practical ethics, 3rd edn. Cambridge University Press, Cambridge. https://doi.org/10.1017/CBO9780511975950

Smye SW, Frangi AF (2021) Interdisciplinary research: shaping the healthcare of the future. Future Healthc J 8(2):e218–e223. https://doi.org/10.7861/fhj.2021-0025

Søgaard Neilsen A, Wilson RL (2019) Combining e-mental health intervention development with human computer interaction (HCI) design to enhance technology-facilitated recovery for people with depression and/or anxiety conditions: an integrative literature review. Int J Ment Health Nurs 28(1):22–39. https://doi.org/10.1111/inm.12527

Tabak RG, Bauman AA, Holtrop JS (2021) Roles dissemination and implementation scientists can play in supporting research teams. Implement Sci Commun 2(1):9. https://doi.org/10.1186/s43058-020-00107-4

Thacker SB, Berkelman RL (1988) Public health surveillance in the United States. Epidemiol Rev 10(1):164–190. https://doi.org/10.1093/oxfordjournals.epirev.a036021

The British Academy (2016) Crossing paths: interdisciplinary institutions, careers, education and applications. The British Academy, London

Thieme A, Belgrave D, Doherty G (2020) Machine learning in mental health. ACM Trans Comput Hum Interact 27(5):1–53. https://doi.org/10.1145/3398069

Torous J, Wisniewski H, Bird B, Carpenter E, David G, Elejalde E, Fulford D, Guimond S, Hays R, Henson P, Hoffman L, Lim C, Menon M, Noel V, Pearson J, Peterson R, Susheela A, Troy H, Vaidyam A, Weizenbaum E, Naslund JA, Keshavan M (2019) Creating a digital health smartphone app and digital phenotyping platform for mental health and diverse healthcare needs: an interdisciplinary and collaborative approach. J Technol Behav Sci 4(2):73–85. https://doi.org/10.1007/s41347-019-00095-w

Torous J, Bucci S, Bell IH, Kessing LV, Faurholt-Jepsen M, Whelan P, Carvalho AF, Keshavan M, Linardon J, Firth J (2021) The growing field of digital psychiatry: current evidence and the future of apps, social media, chatbots, and virtual reality. World Psychiatry 20(3):318–335. https://doi.org/10.1002/wps.20883

Tucker A (2003) A model curriculum for K-12 computer science: final report of the ACM K-12 task force curriculum committee. Association for Computing Machinery, New York. https://doi.org/10.1145/2593247

Tulchinsky TH, Varavikova EA (2014) A history of public health. In: Tulchinsky TH, Varavikova EA (eds) The new public health, 3rd edn. Elsevier, Amsterdam, pp 1–42. https://doi.org/10.1016/B978-0-12-415766-8.00001-X

U.S. Institute of Medicine (1988) The future of public health. National Academy Press, Washington, DC

von Wehrden H, Guimarães MH, Bina O, Varanda M, Lang DJ, John B, Gralla F, Alexander D, Raines D, White A, Lawrence RJ (2019) Interdisciplinary and transdisciplinary research: finding the common ground of multi-faceted concepts. Sustain Sci 14(3):875–888. https://doi.org/10.1007/s11625-018-0594-x

von Zezschwitz F (2020) Neue regulatorische Herausforderungen für Anbieter von Gesundheits-Apps (New regulatory challenges for health app providers). Medizinrecht 38(3):196–201. https://doi.org/10.1007/s00350-020-5482-6

Wagner CS, Roessner JD, Bobb K, Klein JT, Boyack KW, Keyton J, Rafols I, Börner K (2011) Approaches to understanding and measuring interdisciplinary scientific research (IDR): a review of the literature. J Informetr 5(1):14–26. https://doi.org/10.1016/j.joi.2010.06.004

Weisel KK, Fuhrmann LM, Berking M, Baumeister H, Cuijpers P, Ebert DD (2019) Standalone smartphone apps for mental health—a systematic review and meta-analysis. npj Digit Med 2(1):118. https://doi.org/10.1038/s41746-019-0188-8

Wienert J, Zeeb H (2021) Implementing health apps for digital public health—an implementation science approach adopting the consolidated framework for implementation research. Front Public Health 9:610237. https://doi.org/10.3389/fpubh.2021.610237

Williamson T (2007) The philosophy of philosophy. The Blackwell/Brown lectures in philosophy. Blackwell Publishing, Carlton. https://doi.org/10.1002/9780470696675

Wiltsey Stirman S, Beidas RS (2020) Expanding the reach of psychological science through implementation science: introduction to the special issue. Am Psychol 75(8):1033–1037. https://doi.org/10.1037/amp0000774

Winslow C-EA (1920) The untilled fields of public health. Science 51(1306):23–33. https://doi.org/10.1126/science.51.1306.23

Wittenberg-Lyles EM, Gee GC, Oliver DP, Demiris G (2009a) What patients and families don't hear: backstage communication in hospice interdisciplinary team meetings. J Housing Elderly 23(1–2):92–105. https://doi.org/10.1080/02763890802665007

Wittenberg-Lyles EM, Oliver DP, Demiris G, Regehr K (2009b) Exploring interpersonal communication in hospice interdisciplinary team meetings. J Gerontol Nurs 35(7):38–45. https://doi.org/10.3928/00989134-20090527-04

Wong et al. (2022) https://www.thelancet.com/journals/lanepe/article/PIIS2666-7762(22)00009-6/fulltext

World Health Organization (1946) Constitution of the World Health Organization. WHO, New York

World Health Organization (2013a) Mental health action plan 2013–2020. WHO, Geneva

World Health Organization (2013b) Health 2020: a European policy framework and strategy for the twenty-first century. World Health Organization Regional Office for Europe, Copenhagen

Xyrichis A, Lowton K (2008) What fosters or prevents interprofessional teamworking in primary and community care? A literature review. Int J Nurs Stud 45(1):140–153. https://doi.org/10.1016/j.ijnurstu.2007.01.015

Youngwerth J, Twaddle M (2011) Cultures of interdisciplinary teams: how to foster good dynamics. J Palliat Med 14(5):650–654. https://doi.org/10.1089/jpm.2010.0395

Zeeb H, Pigeot I, Schüz B, Leibniz-WissenschaftsCampus Digital Public Health Bremen (2020) Digital Public Health – ein Überblick (Digital public health—an overview). Bundesgesundheitsblatt - Gesundheitsforschung - Gesundheitsschutz 63(2):137–144. https://doi.org/10.1007/s00103-019-03078-7

Open Access This chapter is licensed under the terms of the Creative Commons Attribution 4.0 International License (http://creativecommons.org/licenses/by/4.0/), which permits use, sharing, adaptation, distribution and reproduction in any medium or format, as long as you give appropriate credit to the original author(s) and the source, provide a link to the Creative Commons license and indicate if changes were made.

The images or other third party material in this chapter are included in the chapter's Creative Commons license, unless indicated otherwise in a credit line to the material. If material is not included in the chapter's Creative Commons license and your intended use is not permitted by statutory regulation or exceeds the permitted use, you will need to obtain permission directly from the copyright holder.

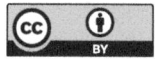

Overarching Issues

Public Health in the Digital Era: Digital Entry Points for Population Health

Tina Jahnel, Benjamin Schüz, and Hajo Zeeb

Abstract In this chapter, we investigate the development and implementation of digital health technologies in public health using the perspective of digital entry points into the overall systems of health determinants. We use current case studies to illustrate how digital technologies can enter and shape the sphere of health and social interventions or—through their post-entry diffusion—lead to positive or adverse consequences. We present digital extensions of widely used socio-ecological models of health that illustrate entry points and interactions and outline strategies for how identified entry points on various levels can be used to develop strategies for wider dissemination of digital approaches for public health, e.g., through participatory research. Further applied examples focusing on co-created tools and interventions to address social media misinformation illustrate some of the analytic and developmental potentials of the perspectives outlined in this chapter.

Keywords Entry points · Socio-ecological model · Social determinants · Diffusion of technology · Participatory design

1 Introduction to concepts of digitalization in Public Health

There is little doubt that information and communication technology has become a permanent and highly dynamic feature of modern social, economic, and cultural life and, at times, even a catalyzing force. Health services, the broader health system,

---

T. Jahnel · B. Schüz
Leibniz ScienceCampus Digital Public Health Bremen, Bremen, Germany

Institute for Public Health and Nursing Research, University of Bremen, Bremen, Germany
e-mail: tina.jahnel@uni-bremen.de; benjamin.schuez@uni-bremen.de

H. Zeeb (✉)
Leibniz ScienceCampus Digital Public Health Bremen, Bremen, Germany

Department of Prevention and Evaluation, Leibniz Institute for Prevention Research and Epidemiology – BIPS, Bremen, Germany
e-mail: zeeb@leibniz-bips.de

and public health, in general, are not exempt from these developments. In fact, they are often at the center of debates and societal arguments about the role, scope, and threats of digital technology, such as in the area of privacy and data protection, especially of highly confidential health data. Digitalization also affects public health through rapid changes in the workplace and the environment, for example, as new jobs emerge and old jobs lose some adverse characteristics but potentially gain new problematic ones. But how can we conceptualize the digitization of public health? Is it a random process in which technologies and their consequences simply arrive on the scene through trial and error? Or are there issues or areas—loosely called "entry points"—that are particularly amenable or open to digitization, for better or worse? We start the discussion with two case studies. They illustrate different arguments:

Case Study 1 The Bottle
In 2021, a bottle filled with what looked like urine became a global symbol of the sometimes horrific conditions under which employees of large online retailers were forced to work in warehouses and delivery trucks (https://www.cbsnews.com/news/amazon-drivers-peeing-in-bottles-union-vote-worker-complaints/). With their workdays and delivery routes meticulously planned and pre-determined by digital optimization algorithms, and then delivered to digital handheld tools (mobile phone apps), these workers had no time to schedule bathroom breaks or, in the case of deliveries, to stop for a bathroom break. Beyond the obvious issues of workers' rights and physical and mental health, digitally mediated working conditions like these are a key factor in explaining the social gradient in health—and how the pervasive digitization of everyday life and working conditions affects population health. There is little doubt that such working conditions are socially unevenly distributed. While the increased convenience of ordering consumer goods online and having them delivered quickly outside of national postal systems may improve the quality of life of customers who can afford to order these goods, those who work under these conditions often have no other choice due to lower educational attainment, structural racism, or the targeting of low-income groups for such jobs.

Case Study 2 The Pill Box
At the beginning of 2023, Germany (which tends to be a bit behind in such matters) faced yet another attempt to introduce digital patient records (also known as electronic patient records or EPR) into the healthcare system. Among other things, digital patient records would allow healthcare professionals (e.g., doctors, pharmacists) to access a patient's medication history and current prescriptions. This, in turn, would allow the assessment of potentially dangerous interactions between prescribed medicines, thus enabling safer and more reliable prescribing. This could provide significant benefits over the status quo and improve population health, particularly for older adults at high risk of multimorbidity and poly-medication. Other advantages of EPR include enabling quick access to patient records for more coordinated, efficient care across different physicians and improving patient and provider interaction and communication. At the same time, concerns and worries about privacy, unauthorized access to health records, data protection, and widespread

distrust of digital tools in health services, together with extensive lobbying by interest groups, have stalled efforts to introduce electronic patient records in Germany since the concept was first discussed in the early 2000s.

These two seemingly disparate case examples highlight that digital technology can affect population health through specific entry points: digital technology has the potential to streamline health services and processes that affect public health, deliver high-quality information or health promotion/prevention content to a wide population, and at the same time serve as a catalyst for social and health inequalities. Clearly, both examples raise more issues, serving to pinpoint the complexity associated with increasing digitalization and its contested effects on population health while very different entry points emerge.

In this chapter, we will attempt a systematic conceptualization of these digital "entry points" into public health. A systematic understanding of how digital technology interacts with known determinants of public health and how it can serve essential public health functions will support the development of effective technology-mediated tools to improve public health. Such an understanding can also improve the identification of potential risks for public health that emerge from an increasing use of digital technologies in everyday life and health settings.

2 Entry Points, Social Determinants, and Digital Rainbows

We use "entry point" to describe interactions between digital technology and processes or services that promote, reconstitute, or in the broadest sense, produce population health. Usually, "entry" or "access" points (Spruce et al. 2020; Walker 1975) describe locations or services through which individuals interact and enter the healthcare system. Here, we draw on a definition often used in computer science where the entry point describes the point in computer code at which a program begins to exert its function (Wikipedia 2023). This helps illustrate at which points and through which processes digital technology affects population health.

We are, of course, aware that speaking of digital entry points falls somewhat short of the actual state of affairs in prevention, health promotion, and health services, where digitalization permeates into applications, interventions, and systems. Nevertheless, identifying and understanding where the digital journey for public health begins and how information and communication technology finds its way into health and social systems and affects the distribution of health outcomes and access to health services is crucial both for analysis and for planning, e.g., of new interventions or services.

To derive and classify entry points of digital technology into population health, we rely on two central socio-ecological frameworks of health, which we extended with a view to digitalization in health. We present a digital adaptation of Dahlgren's and Whitehead's frequently used "rainbow" model of health (Dahlgren and Whitehead 2007; Jahnel et al. 2022) and a digital adaptation of the WHO Social Determinants of Health model (World Health Organization 2023). Social-ecological models outline the determinants of a particular outcome (in our case: health) on various, hierarchically organized levels within which lower levels are (partially) nested. For example, legal determinants for access to digital healthcare solutions might be decided on a state government level but affect the development and distribution of digital healthcare solutions on lower organizational levels such as neighborhoods.

The rationale behind using a social-ecological approach is that because digital technology and digitalization processes affect virtually every aspect of our everyday life in general and interactions with the healthcare system in particular, we can examine how digital technology operates within the suggested levels and processes of these frameworks.

3 (Digital) WHO Social Determinants of Health Model

As indicated above, digital technology and its application in public health are strongly framed and influenced by social and economic conditions. A complex set of links between aspects of digital technology and population health outcomes is thus likely.

The World Health Organization's Commission on the Social Determinants of Health Model is an influential social-ecological framework outlining pathways via which social inequality affects health outcomes, which at the same time outlines entry points of digital technology into public health. In Fig. 1, we provide an adaptation of the model to highlight entry points of digital technology into these social determinants of health and the respective outcomes.

The WHO social-ecological framework outlines three spheres of influences on health, which, in themselves, might operate on multiple environmental levels: (1) a higher-order sphere outlining factors in the socio-economic and political context that affect health, such as economic policies, governance factors, or cultural and social norms; (2) a sphere outlining how these higher-order factors determine an individual's standing within society, for example, through educational attainment that provides an individual with prestige and power, or through prestige assigned to specific occupations, or through societal gender norms (note that no distinction is made according to horizontal or vertical dimensions of inequality); and (3) intermediary and social determinants of health that operate on different levels from more macro-level determinants such as equal access to healthcare to more micro-level determinants such as individual health behaviors.

This distinction of spheres of influence allows the identification of mechanisms through which digital technology might affect public health.

The governance and legislation factors on the higher-order sphere affect the availability and integration of digital technology into the overall provision of health services, determine digital curricula for both health services employees and health services users, determine infrastructural requirements (e.g., building broadband networks, legislation for mobile data services), but also influence overall societal

Public Health in the Digital Era: Digital Entry Points for Population Health

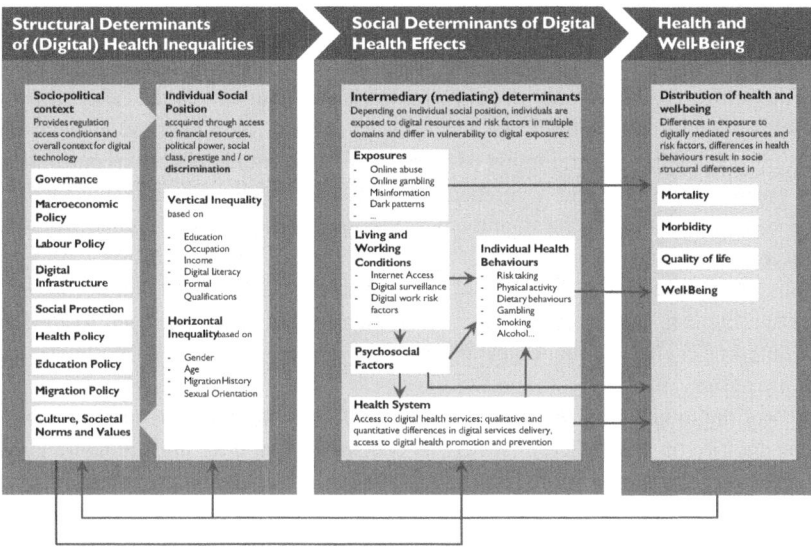

Fig. 1 WHO Social Determinants of Health Model (Source: own figure adapted from Weber 2020) with entry points for digital technology

norms and attitudes towards digital technology. For example, in Germany, a sometimes idiosyncratic interpretation of European data protection law has contributed to an overall climate that is critical of digital health infrastructure. At the same time, Germany has one of the first legislations globally regulating the registration requirements and reimbursement through statutory health insurances for digital health applications prescribed by physicians. The degree to which such applications are accessible to or prescribed to individuals thus depends both on the broader societal and policy frameworks—and on whether the prescribing physicians perceive a patient as a suitable candidate for a digital health application (which in turn is based on the physician's interpretation of the patient's social standing).

Together, these two spheres of broader societal factors and social standing determine an individual's access to (digital) resources and presentation to (digital) exposures in everyday life. The first example case at the beginning of this chapter highlights how occupational standing, affected by, for example, ethnicity or language skills, can increase the risk of being exposed to potentially health-damaging digital technology in the workplace. At the same time, the effects of digital exposures, such as dark patterns (manipulative design features) in websites that increase the likelihood of agreeing to potentially damaging contracts or features, depend on socially determined resources, such as educational attainment and (digital) health literacy. In addition, the risk of being exposed to online abuse increases disproportionally for those such as members of ethnic and sexual minorities, and the risk of acting on health-related misinformation in social media is similarly socially patterned.

4 The (Digital) Rainbow Model

Similar to the WHO Social Determinants of Health Model, the "Rainbow" Model of health inequities is a socio-ecological framework that categorizes the determinants of health into multiple hierarchical levels starting from individual-level determinants such as educational attainment to higher-level determinants such as cultural or policy norms (Dahlgren and Whitehead 2007). Specifically, these levels include general socio-economic, cultural, and environmental conditions, living and working conditions, social and community networks, individual lifestyle factors, and age, sex, and constitutional factors (Fig. 2). Within each level, "positive health factors," "protective factors," and "risk factors" are included that are considered to impact health outcomes. The unequal distribution of these factors may, in turn, determine health inequities.

The original model emphasizes the interactions and interdependent relationships between factors on the different levels as crucial to mapping and understanding health inequities. Since the model's original version in 1991, technological advancements have reshaped and influenced almost all aspects of society and everyday life. These developments in digital technology and digital transformation also imply that the determinants of health and health inequities in the model are undergoing a digital transformation, involving digital technology replacing or complementing existing non-digital systems and creating novel processes. As an addition to the WHO's Social Determinants of Health Model, the Digital Rainbow Model (with its hierarchical levels) serves as a usable framework to describe, examine, and modify digital determinants of health inequities and provides examples for digital entry points (Jahnel et al. 2022).

More importantly, this also allows hypothesizing and examining within-and between-layer interactions. It is possible that digital developments in one particular domain within one layer can buffer or exacerbate the effects of other digital determinants in the same layer or between different levels. For example, public discussion surrounding data protection and data security issues can influence the design of digital public health surveillance systems (an example of a within-layer interaction in the outermost layer "general socioeconomic, cultural and environmental"). Further, public opinion towards the acceptability of such digital public health surveillance systems can also influence the degree to which such tools are likely to be utilized (an example of between-layer interaction between the outermost layer and "Living and working conditions" (Pool et al. 2020)). Another example of between-layer interactions between the outermost layer and "Living and working conditions" lies in the expansion of the digital infrastructure, which determines individual internet access. The degree to which digital access constitutes health-protective or health-risk factors will likely depend on a person's access to tangible and intangible resources. Thus, people living in more deprived areas often lack sufficient internet bandwidth, which in turn influences access to online health information (an example of a between-layer interaction between "Living and working conditions" and "Social and community networks" (Kim et al. 2021)).

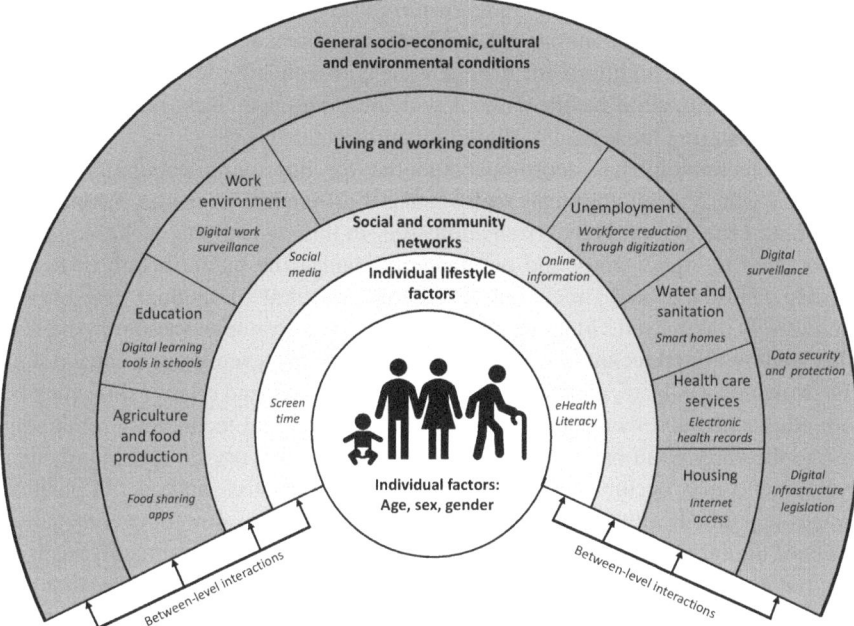

Fig. 2 The Digital Rainbow Model adapted from the original model by Dahlgren and Whitehead. (Source: own figure adapted from Dahlgren and Whitehead 2007)

The degree to which individuals access and utilize online health information is not only likely to depend on a person's internet access but also on how well they understand online health information and technical skills to navigate online health platforms (an example of a between-layer interaction between "Individual lifestyle factors" and "Social and community networks" (Cheng et al. 2020)). Thus, individuals with limited health literacy may be more vulnerable to misinformation, privacy breaches, or cyber attacks (Alvarez-Galvez et al. 2020).

5 From Entry Points to Digital Diffusion

The social-ecological models and examples above have highlighted how and where digital technology interacts with health determinants. The "entry point" metaphor can serve as a tool for understanding and identifying interactions between technology and determinants at different levels.

Here we want to outline a broader understanding of digital technology as a catalyst for the diffusion of health-promoting and preventive content. This understanding can act as an additional, novel component or pathway in the complex relationship between structural and individual aspects that influence health and disease, one that can both moderate other relationships between determinants and outcomes or act as a negative or positive "exposure" in its own right. By understanding entry points—both in terms of potential and as catalysts of inequalities and exposures—we may be able to identify conditions for diffusion and subsequently develop applications that promote population health without widening digital divides, favoring digital natives, or fostering the spread of digital misinformation.

Digital technology has enormous potential for improving population health when and where technology can really make a difference, as in the second case study, once critical issues have been addressed. In this case, digital technology has the potential to significantly and permanently change the public health or health services landscape and many of the structural and individual conditions. Alternatively, taking individual health behaviors as an example, these may be less influenced by digital technology, at least in some groups, even though entry points exist in abundance. Here, existing motivations, conditions, and relationships may be more entrenched and therefore slow to change, with digital technology remaining close to the entry point but not leading to change, or only very slowly. Many other developments may occur, ranging from successful, innovative, and overall positive changes in public health and its determinants to unfavorable, slow, or even negative effects of digital technology. However, where the "entry point" ultimately leads is often not easy to predict and is indeed an open question. To return to the first use case, digital technology may at some point have had some very positive effects on the health of delivery workers by simplifying processes, reducing unnecessary driving time, etc., but the role and influence of digital technology on the health of delivery workers overall are not clear. Therefore, examining digital technologies in the context of health also means looking for potential inflection points where effects and perspectives change.

If we systematically apply entry point knowledge derived from social-ecological models to identify challenges and then use matching knowledge and techniques to address these challenges, such as participatory agile development, digital technology has the potential to diffuse effective health promotion content into the wider population. This means that digital public health technology must perform tasks that are considered relevant by as large a proportion of the population as possible and then perform those tasks in a way that can meaningfully serve as large a proportion of the population as possible. To do this, the needs and preferences of different target groups must be integrated and taken into account in the development of applications.

Here, we explicitly distinguish between the inclusion of target groups in the planning and needs assessment of public health tools and the optimization of developing tools in relation to the preferences of the addressed populations: the former means that needs are actively taken into account already in the planning, and in the formulation of requirements, the latter means that preferences are taken into account later in the process during the design and operation of already developed tools. This can also mean that a certain degree of back-fitting of specialist technologies may be required for implementation if these were initially developed without much target group involvement.

A stepwise procedure (Fig. 3), for example, could suggest identifying the relevant target groups for interventions through systematic research, either using primary or secondary data or published research (step 1). In the second step, strategies can be identified and measures developed to ensure that members of these relevant population segments can be recruited for the development of digital tools. In concrete terms, the question must be answered regarding how such groups can be approached and motivated to participate. In the third step, suitable methods must be developed that enable and encourage active participation by members of the relevant target group, taking into account relevant culturally specific and social characteristics. In the fourth step, the requirements for digital applications can then be specified, e.g., within co-creation workshops, which can then be programmed through the joint development of an initially analog (i.e., non-digital) prototype (wireframe) and later as a digital version. Through suitable studies, which correspond to an iterative-cyclical procedure such as in design-based research, the prototypes of the application can then be further adapted to the needs of the relevant target groups and the fulfillment of central public health functions.

Case Study 3 highlights how entry points for digitally exacerbated inequalities—language and literacy barriers in particular—can be overcome through systematic research and co-creation, thus providing a pathway for the diffusion of digital health promotion content.

Case Study 3 The Chatbot
Informal caregivers of people with dementia are at significantly increased risk of poor mental health compared to the general population. Caregivers often provide care on top of their day jobs and in addition to caring for their own families. This puts them at risk of exhaustion and limits the potential to access both therapeutic and preventive interventions. Informal caregivers from minority groups are at an even greater risk, as the (limited) support structures and interventions available are often not tailored to specific cultural backgrounds or lack multilingual support. In Germany, for example, the largest minority group is Turkish Germans, with significant numbers of first-generation immigrants reaching ages at increased risk of

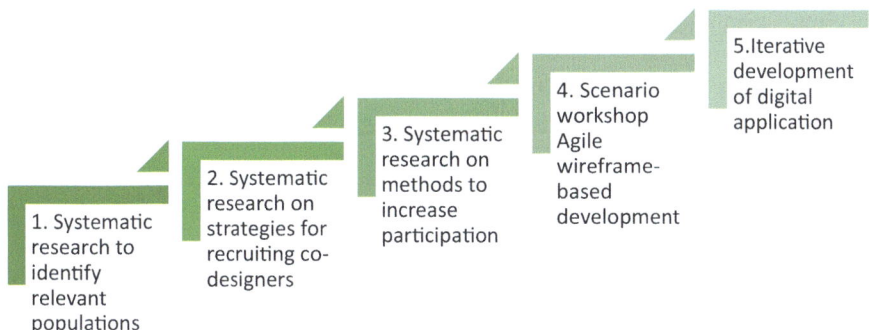

Fig. 3 Stepwise procedure in participatory design for digital public health applications. (Source: own figure)

dementia. At the same time, most support structures for caregivers are only available in German or are provided through non-minority networks (e.g., German-speaking neighborhood centers). In a current intervention development project (M-GENDER; www.m-gender.de), researchers have systematically used participatory co-design techniques to adapt and create intervention content for diverse target groups. A series of qualitative focus groups with Turkish-speaking informal caregivers identified that many caregivers use social media for information and socializing. Also, preferences and needs for specific information and support content were identified. In subsequent co-creation workshops, a social media-based multilingual chatbot was built and tested as a low-threshold access point for intervention content, and specific co-created intervention content (e.g., Turkish language instructions for applying for financial support, language-specific adaptations of evidence-based caregiver support videos) was integrated into this structure.

6 Diffusion Potential as Exposure? Social Media as an Example

At the same time, the diffusion potential of digital technology, such as the potential for enormous reach, can also become a risk factor. For example, during the recent COVID-19 pandemic, a "pandemic of misinformation" was spread mainly through digitally mediated social media. Previous perspectives on social media (Kickbusch 2019; Topol 2013) have highlighted the potential of these platforms to deliver health-promoting content to diverse populations with significant reach and ease of scaling. However, as both the algorithms underlying the promotion of social media posts and human attention and memory processes favor content that elicits strong emotional responses in recipients (and which is more likely to be false (Vosoughi et al. 2018)), the potential for the spread of misinformation becomes more apparent. Most of the algorithms that underpin social media recommendation systems are designed to maximize the amount of time users spend on the site in order to show them more advertisements and generate more advertising revenue. These algorithms take into account the amount of time users spend on a particular piece of content and, based on previously consumed content, serve up more and potentially more highly partisan content. For example, a person who reads posts with anti-vaccine information will be presented with more and more extreme content in their recommendations, with an increasing amount of (deliberate) misinformation in their recommendations. At the same time, the degree to which users are able to distinguish misinformation from factual information is socially stratified and varies by level of digital literacy (Rivera-Romero et al. 2022). Most current attempts to mitigate the effects of misinformation (if platform providers engage in such activities at all) rely on providing corrections to misinformation (so-called de-bunking (Walter et al. 2021)) or alerting users to the fact that they are being exposed to misinformation and providing them with techniques to identify misinformation as well as factual information (so-called pre-bunking (van der Linden et al. 2020)).

Building on our previously established terminology, this would imply that such interventions target known entry points, such as digital literacy. However, if we go beyond entry points and attempt a diffusion perspective, we might consider additional factors relevant to social media. Posting and sharing information on social media is a human behavior—and as a behavior, it can serve specific functions and have determinants that go beyond the mere factual or informational content of social media posts. An important notion here is that engagement with social media, particularly the sharing of posts, is a social behavior that may serve specific social functions. This may include signaling membership of or alignment with particular social groups or value-based communities or may be the result of operant conditioning processes whereby the sharing of specific content is rewarded with social reinforcements such as "likes," "re-shares," or an increasing number of followers.

For example, for a public health researcher, sharing information about the safety of COVID vaccines on social media may not only serve the function of informing other users but also signal specific identity-relevant information, e.g., that the researcher supports evidence-based health interventions and thus shares certain values with their network, or that they disassociate themself from anti-vaccine groups. Similarly, a person who shares vaccine-related misinformation may be signaling to their network that they share certain values with their network. As such, the message is stripped of its actual content but serves primarily as a social identification tool. Similarly, social processes in social networks, such as liking or sharing messages, provide social reinforcement to the person providing or sharing the information. Again, the main purpose of writing or sharing messages in this perspective changes from providing information to gaining reinforcement—making the actual content less relevant to these processes and suggesting that social processes, in addition to content correction, may lead to less misinformation being shared.

Case Study 4 Your Network Does Not Like This
A recent social media-based intervention developed by LSC members (Jones et al. 2023) makes use of the notion that sharing misinformation might also serve a social function. The intervention essentially consists of a balanced feedback tool—i.e., users who share posts do not only receive information on how many other users like or share the message but also information on how many users did *not* like or share the information. Together with information on the veracity or likely veracity of a post (e.g., warnings such as "This information on COVID-19 is misleading" previously implemented on Twitter), this demonstrably reduces the amount of misinformation shared by social media users. In a series of online experiments, the researchers exposed participants to certified (i.e., fact-checked and thus factually incorrect) misinformation on COVID-19 in their Twitter timeline and combined this information with either a label identifying the posts as misinformation, a label with balanced social feedback, both, or no label at all. Participants who saw posts that were accompanied by the combined misinformation and social feedback (see example below) were substantially less likely to share this misinformation than those

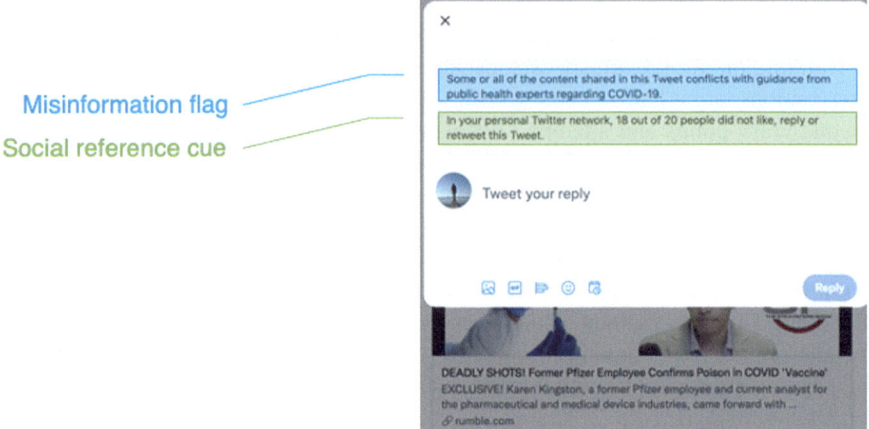

Fig. 4 Example misinformation post with misinformation flag and social reference cue. (Source: Jones et al. 2023)

who saw posts without labels. Importantly, they did not share fewer posts overall, which means that the intervention affected the sharing of misinformation but not the engagement and sharing of other information (Fig. 4).

7 Epilogue: Exit Points or the Reality Check in Non-digital Populations

Whether digital technologies for population health successfully move from just utilizing an entry point to the diffusion stage also depends on issues such as who is driving the idea of using new technologies: are users genuinely demanding digital approaches to improve their health situation, are professionals pushing for more digitalization, or are administrative processes requiring change towards digitalization?

As outlined previously, digital technologies that perform essential public health functions can serve to improve population health. If such essential public health operations are better served by non-digital means, either in whole populations or in specific population segments, effective and successful diffusion may also require analog or face-to-face solutions. If the development and advancement of digital tools in public health are driven primarily by technological advances, more powerful machine learning algorithms, cheaper and more powerful processors, or more easily integrated sensors, we may have a case of solutions in search of problems—rather than an evidence-based decision-making process in which population health needs drive a process for systematically identifying entry points for digital technology in health and scaling technology for population health benefit.

References

Alvarez-Galvez J, Salinas-Perez JA, Montagni I, Salvador-Carulla L (2020) The persistence of digital divides in the use of health information: a comparative study in 28 European countries. Int J Public Health 65:325–333. https://doi.org/10.1007/s00038-020-01363-w

Cheng C, Beauchamp A, Elsworth GR, Osborne RH (2020) Applying the electronic health literacy lens: systematic review of electronic health interventions targeted at socially disadvantaged groups. J Med Internet Res 22:e18476. https://doi.org/10.2196/18476

Dahlgren G, Whitehead M (2007) European strategies for tackling social inequalities in health: levelling up part 2. WHO Regional Office for Europe, Copenhagen

Jahnel T, Dassow H-H, Gerhardus A, Schüz B (2022) The digital rainbow: digital determinants of health inequities. Digit Health 8:20552076221129093. https://doi.org/10.1177/20552076221129093

Jones CM, Diethei D, Schöning J, Shrestha R, Jahnel T, Schüz B. Impact of social reference cues on misinformation sharing on social media: Series of experimental studies. j med internet Res. 2023;25:e45583. https://doi.org/10.2196/45583

Kickbusch I (2019) Health promotion 4.0. Health Promot Int 34:179–181. https://doi.org/10.1093/heapro/daz022

Kim H, Mahmood A, Goldsmith JV, Chang H, Kedia S, Chang CF (2021) Access to broadband internet and its utilization for health information seeking and health communication among informal caregivers in the United States. J Med Syst 45:24. https://doi.org/10.1007/s10916-021-01708-9

Pool J, Akhlaghpour S, Fatehi F (2020) Towards a contextual theory of Mobile Health Data Protection (MHDP): a realist perspective. Int J Med Inform 141:104229. https://doi.org/10.1016/j.ijmedinf.2020.104229

Rivera-Romero O, Gabarron E, Miron-Shatz T, Petersen C, Denecke K (2022) Social media, digital health literacy, and digital ethics in the light of health equity. Yearb Med Inform 31:82–87. https://doi.org/10.1055/s-0042-1742503

Spruce MW, Thomas DM, Anderson JE, Ortega JC, Mortazavi K, Galante JM (2020) Trauma as an entry point to the health care system. JAMA Surg 155:982–984. https://doi.org/10.1001/jamasurg.2020.2178

Topol E (2013) The creative destruction of medicine: how the digital revolution will create better health care. Basic Books, New York

van der Linden S, Roozenbeek J, Compton J (2020) Inoculating against fake news about COVID-19. Front Psychol 11:566790. https://doi.org/10.3389/fpsyg.2020.566790

Vosoughi S, Roy D, Aral S (2018) The spread of true and false news online. Science 359:1146–1151. https://doi.org/10.1126/science.aap9559

Walker LL (1975) The emergency department—entry point into the health care system. J Am Coll Emerg Physicians 4:129–132. https://doi.org/10.1016/S0361-1124(75)80244-4

Walter N, Brooks JJ, Saucier CJ, Suresh S (2021) Evaluating the impact of attempts to correct health misinformation on social media: a meta-analysis. Health Commun 36:1776–1784. https://doi.org/10.1080/10410236.2020.1794553

Weber D (2020) Chancengleichheit in der Gesundheitsförderung und Prävention in der Schweiz. Begriffsklärungen, theoretische Einführung, Praxisempfehlung. GFCH, BAG, GDK, Bern

Wikipedia (2023) Entry point. https://en.wikipedia.org/wiki/Entry_point#. Accessed 1 Jul 2023

World Health Organization (2023) The social determinants of health. World Health Organization, Geneva. https://www.who.int/health-topics/social-determinants-of-health#tab=tab_1. Accessed 12 Mar 2023

Open Access This chapter is licensed under the terms of the Creative Commons Attribution 4.0 International License (http://creativecommons.org/licenses/by/4.0/), which permits use, sharing, adaptation, distribution and reproduction in any medium or format, as long as you give appropriate credit to the original author(s) and the source, provide a link to the Creative Commons license and indicate if changes were made.

The images or other third party material in this chapter are included in the chapter's Creative Commons license, unless indicated otherwise in a credit line to the material. If material is not included in the chapter's Creative Commons license and your intended use is not permitted by statutory regulation or exceeds the permitted use, you will need to obtain permission directly from the copyright holder.

A Framework to Develop and Evaluate Digital Public Health Interventions

Chen-Chia Pan, Núria Pedrós Barnils, Saskia Muellmann, Tina Jahnel, Dorothee Jürgens, Merle Freye, Hans-Henrik Dassow, Wolf Rogowski, and Ansgar Gerhardus

C.-C. Pan
Leibniz Institute for Prevention Research and Epidemiology – BIPS, Bremen, Germany

Department of Prevention and Health Promotion, Institute for Public Health and Nursing Research, University of Bremen, Bremen, Germany
e-mail: pan@leibniz-bips.de

N. Pedrós Barnils · D. Jürgens
Department of Prevention and Health Promotion, Institute for Public Health and Nursing Research, University of Bremen, Bremen, Germany
e-mail: nupedros@uni-bremen.de; doju@uni-bremen.de

S. Muellmann
Leibniz Institute for Prevention Research and Epidemiology – BIPS, Bremen, Germany
e-mail: muellmann@leibniz-bips.de

T. Jahnel
Department for Health Services Research, Institute for Public Health and Nursing Research, University of Bremen, Bremen, Germany

German Centre for Neurodegenerative Diseases e.V, DZNE, Rostock, Germany
e-mail: tina.jahnel@dzne.de

A. Gerhardus (✉)
Department for Health Services Research, Institute for Public Health and Nursing Research, University of Bremen, Bremen, Germany
e-mail: ansgar.gerhardus@uni-bremen.de

M. Freye
Institute for Information, Health and Medical Law, University of Bremen, Bremen, Germany
e-mail: mfreye@uni-bremen.de

H.-H. Dassow
Institute for Philosophy, University of Bremen, Bremen, Germany

Junior professorship for Medical Ethics with a focus on Digitization, Faculty for Health Sciences Brandenburg, University of Potsdam, Potsdam, Germany
e-mail: dassow@uni-potsdam.de

W. Rogowski
Department of Health Care Management, Institute for Public Health and Nursing Research, University of Bremen, Bremen, Germany
e-mail: rogowski@uni-bremen.de

Abstract A rapidly increasing number of digital technologies have emerged with the aim of improving public health. To assess these technologies, a framework is needed that incorporates a public health perspective and takes the complexity of the technology, the context in which it operates, and its implementation into account.

Existing frameworks focus on health technologies, public health, or digital technologies. A framework for digital public health that supports developers, evaluators, policymakers, and researchers in systematically developing and evaluating digital public health interventions is missing.

We combined a scoping review of existing public health and digital health frameworks together with a consensus meeting with multidisciplinary experts. The outcome was a framework (DigiPHrame) that consists of 182 questions, structured by 12 domains: (1) Health Condition and Current Public Health Interventions, (2) Technical Aspects, (3) Usability, (4) Infrastructure and Organization, (5) Implementation, (6) Intended & Unintended Health-related Effects, (7) Social, Cultural, and Intersectional Aspects, (8) Ethics, (9) Legal and Regulatory, (10) Data Security and Data Protection, (11) Cost and Economics, and (12) Sustainability.

Potential users can apply these questions to any digital public health intervention they want to develop and assess. The framework is a living framework that will be constantly revised.

Keywords Digital public health · Health intervention · Framework · Checklist · Guideline · Criteria · Health Technology Assessment · Evaluation

Abbreviations

AI	Artificial Intelligence
CE	Conformité Européene
CEA	Cost-effectiveness analysis
CUA	Cost-utility analysis
HCI	Human-Computer Interaction
IT	Information Technology
LSC	Leibniz Science Campus
OSF	Open Science Framework

1 Introduction

The aim of public health is to promote and improve the health of people and communities through organized efforts of society. In recent years, a rapidly increasing number of health-related digital technologies pursuing these specific goals have emerged with a new concept: digital public health (Zeeb et al. 2020). While digital public health technologies operate in and interact with complex systems, both positive and potential negative effects depend on these interactions (Pan et al. 2024). In order to develop and evaluate digital technologies that incorporate a public health perspective, a systematic framework is needed that takes the complexity of the technology, the context in which the technology is supposed to operate, its implementation, and its varying effects on public health into account. Otherwise, we risk proliferating low-value technologies that are ineffective, burdensome, and reduce both quality and efficiency.

Currently, there are frameworks that analytically assess the use of medical-related technologies, for instance, the Health Technology Assessment Core Model in medical and surgical interventions, pharmaceuticals, and screening and diagnosis technologies (Lampe et al. 2009). A growing body of literature collects and synthesizes theoretical models and conceptual frameworks for either public health or digital health (Bashi et al. 2020; Shahin et al. 2020). However, a research-based framework for the development and evaluation of digital public health interventions is still missing. As such, with the *Leibniz ScienceCampus (LSC) Digital Public Health Intervention Framework*, (DigiPHrame), we aim to fill this research gap. It provides a systematic assessment tool that accounts for aspects such as the context where the technology operates, the stakeholders involved in the process, the complexity and implementation of technologies, and the intervention's intended and unintended societal effects (Pan et al. 2022).

This framework aims to facilitate the systematic development and evaluation of digital public health interventions for developers, evaluators, policymakers, and researchers. We developed a systematic framework with a comprehensive set of criteria framed as open-ended questions clustered within domains that are based on the insights of existing public health and digital health frameworks. That will lead interested parties through a broad spectrum of crucial elements when developing and evaluating digital public health interventions.

In this chapter, we introduce the 1.1 version of the LSC Digital Public Health Framework, DigiPHrame (Pan et al. 2023; Jahnel et al. 2024). Following a brief methods section, all 12 domains will be presented in more detail, including a definition, a justification for their importance, and potential stakeholders and experts to be included in each domain.

2 Methods

We took a mixed methods approach to develop this framework, combining a scoping review of the literature and a scientific consensus meeting with experts. The scoping review protocol is available at Open Science Framework (OSF https://osf.io/ku38m/). The scoping review was designed to (1) identify existing public health and digital health frameworks for developing or evaluating digital public health interventions in primary prevention and health promotion and (2) compile assessment criteria from identified frameworks. The search strategy included an electronic search of bibliographic databases, a hand search of grey literature with guidelines and frameworks, and a screening reference list of relevant reviews. The electronic search was executed on five international literature databases, MEDLINE (via PubMed), Scopus, IEEE, CINAHL (via EBSCO), and PsycINFO (via Ovid), in April 2022. Two researchers screened all references independently. Assessment criteria were extracted from each framework and mapped to the pre-defined domains based on the Health Technology Assessment Core Model (Lampe et al. 2009). For some domains, additional theoretical and conceptual literature was consulted. Criteria and domains were examined, synthesized, and validated during the online consensus meeting with 25 multidisciplinary experts and members of the LSC on the 19th of July, 2022. Domains were re-grouped based on the experts' opinions in order to best adapt to the landscape of digital public health.

3 The Framework

The first version of the *LSC Digital Public Health Intervention Framework* was published on the LSC website in July 2022, the (in 2025) current version 1.1 (Pan et al. 2023) can be downloaded as pdf file at https://www.digital-public-health.de/research/framework.html. In total, the framework consists of 182 questions, structured by 12 domains: (1) Health Condition and Current Public Health Interventions, (2) Technical Aspects, (3) Usability, (4) Infrastructure and Organization, (5) Implementation, (6) Intended and Unintended Health-related Effects, (7) Social, Cultural and Intersectional Aspects, (8) Ethics, (9) Legal and Regulatory, (10) Data Security and Data Protection, (11) Cost and Economics, and (12) Sustainability. The relevance and application of each domain will be summarized in the following sections of this chapter. If you find items missing or questions difficult to understand or operationalize, or if you have applied the framework and would like to share your experiences or have other relevant feedback, please contact us via: framework@lsc-digital-public-health.de.

3.1 Health Condition and Current Public Health Interventions

The domain *Health Condition and Current Public Health Interventions* comprises background information needed for developing and implementing digital public health interventions, the description of characteristics targeted by digital public health interventions, and current public health interventions or common alternatives. As reducing social inequalities in health is a priority for public health, this domain captures health inequities in digital public health interventions. It contains four topics with detailed criteria. This domain requires an extensive public health background.

Firstly, a general description and the number of people affected by the target disease, health condition, or health behavior are considered, followed by the health-related needs and requirements of the population and relevant settings. Components of the target population regarding digital literacy are assessed.

Secondly, target conditions are addressed. Conditions are defined as, for example, diseases, health conditions, or health behaviors described by basic epidemiological assessments. Relevant health determinants and the strength of association with the target conditions are appraised. The impact of the target condition on general society is also considered.

Further, the risk of digital public health interventions to increase health-related inequities between population groups is assessed. Disadvantaged groups can be identified, for instance, by using PROGRESS-Plus characteristics (O'Neill et al. 2014).

Finally, the current management of the health condition in this setting is analyzed, and the effectiveness of alternative public health interventions can be assessed.

3.2 Technical Aspects

We refer to health technologies or digital health technologies as digital technologies for public health interventions (Wienert et al. 2022; National Institute for Health and Care Excellence 2019). A health technology is not necessarily identical to the intervention but is an integral part of it. For example, a fitness tracker is a health technology; it can measure and record a user's physical activity level. However, wearing a device in itself is not a (health) intervention if the user does not interact with it or if the device does not show any results. The actual intervention involves presenting the data collected via the device to the user and providing feedback on or reminders of the daily steps to generate awareness of the inactivity or manage the exercise progress.

The technology elements of the health intervention can be assessed by two closely related domains within our framework, i.e., the *Technical Aspects*, and the *Usability*. In the domain *Technical Aspects*, we focus on the foundational technological components that enable a digital public health intervention. This domain addresses topics on the health technology's features and functions, interoperability across hardware and software systems, data integration capabilities, open-source design, software stability, internet connectivity requirements, and the feasibility of real-world testing. These elements are central because they directly influence the reliability, scalability and public receptiveness of the intervention. The adoption, sustainability, and effectiveness of the intervention in diverse setting can be determined by these technical aspects. Interoperability and data integration, for example, are crucial for ensuring that the intervention can function within existing health systems and data infrastructures as well as across the diverse devices (i.e., different operating systems and mobile devices, e.g., Android vs. Apple devices or Microsoft vs. Linux) within the general public. Open-source standards promote transparency and reproducibility, while considerations around internet dependency address potential accessibility barriers for underserved populations. Given the complexity of these technical aspects, a multidisciplinary team should be involved in this domain. This includes software developers, data engineers, user experience (UX) and user interface (UI) designers, cybersecurity experts, and healthcare information technology (IT) specialists, along with public health practitioners. Their combined expertise ensures that technological decisions align with both public health goals and the needs of the target population.

3.3 Usability

The domain *Usability* addresses how effectively, efficiently, and satisfactorily users can interact with a digital public health intervention. It covers critical issues such as accessibility features, language availability, user interface design, adaptability to users' needs, and co-creation with end users and stakeholders. It also considers user empowerment, trustworthiness of the information provided, and the presence of legal and regulatory transparency. These elements are essential because even the most technically advanced intervention can fail if users find it difficult to understand, navigate, use, or trust it. Usability directly impacts user uptake, adherence, and long-term engagement, which are all key to achieving meaningful public health outcomes. Poor usability can exacerbate digital divides, particularly among populations with lower digital literacy or accessibility needs. To ensure the intervention is inclusive and user-friendly, input from a wide range of stakeholders is necessary. This includes UX and UI designers, accessibility experts, health literacy specialists, software developers, and (representatives from) the target user group. Their collaboration helps ensure that the intervention is not only technically functional but also intuitive, equitable, and tailored to the real-world contexts in which it will be used.

3.4 Infrastructure and Organization

The domain *Infrastructure and Organization* is aimed at analyzing the structural features needed for developing and implementing digital public health interventions, as well as the impact of such interventions on the structure of the health system. Public health professionals are encouraged to address these questions to avoid potential implementation failure.

Firstly, in order to evaluate the structure of the setting where the intervention is taking place, a general assessment of potential barriers and facilitators is necessary. These barriers and facilitators can be found in different contexts, such as the political structure, the distribution of power, the budget allocation, the health system structure, etc. The degree of interaction between these contexts and the digital public health intervention needs to be considered. Further, the degree of flexibility of the intervention to suit the specific setting's local, cultural, and social needs is appraised.

Secondly, aspects relating to the digital public health intervention's stakeholders must be considered. This includes the required capabilities of the stakeholders (e.g., funds, human resources, or skills), the nature of the relationship between stakeholders (e.g., dependency, power structure, the intensity of connection), and the communication between them (e.g., regularity, intensity, mechanisms for conflict management). The study team should consider mechanisms for conflict management alongside examining the degree of alignment between stakeholders (e.g., shared vision, common goals, mutual acceptance).

Finally, this domain accounts for the interaction between digital public health interventions and the health system. The intervention may have an impact on the health system, its organization, and its efficiency.

3.5 Implementation

The domain *Implementation* describes aspects to consider before and during the implementation of the digital public health intervention to ensure that the intervention is delivered properly. Implementation failure (e.g., if the digital public health intervention is not delivered as intended) can result in diminished, unintended, or even adverse intervention effects for the target population. In addition, implementation failure may result in frustration for the intervention deliverers (e.g., health professionals). A public health generalist and individuals responsible for implementing the digital public health intervention are recommended to address this domain.

The implementation of the digital public health intervention is guided by a suitable implementation theory to underpin the implementation process as a priority. The interaction of the implementation theory with the setting, the context, and the digital public health intervention needs to be considered. In addition, the implementation outcomes and structure should be determined before implementing the digital public health intervention. The study team needs to decide on the reported implementation outcomes by being aware of a possible interaction between implementation and intervention outcomes. In order to successfully implement the digital public health intervention, several structural aspects are important:

- Material investments, premises, equipment, and supplies needed for the implementation.
- Data, records, or registries required to monitor the implementation.
- Requirements for qualification and quality assurance process to implement and maintain the intervention.
- Skills or training resources for the implementation personnel.
- Training resources and/or information about the intervention for the target group, their families, the general public, or other affected groups.

During the implementation of a digital public health intervention, several aspects need to be considered, including the stages of the implementation process (which are passed during the implementation), the employed implementation strategy, and the involved implementation agents. To assess the implementation's process, and agents, the interaction with the setting and the context, as well as the digital public health intervention, need to be monitored. Regarding the entire process of implementing the digital public health intervention, considerations must be made for implementation difficulties concerning duration, scope, disruptiveness, centrality, complexity, and the number of steps required.

3.6 Intended and Unintended Health-Related Effects

The main aim of digital public health interventions is to improve the health of individuals and the population. Therefore, the domain of *Intended and Unintended Health-related Effects* is based on a broad understanding of health. It considers the positive and negative, intended and unintended consequences of the digital public health intervention on physical, mental, and social health, quality of life, and well-being. It also includes changes in knowledge, beliefs, and behaviors, which might impact health.

As the domain is extensive and clearly structured, it should help to avoid these typical pitfalls in the assessment of digital public health interventions: (1) often, the intervention only focuses on changes in knowledge and behaviors without explicitly considering the effects on health; (2) even if the focus is on a positive health-related outcome, other outcomes, e.g., unintended negative consequences, might be overlooked; (3) health effects are not limited to physical health but also include effects on social and mental health; (4) while the focus is often on short-term effects, long-term effects may be of greater importance.

This domain distinguishes between mortality, effects on physical, mental, and social health (health effects in a narrow sense), physical and cognitive functionality, quality of life, and well-being. The choice of the most relevant health effects depends on the digital public health intervention.

Besides the direct effects on health, this domain also considers parameters such as knowledge, attitudes, behavior, motivation, and competencies, i.e., factors that might be modified by the digital public health intervention in order to impact health.

When applying this domain, it will first be necessary to identify the most relevant criteria for assessing the digital public health intervention and then operationalize them further.

3.7 Social, Cultural, and Intersectional Aspects

All digital public health interventions are acting within a social and cultural context. The relationship is mutual: The interventions are shaped by it and, at the same time, have an impact on it. For example, a fitness app to count daily steps is designed to improve health. However, it can also turn the activity associated with pleasure (walking) into an activity perceived as a duty (reaching a defined number of steps each day). Contact-tracing apps are designed to decrease the number of transmissions of infections, but they can also be perceived as a tool to control one's movements. Acceptance of a digital intervention may also vary depending on a wide range of socio demographic characteristics, and their intersections (e.g., gender, ethnicity, social class, education).

In this domain, the social, cultural, and intersectional aspects related to societies, communities, and groups of people, e.g., ethnic groups, demographic groups, people sharing the same neighborhood, interests, or a specific physical or mental health condition, are analyzed. Items of this domain include the context in which the digital public health intervention is supposed to be employed, the impact on values, norms, attitudes and perspectives of the community, and the relationship between the existing social groups. It also focuses on the acceptability of the intervention by the community and the role of the stakeholders and community members for the development and implementation of the intervention.

As this domain tackles many different perspectives (social, cultural, and intersectional), it will not be possible to identify one specific expert for an extensive assessment. Instead, it should raise awareness of identifying these perspectives and include at least some representatives from each perspective.

3.8 Ethics

This domain is dedicated to the ethical evaluation of digital public health interventions. It addresses the potential benefits and threats to ethical values that may result from the use of digital public health intervention. The domain is structured by the four ethical principles described by Beauchamp and Childress in their "Principles of biomedical ethics" (Beauchamp et al. 1994; Beauchamp 2019): autonomy, beneficence, non-maleficence, and justice. Detailed evaluation questions resulted from the scoping review, and a framework for the ethical evaluation of digital public health interventions was developed (Marckmann 2020).

The ethical evaluation questions presented are intentionally broad in scope to maintain their applicability in diverse contexts. The diverse contexts in which ethical considerations play a central role in evaluating digital public health interventions are impossible to cover comprehensively with a catalog of set questions. Therefore, experts in the field of ethics must specify the questions for concrete use cases. Empirical scientists should then provide normative fundamental reflection with empirical data in order to arrive at an ethically justifiable judgment for individual cases. Interdisciplinarity is thus a characteristic of the ethics of digital public health. The disciplines to be involved will depend on the specific intervention (see "Why Is It Essential to Address Digital Public Health in an Interdisciplinary Way?" chapter, Maaß et al. in this handbook).

Dealing with ethical conflicts does not usually lead to a solution free of contradictions. A central challenge of ethical evaluation is, therefore, to balance the outcomes of different questions and maybe even the underlying values. It can be necessary to involve relevant groups of the target populations in the ethical deliberation to better integrate their ethical values.

3.9 Legal and Regulatory

The legal and regulatory environment sets a framework of rules. The domain of *Legal and Regulatory* generates awareness about the areas of law that must be considered when developing or evaluating digital public health interventions.

Since the legal framework differs by country, the criteria only support developers and evaluators in deciding which areas of law need attention and whether an additional expert consultation in particular fields is advisable. Detailed legal questions are still left to legal experts. Consequently, this domain takes a meta-perspective: It is not the purpose of the domain to pose every specific legal question that has to be answered to develop or evaluate digital public health interventions. Nor is the domain intended to be final and static, regarding the fact that new regulations for health technology are constantly arising. The following criteria are independent of specific countries and, therefore, internationally adaptable.

As digital public health interventions inevitably process (personal health) data, legal requirements arise with respect to data protection. Depending on the country, there could be national or international laws or a combination of both that are relevant for evaluating or implementing digital public health interventions. Key topics include user information, consent, specific safeguards for data processing, and user rights. Additionally, there might be regulations about specifically dangerous data processing, such as data transfer to third parties or other countries and automated decision-making (e.g., AI). While closely related to data protection and not always clearly distinguishable from it, data security is another field focusing primarily on technological requirements. It might require appropriate technical and organizational measures or provisions for risk management, which is part of the *Data Protection and Data Security* domain.

The predominant user of a digital public health intervention will be an individual person who often is a consumer in a legal sense. Consequently, consumer protection can also affect the implementation and evaluation of a digital public health intervention. There might be requirements for creating terms and conditions and for the process of offering an intervention as a business model.

Additionally, some digital public health interventions fulfill the definition of a medical device and thus are affected by medical device regulation. There might be strict requirements to be fulfilled by those interventions to access the market, and permission (such as a CE-marking) is often mandatory. Closely related to market access, evaluators and developers should consider the possibility of becoming financed by the national health system. Recently, countries like Germany and France started reimbursing specific interventions when they meet national requirements.

3.10 Data Protection and Data Security

This domain provides information relating to data security and data protection. Digital public health interventions inevitably process (personal health) data. Therefore, security and data protection become essential elements when evaluating and implementing such interventions. To decide whether the requirements for data security and data protection are fulfilled, developers and evaluators need support from security experts and experts in data protection.

Data security focuses on the technological protection of data and therefore combines the aspects of data confidentiality, data integrity, data authenticity, data availability, and data controllability. Data protection relates to the processing of personal data. Regarding the principles of data security, such as confidentiality, data integrity, data authenticity, data availability, and data controllability, it is essential to consider their dynamic character: Technology is rapidly developing, and concrete protective measures might soon be outdated. Therefore, the criteria list specific technological measures (logging process, digital signature, security copies) but also refer to more generic measures (e.g., access and unauthorized access, cryptographic measures, protection).

The criteria to ensure data protection are mainly based on data protection laws and therefore require legal knowledge in some instances. Despite this legal background, the criteria do not replace a legal evaluation and should therefore not be perceived as such: Since digital public health interventions differ in functionality and concepts, additional questions in detail might arise from the legal perspective. The questions address universally accepted central principles (purpose limitation, data minimization, storage limitation) and dangerous data processing methods (e.g., processing in another country, third-party access, automated decision-making).

In sum, data security and legal experts should be consulted to ensure both legal and technological protection of the users' data.

3.11 Cost and Economics

Resources for funding digital public health interventions are scarce. Although digital public health interventions may lead to overall cost savings, the benefits they deliver frequently come with additional costs. The question of whether digital public health interventions can be considered a rational use of scarce resources is addressed by the domain of *Costs and Economics* with expertise in health economics.

To address this question, the relevant costs and effects need to be identified, and for which payer these are relevant. Digital public health interventions can be acquired by different payers like private individuals, companies, healthcare reimbursement agencies, or other public bodies. Weighing costs and benefits can be very different exercises depending on the funding body. Individuals who acquire health-related devices like wearable sensors may base their decision on technological fit with other digital tools, personal style, or display preferences. Companies might regard the acquisition as an investment into workplace health promotion which should result in net savings. These considerations differ from public healthcare reimbursement agencies, which are the standard recipient of health economic evidence and are typically interested in the costs of health gains when formally considering economic aspects. Complementary to health care funders, there may also be other public policymakers who may consider further aspects such as education or community building.

Tailored to the decision context, different methods can be used. On the one hand, the cost of illness analysis may shed light on the economic burden of the health condition addressed by the intervention. On the other hand, the intervention's success in alleviating the disease when compared to costs may be more relevant to the decision of whether to adopt it as a digital public health intervention.

The private value individuals place on digital public health interventions is typically measured by their willingness to pay. While individual decisions to acquire digital health technologies have a public health impact, they typically do not involve formal evidence. Nevertheless, manufacturers may elicit a willingness to pay for different device configurations to prepare for entry into the consumer market. Companies that decide on digital public health interventions as investments in workplace health promotion may be interested in return-on-investment analyses for different possible interventions. This typically involves comparing their costs with the potential cost savings from a company perspective, for example, due to reduced absenteeism or presenteeism. The standard case of economically evaluating new digital public health interventions takes a healthcare payers' perspective. It assesses their costs in relation to condition-specific endpoints (cost-effectiveness analysis, CEA) or condition-neutral measures of value (cost-utility analysis, CUA). For CEA and CUA, healthcare payers who consider economic evidence typically provide methodological guidance to ensure that the results are comparable across evaluations. Other public payers can, in principle, compare costs with users' willingness to pay to assess whether the interventions provide value for money even if its acquisition cannot be left to markets and even if health alone is insufficient for capturing the value provided by the digital public health intervention.

Besides the relation of costs and benefits, the impact of implementing a digital public health intervention on the payer's budget may be relevant. Even if budget impact analysis provides no information about the intervention's efficiency, it is still relevant for public decision-makers as it helps to estimate whether the budgets generated by the existing funding mechanisms are large enough to pay for the new intervention.

3.12 Sustainability

This domain focuses on the potential long-term impacts of digital public health interventions on the planet and its resources. Potential unintended and adverse effects on environmental, social, and economic sustainability may be prevented. Public health experts and professionals with sustainability or climate change knowledge may be consulted to address this domain.

Environmental sustainability is addressed following the logic of the life cycle analysis. That is, all resources needed to develop and maintain digital public health interventions and their carbon footprint are assessed. Moreover, several strategies that aim to reduce or mitigate the carbon impact and guarantee the enhancement of the environment ought to be considered when developing and implementing digital public health interventions. In order to be socially sustainable, digital public health interventions need to work towards generating more equitable, connected, diverse, and democratic societies. Additionally, the unintended social impacts of digital public health interventions and their mitigation should be considered, i.e., in order to be socially sustainable, digital public health interventions need to work towards generating more equitable, connected, diverse, and democratic societies. Finally, the potential financial burden, including cost-benefit effects for the upcoming generations, should be assessed.

4 Conclusion

This framework offers a comprehensive set of criteria/questions to support the development and assessment of digital public health interventions.

Users are encouraged to apply these questions to any digital public health intervention they want to develop or assess. Not all questions will be equally important or pertinent for all interventions, and some may not be applicable at all. As digital public health technologies differ widely, it is not possible to suggest a generic prioritization of criteria. Thus, the application of the framework is primarily user-led. At a minimum, it can serve as a checklist that helps to avoid overlooking key issues relevant to the performance of the intervention.

While this framework does not provide methodologies related to the questions, it may be sufficient to use common sense for some questions; specialist expertise will be necessary for others.

The current version of the framework is based on a systematic literature search and a subsequent meeting with interdisciplinary experts. It has also been applied to a few digital public health interventions. We acknowledge the ever-evolving digital world and new digital public health technologies opportunities by continually revising the framework as the digital future emerges.

Thus, the framework will be a living document. If readers are interested in participating as experts, think that some items are missing, find questions difficult to understand or operationalize, or if readers have applied the framework and would like to share their experience, they may contact the authors via email: framework@lsc-digital-public-health.de.

References

Bashi N, Fatehi F, Mosadeghi-Nik M, Askari M, Karunanithi M (2020) Digital health interventions for chronic diseases: a scoping review of evaluation frameworks. BMJ Health Care Inform 27(1):e100066. https://doi.org/10.1136/bmjhci-2019-100066

Beauchamp TL (2019) In: Childress JF (ed) Principles of biomedical ethics. Oxford University Press, New York, NY

Beauchamp TL, Beauchamp TA, Childress JF (1994) Principles of biomedical ethics. Edicoes Loyola

Jahnel T, Pan CC, Pedros Barnils N, Muellmann S, Freye M, Dassow HH, Lange O, Reinschluessel AV, Rogowski W, Gerhardus A (2024) Developing and Evaluating Digital Public Health Interventions Using the Digital Public Health Framework DigiPHrame: A Framework Development Study. Journal of Medical Internet Research 26e54269-10.2196/54269

Lampe K, Mäkelä M, Garrido MV, Anttila H, Autti-Rämö I, Hicks NJ, Hofmann B et al (2009) The HTA core model: a novel method for producing and reporting health technology assessments. Int J Technol Assess Health Care 25(S2):9–20

Marckmann G (2020) Ethische fragen von digital public health. Bundesgesundheitsblatt-Gesundheitsforschung-Gesundheitsschutz 63(2):199–205

National Institute for Health and Care Excellence (2019) Evidence standards framework for digital health technologies. National Institute for Health and Care Excellence, London

O'Neill J, Tabish H, Welch V, Petticrew M, Pottie K, Clarke M, Evans T et al (2014) Applying an equity lens to interventions: using PROGRESS ensures consideration of socially stratifying factors to illuminate inequities in health. J Clin Epidemiol 67(1):56–64

Pan CC, Pedros Barnils N, Juergens D, Muellmann S, Janetzki S, Kolschen J, Freye M, Dassow HH, Lange O, Rogowski W, Reinschluessel A, Forberger S, Jahnel T, Schuez B, Gerhardus A. (2023) Developing and Assessing Digital Public Health Interventions: A Digital Public Health Framework (DigiPHrame) Version 1.1. Leibniz ScienceCampus Digital Public Health, Bremen. https://doi.org/10.17605/OSF.IO/UB3W4

Pan CC, Urban M, Schuez B (2024) Unintended Consequences of Digital Behavior Change Interventions: A Social–Ecological Perspective. European Journal of Health Psychology, 31(3), 141–149. https://doi.org/10.1027/2512-8442/a000149

Shahin Z, Messick A, Harris J, Waterfield KC, Shah GH (2020) A scoping review of theoretical models and conceptual frameworks used in Public Health Services and Systems Research (PHSSR) literature. Glob J Med Public Health 9(1):1

Wienert J, Jahnel T, Maaß L (2022) What are digital public health interventions? First steps toward a definition and an intervention classification framework. J Med Internet Res 24(6):e31921

Zeeb H, Pigeot I, Schüz B (2020) Digital Public Health–ein Überblick. Bundesgesundheitsblatt-Gesundheitsforschung-Gesundheitsschutz 63(2):137–144

Open Access This chapter is licensed under the terms of the Creative Commons Attribution 4.0 International License (http://creativecommons.org/licenses/by/4.0/), which permits use, sharing, adaptation, distribution and reproduction in any medium or format, as long as you give appropriate credit to the original author(s) and the source, provide a link to the Creative Commons license and indicate if changes were made.

The images or other third party material in this chapter are included in the chapter's Creative Commons license, unless indicated otherwise in a credit line to the material. If material is not included in the chapter's Creative Commons license and your intended use is not permitted by statutory regulation or exceeds the permitted use, you will need to obtain permission directly from the copyright holder.

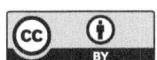

Participatory Approaches for Digital Public Health: Giving Voice to Values

Rehana Shrestha, Anke V. Reinschluessel, and Jasmin Niess

Abstract This chapter discusses the need for community involvement and stakeholder engagement in the development and implementation of digital public health tools. The advent of digitalization in public health has necessitated an exploration of how to design tools that meet the needs of the community they serve. This can be achieved through a participatory approach that incorporates the voices and perspectives of all stakeholders in a democratic manner. Specifically, this chapter discusses two participatory approaches: participatory design and participatory research. These approaches originate from different intellectual traditions but share a vision of incorporating everyone from the community affected by the intervention or technology. Additionally, this chapter presents application examples from the literature on how the development of health-related applications benefited from participatory research and participatory design to illustrate the added value of integrating these approaches.

Keywords Participation · Digital public health · Participatory design · Participatory research

---

R. Shrestha (✉)
University of Bremen, Social Epidemiology, Bremen, Germany

Leibniz ScienceCampus Digital Public Health Bremen, Bremen, Germany
e-mail: rehana@uni-bremen.de

A. V. Reinschluessel
Leibniz ScienceCampus Digital Public Health Bremen, Bremen, Germany

University of Bremen, Digital Media Lab, Bremen, Germany

HCI Group, University of Konstanz, Konstanz, Germany
e-mail: anke.reinschluessel@uni-konstanz.de

J. Niess
Leibniz ScienceCampus Digital Public Health Bremen, Bremen, Germany

Design of Information Systems (DESIGN), University of Oslo, Oslo, Norway
e-mail: jasminni@uio.no

© The Author(s) 2025
H. Zeeb et al. (eds.), *Digital Public Health*, Springer Series on Epidemiology and Public Health, https://doi.org/10.1007/978-3-031-90154-6_4

Abbreviations

DEMOS	DEMOkratiske Styringsssstemer
DHIS	District Health Information Software
d-MH	Digital mental health
d-SWEB	Digital social and emotional well-being
DUE	Demokrati Udvikling og Edb
HCI	Human-Computer Interaction
HISP	Health Information Systems Program
IAP	International Association of Public Participation
NHS	National Health Service
PLWH	People living with HIV
SES	Socio-economic status
WHO	World Health Organization

1 Introduction

In this chapter, digital public health is defined as using digital technologies to work towards achieving public health goals (Iyamu et al. 2021; Odone et al. 2019). Thus, digital technologies and concepts can be applied to restructure and reimagine processes and knowledge acquisition and distribution in the context of digital public health. For example, the health data collected by fitness trackers (e.g., heart rate, steps taken) can be used to inform public health policies or personalize public health interventions. Both policymakers and researchers argue for the potential that digital public health holds. However, despite the increasing interest in digital public health, open challenges such as ethical questions, a lack of clear standards regarding the design of digital public health interventions, and challenges concerning access to technologies remain (Iyamu et al. 2022). To illustrate, not everyone in the world has the same access to digital public health interventions and has comparable technical infrastructures available. This, in turn, can lead to or exacerbate health inequalities. For instance, people in rural or low socio-economic status (SES) areas may not have access to (high-speed) internet or smartphones, which will naturally limit their ability to access and use digital health technologies. Consequently, this potentially reinforces inequalities as it gives people different levels of access to health information and resources than people in more affluent areas.

To address open challenges in digital public health and establish structures that facilitate societies' long-term health and well-being, the participation of all stakeholders is crucial. Participation of the community, as well as other stakeholders, including consumers and end-users, youth, individuals from marginalized communities, developers, and practitioners, among others, is widely recognized as essential for building a healthier society. The World Health Organization (WHO) regards participation as a "means of organizing action and motivating individuals and communities" to "shape policies and projects to meet their priorities" (World Health Organization 1992). On another note, the importance of community participation in health research was formally recognized by the 1986 Ottawa Charter, which defines health promotion as "the process of enabling people to increase control over and to improve their health" (World Health Organization 1986). Emphasizing community participation as a cornerstone to achieve health for all and reduce health inequalities, the Charter indicates "working through concrete and effective community action in setting priorities, making decisions, planning strategies, and implementing them to achieve better health" (World Health Organization 1986). "Increasing control over one's health" includes control over digital public health strategies, initiatives, personal health technologies, and digital public health systems.

In other words, in the context of digital public health, participation can foster a closer fit to user needs, improved service experiences, integration of values, facilitating change from within, and supporting uptake and long-term use of the digital public health system.

Although participatory approaches have a high potential to promote and support digital public health in a meaningful way, the concrete ways to actually apply them in digital public health contexts are still underexplored. Along similar lines, participatory approaches are not yet widely used in Europe (with a few notable exceptions). Whereas participatory approaches are already frequently applied in smaller (research) projects focusing on the participatory development of health applications for individuals or small groups, participatory approaches in the area of public health are rarely observed on a societal level. This chapter aims to discuss the potential of participatory approaches for digital public health. Positive examples are used to illustrate the potential of participatory approaches in this context. However, challenges and potential conceptual ambiguities will also be discussed, which can be partly attributed to the inter- and multidisciplinarity in the field of digital public health.

Consequently, this chapter aims to discuss definitions and approaches of participation and their relevance to the digital public health field. It is important to note that this chapter is not meant to be a complete account of all existing participatory approaches. Instead, it is intended (with the help of examples) to provide inspiration and starting points for interested readers and to demonstrate the potential of participatory approaches for the field of digital public health. The structure of this chapter is as follows: First, it will give an account of participatory approaches such as participatory research and participatory design. Then, it will outline a few cases of participatory approaches in the context of digital public health. The chapter then concludes with a short summary and outlook.

2 Participatory Approaches

When conceptualizing, designing, evaluating, and refining digital public health interventions, many different groups are involved (e.g., designers and end users). This is the case for the majority of technologies developed and available today. In the field of digital public health, however, the situation is somewhat more complex since several different users can potentially be counted towards the group of end users (e.g., patients, clinicians, and politicians). There are efforts and a demand to integrate all relevant groups into the design and research process of digital public health interventions. However, in practice, there is still considerable potential for improvement (Mucha et al. 2022). To address the needs of relevant stakeholder groups in designing solutions, two different participatory approaches have emerged in different intellectual traditions. On the one hand, *Participatory Research* is emerging from Kurt Lewin's "northern tradition" of social action research and Paulo Friere's "southern tradition" of emancipatory theory and practice (Macaulay 2016) and on the other hand, there is *Participatory Design*, which has its roots in Scandinavian action research and what was then often called cooperative design (Bødker and Kyng 2018). These approaches have some similarities and differences. In the following sections, we describe both approaches briefly and highlight their similarities and differences.

2.1 Participatory Research

Participatory research finds its origins in social action research and emancipatory philosophy, thereby promoting that research be undertaken with or by society's marginalized people, or having people as full participants in inquiry, enabling them to determine their own needs to improve their own lives (Macaulay 2016). It is considered a research-to-action approach that engages those who are usually not trained in research. Vaughn and Jacquez (2020) defined participatory research as an umbrella term for "research designs, methods, and frameworks that use systematic inquiry in direct collaboration with those affected by the issue being studied for the purpose of action or change." The main premise of participatory research is to ensure the active roles of stakeholders, community members, and end users in the research process and shared decision-making while also including those with insider knowledge and lived experience or those belonging to or representing the interests of the people who are the focus of the research (Jagosh et al. 2012). As pointed out by Cook (2012), participatory approaches do not merely ask participants to comment on what "is" but engage them to work together to design what "could be." As such, the approach intends to build positive working relationships and meaningful interactions to harness the dynamic interchange of knowledge and understanding, bringing together contextualized understanding, practical experience, wisdom, and reasoning.

Many variations of participatory research are used across disciplines (see Vaughn and Jacquez 2020 for an overview). Among the approaches included within the field of public health are, for instance, community-based participatory research (Minkler and Wallerstein 2011), participatory action research (Kemmis 2006), participatory rural appraisal (Chambers 1994), cooperative inquiry (Reason 1999), participatory evaluation (Cousins and Whitmore 1998), etc. As suggested by Vaughn and Jacquez (2020), the breadth of terms describing the participatory research orientation is vast, spreading across disciplines. Nonetheless, they share a common mission of inclusivity, valuing the direct engagement of those who are beneficiaries, users, and stakeholders of the research rather than considering them mere subjects of the research. This integrates researchers' theoretical and methodology expertise with nonacademic participants' real-world knowledge and experiences (Balazs and Morello-Frosch 2013; Cargo and Mercer 2008; Vaughn and Jacquez 2020). Thus, participatory research is an orientation rather than a method, and research designs and methods used in participatory research are highly diverse, including both qualitative and quantitative methods. Instead of single-event data collection methods, participatory research uses methods that engage people in each step of the research process. These methods include tools, tasks, structured activities, networks, that facilitate shared decision-making, and mutual learning. In this respect, Duea et al. (2022) provide an overview of participatory research methods that are organized into five domains: (1) engagement and capacity building, (2) exploration and visioning, (3) visual and narrative, (4) mobilization, and (5) evaluation. Rather than supporting a specific stage in the research process, these categorizations intend to link each method to a collaborative goal.

Participatory research approaches are suggested to have a direct effect on both participants as well as researchers. In the case of participants, the approach holds the possibility to shape their thoughts, knowledge, and practices, whereas researchers are influenced by making them to reflect on the theories they draw upon, the design, rigor, and trustworthiness of the process that is adopted, as well as knowledge about practice and policy (Cook 2012). Thus, according to Cargo and Mercer (2008) the presence of mutual respect and trust among those involved in participatory research is essential to support capacity building, empowerment, and ownership, and these are the aspects that separate participatory research from other forms of research that are collaborative or action-oriented but not participatory.

Similarly, Bergold and Thomas (2012) propose fundamental principles or distinctive features of participatory research that guide researchers to make greater use of participatory research elements. These principles include (1) democracy as a precondition, (2) creating a "safe space," (3) defining "community," and (4) determining degrees of participation. As participatory research aims at an equitable research process for both the participants and researchers, forging a democratic working process is one of the key aspects. Achieving such a democratic working process, however, demands a higher level of involvement of participants as co-researchers (Unger 2013). Creating a "safe space" is another crucial aspect that needs consideration, especially while working with vulnerable groups (Duarte et al. 2018). Since participatory research requires a strong willingness on the part of participants to contribute their personal views, opinions, and experiences, a sufficient degree of openness and trust between researchers and participants is necessary for participants to dare to share their thoughts. Such a "safe space" becomes even more important in a participatory research process seeking to co-produce knowledge amidst dissenting views. Instead of creating a conflict-free space, ensuring a space where such conflicts can be jointly discussed, solved, or at least accepted as different positions can bring different perspectives on the subject under study (Bergold and Thomas 2012). Another vital element to be considered in participatory research is defining the "community" or, in other words, identifying groups to be involved. Bergold and Thomas (2012) put forward two fundamental dichotomies observed in participatory research. While there are a number of studies in which researchers and practitioners collaborate and in which practitioners are either involved, or they themselves carry out research with the support of researchers, several other studies directly involve the affected groups in research. The former category of studies has been referred to as "practice-partners" and the latter as "community-partners" research (Von Unger et al. 2012). Nonetheless, it remains rather challenging to define, identify, and include representatives of all groups affected by a problem, and, as suggested by Le Dantec and Fox (2015), the decision on who is involved should be made at the beginning of the research.

Following the question of which groups will be collaborators, another question arises as to what degree these groups should be involved, i.e., the degree of participation. Discussions are ongoing regarding which activities or research processes the participants should be involved in and whether there should be different degrees of participation for different groups. To determine the degree of participation, several participation models exist currently, such as the model developed by Wright et al. (2010), and by the International Association of Public Participation (IAP2) (IAP 2014), all drawing upon the seminal work of Arnstein's "ladder of participation" (Arnstein 1969). Ideally, as mentioned above, to achieve a democratic working process, it is suggested to involve participants in all stages of the research process as equal partners, such as research design, data collection, and data analysis. Yet, the degree of participation may vary depending on their particular situation and interest (Duarte et al. 2018). While on the one hand, Unger (2013) suggests involving at least some members of all affected groups across all stages of the research process with sufficient flexibility according to the conditions, Wright et al. (2010), on the other hand, do not demand the involvement of the same group across all stages. In this respect, as Bergold and Thomas (2012) suggested, it is important to specify "who, with what rights, at what point in time, and with regard to what theme" can participate in a decision. For example, in the development of community-based digital mental health (see Sect. 3), the researchers seek to involve local indigenous community members, organizational representatives, researchers, and others in all elements of a research project from the outset of the project. Through this, the researchers aim to develop culturally relevant digital health interventions. Whereas in most participatory sensing research (see Sect. 3), researchers often seek to integrate the participants' subjective perception, thereby engaging participants during the data collection phase.

2.2 Participatory Design

As mentioned in the introduction of this section, one way to integrate the user directly into the design process is through *participatory design* (Simonsen 2013). The field of Human-Computer Interaction (HCI) generally centers the user in its research and development. Therefore, concepts like human-centered and user-centered design exist, which consider the users' needs and capabilities. Nevertheless, the users do not actively participate in each stage of the design process. They are "simply" kept in mind when designing interfaces and tools. In contrast to this, in participatory design, users are "active, first-class members of the product design team" (Shneiderman et al. 2018), meaning participatory design is used to gain insights into the user's tasks and work life, inviting them to take on the role of the designer themselves (Muller and Druin 2012; Dix et al. 2004). Therefore, they *participate* in the design process by taking an active role in the overall process. Simonsen (2013) defines it in their handbook of participatory design as the following:

> a process of investigating, understanding, reflecting upon, establishing, developing, and supporting mutual learning between multiple participants in collective 'reflection-in-action'. The participants typically undertake the two principal roles of users and designers where the designers strive to learn the realities of the users' situation while the users strive to articulate their desired aims and learn appropriate technological means to obtain them.

In this context, 'users' are the participants who will interact with the technologies of interest, and the 'designers' are professionals responsible for the design. Yet, these roles are simplified because many more stakeholders are involved in a participatory design process (as mentioned in the beginning of this section), and the distinction between them blurs throughout the application of participatory design (Simonsen 2013).

Participatory design, then often referred to as cooperative design, emerged from Scandinavian action research in the early 1970s when computers were slowly integrating into everyday work life (Bødker and Kyng 2018). Bødker and Kyng (2018) describe three projects that can be seen as the first participatory design projects: the first is the *NJMF*, which was initiated by and named after the Norwegian Iron and Metal Workers' Union; the second is the Swedish *DEMOS* project (DEMOkratiske Styringssystemer); and the third is the Danish *DUE* project (Demokrati, Udvikling og Edb) (Bjerknes and Bratteteig 1995). The early projects all shared the goal and ideal of "promoting visions of democracy" as part of the joint effort in the research projects. According to the authors, the aspect of (workplace) democracy and changing the practice was one core element of participatory design—also because the first projects were initiated and executed together with trade unions, who wanted to contribute to a more democratic society.

In line with this vision, Simonsen (2013) states that participatory design has four central concepts: (1) take a stand, (2) participation, (3) practice, and (4) design. As participatory design prioritizes human action and people's right to participate in creating the world they will live in, one crucial aspect is always where they *take a stand* in designing their future. Therefore, in the methodology of participatory design, there is the understanding that design has to be ethical as it is accountable for the design of the world it creates and the lives of those who inhabit it. With *participation* being the core aspect of participatory design, it asks for integrating the participants (or 'users') into the design process on an equal level as the designers and other stakeholders. This form of end-user participation requires acknowledging the users' interests as fully legitimate elements of the overall design process. The concept of *practice* is important to participatory design, as there tends to be a difference between how people really work—how their practice actually is—and how others describe the work or, how the work processes are designed in the form of workflow diagrams and similar representations. Therefore, understanding practice is inevitable for a successful participatory design process.

The last central concept is *design*. In the early days, participatory design was primarily used for small-scale and custom-made systems, but since technology use has grown and off-the-shelf systems have become more configurable, the application area of participatory design has expanded. The availability of technology to use during the system design made it possible not just to investigate anticipated use but also unanticipated, unforeseen use. This also incorporates the so-called "designing for design after design," which refers to the fact that the design explicitly supports the potential for unanticipated use.

When applying participatory design, researchers and designers have many methods available to engage users in the design process encompassing dramatic performances, photography exhibits, games, or sketches and written scenarios (Shneiderman et al. 2018). Among those methods are paper prototyping, sketching interfaces, and creating low-fidelity prototypes with the material at hand, e.g., paper, pieces of plastic, and tape. Furthermore, a scenario walk-through using high-fidelity prototypes or simulation can also help elicit user requirements. Further methods to engage the users as active collaborators include workshops, in which (future) users take part in the design process and actively contribute to shaping representations of their tasks and work-life (Dix et al. 2004). The method of providing sketches was used, for example, by Wadley et al. (2013). They created four different design sketches of an online platform to deliver therapy content and support therapies and used them during a co-design workshop to seed discussions.

2.3 Summarizing Participatory Design and Participatory Research

Participatory research and participatory design share a similar ideological stance in incorporating the participants' perspectives and promoting empowerment, democracy, inclusivity, and equality. Both approaches stress that incorporating stakeholders is essential to create a beneficial outcome for everyone. As the approaches originate from different backgrounds, they differ slightly in their methods and dominant application areas. This is particularly visible in the way technology is incorporated into both approaches. Participatory design emerged as the advancements in technology slowly but significantly integrated and changed the work life of many, with a strong focus on supporting worker in shaping how these technologies were introduced and used. Therefore, most participatory design approaches have some form of technology (design and use) as one of their main objectives. Participatory research, by contrast, was developed to engage all types of stakeholders in the research process. It highly values the community's involvement, independent of the research objective. It emphasizes the collaboration between researchers and practitioners, allowing them to develop and adapt specific research elements, e.g., research questions, objectives, methods, data analysis, and outcomes. As technology is becoming omnipresent, participatory research also adapts technology-focused methods, and both approaches show more and more similarities; however, due to their significantly different origins, both stand on their own as useful approaches to foster participation.

3 Participatory Research and Participatory Design in the Context of Digital Public Health

In this section, we will present how participatory research and participatory design can be and are used in the context of digital public health. We will offer insights on how technology is integrated into participatory research and report on application examples from the literature where participatory design was employed to develop and advance the knowledge and the applications for digital public health.

3.1 Participatory Research

Digital technologies change how researchers engage participants in participatory research to collect more adequate and relevant data. Similarly, participatory research is also being increasingly applied to engage participants in the development of digital public health interventions tailored to the community. In the following sections, we present these two strands of participatory research where (1) digital technologies are applied to engage participants in the research process and (2) a participatory research approach is employed to develop digital public health interventions.

3.1.1 Application Example 1: Community-Based Digital Mental Health Program

Bennett-Levy et al. (2021) demonstrate how bottom-up community-guided processes and locally-generated advocacy played a key role in developing and implementing digital mental health training programs into training that was far more culturally relevant, thus impacting not only locally but nationally in Australia. This has been possible through grounding community-based participatory research from its inception. The project opted to involve local indigenous community members, organizational representatives, researchers, and others in all elements of a research project in collaborative and equitable partnerships from the outset. Thus, it proved useful in building indigenous capacity from the outset and enhancing community confidence in the project. The authors further describe how local indigenous guidance on re-framing the project from a mere focus on digital mental health to encompassing the indigenous Australian framework of social and emotional well-being led to the transformation of the project from a "top-down" government-funded project into a community-guided bottom-up project. By doing so, the project reported several unexpected and notable outcomes. At the beginning of the project, digital mental health (d-MH) was limited to the conventional understanding that it consisted of evidence-based online therapy programs. However, the iterative reflective processes of the learning circles and constant feedback from participants ensured that initially conceived non-indigenous d-MH programs were culturally inappropriate. This led to the development of indigenous-specific digital social and emotional wellbeing (d-SEWB) and digital mental health (d-MH) resources that were culturally relevant. The d-SEWB adopted a multidimensional concept of health that includes not only mental health but encompasses domains of health and well-being as the connection to land or "country," culture, spirituality, ancestry, family, and community and is firmly grounded in the impact of colonization on the well-being of Indigenous Australians through political, historical, social and cultural factors. As a result, the original d-MH program underwent significant expansion and was included as a subset in the d-SEWB, which included different types of digital resources across a wide range of cultural domains from indigenous connection to land and sea, community and kin, as well as the individual domains of body, mind, and emotions. Additionally, the project was able to successfully advocate for an Aboriginal-specific online therapy program and the development of a dedicated one-stop-shop d-SEWB website, Wellmob. Thus, in this project, a participatory research approach such as a community-based participatory research approach is especially valued for promoting equitable partnerships with community members in defining problems and seeking solutions, focusing on public health concerns within a local context, disseminating knowledge and sustainable support for interventions, and focusing on how race, ethnicity, racism, and class shape health outcomes.

3.1.2 Application Example 2: Participatory Sensing in Environmental Health Research

Increasing participatory research in the public health field nowadays employs digital methods to engage participants in certain stages of research, particularly to collect more adequate and relevant data for them. Such use of digital technologies is vivid in participatory sensing in environmental health research. The emergence of environmental monitoring and mapping technologies, the increasing use of mobile devices, and the growth of online data-sharing platforms are now supporting the involvement of diverse citizens and communities in participatory research approaches, such as citizen science and crowd-sourced science. These approaches are increasingly reliant on digital technologies such as smartphone-based apps and sensor technologies as research instruments to promote community/citizen involvement in neighborhood documentation and representation, foster greater data accessibility, democratize science, and mobilize diverse people and communities. For example, a smartphone-based assessment was developed within the CITI-SENSE project to study the acoustic environment of urban spaces (Aspuru et al. 2016). The project is based on three fundamental concepts: (1) technological platforms for distributed monitoring, (2) information and communication technologies, and (3) societal involvement. The solution comprises a smartphone allowing the post-processing of acoustic signals, an external microphone for measuring noise levels, a smartphone app with an embedded questionnaire that allows citizens to provide their perception of the area, and a protocol for making the observations that includes clear instructions for the participants.

Overall, the project intended to empower citizens to collect and share perceptual analysis of the surrounding acoustic environment, thereby promoting citizens' contributions as active participation in environmental governance.

The participants involved were the general public, who were contacted through civic associations. Within the project, they received the smartphone and instructions to perform the observations, including both the acoustic measurement and the questionnaire to be filled in. Before the launch of the observation event, participants were invited to a specific workshop where the objectives of the exercise, the tool, and the protocol were presented, and attendees' expectations were noted concerning the observations of urban places and initiatives. Those participants engaged in making the observations were then provided with a training workshop on how to use the CITI-SENSE kit that included the tool and protocol for making observations. The observations for four places were made for 1.5 weeks. In the end, participants were invited to the feedback workshop, where they were asked to identify areas and provide suggestions for improvement. Furthermore, they assessed their experiences of using the tool and protocol for evaluating environmental quality in urban areas. One of the aims of this project was the simultaneous collection of objective and subjective data on-site and the empowerment of participants as active citizens in environmental governance. In this line, participants found the project and its results useful to educate and raise awareness of these issues and the importance of improving comfort in public spaces. However, some doubts and difficulties in generalizing the use of devices were raised as they are not available to a significant number of people. Moreover, an evaluation of technical solutions showed that while older participants thought the tool and protocol were complex, younger people considered them to be practical, user-friendly, manageable, and intuitive. Nonetheless, researchers argue that such solutions can be applied to develop empowerment initiatives such as evaluating quiet areas and collecting ideas for their improvement, identifying priorities for Noise Action Plans, including citizen perception, and participatory co-design of action within the Noise Action Framework.

3.1.3 Application Example 3: Digitalization of Participatory Research Methods

The use of visual methods in the form of photo and video-voice is a commonly practiced research method in participatory research. Major benefits related to such methods in participatory research in health include (1) enhanced community engagement in action and advocacy, (2) improved understanding of community needs and assets, which in turn could have community or public health benefits, and (3) increased individual empowerment (Catalani and Minkler 2010). The adoption of smartphones and social media has further changed the way these visual methods can be used innovatively for engaging participants in collecting and sharing photographs and videos for research purposes. For instance, Earnshaw et al. (2022) demonstrate how the online asynchronous photovoice method presents a promising alternative to work with key populations such as transgender women, female sex workers, and people living with HIV (PLWH). Their research project focused on understanding key populations' and PLWH's experiences of stigma in healthcare settings in Malaysia. Photovoice projects traditionally involve in-person, synchronous interactions between facilitators, participants, and other stakeholders such as community members and policymakers. Yet, this format may not always be feasible and acceptable due to participant locations and, importantly, concerns related to confidentiality (e.g., in places with strong HIV-related stigma) or safety (e.g., during COVID-19 surges). Thus, a project website was set up that facilitated the project introduction to participants and an informed consent process, provided photography skills and an understanding of visual literacy, and enabled the collection of photovoice submissions from participants. The authors leveraged online and asynchronous photovoice methods via the website, which could be accessed online at any time, as an alternative to engage more members of key populations and PLWH confidentially and safely. The results suggest the feasibility and acceptability of online, asynchronous photovoice methods to engage with key populations and PLWH in research. Amongst a number of positive comments, participants especially enjoyed expressing themselves through photography, learning new skills, and the anonymity maintained by the website. One participant even stated that they appreciated "expressing who we are without revealing ourselves." In this line, the authors argue that online, asynchronous photovoice methods may enhance participant safety and address confidentiality concerns in a case study context with pronounced stigma towards key populations and PLWH, as in this project. As the methods do not require participants to physically gather at a study site, they can remain anonymous to other participants. In another example, Volpe (2019) argues that the use of mobile phones among young people is increasing, and they are already engaged in showing and sharing their pictures or videos on social media. Thus, these actions can provide insights into the movements and mobilities of young people in online spaces, creating "digital diaries" of the "everydayness" of their lives through the pictures and videos they share on social media. As young people are already producing digital representations of their real, lived experiences, with participants' permission, they can provide a diarized inspection of their daily lives

(Volpe 2019). Not only does it produce rich visual and narrative data on experiences of participants guided by participants' interests and priorities, but it also puts the methods in the hands of the participants.

3.2 Participatory Design

Participatory design has a stronger focus on technologies as it emerged when computers became more common in the workplace (see Sect. 2.2). In participatory design, all parties are influenced by the technology—e.g., the users—or can influence the technology either because they are designers, for example, or hold a position—e.g., in a government—that impacts the rules and the roll-out of the technology. There are various examples throughout research where participatory design was used in a health context, such as the work by Wadley et al. (2013), van Hierden et al. (2021), Bowen et al. (2013), Reeder et al. (2014), and Schmitt and Yarosh (2018).

Bowen et al. (2013) worked with nurses in the UK National Health Service (NHS) to understand and develop participatory methods for designing health services for the NHS. Reeder et al. (2014) followed a participatory design approach to engage public health nurses and nurse managers in the design process of an information system to enable analysis, visualization, and sharing of data between and across public health jurisdictions for different stakeholders to support public health work. Wadley et al. (2013), Schmitt and Yarosh (2018), and van Hierden et al. (2021) focused more on applications for supporting individuals with drug problems and mental health issues. Some of these projects would be described by Bødker and Kyng (2018) as focusing on the "small issues." They use participatory design mainly to facilitate direct collaboration between users and designers through co-design and being able to "engage with everyday issues of use, through technology", rather than aiming for broader or systemic transformation in practices or institutions.

In the following two sections, we will present two examples of participatory design, one by Wadley et al. (2013) focusing on designing an online therapy platform in Australia and the other being the Health Information Systems Program (HISP) project (Braa and Sahay 2012; Bødker and Kyng 2018), which started in 1994 in South Africa, and aimed to provide equity in health service delivery.

3.2.1 Application Example 4: Designing an Online Therapy Platform

In this section, we will briefly describe the work of Wadley et al. (2013), who used participatory design to design a platform for adolescents between 15 and 25 years old who received treatment at a local clinic. They describe how they ran co-design workshops with potential users of an online therapy platform, which included patients of a collaborating clinic and the clinicians of the same clinic, as treatment involves both parties. They used sketches and mock-ups of the potential online platform to spark and facilitate discussions in the co-design workshops.

Generally, the feedback on an online therapy platform was positive. However, the potential for (increased) anxiety was also mentioned, as reading about psychosis online can trigger an individual's anxieties. One reported benefit was the exchange of experiences among patients with similar experiences on digital platforms such as social networks (e.g., Facebook). The digital format of an online therapy platform was also perceived as possibly helpful as long as there were no "'corny' computer-generated messages." The workshop with the clinicians revealed that they were concerned that socio-economic factors could impact the accessibility of an online therapy platform and that some patients may benefit from actually leaving their homes to attend face-to-face therapy. Also, they mentioned that direct communication between patients could be helpful but should be moderated and thus wondered about the availability of the required human resources.

The three main design decisions resulting from the workshops are, first, that the platform will feature psychoeducational content accessible to the clients at times, places, and at a pace that is convenient to them. Second, it will allow for peer-to-peer social interaction inspired by social media. And last, the client interaction will be moderated by professional clinical staff who can also provide advice.

Based on the insights provided by the participants, the researchers developed the platform and refined it during sessions with the participants. After this step was finished, they started a trial run with clinicians and patients of the collaborating clinic and did post-trial interviews with the participants to understand the use of the platform. Based on the results, such as that the patients wanted to have more freedom in selecting therapy modules, the researchers proposed various changes to their system, which was planned to be tested in a larger trial. Still, the researchers already found a positive impact on the participants' mental health within the 6 weeks trial phase. For further details, we refer to the publication by Wadley et al. (2013).

3.2.2 Application Example 5: The HISP Project

In contrast to the relatively small scope of the presented study in the section above, the *HISP project*— "HISP" stands for Health Information Systems Program (Braa and Sahay 2012)—has lasted for several decades and has expanded to other communities. The HISP project started as an initiative in South Africa. It was initiated in 1994, just after apartheid ended. Among its aims was to provide equity in health service delivery and to develop and empower those communities and groups that were most disadvantaged under apartheid. The project aimed to build a flexible local data processing system enabling a local collection and delivery of health data requested from various health care providers such as hospitals, clinics, school health, or NGOs (nongovernment organizations). Due to political changes, the focus shifted slightly during the early phase of the project, and the goal to integrate the processes and information systems from the Department of Health was added to the original list of objectives. The software developed in the HISP project is the District Health Information Software (DHIS). It allows its users to access their information immediately. During the pilot phase, the software was developed and piloted at two universities in Cape Town and three health districts nearby (Braa and Hedberg 2002). University staff, activists from the health sectors and NGOs, and two Norwegian researchers built a team to identify information needs and support the interim district management teams. By providing this, it was possible to implement and test the "information cycle" hands-on, leading to further improvements as users urged for "better information, analytical tools, and graphs." This shows that if participatory design is deeply integrated into all processes, there exists an ever-changing system that will constantly adapt to the requirements and therefore is never 'finished.'

One of the benefits of the HISP project is its linking of the South African community with the University of Oslo, where educational programs helped disseminates the participatory design approach on which the project was based. HISP has been successfully expanded to various countries, such as Cuba, India, and Mozambique, in the first phase of expansion. Thereby the team of developers, health professionals, and government officials working on and informing the project has increased. The expansion also led to the network becoming even more extensive, creating linkages for more collaboration in health information system development, implementation, and scaling.

Following this first expansion, the HISP project underwent some major concept changes, such as explicitly changing from a standalone application to a networked application within the health systems of developing countries. Furthermore, as the open-source technologies were gaining momentum, the technologies had matured enough that "the entire web-based technology stack could be provided as Free and Open-Source Software." Following this change, after the civil war in Sierra Leone ended in 2002, their health systems needed extensive rebuilding, and in 2008 DHIS (in version 2) was introduced there. Participatory design was and is still a core element. The general process followed is, first, to implement the software as it is and enrich it with datasets to enable a hands-on experience for its users. In a second step, this allows users to prototype *their* version of the software and discuss what the revised system should look like. As a third and last step, the original system is adjusted to meet the users' needs, which includes paper forms and data standards. In Sierra Leone, the traditional chiefdoms were facing systemic disadvantages and were eager to use the new system to demonstrate this. Therefore, they were part of the design process and even competed to produce "the best-quality data on health services and produce tables ranking their achievements, in both their local and their national contexts." The HISP project continues, and with participatory design at its core, it confidently faces new challenges like the rapid improvement of mobile networks, enabling many online web-based services and cloud computing in developing countries.

Bødker and Kyng (2018) highlight the HISP project as one of the projects that inspired a "new" participatory design in the spirit of its roots. It is a long-sustained project (running for 20+ years now), and it has kept its continued focus on developing approaches to collecting and using data while supporting local action. Furthermore, it contributed to an ongoing participatory process of data standardization to support cooperation on a local-to-local and local-to-central level, including the scaling up. They also highlight that HISP has created a "self-sustaining organizational network which handles the technological core and the processes of continued development, deployment, and use."

4 Outlook

As digitization is advancing in nearly all areas of life, it also gets integrated into the domain of public health, thereby offering considerable potential to support and improve various health issues such as mental health, obesity, and chronic diseases. Despite the possibilities, research mentions significant challenges regarding the uptake of or adherence to digital interventions. The failure to ensure culturally and logistically appropriate digital public health interventions has been reported, among other reasons. In our understanding, the integration of participatory approaches, such as participatory research and participatory design, can address these reasons for failure.

The research presented in the previous section shows that participatory research and participatory design are valuable approaches for designing, developing, and implementing technologies and interventions for the health domain. In the examples mentioned, different methods were used to engage the users, such as focus groups, co-design workshops, cultural probes such as photos or videos, diaries, smartphone recordings, and questionnaires. The application examples are similar in that they want the development or research to be undertaken with or by society's marginalized people, thereby having people as full participants involved throughout the process to determine their own needs to improve their own lives. This highlights that although participatory research and participatory design have different historical origins, they share similar ideologies of empowerment, democracy, and inclusivity.

Participatory research has a strong focus on the research process itself. It may focus on establishing an equitable community partnership process to design digital interventions to develop co-ownership and co-decision-making (cf. Application Example 1). Sometimes participatory research may be limited to just documenting or studying a problem or the needs and requirements of a community by involving participants in certain stages of research activity. In this case, digital technologies provide a research instrument for involving participants in research activity (cf. Application Example 2). Furthermore, the ubiquitous use of digital technologies such as smartphones, online platforms, and social media is opening up new possibilities and new ways to utilize existing participatory methods to involve research participants, especially in data collection processes (cf. Application Example 3).

While participatory research helps to understand the circumstances and context of the user group by involving them into the process, participatory design can help design and understand newly developed technical aspects brought into society. With its history of giving a voice to the people affected by the beginning of the digital age, participatory design can be a useful tool in supporting the design, development, and integration of technology into the public health context. Among the most important questions for new technology—be it a device or a piece of software—are the questions "Is this useful and usable for the target group?" and "Does this meet the needs of the target group?" This was nicely illustrated by Application Example 5— where the requested features of the HISP project and resulting software changed several times over the course of its long-term development. It was designed hand in hand with its users and the relevant stakeholders and thereby focused on their needs.

Overall, the objectives of participatory research and participatory design complement each other well. Thus, harnessing the strengths of participatory research and participatory design not only improves the functionality of technologies used by participants but might also ensures that participants use these technologies more effectively in research and practice to improve health and well-being. Their vision of empowering the people affected, establishing a democratic process, and striving for inclusivity is highly relevant for creating a future in which digital public health is accessible and beneficial for everyone.

References

Arnstein SR (1969) A ladder of citizen participation. J Am Inst Plann 35(4):216–224
Aspuru I, García I, Herranz K et al (2016) Citi-sense: methods and tools for empowering citizens to observe acoustic comfort in outdoor public spaces. Noise Mapp 3(1)
Balazs CL, Morello-Frosch R (2013) The three Rs: how community-based participatory research strengthens the rigor, relevance, and reach of science. Environ Justice 6(1):9–16
Bennett-Levy J, Singer J, Rotumah D et al (2021) From digital mental health to digital social and emotional wellbeing: how indigenous community-based participatory research influenced the Australian government's digital mental health agenda. Int J Environ Res Public Health 18(18):9757
Bergold J, Thomas S (2012) Participatory research methods: a methodological approach in motion. Hist Soc Res 37(4):191–222
Bjerknes G, Bratteteig T (1995) User participation and democracy: a discussion of Scandinavian research on system development. Scand J Inf Syst 7(1):1
Bødker S, Kyng M (2018) Participatory design that matters—facing the big issues. ACM Trans Comput Hum Interact 25(1):1–31. https://doi.org/10.1145/3152421
Bowen S, McSeveny K, Lockley E et al (2013) How was it for you? Experiences of participatory design in the UK health service. CoDesign 9(4):230–246
Braa J, Hedberg C (2002) The struggle for district-based health information systems in South Africa. Inf Soc 18(2):113–127
Braa J, Sahay S (2012) Health information systems programme: participatory design within the HISP network. In: Routledge international handbook of participatory design. Routledge, London, pp 235–256
Cargo M, Mercer SL (2008) The value and challenges of participatory research: strengthening its practice. Annu Rev Public Health 29:325–350
Catalani C, Minkler M (2010) Photovoice: a review of the literature in health and public health. Health Educ Behav 37(3):424–451
Chambers R (1994) The origins and practice of participatory rural appraisal. World Dev 22(7):953–969. https://doi.org/10.1016/0305-750X(94)90141-4, https://www.sciencedirect.com/ science/article/pii/0305750X94901414

Cook T (2012) Where participatory approaches meet pragmatism in funded (health) research: the challenge of finding meaningful spaces. Forum: Qualitative Social Research, Forum Qualitative Sozialforschung 13(1):Art–18

Cousins JB, Whitmore E (1998) Framing participatory evaluation. N Dir Eval 80:5–23. https://doi.org/10.1002/ev.1114

Dix A, Finley J, Abowd GD et al (2004) Human-computer interaction, 3rd edn. Pearson, London

Duarte AMB, Brendel N, Degbelo A et al (2018) Participatory design and participatory research: an HCI case study with young forced migrants. ACM Trans Comput Hum Interact 25(1):1–39

Duea SR, Zimmerman EB, Vaughn LM et al (2022) A guide to selecting participatory research methods based on project and partnership goals. J Participatory Res Methods 3(1):32605

Earnshaw VA, Cox J, Wong PL et al (2022) Acceptability and feasibility of online, asynchronous photovoice with key populations and people living with HIV. AIDS Behav 27(7):2055–2069

IAP (2014) Public participation spectrum. International Association for Public Participation-IAP2 Federation, Wollongong

Iyamu I, Xu AX, Gómez-Ramírez O et al (2021) Defining digital public health and the role of digitization, digitalization, and digital transformation: scoping review. JMIR Public Health Surveill 7(11):e30399

Iyamu I, Gómez-Ramírez O, Xu AX et al (2022) Challenges in the development of digital public health interventions and mapped solutions: findings from a scoping review. Digit Health 8:20552076221102255

Jagosh J, Macaulay AC, Pluye P et al (2012) Uncovering the benefits of participatory research: implications of a realist review for health research and practice. Milbank Q 90(2):311–346

Kemmis S (2006) Participatory action research and the public sphere. Educ Action Res 14(4):459–476

Le Dantec CA, Fox S (2015) Strangers at the gate: gaining access, building rapport, and co-constructing community-based research. In: Proceedings of the 18th ACM conference on computer supported cooperative work & social computing, pp 1348–1358

Macaulay AC (2016) Participatory research: what is the history? Has the purpose changed? Fam Pract 34(3):256–258. https://doi.org/10.1093/fampra/cmw117. https://arxiv.org/abs/https://academic.oup.com/fampra/article-pdf/34/3/256/17695896/cmw117.pdf

Minkler M, Wallerstein N (2011) Community-based participatory research for health: from process to outcomes. John Wiley & Sons, New York

Mucha H, de Barros AC, Benjamin JJ et al (2022) Collaborative speculations on future themes for participatory design in Germany. i-com 21(2):283–298. https://doi.org/10.1515/icom-2021-0030

Muller MJ, Druin A (2012) Participatory design: the third space in human–computer interaction. In: The human–computer interaction handbook. CRC Press, Boca Raton, pp 1125–1153

Odone A, Buttigieg S, Ricciardi W et al (2019) Public health digitalization in Europe: Eupha vision, action and role in digital public health. Eur J Pub Health 29(Suppl 3):28–35

Reason P (1999) Integrating action and reflection through co-operative inquiry. Manag Learn 30(2):207–225

Reeder B, Hills RA, Turner AM et al (2014) Participatory design of an integrated information system design to support public health nurses and nurse managers. Public Health Nurs 31(2):183–192

Schmitt Z, Yarosh S (2018) Participatory design of technologies to support recovery from substance use disorders. Proc ACM Hum Comput Interaction 2(CSCW):1–27

Shneiderman B, Plaisant C, Cohen M, et al (2018) Designing the user interface: strategies for effective human-computer interaction, Global edn. Pearson Deutschland. https://elibrary.pearson.de/book/99.150005/9781292153926

Simonsen J (2013) Routledge international handbook of participatory design, vol 711. Routledge, London

Unger H (2013) Partizipative Forschung: Einführung in die Forschungspraxis. Springer, Berlin van Hierden Y, Dietrich T, Rundle-Thiele S (2021) Designing an eHealth wellbeing program: a participatory design approach. Int J Environ Res Public Health 18(14):7250

Vaughn LM, Jacquez F (2020) Participatory research methods–choice points in the research process. J Participatory Res Methods 1(1):13244

Volpe CR (2019) Digital diaries: new uses of photovoice in participatory research with young people. Childrens Geogr 17(3):361–370

Von Unger H et al (2012) Participatory health research: who participates in what? Forum Qual Soc Res 13(1)

Wadley G, Lederman R, Gleeson J, et al (2013) Participatory design of an online therapy for youth mental health. In: Proceedings of the 25th Australian computer-human interaction conference: augmentation, application, innovation, collaboration, OzCHI'13. Association for Computing Machinery, New York, pp 517–526. https://doi.org/10.1145/2541016.2541030

World Health Organization (1986) Ottawa charter for health promotion, 1986. Tech. rep. World Health Organization. Regional Office for Europe

World Health Organization (1992) Our planet, our health: report of the WHO Commission on Health and Environment. World Health Organization, Geneva

Wright MT, Von Unger H, Block M (2010) Partizipation der zielgruppe in der gesundheitsförderung und prävention. Partizipative Qualitätsentwicklung in der Gesundheitsförderung und Prävention 1:35–52

Open Access This chapter is licensed under the terms of the Creative Commons Attribution 4.0 International License (http://creativecommons.org/licenses/by/4.0/), which permits use, sharing, adaptation, distribution and reproduction in any medium or format, as long as you give appropriate credit to the original author(s) and the source, provide a link to the Creative Commons license and indicate if changes were made.

The images or other third party material in this chapter are included in the chapter's Creative Commons license, unless indicated otherwise in a credit line to the material. If material is not included in the chapter's Creative Commons license and your intended use is not permitted by statutory regulation or exceeds the permitted use, you will need to obtain permission directly from the copyright holder.

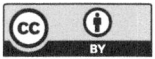

Open Data for DiPH Research Versus Data Protection

Merle Freye and Benedikt Buchner

Abstract Research in public health is particularly dependent on the unrestricted use of data. The processing of personal health data can serve health-related public interests and bring significant benefits to individuals and society (https://www.oecd.org/health/ministerial-statement-2017.pdf). In contrast, data protection law aims to protect personal data and is consequently based on the prohibition principle and the principle of purpose limitation. Although the General Data Protection Regulation (GDPR) also contains research-friendly approaches and provides the possibility of privileging research data processing at various points, in practice, data protection still poses challenges to research for public health purposes. The concept of consent is questionable, and—especially in Germany—many uncertainties arise from the complex patchwork of state-specific regulations. New concepts such as "broad consent," "dynamic consent," "no consent," and "synthetic data" are intended to facilitate the processing of data for research purposes in line with data protection law. Fueled by these debates, national and international data protection laws will inevitably have to face changes in the near future.

Keywords Anonymization of data · Broad consent · Data protection law · Dynamic consent · GDPR · Medical confidentiality · Synthetic data

---

M. Freye (✉)
Faculty of Law, Institute for Information, Health and Medical Law (IGMR), University of Bremen, Bremen, Germany

Leibniz Science Campus Digital Public Health (LSC DiPH), Bremen, Germany
e-mail: mfreye@uni-bremen.de

B. Buchner
Faculty of Law, Institute for Bio, Health and Medical Law (IBGM), University of Augsburg, Augsburg, Germany
e-mail: benedikt.buchner@jura.uni-ausgburg.de

Abbreviations

BCS70	British Cohort Study
BDSG	German Federal Data Protection Act
DGA	Data Governance Act
DSK	Data Protection Conference
EDPB	European Data Protection Board
EU	European Union
FOG	Forschungsorganisationsgesetz
GDPR	General Data Protection Regulation
GNC	German National Cohort
MII	Medical Informatics Initiative
SOEP	Socio-Economic Panel
StGB	German Criminal Code
UAC	Use-and-access-committees

1 Introduction

As an empirical science, public health is particularly dependent on the unrestricted use of data. Whether it is research into the conditions for health and disease, the interaction between people and their environment, or the evaluation of health system performance: all these public health objectives can only be achieved if as much data as possible are freely available and can be easily linked and tracked over the long term.

The Corona pandemic has emphatically shown us the importance of and dependence on a sufficient database for health sciences. The fact that even after more than 2 years of the pandemic, the Corona Expert Council set up by the German government was still unable to assess the suitability of individual protective measures *due to a lack of data* reveals that Germany is dealing with a structural data problem. During the Corona pandemic, data protection was identified as one of the main culprits for this structural data problem. It is undoubtedly true that the philosophy of Open Data contradicts the basic principles of data protection: in "Big Data," data can "be freely accessed, used, modified, and shared by anyone for any purpose" (FIT4RRI and Foster 2023), on the contrary, data protection law is based on the prohibition principle and strict purpose limitation of data processing.

Nevertheless, the European data protection law is, in theory, not as inflexible as frequently thought since the General Data Protection Regulation (GDPR) was designed to be research-friendly. Accordingly, the GDPR provides special regulations appropriate to research in all central legal questions, which are intended to harmonize the protection of informational self-determination with the special interests and needs of research.

However, the legislator's good intentions cannot overcome the fact that there are still considerable uncertainties in research practice about the application and interpretation of the regulations (Cepic 2021). Data protection and scientific research are often conflicting (Roßnagel 2019a): On the one hand, "access to, and the processing of personal health data can serve health-related public interests and bring significant benefits to individuals and society [...]" (OECD 2017). On the other hand, data protection law aims to protect personal data and thus does not release institutions from their responsibility. Additionally, legal restrictions impeding everyday research may be imposed by national regulations in the member states and consequently challenge the research-friendly setting of the GDPR in practice. Some of these national regulations are general, and others are sector-specific, resulting in an impenetrable jungle of rules. Whether national or international, sector-specific or general—discussion for research primarily revolves around the question of consent. Particularly in large-scale epidemiological studies or genetic studies, the classic concept of (informed) consent is not the most appropriate legal basis (Directorate-General for Health and Food Safety 2021; Chico 2018; Dove 2018). It raises the question of new models of consent and more suitable approaches such as "data donation," "dynamic consent," and "no consent." Although solutions constantly arise, they cannot keep up with technological developments, leading to further uncertainties. For example, the relatively new technical procedure of synthesizing data to generate realistically simulated data from original patient data has recently imposed new challenges for data protection law. The following chapter will discuss whether the current data protection law is sufficient on a national and international level or whether new regulations are inevitable for public health research.

2 Research-Friendly Design of the GDPR

Although data protection was identified as one of the main culprits for the absence of a reliable data basis during the Corona pandemic, this argumentation does not correspond to the concept of GDPR, which is consistently designed to be research-friendly and provides the possibility of privileging research data processing at various points (Buchner 2022).

To begin with, there are exceptions for research projects affecting the two main principles of the GDPR: the purpose limitation principle and the principle of storage limitation. According to the principle of purpose limitation, personal data shall be collected for specified, explicit, and legitimate purposes and not further processed in a manner that is incompatible with those purposes. In deviation from the purpose limitation principle, further processing of data for scientific research purposes is not considered to be incompatible with the original data processing purposes (Art. 5 (1) (b) GDPR). Additionally, the storage limitation principle states that personal data shall be kept in a form that permits the identification of data subjects for no longer than is necessary for the purposes for which the personal data were processed. The exception for research projects is that personal data may be "stored longer" if processed exclusively for research purposes (Art. 5 (1) (e) GDPR).

Moreover, the European legislator enshrined another privilege for research data processing with regard to divergent laws in European countries. According to Art. 9 (2) (j) GDPR, national legislators of the European member states are allowed to adopt national rules that legitimize the processing of sensitive data in as far as it is necessary for research purposes.

In addition, the GDPR contains exceptions to the rights of data subjects since some rights are not feasible in the research context and would unduly complicate research. When informing the data subject about data processing proves impossible or would involve a disproportionate effort, information shall not be provided (Art. 14 (5) (b) GDPR). For the same reason, the right to erasure does not apply in so far as the right is likely to render impossible or seriously impair the achievement of the objectives of that processing (Art. 17 (3) (d) GDPR). With regard to national law in Europe, member states may provide derogations from data subject rights in their national laws in so far as such rights are likely to render impossible or seriously impair the achievement of the specific purposes, and such derogations are necessary for the fulfillment of those purposes, Art. 89 (2) GDPR.

Lastly, an essential privilege of research is located in Recital 33 GDPR and introduces the concept of "broad consent." In practice, broad consent is the central issue, dominating the discussion about data protection in research practice.

The given examples emphasize that the GDPR provides special regulations appropriate for research concerning all the central legal issues (consent, legal permissions, general data processing principles, data subject rights), which are intended to balance the protection of informational self-determination with the special interests and needs of research (Buchner 2022).

3 Central Role of Consent

Mainly driven by the exception of broad consent noted above, research for public health purposes in practice is primarily based on consent. In addition to broad consent, another model was developed for research with biobanks: dynamic consent. Consequently, consent plays a central role in research practice. The essential position of consent is not an end in itself since it is also deeply rooted in the ethical principle of autonomy (Beauchamp and Childress 2019): Despite the potential benefits of research for public health purposes to the *public*, the autonomy of the *individual* participant must also be respected. Nevertheless, broad consent and dynamic consent models are not the panaceas they seem to be.

3.1 New Consent Models in Practice...

Consent is one of the lawful grounds on which personal data processing may be based, pursuant to Article 6 of the GDPR. In order to obtain valid consent, certain requirements must be met. Article 4 (11) GDPR stipulates that:

> 'consent' of the data subject means any freely given, specific, informed and unambiguous indication of the data subject's wishes by which he or she, by a statement or by a clear affirmative action, signifies agreement to the processing of personal data relating to him or her.

Research for public health purposes poses the main challenge that objectives and duration are often not clearly definable or foreseeable at the beginning of the project. Hence, specific information about the planned data processing is not always possible. Broad consent addresses this problem by creating exceptions to the element of "specific" consent. Instead of consenting to specific purposes of data processing, participants consent to broadly defined areas of scientific research or parts of research projects (Raum 2018, marginal no. 35; Caspar 2019, marginal no. 37; Eichler 2023b, marginal no. 2a). Consequently, the exact objective of research projects does not have to be precisely defined from the outset when consent is given; rather, it can be "broader" in the sense of being vaguer.

In Germany, the Medical Informatics Initiative (MII) developed a sample text for a uniform patient information and consent form in close consultation with the Data Protection Conference (DSK) (MII 2020a). The form aims to ensure patient data from care and research are available in an integrated manner at all university hospitals in Germany for direct care and medical research (MII 2020b). Consequently, the sample text affects research for public health purposes that takes part at university hospitals in Germany. Nevertheless, the form has not only gained applause but was also met with severe criticism from the perspective of data protection law (Fröhlich and Spiecker gen. Döhmann 2022). Although this criticism is partly justified, the current version of MII's form is only one national approach to provide guidance on broad consent and is, therefore, not representative of broad consent approaches in Europe. Interestingly, broad consent is also a subject of new European legislative initiatives. Recently, the dazzling notion of "data altruism" in the Data Governance Act (DGA) of 2022 refers to broad consent: According to Art. 2 (16) DGA, so-called data altruism is also based on consent. Recital 50 sentence 5 suggests that data subjects could also consent to certain areas of research or parts of research project. In Austria, broad consent is explicitly named in § 2d (3) FOG (Forschungsorganisationsgesetz), according to which "the indication of a purpose may be made by indicating a research area or several research areas or research projects or parts of research projects ("broad consent")."

In addition to broad consent, dynamic consent has been developed for biobanks. Dynamic consent consists of accompanying permanent information: When new research purposes are determined, new consent forms will be offered (Raum 2018, marginal no. 36; Caspar 2019, marginal no. 41; Eichler 2023b, marginal no. 2d). As soon as the research purpose can be concretized factually and institutionally over time, consent progresses dynamically in parallel (Spitz and Cornelius 2022). Unlike broad consent, dynamic consent thus represents a stretching of the consent process but is not necessarily an exception to specific consent: Essential to this concept is an individual interface or interactive platform tailored to the user's needs. Users can choose how and whether they want to be contacted for new consent and what information they are interested in (Kaye et al. 2015). Consequently, dynamic consent can also integrate broad consent if subjects initially specify that they do not want to be informed dynamically but only once by using broad consent. Dynamic consent has drawn the attention of the German Data Ethics Commission (Datenethikkommission 2019) and the European Data Protection Board (EDPB). According to EDPB, innovative forms of consent in research activities, like dynamic consent, are promising practices that should be further encouraged and developed (European Data Protection Supervisor 2020).

3.2 ...Old Questions

As innovative as broad consent and dynamic consent might appear, both models do not eliminate all the concerns that necessarily accompany consent in public health research projects.

Consent—whether broad or dynamic—is inevitably accompanied by the disadvantage of excluding data processing for which no consent has been given. It is, therefore, questionable whether and to what extent consent-based research data processing can guarantee a database that is representative and free of systematic bias (MII 2020b).

Furthermore, consent comes with a series of deficits that generally call into question the legitimacy of consent as a legal basis for data processing. Regarding the form of MII, subjects still obtain 7 pages of information and, in addition, a 3-page consent text (Sachverständigenrat 2021). Whether and to what extent research subjects are actually (broadly) informed seems at least questionable, given the already very complex daily treatment routine from the patient's point of view. Even dynamic consent only partially solves the information problem. On the one hand, participants obtain information piece by piece, and thus the amount of information per stage decreases. On the other hand, there is no common understanding of informing patients in dynamic consent models, and information thus might be as complex as with broad consent.

When the individuals concerned are patients, the voluntary nature of consent could also be particularly problematic in medical research projects since patients might assume that consent is a prerequisite for treatment. Therefore, the MII Consent Handout states that consent documents should not be presented as part of the admission contract or otherwise suggest to the patient that signing the patient consent would be a prerequisite for treatment. Nevertheless, the MII Consent Handout also recommends asking for consent as early as possible, i.e., before treatment begins or at the start of the treatment process. Hence, the MII Consent Handout itself is not clear on whether, in practice, the consent process is actually "decoupled" from the administrative admission process (MII 2020b). The current concept of broad consent cannot guarantee that patients are not under any perceived pressure to consent. Equally, there is no concept for ensuring the voluntary nature of consent in dynamic consent either.

Another unsolved question relates to the withdrawal of consent. According to the concept of consent, data subjects shall have the right to withdraw their consent at any time, Art. 7 (3) GDPR. Therefore, separate mechanisms must always be provided if data subjects may revoke their consent in the future and thus withdraw the legitimacy basis for further data processing. In practice, this leads to considerable implementation difficulties and jeopardizes a stable data basis for research which is crucial, especially for epidemiological analysis.

Another disadvantage of consent evolves when examining the interaction of consent with the release from confidentiality. Independent from data protection law, Section 203 of the German Criminal Code (StGB) regulates the duty of confidentiality for healthcare professionals. Therefore, a release from the duty of confidentiality must be obtained in order to process health data when a named healthcare professional is involved. This release is different from consent in data protection law. Regarding the data processing by specialized personnel with an obligation of professional secrecy, data protection and medical law lead to a so-called "two-barrier principle" (March et al. 2019; Weichert 2020, marginal no. 138). Consequently, when data processing gains valid consent under data protection law but simultaneously violates a professional secret, the data processing becomes unlawful as a whole (Weichert 2020, marginal no. 146). Although consent under data protection law and medical confidentiality are legally independent, they can still be declared together. This situation potentially overloads patients with information since they must agree twice. Patients may be under the impression that they are asked to make the same legally relevant declaration twice since the requirements of consent and release from the duty of confidentiality are partially similar: they both require the patient's free will and decision, either expressly or impliedly (Bundesärztekammer and Kassenärztliche Bundesvereinigung 2021). While the data subjects shall have the right to withdraw their consent at any time in data protection law, the release from a professional duty of confidentiality can also be revoked at any time with effect for the future (Oberlandesgericht München 2013). Moreover, blanket consents are invalid in both cases (Bundesärztekammer and Kassenärztliche Bundesvereinigung 2021). In conjunction with consent under data protection law, the release from the duty of confidentiality creates a consent bureaucracy that virtually crushes the respective subjects with extensive information. In this situation, it is highly questionable whether patients are adequately informed. Consent plays a central role in research data protection; nevertheless, this primacy should not obscure the fact that consent is not without criticism.

4 Anonymization: Threat or Tool?

Regarding the insufficient concept of consent in the field of research for public health purposes, the question arises whether the solution to the problem lies in anonymizing data. As depicted in Fig. 1, anonymized data must be distinguished from personal data and pseudonymized data.

4.1 Anonymized Data

The GDPR is only applicable to the processing of personal data. According to Art. 4 (1) GDPR, "personal data are any information relating to an identified or identifiable natural person. An identifiable natural person is one who can be identified,

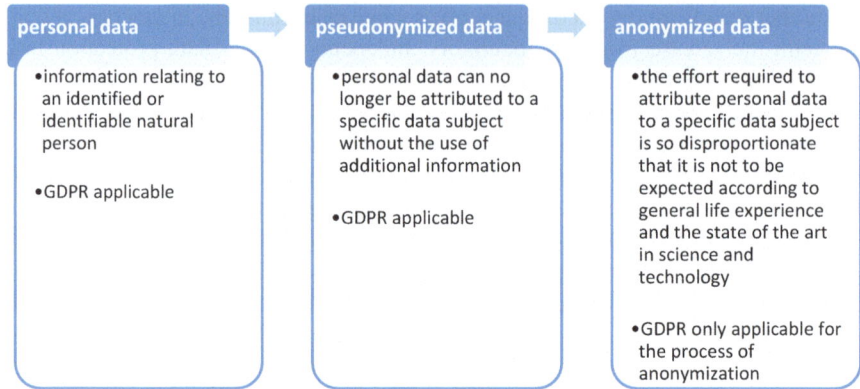

Fig. 1 From personal data to anonymized data. (Source: own figure)

directly or indirectly, in particular by reference to an identifier (such as a name, an identification number, location data, an online identifier or to one or more factors specific to the physical, physiological, genetic, mental, economic, cultural or social identity of that natural person)."

Due to data anonymization, subjects become unidentifiable, and consequently, a legal basis for processing this data is not necessary either. Therefore, Recital 26 states that the GDPR does not concern the processing of anonymous information.

Two different theories are discussed in data protection law to decide whether data "relate to an identifiable person." The absolute theory asks if it is impossible *for anyone* to assign an individual information item to a specific person (Schmidt 2022, marginal no. 7). In contrast, the relative theory only considers the means of identification available *to the respective controller in the specific individual case* to establish the personal reference (Roßnagel 2019b, marginal no. 59). The relative theory is not only widely used in academic literature but can also be found in the European Court of Justice decision Breyer v. Germany (European Court of Justice 2016). However, given the constantly evolving technical possibilities, there is no absolute and incontrovertible anonymity of data (Roßnagel 2021). Hence, the idea of absolute anonymization is outdated and does not reflect reality (Hackenberg 2022, marginal no. 53). In contrast to this, the relative approach requires a risk prognosis and determines whether re-identification should be expected according to general life experience and the state of the art in science and technology. This includes the controller's existing or acquirable additional knowledge, current and future technical possibilities for processing, and the possible effort and available time (Roßnagel and Geminn 2021).

With regard to the re-identification risk of research data, it should be noted that the rarer a clinical picture and the smaller a group of subjects, the less anonymity of datasets can be assumed. The re-identification risk is likely to increase significantly, especially in small groups of persons with rare diseases (Conrad and Treeger 2019, § 34, marginal no. 106). Irrespective of this, anonymization does not exempt from all obligations under data protection law: even if the anonymity of the processed data is assumed, data protection obligations still exist since data protection also protects against possible de-anonymization of data files. Therefore, necessary measures must be taken to reduce this risk as far as possible, including the selection of a sufficiently secure technical procedure for data anonymization and the continuous monitoring and consideration of technical developments (Bundesbeauftragte für den Datenschutz und die Informationsfreiheit 2020).

Although anonymization can be less bureaucratic than obtaining consent in individual cases, in the end, anonymization is still not as straightforward as it seems at first glance. Additionally, the process of anonymization itself constitutes data processing and thus requires a legal basis.

4.2 Pseudonymized Data

Pseudonymization is closely related to anonymization. When anonymization is not possible, the GDPR requires pseudonymization as a legal safeguard for the processing of data for research purposes (Art. 89 (2) GDPR). According to Art. 4 (5) GDPR, "pseudonymization means the processing of personal data in such a manner that the personal data can no longer be attributed to a specific data subject without the use of additional information, provided that such additional information is kept separately and is subject to technical and organizational measures to ensure that the personal data are not attributed to an identified or identifiable natural person."

Consequently, the additional information must be kept separately and be subject to technical and organizational measures to ensure that personal data are not attributed to an identified or identifiable natural person. In scientific studies, pseudonymization is convincing when it is essential to be able to contact the individual subject for queries or for information on any medical conditions and diagnoses that may have been determined (Weichert 2022). For example, frequently contacting the participants becomes essential in long-term studies that are based on a follow-up concept, such as the German National Cohort (GNC) or the Socio-Economic Panel (SOEP), and the British Cohort Study (BCS70).

4.3 Synthetic Data

The relatively new technical procedure of synthesizing data has recently raised debates from the perspective of data protection law spinning around the question of anonymization. In 2019, the German Data Ethics Commission recognized the potential of synthetic data—particularly for simulations—and recommended further exploring the generation and use of synthetic data (Datenethikkommission 2019).

In synthesizing data, an AI-supported learning algorithm generates realistically simulated data from original patient data. For this purpose, a dataset's statistical information and structures are machine-learned in the technical process and "synthesized" with the help of the algorithm (Wegner 2021, Part 6.5, marginal no. 1 ff.). Consequently, personal data are not merely cleansed of identification features according to an anonymization technology, but an entirely new dataset is technically generated based on the trained understanding of an original dataset. With synthesizing, data become more easily accessible to researchers.

From the data protection law perspective, the question arises whether generating synthetic data is an anonymization technique. In this case, the data processing would no longer be subject to the strict limitations of the GDPR due to the lack of personal data processing (Eichler 2023a, marginal no. 27b; Ernst 2021, marginal no. 48). According to the relative approach, a risk prognosis is necessary that focuses on the probability of re-identification risks (Eichler 2023a, marginal no. 15a; Bischoff 2020). To ascertain whether it is likely that the natural person may be identified, all objective factors should be taken into account, such as the costs of and the amount of time required for identification, taking into consideration the available technology at the time of the processing and technological developments (Recital 26 GDPR). At present, a risk analysis for synthetic data production is likely to conclude that establishing a personal reference requires too much effort. Following the relative anonymization approach, there would be no personal reference. In order to exclude a personal reference of the AI models, differential privacy could also be considered as an additional step in the generating of synthetic data (Kaulartz and Braegelmann 2020, Chapter 8.9, marginal no. 25). Nevertheless, synthetic data are as yet largely unexplored by legal scholars, and there is no judicial or regulatory practice of application and interpretation. Therefore, no general statement can be made about the anonymity of synthetic data. In individual cases, synthetic data may be personally identifiable, especially in the case of training data that are few in number or highly personalized (Kaulartz and Braegelmann 2020, Chapter 8.9, marginal no. 24).

Synthetic data illustrate that the question of anonymization remains highly contemporary in the end: Whereas new technologies might be a tool for anonymization when they arise, over time, these former novelties rapidly become state of the art, and there might be no absolute and incontrovertible anonymity of data anymore. Consequently, new technologies turn from tools to threats.

5 No Consent

In light of the fact that data anonymization is not always possible and consent is central but not without criticism, the question arises whether data protection knows a path between consent and anonymization that respects the value of public health research for society. According to the GDPR, all processing of personal data is prohibited and requires a legal basis. Besides consent, the European legislature allows other legal bases of equal importance. For example, when processing health data for research purposes, Art. 9 (2) (j) GDPR enables the European member states to create a legal basis in their national laws and thus offers a legal alternative to consent. In Germany, the legislature made use of this so-called opening clause by creating § 27 of the German Federal Data Protection Act (BDSG): a legal basis for data processing in research without consent. Accordingly, the processing of special categories of personal data shall also be permitted without consent for scientific or historical research purposes or statistical purposes if such processing is necessary for these purposes and the interests of the controller in processing substantially outweigh those of the data subject in not processing the data. This "no consent approach" takes on new relevance as data subjects do not appear to be in favor of consent. According to a Forsa-survey in Germany, only 27% of respondents wanted to be asked for their consent for every new research project (Semler 2019).

Although § 27 BDSG does not require consent and is therefore not subject to the criticism mentioned above, the application of this provision is not trivial either. Instead, the interplay of § 27 BDSG with the data protection laws of the German federal states is highly complex, making it a challenging task to identify the applicable law. So far, Germany's federal and state legislators have failed to create a uniform, practicable, and legally secure legal basis for research data processing. Instead, German law is still characterized by a patchwork of individual regulations that do not reveal any uniform legal concept. For instance, public bodies of the German states can be affected by special laws of the German states, which take precedence over § 27 BDSG. Additionally, there are special laws for hospitals in the federal states and special laws for hospitals under church sponsorship. Due to the legal fragmentation in Germany, it can be complex to determine whether research institutes come under the scope of § 27 BDSG or another law of a federal state.

If § 27 BDSG is applicable, the key question is whether the controller's interests in processing substantially outweigh those of the data subject. On the one hand, this balancing of interest leaves space for the individual circumstances of the specific research project. On the other hand, it leads to legal uncertainty. The fact that a research project concentrates on public health purposes can be a relevant factor in balancing interests. For example, Recital 54 describes that the processing of personal data may be necessary for reasons of public interest in the areas of public health and may be done without consent. Ultimately, it is up to the researchers to ensure that the interests of the persons affected by the data processing are only given a low weight by ensuring the best possible data protection through safeguards and protective measures. For this purpose, researchers have extensive options of guarantees and safeguards, such as anonymization, pseudonymization, and encryption of data, trust and escrow offices, closed data rooms, secure access solutions, and finally also, use-and-access-committees (UAC), which decide on the release of data and ensure compliance with all regulations (Weichert and Krawczak 2019). These and many other instruments not only ensure the highest possible level of data protection in research data processing but simultaneously enable researchers to manage a legally secure balancing of interests in their favor (Buchner 2022). The hurdles for justifying data processing for research purposes without consent are thus not insurmountable.

Besides this "no consent" approach, the opening clause of Art. 9 (2) (j) GDPR allows for a combination of different types of consent with further requirements of another legal basis when processing data for research purposes. In these cases, the primary legal basis is not consent but consent becomes a safeguard. Different types of consent could be the classic informed consent in the GDPR sense but also broad consent as an exception from specific consent. It is important to note that the European Union (EU) countries do not always refer to the same type of consent when discussing data processing for research. Consequently, understanding of consent can vary significantly across EU member states (Directorate-General for Health and Food Safety 2021). For example, the Austrian law (§ 2d (3) FOG) combines broad consent with other prerequisites. In France, consent is required not in a GDPR sense but rather as a national safeguard for the participation of individuals in research (Directorate-General for Health and Food Safety 2021). In the German § 75 SGB X, consent in a GDPR sense is merged with other requirements. Additionally, the buzzword "data donation" (Deutscher Ethikrat 2018; Strech et al. 2020) has started discussions on a new type of legal action in Germany: the so-called "agreement" of the patient. According to the proposal, the agreement is one requirement among others, but it is not equal to consent in GDPR terms since the agreement does not necessarily fulfill the conditions of consent (Strech et al. 2020; Schildbach 2022). Despite all these new consent models, it is not yet foreseeable how the future of data processing for public health research will turn out. To summarize, the GDPR is not only flexible enough to allow for data processing with and without consent but also leaves room for developing new types of consent where the traditional concept of consent no longer appears appropriate.

6 Conclusion

The current legal situation gives rise to considerable practical problems in implementing public health research projects. Although the GDPR theoretically contains several privileges for research, the solutions are still insufficient in practice. Additionally, German law remains a patchwork of individual regulations that do not reveal any uniform legal concept. Partners of joint research projects often belong to different areas with different data protection law requirements, and a distinction must be made between public bodies and private entities. Consent becomes indispensable as the only manageable basis of legitimacy for data processing: To date, practice in public health research is not based on legal privileges but on consent, leading to the fact that consent is central to data processing and perceived as a "silver bullet." However, consent is not without criticism since its conditions are not always fulfilled when the objectives and duration of a project are not definable or foreseeable at the beginning of the project. Although there are approaches for improving consent mechanisms with broad and dynamic designs, the conditions of consent, such as "informed," "voluntarily," and "revocable," are still challenging. Additionally, the interplay of data protection law with medical confidentiality complicates the consent process. In the end, consent is a stopgap rather than a silver bullet.

Three aspects need attention to overcome these structural difficulties and to realize the potential benefits of public health research for society. First, anonymization processes relating to synthetic data should be further developed and evaluated since they are a promising possibility for processing huge amounts of data, including their scientific reuse. Second, new approaches focusing on a legal basis instead of consent need more attention from international and national perspectives. Whether "no consent approaches" comply with current data protection law is still questionable and therefore demands a clear point of view. Last but not least, the harmonization of research data protection is overdue. Politicians and legislators—at both national and European levels—have put the compatibility of data use and data protection on their agendas and are striving to create a legal framework, particularly for the healthcare sector, that will significantly facilitate data use in the future. In line with the European strategy for data, the EU Digital Governance Act and the EU Data Act aim to make the EU a leader in our data-driven society. Explicitly focusing on the regulation of health data, the European Health Data Space has recently come into force, which aims, among other objectives, to support the use of health data for better healthcare delivery, research, innovation, and policy-making.

References

Beauchamp TL, Childress JF (2019) Principles of biomedical ethics. Oxford University Press, New York

Bischoff C (2020) Pseudoymisierung und Anonymisierung von personenbezogenen Forschungsdaten im Rahmen klinischer Prüfung von Arzneimitteln (Teil I) – Gesetzliche Anforderungen. Pharma Recht 4:309–315

Buchner B (2022) Forschungsdaten effektiver nutzen. Datenschutz und Datensicherheit 9:555–560

Bundesärztekammer, Kassenärztliche Bundesvereinigung (2021) Bekanntmachung: Hinweise und Empfehlungen zur ärztlichen Schweigepflicht, Datenschutz und Datenverarbeitung in der Arztpraxis. https://www.kbv.de/media/sp/Empfehlungen_aerztliche_Schweigepflicht_Datenschutz.pdf. Accessed 10 Feb 2023

Bundesbeauftragte für den Datenschutz und die Informationsfreiheit (2020) Positionspapier zur Anonymisierung unter der DSGVO unter besonderer Berücksichtigung der TK-Branche. https://www.bfdi.bund.de/SharedDocs/Downloads/DE/Konsultationsverfahren/1_Anonymisierung/Positionspapier-Anonymisierung.pdf?__blob=publicationFile&v=4. Accessed 10 Feb 2023

Caspar J (2019) Art. 89 DSGVO. In: Simitis S, Hornung G, Spiecker gen. Döhmann I (eds) Datenschutzrecht: DSGVO mit BDSG. Nomos, Baden-Baden

Cepic M (2021) Broad Consent: Die erweiterte Einwilligung in der Forschung. Zeitschrift für Datenschutz-Aktuell 10:05214

Chico V (2018) The impact of the General Data Protection Regulation on health research. Br Med Bull 128:109–118

Conrad I, Treeger C (2019) § 34 Recht des Datenschutzes. In: Auer-Reinsdorff A, Conrad I (eds) Handbuch IT- und Datenschutzrecht, 3rd edn. C.H. Beck, München

Datenethikkommission (2019) Gutachten der Datenethikkommission. https://www.bmi.bund.de/SharedDocs/downloads/DE/publikationen/themen/it-digitalpolitik/gutachten-datenethikkommission.pdf;jsessionid=F1C29557CCDB4CB6F3EC21BCC60A379A.1_cid340?__blob=publicationFile&v=7. Accessed 10 Feb 2023

Deutscher Ethikrat (2018) Stellungnahme: Big Data und Gesundheit – Datensouveränität als informationelle Freiheitsgestaltung. https://www.ethikrat.org/fileadmin/Publikationen/Stellungnahmen/deutsch/stellungnahme-big-data-und-gesundheit.pdf. Accessed 10 Feb 2023

Directorate-General for Health and Food Safety (2021) Assessment of the EU member states' rules on health data in the light of GDPR. https://health.ec.europa.eu/system/files/2021-02/ms_rules_health-data_en_0.pdf. Accessed 10 Feb 2023

Dove E (2018) The EU General Data Protection Regulation: implications for international scientific research in the digital era. J Law Med Ethics 46:1013–1030

Eichler C (2023a) Art. 4 DSGVO. In: Wolff H, Brink S (eds) BeckOK Datenschutzrecht, 44th edn. C.H. Beck, München

Eichler C (2023b) Art. 89 DSGVO. In: Wolff H, Brink S (eds) BeckOK Datenschutzrecht, 44th edn. C.H. Beck, München

Ernst S (2021) Art. 4 DSGVO. In: Paal B, Pauly D (eds) DSGVO BDSG, 3rd edn. C.H. Beck, München

European Court of Justice (2016) Judgment of the Court (Second Chamber) of 19 October 2016 Patrick Breyer v Bundesrepublik Deutschland. https://eur-lex.europa.eu/legal-content/EN/TXT/HTML/?uri=CELEX:62014CJ0582&from=EN. Accessed 10 Feb 2023

European Data Protection Supervisor (2020) A preliminary opinion on data protection and scientific research. https://edps.europa.eu/sites/edp/files/publication/20-01-06_opinion_research_en.pdf. Accessed 10 Feb 2023

FIT4RRI, Foster (2023) Open and FAIR research data: what is open data and what is FAIR data? https://www.fosteropenscience.eu/learning/open-and-fair-research-data/#/id/5e3741af3ccdf1010dbc6f26. Accessed 10 Feb 2023

Fröhlich W, Spiecker gen. Döhmann I (2022) Die breite Einwilligung (Broad Consent) in die Datenverarbeitung zu medizinischen Forschungszwecken – der aktuelle Irrweg der MII. GesundheitsRecht 6:346–353

Hackenberg W (2022) Teil 15.2 Big Data und Datenschutz. In: Hoeren T, Sieber U, Holznagel B (eds) Handbuch Multimedia Recht, 58th edn. C.H. Beck, München

Kaulartz M, Braegelmann T (2020) Kapitel 8.9 Personenbezug von KI-Modellen. In: Rechtshandbuch Artificial Intelligence und Machine Learning. C.H. Beck, München

Kaye J, Whitley E, Lund D, Morrison M, Teare H, Melham K (2015) Dynamic consent: a patient interface for twenty-first century research networks. Eur J Hum Genet 23:141–146

March S, Andrich S, Drepper J, Horenkamp-Sonntag D, Icks A, Ihle P, Kieschke J (2019) Gute Praxis Datenlinkage (GPD). Gesundheitswesen 81:636–650

Medizininformatik-Initiative (MII) (2020a) Arbeitsgruppe Consent Mustertext Patienteneinwilligung. Version 1.6d as of 16.4.2020. https://www.medizininformatik-initiative.de/sites/default/files/2020-04/MII_AG-Consent_Einheitlicher-Mustertext_v1.6d.pdf. Accessed 10 Feb 2023

Medizininformatik-Initiative (MII) (2020b) Handreichung zur Anwendung der national harmonisierten Patienteninformations- und Einwilligungsdokumente zur Sekundärnutzung von Patientendaten. Version 0.9d as of 16.4.2020. https://www.medizininformatik-initiative.de/sites/default/files/2020-04/MII_AG-Consent_Handreichung_v0.9d.pdf. Accessed 10 Feb 2023

Oberlandesgericht München (2013) Arzthaftung: Widerruf der Einwilligung zur Einsichtnahme in Patientenakte. GesundheitsRecht 8:471–475

Organization for Economic Co-operation and Development (OECD) (2017) Ministerial statement. https://www.oecd.org/health/ministerial-statement-2017.pdf. Accessed 10 Feb 2023

Raum B (2018) Art. 89 DSGVO. In: Ehmann E, Selmayr M (eds) DSGVO, 2nd edn. C.H. Beck, München

Roßnagel A (2019a) Die neuen Datenschutzregelungen in der Forschungspraxis von Hochschulen. Zeitschrift für Datenschutz 4:157–164

Roßnagel A (2019b) Art. 4 DSGVO. In: Simitis S, Hornung G, Spiecker gen. Döhmann I (eds) Datenschutzrecht: DSGVO mit BDSG. Nomos, Baden-Baden

Roßnagel A (2021) Datenlöschung und Anonymisierung. Zeitschrift für Datenschutz 4:188–192

Roßnagel A, Geminn C (2021) Vertrauen in Anonymisierung. Zeitschrift für Datenschutz 9:487–490

Sachverständigenrat (2021) Gutachten: Digitalisierung für Gesundheit – Ziele und Rahmenbedingungen eines dynamisch lernenden Gesundheitssystems. https://www.svr-gesundheit.de/fileadmin/Gutachten/Gutachten_2021/SVR_Gutachten_2021.pdf. Accessed 10 Feb 2023

Schildbach R (2022) Zugang zu Daten der öffentlichen Hand und Datenaltruismus nach dem Entwurf des Daten-Governance-Gesetzes. Zeitschrift für Datenschutz 3:148–153

Schmidt B (2022) Art. 2 DSGVO. In: Taeger J, Gabel D (eds) DSGVO – BDSG – TTDSG, 4th edn. dfv, Frankfurt am Main

Semler S (2019) "Datenspende" für die medizinische Forschung: Ergebnisse einer Forsa-Umfrage im Auftrag der Technologie- und Methodenplattform für die vernetzte medizinische Forschung e. V. (TMF). https://www.tmf-ev.de/News/articleType/ArticleView/articleId/4456.aspx. Accessed 10 Feb 2023

Spitz M, Cornelius K (2022) Einwilligung und gesetzliche Forschungsklausel als Rechtsgrundlagen für die Sekundärnutzung klinischer Daten zu Forschungszwecken. Medizinrecht 40:191–198

Strech D, Kielmansegg S, Zenker S, Krawczak M, Semler S (2020) Wissenschaftliches Gutachten „Datenspende"– Bedarf für die Forschung, ethische Bewertung, rechtliche, informationstechnologische und organisatorische Rahmenbedingungen. https://www.bundesgesundheitsministerium.de/fileadmin/Dateien/5_Publikationen/Ministerium/Berichte/Gutachten_Datenspende.pdf. Accessed 10 Feb 2023

Wegner S (2021) Teil 6.5 Synthetische Daten. In: Leupold A, Wiebe A, Glossner S (eds) IT-Recht – Recht, Wirtschaft und Technik der digitalen Transformation, 4th edn. C.H. Beck, München

Weichert T (2020) Art. 9 DSGVO. In: Kühling J, Buchner B (eds) DSGVO BDSG, 3rd edn. C.H. Beck, München

Weichert T (2022) Datenschutzrechtliche Rahmenbedingungen medizinischer Forschung: Vorgaben der EU-Datenschutz-Grundverordnung und national geltender Gesetze. MWV Medizinisch Wissenschaftliche Verlagsgesellschaft mbH & Co. KG, Berlin

Weichert T, Krawczak M (2019) Vorschlag einer modernen Dateninfrastruktur für die medizinische Forschung in Deutschland. GMS Medizinische Informatik, Biometrie und Epidemiologie 15(1):Doc03

Open Access This chapter is licensed under the terms of the Creative Commons Attribution 4.0 International License (http://creativecommons.org/licenses/by/4.0/), which permits use, sharing, adaptation, distribution and reproduction in any medium or format, as long as you give appropriate credit to the original author(s) and the source, provide a link to the Creative Commons license and indicate if changes were made.

The images or other third party material in this chapter are included in the chapter's Creative Commons license, unless indicated otherwise in a credit line to the material. If material is not included in the chapter's Creative Commons license and your intended use is not permitted by statutory regulation or exceeds the permitted use, you will need to obtain permission directly from the copyright holder.

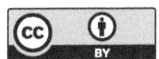

Evidence-Based Approaches in Digital Public Health

Joanna Albrecht, Pinar Tokgöz, and Christoph Dockweiler

Abstract Rapid innovation in technology as well as an increase in its availability for health promotion and care, have revolutionized health service delivery today. Further, this has a maximum impact on developing and improving public health interventions and evidence-based approaches in digital public health. The collection and analysis of user-generated data (real-world evidence) created opportunities for both individual health promotion and the potential to improve and optimize healthcare delivery. However, the development and evaluation of digital health interventions also offer complex challenges. These include, among others: Uncertain dynamics in technology development, intricacies of data analysis methods under data security concerns, and the complexity of personalized health promotion or medicine. To address these challenges, an application-oriented systematization of evidence-based approaches is needed for specific areas of digital public health.

Keywords eHealth · Evidence-based · Digital health intervention · Evaluation · Implementation

Abbreviations

AR	Augmented reality
BZgA	German Federal Centre for Health Education
DHS	Digital health solutions
DHT	Digital health technology
DiPH	Digital public health
DVG	Digital Care Act
EBM	Evidence-based medicine
EBPH	Evidence-based public health

J. Albrecht (✉) · P. Tokgöz · C. Dockweiler
Chair of Digital Public Health, Department of Social Sciences,
Faculty of Arts and Humanities, University of Siegen, Siegen, Germany
e-mail: joanna.albrecht@uni-siegen.de; christoph.dockweiler@uni-siegen.de

eHealth	Electronic health
EHR	Electronic health records
FDA	Food and Drug Administration
IQVIA	Institute for Human Data Science
mHealth	Mobile health
NICE	National Institute for Health and Care Excellence
RCT	Randomized controlled trials
RWD	Real-world data
RWE	Real-world evidence
VR	Virtual reality

1 Introduction

New collection and analysis possibilities for complex data sets in public health have changed existing evidence-based approaches or developed new ones (Meyer 2021). Digital technologies like smartphones and apps, for example, can be used to monitor, measure and analyze the effects of public health interventions. The collection, analysis, and use of (health) data allow a better understanding and promotion of health at the individual and population levels. For example, digital technologies enable networking and communication among healthcare professionals or new ways of designing health promotion and prevention interventions by incorporating digital technologies into the planning, implementation, and evaluation phases (Rossmann and Krömer 2016; Fischer and Dockweiler 2019; Zeeb et al. 2020). On the contrary, integrating digital technologies increased the intricacies of public health interventions, making it more challenging to conduct evidence studies (Brandes et al. 2021).

These challenges must be discussed and addressed to fully exploit the benefits of evidence-based approaches in digital public health (DiPH). This chapter highlights changes in implementation and requirements as well as challenges of evidence-based approaches in DiPH. In this context, it will be demonstrated how digitalization has changed the generation of evidence in public health. Through this, exemplary approaches, methods, and implementation factors for evidence generation in DiPH will be presented.

2 Approaches of Evidence Generation in Digital Public Health

In general, public health interventions should be carefully designed and implemented, considering the benefits and unintended consequences for individuals and population groups. Further, they should be tested under real-world conditions in their respective settings (Brownson et al. 2009).

Evidence-based public health (EBPH) refers to making public health-related decisions using the best available scientific knowledge, the expertise of relevant experts and stakeholders, and the values and preferences of the affected population (Von Philipsborn and Rehfuess 2021). This is vital in developing public health interventions. An evidence-based approach is increasingly seen as a quality criterion in public health, even though there is no standardized procedure for researchers, policymakers, and public health practitioners of evidence generation in public health in Germany or across other countries (Gerhardus et al. 2008; Brownson et al. 2009; Rehfuess et al. 2021; Bennet and Mageras 2021). In Germany, for instance, health promotion and prevention stakeholders refer to the *Memorandum on Evidence-Based Prevention and Health Promotion* of the German Federal Centre for Health Education (BZgA) as their process. Since 2020 this Memorandum has operationalized the understanding and implementation of evidence-based practices in health promotion and prevention (De Bock et al. 2020). In the context of care provision, the German Social Law Code provides a framework for developing healthcare services by statutory health insurance. To be eligible for reimbursement, these services are evaluated according to evidence-based medicine (EBM) principles (Rehfuess et al. 2021). Despite the legal anchoring of EBPH in certain areas of public health, there is no consensus in recent literature on whether potential evidence in public health has been fully exploited yet (Brownson et al. 1999, 2009; Rychetnik et al. 2012; Rehfuess et al. 2021).

As previously mentioned, there is also a high demand for evidence generation in the field of DiPH. This can be observed in the evidence gaps in effectiveness, acceptance, user orientation, health impact assessment, cost-effectiveness, and quality of reporting (Wong and Rigby 2022). As outlined by Wienert et al. (2022) DiPH refers to the use of digital technologies and methods to improve the health and well-being of populations: "A digital public health intervention addresses at least one essential public health function through digital means. Applying a framework for functional classification and stratification categorizes its interaction level with the user. The developmental process of a digital public health intervention includes the user perspective by applying participatory methods to support its effectiveness and implementation to achieve a population health impact" (Wienert et al. 2022, p. 9). It encompasses a range of approaches, such as the development of digital health applications, the use of social media for health communication, the analysis of large data sets for monitoring health trends, and the use of digital technologies for delivering healthcare services (Wienert and Zeeb 2021). DiPH interventions aim to improve healthcare, enhance health outcomes, promote patient engagement, and increase access to healthcare services (Zeeb et al. 2020; Brandes et al. 2021).

2.1 Principles and Processes of Evidence-Based Decision-Making in Public Health

The development and implementation of evidence-based approaches require reference to public health principles and practices. For evidence-based decision-making in public health, De Bock et al. (2020) developed the STIIP principles, which are:

(1) Systematization, (2) Transparency in dealing with uncertainty, (3) Integration and participation, (4) Handling of conflicts of interest, and (5) Structured and reflective process (ibid.; see Table 1). Rehfuess et al. (2021) noted that these principles apply to both health promotion-specific and broader public health perspectives.

Table 1 STIIP principles and methods of evidence-based decision-making in public health (Source: own source based on De Bock et al. 2020, p. 13)

Principle	Explanation	Approaches and methods of implementation
Systematization	A systematic review, evaluation, and synthesis of the best available scientific evidence on a topic are crucial for evidence-based decision-making. Decisions based on one study only or selective study results contradict the principle of systematization	• Systematic reviews • Rapid reviews, evidence mapping, or overviews of systematic reviews
Transparency in dealing with uncertainty	Transparency of the underlying approach allows the reconstruction and critical examination of potential uncertainties, the decision-making process, and the credibility of the evidence used	• Implementing explicit processes for decision-making, such as through guidelines • Establishing a clear methodology for synthesizing scientific evidence and evaluating the quality of studies, particularly in the context of systematic reviews • Conducting systematic and transparent assessments of uncertainty in the evidence used
Integration and participation	In addition to scientific characteristics, in evidence-based decisions, there should be a participatory inclusion of the expertise and experience of those responsible, as well as the values and preferences of those affected. This often involves a diversity of stakeholder groups (sponsors, practitioners, (indirect) recipients of the measure) represented in different societal sectors that need to be considered	• Shared decision-making: involves the active participation of both healthcare providers and patients in the decision-making process, (e.g., through various forms of engagement such as representative surveys, consultations, or direct involvement)
Handling conflicts of interest	In public health decision-making, various legitimate interests must be brought into alignment. Therefore, the role of different interests in decision-making processes should be made transparent	• Disclosure of financial, institutional, familial, and other interests including conflicts of interest • Managing conflicts of interest by scientific rules (e.g., minimizing conflicts of interest that significantly increase the risk of a systematically distorted assessment of evidence, and excluding responsible parties from the decision-making process in cases of serious conflicts of interest to resolve them)

(continued)

Table 1 (continued)

Principle	Explanation	Approaches and methods of implementation
Structured reflective processes	Evidence generation is characterized by a five-step process, which should be considered by the researchers	• Step 1: Formulation of a clear research question • Step 2: Searching for the best evidence available • Step 3: Critical examination of scientific findings in terms of credibility and relevance • Step 4: Application of the evidence (e.g. in the development of a health promotion measure or in the context of a health policy decision) • Step 5: Evaluation of implementation (e.g. through critical reflection or accompanying evaluation)

The first principal *systematization* refers to the requirement of public health professionals to ensure that decisions and interventions are based on the current state of research by systematically reviewing existing literature. Furthermore, ensuring that the methods used, and results obtained, are transparent and accountable is essential throughout the process. This assures integrity in decision-making and the development of public health interventions. Additionally, the decision-making process is also presented in a way that is understandable to other stakeholders, e.g., those who finance, implement, or are affected by the intervention. Regarding the design of the decision-making process and implementation of public health interventions, the participation of relevant interest groups through various forms is highly important (De Bock et al. 2020). Shrestha et al. provide more detailed information on the participatory forms of involvement of stakeholders in their contribution to this compilation (see "Participatory Approaches for Digital Public Health: Giving Voice to Values" chapter, in this handbook).

EBPH is understood as a structured and reflective process (Brownson et al. 1999; Satterfield et al. 2009; Rehfuess et al. 2021), which should be maintained throughout. This requires ensuring the relevance and applicability of decisions and interventions for the target group. Consequently, public health decisions and interventions must be reviewed and evaluated regularly and adapted to changes in the population and the current state of research. In implementing EBPH, it is crucial to identify and resolve conflicts between interest groups or at least make them transparent.

The evidence-based approach to public health interventions is characterized by a structured and reflective process based on solid methodologies for collecting and evaluating evidence and establishing decision-making procedures. This process includes steps such as convening a panel, disclosing and managing conflicts of interest, scoping recommendations, agreeing on and setting criteria for decision-making, formulating specific research questions, collecting and evaluating evidence, making recommendations based on the evidence, and establishing standards. These steps should be explicitly presented, and uncertainties regarding the evidence and recommendations should be disclosed to ensure transparency in dealing with uncertainty. At the same time, EBPH faces the challenge of providing scientific evidence for the effectiveness of individual interventions and ensuring a high degree of relevance to practice achieving higher acceptance and utilization (Jahnel and Schüz 2020).

To meet the requirements of EBPH, it is necessary to systematize evidence-based processes. Basic process elements include involving the community in evaluation and decision-making or systematically using data and information systems. Further, decisions should be made based on the best available expert-reviewed knowledge (both quantitative and qualitative). Additionally, frameworks should be applied for program planning (often based on health behavior theory), thorough evaluations conducted, and the knowledge gained disseminated (Brownson et al. 2009). When choosing the theoretical basis for the research, EBPH prerequisites investigate how existing theories and models can be built upon. Due to the interdisciplinary nature of public health, EBPH requires the cooperation of experts from various fields to collect and use the best possible evidence. Therefore, it is essential to identify and involve these experts in the research topic. Reflecting societal aspects in implementing EBPH is a further necessity due to interdisciplinarity. EBPH decisions and interventions must consider social, cultural, and economic factors to ensure they are relevant, ethically justifiable, and feasible for the affected population. Due to the high context-dependency of societal transformation processes, EBPH must be highly willing to review and adjust decisions and public health interventions in light of new evidence (De Bock et al. 2020).

Gerhardus et al. (2008) also emphasize the importance of addressing non-medical issues, such as ethical, socio-cultural, or organizational matters, when generating evidence in public health. According to this, values and interests influence the decision-making process, the generation of evidence, and the negotiation process (ibid.). Also, the authors propose a three-phased model on how to generate evidence in public health: (1) Deciding and Implementing, (2) Exchanging and Acting, (3) Developing Evidence. The *Deciding and Implementing* segment comprises the decision of which public health problem is of interest for research and the implementation of an intervention for this problem, with the latter being developed in the research process. *Exchanging and Acting* involves translating the public health problem into research questions or developing recommendations for action based on the research findings. Lastly, *Developing Evidence* selects the most appropriate methods to answer the research questions, and the research process is conducted using these methods (ibid.).

2.2 Methods of Evidence Generation in Public Health and Digital Public Health

As already illustrated, systematic screening, evaluation, and summarization of the best available scientific knowledge on a topic are crucial for evidence-based decision-making. Various methods can be applied to generate different levels of evidence depending on the research subject. Fundamental for generating evidence in public health are literature reviews, such as systematic reviews, rapid reviews, evidence mapping, or overviews of systematic reviews to summarize and evaluate current literature on a specific topic. Additionally, there are various study designs in public health, such as experimental and non-experimental or qualitative and quantitative social research methods (Lomas et al. 2005; Von Philipsborn and Rehfuess 2021).

Quantitative approaches include clinical studies that evaluate the effectiveness and safety of treatments and interventions. Surveys are also quantitative approaches, which quantify population groups' opinions, attitudes, and behaviors on particular health topics. Another approach includes analyzing health data (such as mortality rates, hospital stays, and vaccination rates) to identify health trends and risk factors. Overall, qualitative techniques include methods that allow for a deeper analysis of the research subject and, thus, the generation of hypotheses. For example, observational studies are conducted to capture relevant processes, relationships, or developments and to monitor the impact of developed interventions on a specific population over time. This also includes individual and group interviews, which are used to capture population groups' opinions, attitudes, and behavior on specific health topics (Von Philipsborn and Rehfuess 2021).

One way to measure the strength and reliability of evidence is the Grading of Recommendations Assessment, Development, and Evaluation (GRADE) instrument of the World Health Organization (WHO) and Cochrane. This instrument assigns high, moderate, low, and very low reliability on a step-by-step basis and allows for an assessment based on this (Guyatt et al. 2008).

Similar to evidence generation in public health, evidence generation in DiPH is also possible as a multi-stage process involving various methods and data sources and can be conducted via multiple approaches. The World Health Organization (2016) has compiled various techniques for this purpose, which are particularly related to evaluations in digital health interventions (see Table 2).

The gold standard of generating evidence through digital health interventions is—as with public health interventions—implementing (multicenter) RCTs (good to excellent evidence strength). Other essential approaches with good strength of evidence are the implementation of non-randomized trials and other systematic and empirical studies, such as observational studies (cohort and case-control studies). Expert opinion can be a vital contributor to evidence generation, especially when dealing with complex or controversial issues related to digital health intervention for which limited empirical evidence is available. Health data analytics is cited as a relatively new approach to evidence generation. This approach uses large amounts of electronic health (eHealth) data points to identify health-related patterns and relationships between factors and underlying conditions. For data collection itself, participatory approaches to evidence generation are often developed so that there is a collaboration between researchers, patients, practitioners, and other stakeholders to collectively formulate questions, collect data and interpret the results (World Health Organization 2016).

Guo et al. (2020) also argue for more innovative methods. They emphasize the limitations of traditional study designs and methods in evaluating digital

Table 2 Hierarchy of evidence by stage of evaluation of digital health interventions (Source: based on World Health Organization 2016, p. 70, 73)

		Suitable study designs
Confidence in the strength of evidence	Excellent	Multicenter randomized controlled trials (RCTs) (a planned experiment designed to assess the efficacy of an intervention in human beings by comparing the intervention to a control condition; implemented with cluster randomized trials such as parallel/crossover or stepped-wedge)
	Good	RCTs
		Non-randomized trials
		Cohort studies (longitudinal study, measures events in chronological order, used to study disease incidence, causes, and prognosis)
		Case-control studies (retrospective studies in which two groups differing in an outcome are identified and compared based on a supposed causal attribute)
	Fair	Cross-sectional studies (examines the relationship between a characteristic of interest and other variables as they exist in a defined population at one single time point)
	Poor	Case studies (report of an event, unusual disease, or association which aims to prompt future research using more rigorous study designs)
		Case reports (aggregates individual cases in one report)

technologies and interventions, such as the length of studies and delayed publication of results. An appropriate method to generate more extensive evidence is the use of real-time data and the linking of data sources in the context of simulations. Furthermore, various approaches to simulation could be applied in combination with traditional study designs to evaluate digital solutions, such as computational simulation, system simulation, and clinical simulation. For instance, clinical simulation-based studies with micro-randomization design can serve as a potent and pragmatic methodology for assessing digital technologies comprising multiple components during the initial stages of product development (ibid.).

Accordingly, digital technologies and generating evidence are rapidly reciprocally evolving areas in public health, with digital data generating evidence and evidence driving further digital technologies and acceptance (Stern et al. 2022). When examining the intersection between digital health and evidence, there are significant stages in the evidence value chain that are instrumental in generating evidence. Figure 1 illustrates that patients, as a primary source of information, represent the starting point from which data is collected. Following this, the data is stored and transmitted, facilitating its aggregation with data from other patients. Ultimately, the data is analyzed to generate evidence that can be utilized by stakeholders (Khosla et al. 2021).

The differentiation between real-world evidence (RWE) and real-world data (RWD) is crucial in this context. The Food and Drug Administration (FDA) defines RWD as "data relating to people's health status and/or the delivery of health care

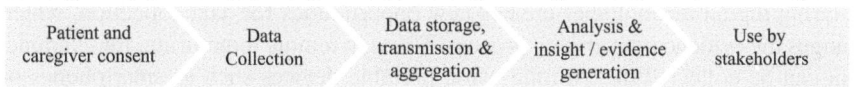

Fig. 1 Stages in the real-world evidence (RWE) value chain. (Source: Khosla et al. 2021)

routinely collected from a variety of sources" and RWE as "the clinical evidence regarding the usage and potential benefits or risks of a medical product derived from analysis of RWD" (US Food and Drug Administration 2023, w. p.). Both concepts are highly relevant to DiPH. Current applications of RWE include demonstrating safety and value, pricing and market access, and enhancing the clinical development process (Hughes et al. 2016; Bennet and Mageras 2021). RWE and RWD are essential tools in DiPH. They refer to data and evidence collected from real-world settings, such as clinical practices, Electronic Health Records (EHRs), claims databases, and patient-generated data, rather than controlled clinical trials (Magalhães et al. 2022).

An additional aspect is using DiPH technologies to deliver interventions and generate data. Evaluating digital health technologies (DHTs) necessitates evidence generation. To structure this evaluation, the National Institute for Health and Care Excellence (NICE) developed the evidence standards framework. This framework includes a total of 21 standards divided into 5 evidence groups: (1) Design factors, (2) Describing value, (3) Demonstrating performance, (4) Delivering value, and (5) Deployment considerations. The listed standards are intended to ensure that DHTs can be evaluated and effectively integrated into public healthcare. This should facilitate the incorporation of safe, effective and public health-relevant DHTs into healthcare that are acceptable to a diverse range of users, scalable, environmentally sustainable, address health inequalities, comply with safety standards and provide reliable health information (National Institute for Health and Care Excellence 2019).

2.3 Examples of Changes in Evidence-Based Approaches in Digital Public Health

The incorporation of new methods for data collection, analysis, and participation characterizes evidence-based approaches in DiPH. This is achieved using scientifically grounded methods and data points that are used in the process of evidence-based decision-making and for developing, implementing, and evaluating digital health solutions or interventions. These changes include the integration of new data collection methods, the consideration of new data collection concepts, and the implementation of new methods of data analysis. Additionally, participation opportunities are transformed into evidence-based approaches in DiPH. The nature and extent of these changes will be illustrated below.

Using digital technologies creates new opportunities for data collection, which changes the evidence-generation process. Through remote monitoring, for example, data can be collected in real-time using portable devices such as smartphones or wearables, and connected health apps or digital health applications can be monitored and processed accordingly (de Farias et al. 2020; Peyroteo et al. 2021). In rehabilitation, new digital-based therapy methods and evidence-based approaches are emerging to make data-based recommendations for improving or restoring motor function in various patient groups. Examples of this include robot-assisted movement training applications (Kahn et al. 2006) or immersive and sometimes playful learning environments using virtual reality (VR) and augmented reality (AR) (Levin et al. 2015). As part of evidence-based rehabilitation, various evidence-based approaches have been developed based on innovative data collection methods. For example, Proffitt and Lange (2015) provide a progressive process that involves the development of interventions based on evidence-based principles and using standardized measurement instruments. The effectiveness of VR interventions can then be evaluated by effectiveness and efficacy studies (ibid.). Baran et al. (2015) advocate an interdisciplinary and coherent approach to developing and using scalable interactive neurorehabilitation systems for managing upper extremities in stroke patients (ibid.). Despite the potential of interactive data collection in the field of rehabilitation and health behavior, there are still gaps in research about how these technologies could be used to improve and address the needs of patients on a broad basis as well as reduce chronic diseases and impairments (Proffitt and Lange 2015).

The integration of digital technologies in the process of evidence generation yields new forms of collected data. For example, self-tracking allows individuals to collect and monitor their health data through digital devices such as smartphones, wearables, or VR and AR technologies. This enables real-time feedback options and visualized data processing, mainly through AR-based innovations in immersive data visualization (Butscher et al. 2018). The self-collected health data allows for the individualization of prevention and care concepts, improving quality and efficiency in service delivery (Schnell 2018). Additionally, self-tracked data can provide added value to society through data donation, which can be used in research to gain insights for developing new drugs, faster diagnoses of rare diseases, or better treatment of chronic diseases (Pilgrim and Bohnet-Joschko 2022). This capability of digital data collection facilitates the generation of RWE, which aims to assess the effectiveness and safety of treatments and interventions in real-world settings. However, it is also essential to consider the potential impact of self-health tracking on the user's mental health and perception of illness and whether it may exacerbate cyberchondria (White and Horvitz 2009).

Using new data analysis methods in the evidence-generation process, e.g., Big Data analysis, allows for the processing and filtering of vast amounts of data. This enables insights to be gathered and analyzed quickly and accurately from various data sources, such as electronic medical records, social media, and tracking sensors. For instance, utilizing Artificial Intelligence (AI) is becoming increasingly important in data analysis. It is employed to identify health trends and risk factors for specific health problems (Karpathakis et al. 2021), to track disease spread, to evaluate treatment and preventive intervention effectiveness (Brandes et al. 2021), or to incorporate cloud-based decision support systems in healthcare decision-making (Moutselos and Maglogiannis 2020). Interactive platforms to capture and analyze data in DiPH during the COVID-19 pandemic are also developed. However, there is a lack of studies examining the practical implications of technology and Big Data on "intelligent" DiPH management and its implications and consequences (Popkova and Sergi 2022).

The integration of digital technologies in EBPH research also changes the consideration of participatory engagement of stakeholders (Hochmuth et al. 2020; Jahnel and Schüz 2020; Brandes et al. 2021; Ledel Solem et al. 2020; Karpathakis et al. 2021; van Kessel et al. 2022) and, therefore, requirements for qualitative research methods. Increasing inclusive and participatory approaches to evidence generation are being proposed to meet the demands of interdisciplinary development and testing of DiPH interventions and the associated process complexity. Often, these are based on qualitative methods (Hochmuth et al. 2020). Participatory processes in the design, development, and implementation of digital technologies in public health can improve user orientation and acceptance and the effectiveness of the intervention (Jahnel and Schüz 2020; van Kessel et al. 2022).

There is a growing need for evidence-based approaches to prove the effectiveness of digital interventions in prevention and health promotion while incorporating unique participation demands in primary prevention and health promotion. In research consortia, non-academic and civil society actors (such as professionals from prevention and health promotion, policymakers, and target groups of public health interventions) and users are involved in research work with varying degrees of participation. This allows non-academic, civil society actors and users to jointly develop, implement and evaluate effective public health interventions (Fischer 2020; Stark et al. 2022).

The pre-established participatory evidence generation in public health is thus being altered by integrating digital technologies into participatory methods. Furthermore, new demand for the participatory involvement of stakeholders in the development process of DiPH interventions has arisen. Thus, digital technologies can pave new ways of participation for stakeholders. For example, the *Healthy Neighborhood Discovery Tool* allows participants to digitally record and photograph their perceptions of health-related features (e.g., the built environment and physical activity friendliness of the neighborhood) and provide the collected data for collaborative analysis and development of more physical activity-friendly interventions (Buman et al. 2013).

The utilization of DiPH technologies depends on the individual preferences and needs of potential users. To increase the usage and acceptance of mobile health (mHealth) as a DiPH intervention, user groups should be involved in the development process of applications for coping with illness and promoting healthy lifestyles (Jahnel and Schüz 2020; van Kessel et al. 2022). There are already various iterative, user-centered design approaches that lack proper systematization. Jahnel and Schüz (2020), therefore, propose developing a method and process catalog for systematically incorporating users in evidence-based techniques and a taxonomy of participation processes and models for technology developers to systematically involve user groups in all phases of digital technology development. Active involvement could be achieved through co-design concepts. For example, workshops during the certification and testing process (Jahnel and Schüz 2020) and user councils or steering committees with representatives of interest groups can be established to develop strategies for overcoming obstacles or conflicts during implementation (Blackmore et al. 2022). Such approaches can be iterative, allowing for the identification and reflection of new challenges, problems, and opportunities from a shared perspective of academic disciplines, civil society user groups, and technology developers on an ongoing basis (Karpathakis et al. 2021). The design and development process of DiPH interventions should aim to combine known evidence-based concepts with input from interest groups beyond the actual requirements for participatory development processes. eHealth interventions' design and development process should strive to merge established evidence-based principles with feedback from stakeholders beyond the essential prerequisites for participatory development processes (Ledel Solem et al. 2020).

3 Examples of Challenges of Evidence Generation in Digital Public Health

Overall, RWE and RWD can potentially improve the efficiency, effectiveness, and quality of DiPH interventions and services. However, the pathways of evidence-based DiPH lead to various challenges in developing and implementing evidence-based approaches to DiPH.

3.1 Non-technical Challenges

Non-technical challenges for the integration of DiPH interventions affect multiple levels. One of the most prominent challenges in many public health areas is the systematization principle in evidence generation. There is a lack of systematic approaches or guidelines that assess the effectiveness, usability, and quality of DiPH interventions and the digital technologies used (Fernandez-Luque et al. 2020; Balcombe and de Leo 2022). Developing evidence-based guidelines for the systematic design and use of digital health solutions is urgently needed. It is, however, particularly challenging to keep the development of evaluation methods on pace with rapid technological advancement (Malvey and Slovensky 2014). Furthermore, the procedures for developing evidence-based guidelines are relatively complex and time-consuming due to multidisciplinary considerations (Fernandez-Luque et al. 2020). As an example, the Institute for Human Data Science (IQVIA) developed a digital health evidence generation strategy for digital health solutions (DHS). This strategy addresses the challenges outlined in developing and implementing DHS (Bennet and Mageras 2021). According to this strategy, at first defining the DHS scope is of importance. Related to this, hypotheses based on the initial understanding of the external landscape and internal objectives as well as the target use case and key stakeholders should be defined. This is followed by the phase of exploring. In this phase, it is important to first build a fact base and gather information to test the initial hypotheses. Then evidence requirements should be identified and established to answer key research questions for evidence generation in collaboration with stakeholders and funding routes. The last phase consists of the definition of an evidence generation roadmap and the planning and deploying of it. For this purpose, key activities and milestones for evidence generation and dissemination should be defined and established as a roadmap. Additionally, a study concept including timeline, costs and internal as well as external stakeholder engagement should be created to realize the roadmap (Bennet and Mageras 2021, p. 1).

Digitalization leads to new requirements for DiPH interventions. The already existing complexity in the development of evidence and the consideration of general societal aspects (De Bock et al. 2020), is further increased by the additional component of digital technologies. This creates further non-technological challenges in considering the complexity of broader societal aspects, such as ethics, sociotechnology, privacy, equity, and quality of evidence, resulting in an increase in the complexity of equity discourse through digitalization (Iyamu et al. 2022). Thus, the discourse around equity becomes more complex through digitalization. The use of digital health interventions opens up new questions about the promotion and reduction of health inequalities, which interact with social and health inequality formation in society and thus also need to be reflected in their interaction (Dockweiler and Hochmuth 2019).

To develop evidence-based DiPH interventions under the premise of reducing or at least not increasing inequalities in society, aspects such as acceptance of the intervention in the population, feasibility and costs of implementation, as well as effects on health equity and the environment, must be taken into account (De Bock et al. 2020). It can be assumed that, in addition to a lack of access to and use of digital (health) technology, insufficiently available resources (e.g., skills, financial resources, social support) have a significant influence on the uptake and effective use of digital care and prevention services (Cornejo Müller et al. 2020).

Some populations have unequal access to and use of necessary technologies and data to benefit from DiPH intervention approaches, which can lead to social inequities (van Kessel et al. 2022). There is a growing risk that health inequalities of specific population groups will exacerbate further if some comprising individuals or groups cannot participate due to a lack of prerequisites. It is, therefore, essential to increase social, cultural, and economic equity of access. However, social differences do not only refer to access and availability but also differences in eHealth literacy. Current studies in this area are rudimentary, so further scientific evidence on health inequalities (Cornejo Müller et al. 2020) and eHealth literacy (El Benny et al. 2021) is required. To assure the safe and responsible use of digital (health) technologies and the ability to maximize the trustworthiness of information on the internet, it is advocated that future digital health interventions comprehensively incorporate models of eHealth literacy. This will allow the development and evaluation process of digital health interventions to understand contexts, what competencies are needed, and how and why interventions can be effective (El Benny et al. 2021). The topics of digital health inequalities and the digital divide are discussed in more detail in this compilation in the contribution by Brand et al. (see "Digital Health Inequalities" chapter) and Zeeb and Dratva ("Digital Health Literacy" chapter) in this handbook.

Participatory methods are particularly suitable for discussing the impact of DiPH interventions on socially relevant factors. However, the digitally supported participation methods have not been tested for all population groups. There is a lack of other strategies and evidence to address and demonstrate digital interventions' safety and clinical effectiveness for digitally excluded populations (Sheehan and Hassiotis 2017; Herman et al. 2023). For instance, Sheehan and Hassiotis (2017) emphasize this necessity in mental health for individuals with and without intellectual disabilities. An explicit digital inclusion strategy tailored to the requirements of people with intellectual disabilities would foster more significant equity in DiPH (ibid.). In evidence-based health promotion, Herman et al. (2023) present the *Inclusive Community Implementation Process* as an example of implementing the inclusion of people with disabilities in all policy planning and implementation and reducing barriers to access and use of evidence-based health promotion programs (ibid.).

Another challenge is the complexity of evidence generation in digital technology integration, as described earlier. This results, among other things, from the often multimodal and heterogeneous application possibilities of digital technologies, which further intensifies existing difficulties in the evaluation of public health measures (Fischer 2020; Brandes et al. 2021). The additional complexity in development and evaluation of digital technologies can arise from interactions between technical components (e.g., sensors for data collection), different requirements for users when implementing the intervention (e.g., knowledge about data security), involvement of other groups or organizational levels (e.g., patients or researchers), or the degree of adaptation or flexibility of the intervention (e.g., further agile development through software updates) (Hochmuth et al. 2020).

One consequence of the complexity of evidence generation is the challenge of transferring evidence-based findings into practice. Two obstacles can currently be identified. Digital technologies have been hastily introduced into healthcare due to a lack of evidence-based strategies in DiPH. During the COVID-19 pandemic, numerous digital health interventions were expeditiously implemented in healthcare settings, often without first having undergone evidence-based evaluation. For example, in mental healthcare, digital alternatives were designed as a short-term solution to respond to interventions of physical distancing, quarantine, and social contact restrictions. Strategies that generate evidence on process quality, cost-effectiveness, and long-term impact need to be developed to harness the potential of DiPH interventions, which have already been demonstrated in many public health settings (Rauschenberg et al. 2021). Remote technologies in primary care (Peek et al. 2020) and telemedicine (de Farias et al. 2020; Wong and Rigby 2022; Gerli et al. 2021) are also under-researched and possess potential safety concerns without evidence.

A second related obstacle is the developmental dynamics of digitalization, which counteracts the complex process of evidence-based DiPH. Evidence-based DiPH is subject to considerable developmental dynamics, which can be attributed to the rapid development of technology, the amount and processing of data, including data security, and the design of personalization of measurement and interventions (Fleming et al. 2020).

3.2 Technical Challenges

In addition to the non-technological challenges, evidence-based approaches in DiPH also face technological challenges. These include fragmented and unsustainable systems, a lack of clear standards, unreliable data and infrastructure gaps. There are also challenges in terms of hardware and software, internet connectivity and computing power (Vajawat et al. 2021). Another key problem is the quality, origin and validity of the health data collected (Vajawat et al. 2021; Meyer 2021; Iyamu et al. 2022). Data sources are often incomplete or inconsistent, which significantly limits the validity and comparability of the results. In order to improve the evidence base of digital health technologies, targeted measures are therefore needed to ensure data quality as well as better access and more effective use of existing data (Meyer 2021). Data protection and data security issues also remain key challenges - for example in connection with digital self-measurement technologies, which are often used without sufficient transparency. Users usually have no clear idea of how their data is processed (Kramer et al. 2019), and there is a lack of validated standards for assessing the informative value of such technologies (Iyamu et al. 2022). The German Digital Care Act (DVG), which has been in force since 2020, already provides a legal framework to ensure the testing of health apps for effectiveness, data security, and data protection (Bundeministerium für Gesundheit 2019). Nevertheless, both developers and users continue to face considerable problems implementing data protection-compliant designs for digital health applications (Iyamu et al. 2022).

4 Conclusion

Digital transformation implies the integration of digital technology into every area of life. The effects of digital technologies as determinants of health are essential to consider, and their influence on other determinants is crucial to address. We must ensure that this fundamental change in all fields is healthy, sustainable and can reduce inequalities instead of becoming another reason people are left behind.

Therefore, generating evidence is key. In summary, approaches to evidence generation in DiPH are highly complex and require an interdisciplinary approach to meet the demands and challenges presented. Due to the dynamic nature of digitalization, DiPH interventions are constantly changing and should be regularly evaluated for relevance and timeliness.

Even though there are various approaches to producing evidence and similarities to evidence-generation methodology in public health, a structural framework outlining the requirements for evidence-based DiPH is missing. Such a framework is necessary to conceptualize, implement, and evaluate the aspects of continuously changing DiPH interventions. It further enables the thorough consideration of socially relevant elements. It will therefore be crucial to build partnerships in DiPH and implementation research with potential users so that together, we can ensure we develop evidence-based DiPH innovations, programs, and policies that value all voices in society and promote health and well-being. In other words, we need digital technologies that effectively address the needs of healthcare while also addressing the underlying factors that affect health.

There can be no evidence-based DiPH without policies accelerating education and raising awareness among health professionals and policymakers. Training programs must include updates on evidence-based technologies in public health. More generally, they must build digital skills for health professionals by equipping them with the necessary capabilities to provide evidence-based, more patient-focused care.

References

Balcombe L, de Leo D (2022) Evaluation of the use of digital mental health platforms and interventions: scoping review. Int J Environ Res Public Health 20(1):362. https://doi.org/10.3390/ijerph20010362

Baran M, Lehrer N, Duff M, Venkataraman V, Turaga P, Ingalls T et al (2015) Interdisciplinary concepts for design and implementation of mixed reality interactive neurorehabilitation systems for stroke. Phys Ther 95(3):449–460. https://doi.org/10.2522/ptj.20130581

Bennet K, Mageras N (2021) Digital health evidence generation strategy. https://www.iqvia.com/-/media/iqvia/pdfs/uk/fact-sheets/digital-health-evidence-generation-strategy-dig-ltr.pdf. Accessed 15 Feb 2023

Blackmore R, Boyle JA, Gray KM, Willey S, Highet N, Gibson-Helm M (2022) Introducing and integrating perinatal mental health screening: development of an equity-informed evidence-based approach. Health Expect 25(5):2287–2298. https://doi.org/10.1111/hex.13526

Brandes M, Muellmann S, Allweiss T, Bauer U, Bethmann A, Forberger S et al (2021) Evidenzbasierung in Primärprävention und Gesundheitsförderung: Methoden und Vorgehensweisen in 5 Forschungsverbünden. Bundesgesundheitsblatt Gesundheitsforschung Gesundheitsschutz 64(5):581–589. https://doi.org/10.1007/s00103-021-03322-z

Brownson RC, Gurney JG, Land GH (1999) Evidence-based decision making in public health. J Public Health Manag Pract 5(5):86–97. https://doi.org/10.1097/00124784-199909000-00012

Brownson RC, Fielding JE, Maylahn CM (2009) Evidence-based public health: a fundamental concept for public health practice. Annu Rev Public Health 30:175–201. https://doi.org/10.1146/annurev.publhealth.031308.100134

Buman MP, Winter SJ, Sheats JL, Hekler EB, Otten JJ, Grieco LA, King AC (2013) The Stanford healthy neighborhood discovery tool: a computerized tool to assess active living environments. Am J Prev Med 44(4):e41–e47. https://doi.org/10.1016/j.amepre.2012.11.028

Bundeministerium für Gesundheit (2019) Ärzte sollen Apps verschreiben können: Gesetz für eine bessere Versorgung durch Digitalisierung und Innovation. https://www.bundesgesundheitsministerium.de/digitale-versorgung-gesetz.html. Accessed 15 Jan 2023

Butscher S, Hubenschmid S, Müller J, Fuchs J, Reiterer H (2018) Clusters, trends, and outliers. In: Mandryk R, Hancock M, Perry M, Cox A (eds) CHI'18: CHI conference on human factors in computing systems; Montreal QC Canada, 21-26 April 2018. ACM, New York, pp 1–12. https://doi.org/10.1145/3173574.3173664

Cornejo Müller A, Wachtler B, Lampert T (2020) Digital Divide – Soziale Unterschiede in der Nutzung digitaler Gesundheitsangebote. Bundesgesundheitsblatt Gesundheitsforschung Gesundheitsschutz 63(2):185–191. https://doi.org/10.1007/s00103-019-03081-y

De Bock F, Dietrich M, Rehfuess E (2020) Evidenzbasierte Prävention und Gesundheitsförderung. Memorandum der Bundeszentrale für gesundheitliche Aufklärung. https://www.bzga.de/fileadmin/user_upload/Studien/PDF/BZgA_Memorandum_Evidenzbasierung.pdf. Accessed 15 Feb 2023

de Farias FAC, Dagostini CM, Bicca YA, Falavigna VF, Falavigna A (2020) Remote patient monitoring: a systematic review. Telemed J E Health 26(5):576–583. https://doi.org/10.1089/tmj.2019.0066

Dockweiler C, Hochmuth A (2019) Digital, gesund und sozial? Zusammenhänge und Einflussfaktoren sozialer, gesundheitlicher und digitaler Ungleichheit in der Bevölkerung. Das Gesundheitswesen 81(8):672–673. https://doi.org/10.1055/s-0039-1694381

El Benny M, Kabakian-Khasholian T, El-Jardali F, Bardus M (2021) Application of the eHealth literacy model in digital health interventions: scoping review. J Med Internet Res 23(6):e23473. https://doi.org/10.2196/23473

Fernandez-Luque L, Kushniruk AW, Georgiou A, Basu A, Petersen C, Ronquillo C et al (2020) Evidence-based health informatics as the foundation for the COVID-19 response: a joint call for action. Methods Inf Med 59(6):183–192. https://doi.org/10.1055/s-0041-1726414

Fischer, F, Dockweiler, C (2019) ePublic Health: Einführung in ein neues Forschungs-und Anwendungsfeld. Hogrefe AG

Fischer F (2020) Digitale Interventionen in Prävention und Gesundheitsförderung: Welche Form der Evidenz haben wir und welche wird benötigt? Bundesgesundheitsblatt Gesundheitsforschung Gesundheitsschutz 63(6):674–680. https://doi.org/10.1007/s00103-020-03143-6

Fleming GA, Petrie JR, Bergenstal RM, Holl RW, Peters AL, Heinemann L (2020) Diabetes digital app technology: benefits, challenges, and recommendations. A consensus report by the European Association for the Study of Diabetes (EASD) and the American Diabetes Association (ADA) Diabetes Technology Working Group. Diabetes Care 43(1):250–260. https://doi.org/10.2337/dci19-0062

Gerhardus A, Breckenkamp J, Razum O (2008) Evidence-based Public Health. Prävention und Gesundheitsförderung im Kontext von Wissenschaft, Werten und Interessen. Med Klin (Munich) 103(6):406–412. https://doi.org/10.1007/s00063-008-1060-9

Gerli P, Arakpogun EO, Elsahn Z, Olan F, Prime KS (2021) Beyond contact-tracing: the public value of eHealth application in a pandemic. Gov Inf Q 38(3):101581. https://doi.org/10.1016/j.giq.2021.101581

Guo C, Ashrafian H, Ghafur S, Fontana G, Gardner C, Prime M (2020) Challenges for the evaluation of digital health solutions—a call for innovative evidence generation approaches. NPJ Digit Med 3:110. https://doi.org/10.1038/s41746-020-00314-2

Guyatt GH, Oxman AD, Vist GE, Kunz R, Falck-Ytter Y, Alonso-Coello P, Schünemann HJ (2008) GRADE: an emerging consensus on rating quality of evidence and strength of recommendations. BMJ 336(7650):924–926. https://doi.org/10.1136/bmj.39489.470347.AD

Herman C, Eisenberg Y, Vanderbom K, Tempio D, Gardner J, Rimmer J (2023) Feasibility of implementing disability inclusive evidence-based health promotion. J Public Health Manag Pract 29(1):82–92. https://doi.org/10.1097/PHH.0000000000001671

Hochmuth A, Exner A-K, Dockweiler C (2020) Implementierung und partizipative Gestaltung digitaler Gesundheitsinterventionen. Bundesgesundheitsblatt Gesundheitsforschung Gesundheitsschutz 63(2):145–152. https://doi.org/10.1007/s00103-019-03079-6

Hughes B, Kessler M, McDonell A (2016) Breaking new ground with RWE. https://www.iqvia.com/-/media/quintilesims/pdfs/qims_breaking_new_ground_with_rwe_whitepaper.pdf. Accessed 21 Feb 2023

Iyamu I, Gómez-Ramírez O, Xu AX, Chang H-J, Watt S, Mckee G, Gilbert M (2022) Challenges in the development of digital public health interventions and mapped solutions: findings from a scoping review. Digit Health 8:20552076221102255. https://doi.org/10.1177/20552076221102255

Jahnel T, Schüz B (2020) Partizipative Entwicklung von Digital-Public-Health-Anwendungen: Spannungsfeld zwischen Nutzer*innenperspektive und Evidenzbasierung. Bundesgesundheitsblatt Gesundheitsforschung Gesundheitsschutz 63(2):153–159. https://doi.org/10.1007/s00103-019-03082-x

Kahn LE, Lum PS, Rymer WZ, Reinkensmeyer DJ (2006) Robot-assisted movement training for the stroke-impaired arm: does it matter what the robot does? J Rehabil Res Dev 43(5):619–630. https://doi.org/10.1682/JRRD.2005.03.0056

Karpathakis K, Libow G, Potts HWW, Dixon S, Greaves F, Murray E (2021) An evaluation service for digital public health interventions: user-centered design approach. J Med Internet Res 23(9):e28356. https://doi.org/10.2196/28356

Khosla S, Tepie MF, Nagy MJ, Kafatos G, Seewald M, Marchese S, Liwing J (2021) The alignment of real-world evidence and digital health: realising the opportunity. Ther Innov Regul Sci 55(4):889–898. https://doi.org/10.1007/s43441-021-00288-7

Kramer U, Borges U, Fischer F, Hoffmann W, Pobiruchin M, Vollmar HC (2019) DNVF-Memorandum – Gesundheits- und Medizin-Apps (GuMAs). Gesundheitswesen 81(10):e154–e170. https://doi.org/10.1055/s-0038-1667451

Ledel Solem IK, Varsi C, Eide H, Kristjansdottir OB, Børøsund E, Schreurs KMG et al (2020) A user-centered approach to an evidence-based electronic health pain management intervention for people with chronic pain: design and development of EPIO. J Med Internet Res 22(1):e15889. https://doi.org/10.2196/15889

Levin MF, Weiss PL, Keshner EA (2015) Emergence of virtual reality as a tool for upper limb rehabilitation: incorporation of motor control and motor learning principles. Phys Ther 95(3):415–425. https://doi.org/10.2522/ptj.20130579

Lomas J, Culyer T, Mccutcheon C, Mcauley L, Law S (2005) Conceptualizing and combining evidence for health system guidance. https://savoir-sante.ca/en/content_page/download/116/222/21?method=view. Accessed 15 Feb 2023

Magalhães T, Dinis-Oliveira RJ, Taveira-Gomes T (2022) Digital health and big data analytics: implications of real-world evidence for clinicians and policymakers. Int J Environ Res Public Health 19(14):8364. https://doi.org/10.3390/ijerph19148364

Malvey D, Slovensky DJ (2014) Research evidence and other information sources. In: Malvey D, Slovensky DJ (eds) mHealth. Springer US, Boston, pp 169–185. https://doi.org/10.1007/978-1-4899-7457-0_8

Meyer I (2021) Die Nutzbarmachung von Daten für Public Health und Gesundheitsversorgung – ein gemeinsames Ziel der EU-Mitgliedsstaaten. Bundesgesundheitsbl 64(5):610–615. https://doi.org/10.1007/s00103-021-03317-w

Moutselos K, Maglogiannis I (2020) Evidence-based public health policy models development and evaluation using big data analytics and web technologies. Med Arch 74(1):47–53. https://doi.org/10.5455/medarh.2020.74.47-53

National Institute for Health and Care Excellence (2019) Evidence standards framework for digital health technologies. https://www.nice.org.uk/corporate/ecd7/resources/evidence-standards-framework-for-digital-health-technologies-pdf-1124017457605. Accessed 17 Feb 2023

Peek N, Sujan M, Scott P (2020) Digital health and care in pandemic times: impact of COVID-19. BMJ Health Care Inform 27(1):e100166. https://doi.org/10.1136/bmjhci-2020-100166

Peyroteo M, Ferreira IA, Elvas LB, Ferreira JC, Lapão LV (2021) Remote monitoring systems for patients with chronic diseases in primary health care: systematic review. JMIR mHealth uHealth 9(12):e28285. https://doi.org/10.2196/28285

Pilgrim K, Bohnet-Joschko S (2022) Effectiveness of digital forced-choice nudges for voluntary data donation by health self-trackers in Germany: web-based experiment. J Med Internet Res 24(2):e31363. https://doi.org/10.2196/31363

Popkova EG, Sergi BS (2022) Digital public health: automation based on new datasets and the Internet of Things. Socio Econ Plan Sci 80:101039. https://doi.org/10.1016/j.seps.2021.101039

Proffitt R, Lange B (2015) Considerations in the efficacy and effectiveness of virtual reality interventions for stroke rehabilitation: moving the field forward. Phys Ther 95(3):441–448. https://doi.org/10.2522/ptj.20130571

Rauschenberg C, Schick A, Hirjak D, Seidler A, Paetzold I, Apfelbacher C et al (2021) Evidence synthesis of digital interventions to mitigate the negative impact of the COVID-19 pandemic on public mental health: rapid meta-review. J Med Internet Res 23(3):e23365. https://doi.org/10.2196/23365

Rehfuess EA, Zhelyazkova A, von Philipsborn P, Griebler U, de Bock F (2021) Evidenzbasierte Public Health: Perspektiven und spezifische Umsetzungsfaktoren. Bundesgesundheitsblatt Gesundheitsforschung Gesundheitsschutz 64(5):514–523. https://doi.org/10.1007/s00103-021-03308-x

Rossmann C, Krömer N (2016) mHealth in der medizinischen Versorgung, Prävention und Gesundheitsförderung. In: Fischer F, Krämer A (eds) eHealth in Deutschland. Springer, Berlin, pp 441–456. https://doi.org/10.1007/978-3-662-49504-9_24

Rychetnik L, Bauman A, Laws R, King L, Rissel C, Nutbeam D et al (2012) Translating research for evidence-based public health: key concepts and future directions. J Epidemiol Community Health 66(12):1187–1192. https://doi.org/10.1136/jech-2011-200038

Satterfield JM, Spring B, Brownson RC, Mullen EJ, Newhouse RP, Walker BB, Whitlock EP (2009) Toward a transdisciplinary model of evidence-based practice. Milbank Q 87(2):368–390. https://doi.org/10.1111/j.1468-0009.2009.00561.x

Schnell MW (2018) Ethik der digitalen Gesundheitskommunikation. In: Pundt J, Scherenberg V (eds) Digitale Gesundheitskommunikation: Zwischen Meinungsbildung und Manipulation. APOLLON University Press, pp 277–292

Sheehan R, Hassiotis A (2017) Digital mental health and intellectual disabilities: state of the evidence and future directions. Evid Based Ment Health 20(4):107–111. https://doi.org/10.1136/eb-2017-102759

Stark AL, Geukes C, Dockweiler C (2022) Digital health promotion and prevention in settings: scoping review. J Med Internet Res 24(1):e21063. https://doi.org/10.2196/21063

Stern AD, Brönneke J, Debatin JF, Hagen J, Matthies H, Patel S et al (2022) Advancing digital health applications: priorities for innovation in real-world evidence generation. Lancet Digit Health 4(3):e200–e206. https://doi.org/10.1016/S2589-7500(21)00292-2

US Food and Drug Administration (2023) Real-world evidence. https://www.fda.gov/science-research/science-and-research-special-topics/real-world-evidence. Accessed 15 Feb 2023

Vajawat B, Varshney P, Banerjee D (2021) Digital gaming interventions in psychiatry: evidence, applications and challenges. Psychiatry Res 295:113585. https://doi.org/10.1016/j.psychres.2020.113585

van Kessel R, Hrzic R, O'Nuallain E, Weir E, Wong BLH, Anderson M et al (2022) Digital health paradox: international policy perspectives to address increased health inequalities for people living with disabilities. J Med Internet Res 24(2):e33819. https://doi.org/10.2196/33819

Von Philipsborn P, Rehfuess E (2021) Evidenzbasierte Public Health. In: Schmidt-Semisch H, Schorb F (eds) Public health. Springer Fachmedien Wiesbaden, Wiesbaden, pp 303–329. https://doi.org/10.1007/978-3-658-30377-8_17

White RW, Horvitz E (2009) Cyberchondria. ACM Trans Inf Syst 27(4):1–37. https://doi.org/10.1145/1629096.1629101

Wienert J, Zeeb H (2021) Implementing health apps for digital public health—an implementation science approach adopting the consolidated framework for implementation research. Front Public Health 9:610237. https://doi.org/10.3389/fpubh.2021.610237

Wienert J, Jahnel T, Maaß L (2022) What are digital public health interventions? First steps toward a definition and an intervention classification framework. J Med Internet Res 24(6):e31921. https://doi.org/10.2196/31921

Wong ZS-Y, Rigby M (2022) Identifying and addressing digital health risks associated with emergency pandemic response: problem identification, scoping review, and directions toward evidence-based evaluation. Int J Med Inform 157:104639. https://doi.org/10.1016/j.ijmedinf.2021.104639

World Health Organization (2016) Monitoring and evaluating digital health interventions: a practical guide to conducting research and assessment. World Health Organization, Geneva. Licence: CC BY-NC-SA 3.0 IGO. https://apps.who.int/iris/bitstream/handle/10665/252183/?sequence=1. Accessed 15 Jan 2023

Zeeb H, Pigeot I, Schüz B (2020) Digital Public Health – ein Überblick. Bundesgesundheitsblatt Gesundheitsforschung Gesundheitsschutz 63(2):137–144. https://doi.org/10.1007/s00103-019-03078-7

Open Access This chapter is licensed under the terms of the Creative Commons Attribution 4.0 International License (http://creativecommons.org/licenses/by/4.0/), which permits use, sharing, adaptation, distribution and reproduction in any medium or format, as long as you give appropriate credit to the original author(s) and the source, provide a link to the Creative Commons license and indicate if changes were made.

The images or other third party material in this chapter are included in the chapter's Creative Commons license, unless indicated otherwise in a credit line to the material. If material is not included in the chapter's Creative Commons license and your intended use is not permitted by statutory regulation or exceeds the permitted use, you will need to obtain permission directly from the copyright holder.

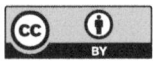

Digital Interventions for Public Health: A Systematic Planning Approach

J. Bruinsma and R. Crutzen

Abstract This chapter outlines the Intervention Mapping (IM) approach, a planning framework for the systematic development, implementation, and evaluation of health promotion interventions. IM is a comprehensive approach to intervention development in general. This chapter describes the six steps of IM and emphasizes using it for digitally supported interventions within the context of public health specifically. The chapter starts by describing Core Processes, a systematic way of answering planning questions to safeguard the use of available evidence and insights from theory. Subsequently, this chapter zooms in on understanding behavior as this is key during the development of health-promoting interventions that aim to establish behavior change. Successively, the steps of IM are discussed separately and illustrated by examples of interventions that use digital technology in the context of public health. This chapter guides readers through the six IM steps and hopes to inspire them to learn more about IM and behavior change principles and their use for digital interventions.

Keywords Intervention development · Behavior change · Digital interventions

1 Introduction

This chapter is about planning health promotion interventions in a systematic way by means of the Intervention Mapping (IM) approach. Intervention Mapping is a versatile planning framework used for intervention development and anticipates implementation and evaluation during the development process (Bartholomew Eldredge et al. 2016; Kok et al. 2016). It can be applied in a wide variety of contexts and settings to address health and societal problems on both individual and population levels (Garba and Gadanya 2017). For instance, the IM approach has been used

---

J. Bruinsma (✉) · R. Crutzen
Department of Health Promotion of the Care and Public Health Research Institute, Maastricht University, Maastricht, The Netherlands
e-mail: jeroen.bruinsma@maastrichtuniversity.nl; rik.crutzen@maastrichtuniversity.nl

to address many different specific public health problems (Bartholomew Eldredge et al. 2016; Garba and Gadanya 2017) but also to increase employability in low-skilled jobs (Hazelzet et al. 2022) or to tackle stigma (Stutterheim et al. 2025). By following a stepwise approach, IM provides a blueprint to achieve outcomes by incorporating behavior change methods into intervention materials. In this regard, digital technologies offer opportunities in terms of the delivery of the intervention materials and allow for innovative ways to embed behavior change methods in the materials. In this chapter, particular emphasis is placed on using IM to leverage these digital aspects to enhance interventions that promote public health.

IM is a problem-driven approach because it aims to address real-world health challenges by embedding procedures that allow it to work in an evidence-based manner (Bartholomew Eldredge et al. 2016; Ruiter and Crutzen 2020). In other words, the point of departure is a specific (public health) problem that is addressed by answering planning questions. Therefore, this chapter starts by discussing Core Processes—a helpful and systematic way to answer planning questions within the six steps of IM (Fig. 1) (Ruiter and Crutzen 2020). Subsequently, this chapter zooms in on understanding behavior as this is key during the development of health-promoting interventions (i.e., steps 1–4). Specifically, IM focuses on improving health outcomes by encouraging actions that are beneficial for health. To achieve this, it is essential to change the behavior of the priority population as well as the behavior of individuals who have control over the environment (so-called environmental agents) where actions that promote health take place. Successively, the steps of IM are discussed separately and illustrated by examples of interventions that use digital technology in the context of public health.

Planning interventions is complex, and IM is not the only framework available. It is, however, the most comprehensive as it guides health promoters through the complexity of developing, implementing, and evaluating interventions (O'Cathain et al. 2019). Although the use of IM is no magic bullet, it maximizes the likelihood

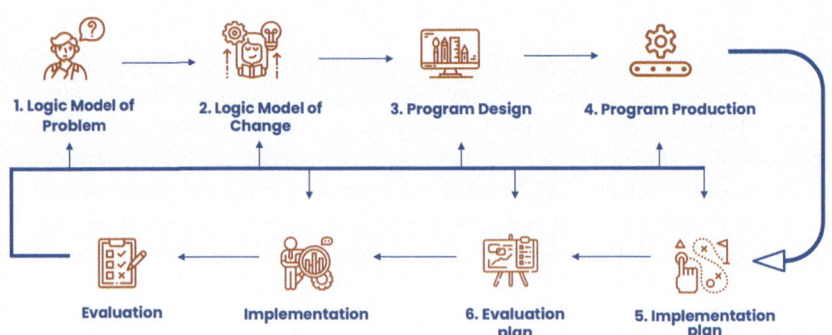

Fig. 1 An overview of Intervention Mapping has been created by Dr. I. Moafa. (Source: based on Moafa 2022, Freepik Licensee: moafaalaa; the icons used in this figure are made by Eucalyp, Freepik, ultimatearm and xnimrodx, all from www.flaticon.com)

of developing an effective intervention. We hope this chapter is a stepping stone that inspires the reader to learn more about this approach.

In short, this chapter is a high-speed training about the systematic planning that is part and parcel of health promotion. Since this book already incorporates detailed sections about co-creation (see "Participatory approaches for digital public health—giving voice to values" chapter, Shrestha et al. in this handbook) and intervention evaluation (see "Evaluation of Digital Public Health Interventions" chapter, Lange et al. in this handbook), these topics are relatively shortly addressed in this chapter despite being a fundamental part of IM.

2 Core Processes

In each step of IM, there are multiple planning questions that need to be answered, and based on these answers, specific decisions need to be made regarding the intervention at hand (Bartholomew Eldredge et al. 2016). The use of Core Processes ensures that these decisions make use of available evidence and insights from theory (Ruiter and Crutzen 2020). In a nutshell, Core Processes guide intervention developers through the process of posing questions, brainstorming, reviewing earlier research, using theory, and—if needed—conducting new research to bridge knowledge gaps. Applying this in a structured manner is useful throughout all IM steps (i.e., from the needs assessment to the evaluation plan). Core Processes have a fixed order. Sticking to this order guarantees that the knowledge available to answer planning questions is optimally used and that new research is both relevant and informative.

2.1 Posing Questions

Each IM step provides planning questions that need to be answered. In step 1, questions revolve around the health problem (i.e., "What is the health problem?", "Who are involved?", and "What aspects of the environment contribute to the problem?"). The digital environment can be an essential part of assessing needs because it has an increasing influence on many health behaviors. In step 2, questions are about the intended outcomes (i.e., "What behavior change is desired?" or "What needs to change in the environment?"), whereas step 3 narrows down on behavior changes (i.e., "What methods can be used to reach the outcomes?" and "How can these methods be delivered?"). In step 4, the questions are focused on the intervention plan and its requirements (i.e., "How long will the intervention last?", "What materials are needed?", and "How do we ensure these materials meet the needs of the priority population?"). Digital technology can provide novel opportunities to reach the intended outcomes. For example, a web-based triage tool can reduce the telephone load in hospital emergency rooms by providing valid health information about if and when patients have to call or whether they can call their general practitioner during office hours.

2.2 Brainstorming Provisional Answers

Answering the questions starts with brainstorming about answers. Essential is that a planning group (i.e., a group of important stakeholders identified in step 1; see Sect. 4.1.1) take part in brainstorming about the questions. This allows them to use their knowledge, experience, and wisdom to formulate provisional answers. Brainstorming is a creative process geared toward generating as many ideas as possible. Ideas that are poorly supported can later be disregarded.

2.3 Reviewing Published Research

Systematically reviewing existing research findings helps ensure that the provisional answers are supported by evidence. This allows those involved in planning to learn from previous research and prevents re-inventing the wheel.

2.4 Using Theory

Theories are useful to thoroughly understand a problem and identify potential solutions. A wide variety of theories are helpful throughout the different steps of IM. For example, theories on quality of life (step 1), behavior change (step 2), communication (step 3), information processing (step 4), or planning the implementation (step 5). We want to reiterate that Core Processes should be followed in this order. For example, it is unwise to use general theories aimed at explaining behavior if there is ample evidence available on determinants regarding the specific behavior of interest. A useful theory to understand technology-related behavior is, for example, the extended Unified Theory of Acceptance and Use of Technology (UTAUT-2) (Tamilmani et al. 2021). That being said, looking at available evidence regarding determinants to use a specific technology first is warranted.

2.5 Conducting New Research

Knowledge gaps might be identified after reviewing existing research and applying theory to answer the planning questions. Then, new research may be needed to bridge this gap. The previous Core Processes help identify specific gaps in currently available evidence and theories.

2.6 Compose a Working List of Answers

After all these tasks, the planning group is ready to summarize and complete the provisional list of answers into a working list for which the theoretical and empirical evidence is evaluated as sufficient.

3 Understanding Behavior (Change)

Health promotion includes intervening on various environmental levels because individuals are part of multiple environments (i.e., interpersonal, organizational, cultural, and political) that have an impact on their behavior (World Health Organization 1986). This also includes the digital space, for example, the availability of misinformation about vaccines or the digital infrastructure available to support remote healthcare services. These examples illustrate that environmental conditions often fall beyond the personal influence of the members of the priority population and are affected by other individuals (i.e., environmental agents such as managers or policymakers). Changing the environment, therefore, requires changing the behavior of these agents. Regardless of whether it concerns the behavior of members of the priority population or agents in their environment, changing their behavior is a complex, multifaceted process that starts with an adequate understanding of the behavior that needs to be changed (Hilliard et al. 2018).

3.1 Understanding Behavior Is Easier Said Than Done

Understanding behavior is crucial to plan intervention activities that aim to change behavior. This is complex because behavior can be reasoned or unreasoned, rational or irrational, or mixtures of both (Strack and Deutsch 2004). Theories provide instrumental frameworks that contain determinants (i.e., key factors) to explain or change behavior.

Most theories consider intention, an individual's conscious plan to perform a behavior, as the strongest predictor of reasoned behavior (Fishbein and Ajzen 2011). In turn, intention is influenced by other determinants of behavior. The following example illustrates this process by describing the determinants of smartphone use while driving a car (Eren and Gauld 2022). This is a pressing public health issue because smartphone use distracts drivers and increases their risk of causing car accidents. This negatively affects overall road safety and poses risks for other drivers or pedestrians.

3.2 Using a Smartphone Behind the Wheel

The Reasoned Action Approach (Fishbein and Ajzen 2011) is a commonly used theory in health promotion. It considers that the intention to perform a behavior is influenced by three key determinants:

- Attitudes (i.e., a latent disposition or tendency to respond with some degree of favorableness or unfavorableness to a behavior)
- Perceived norms (i.e., the perceived social pressure to perform (or not perform) a behavior)
- Perceived behavioral control (i.e., the perceived degree of being capable of, or having control over, performing a behavior)

Eren and Gauld (2022) used these and other constructs to understand why adolescents use smartphones while driving in a car. They demonstrated that adolescents have stronger intentions towards using a smartphone if they are positive about it (attitude), feel others approve (perceived norm), and are confident about using a phone behind the wheel (perceived behavioral control). Understanding these determinants provides valuable insights that help design public health messages that aim to discourage smartphone use while driving. Of course, the findings of Eren and Gauld (2022) do not rule out that this smartphone use while driving is fully reasoned behavior—it might be partly unreasoned. Therefore, insights from multiple theories are often needed to understand public health problem.

3.3 Determinants from Multiple Theories and Models

The provided example is intentionally simplified because its purpose is to explain how determinants influence intentions and behavior. The reality is often more complex. Therefore, in a problem-driven context, it is necessary to combine determinants and insights from multiple theories to get a comprehensive understanding of a specific behavior (Peters and Crutzen 2017). Some theories emphasize understanding behavior, whereas others provide directions to change health behavior. An illustration of the latter is the Health Belief Model, which suggests individuals are likely to change if they (a) perceive themselves as susceptible to a threat and believe the threat has severe consequences, (b) perceive more benefits than barriers, and (c) are exposed to cues to initiate action (Bartholomew Eldredge et al. 2016). Although these theories are useful, additional determinant research is often needed to identify and select the most relevant determinants for specific behaviors in a specific priority population. Furthermore, it has been demonstrated that intuitively selecting determinants of behavior is nearly impossible, even for behavior change experts (Crutzen and Peters 2023).

Interesting Fact

PsyCore (www.psycore.one) is a repository containing construct definitions and qualitative and quantitative measurement instructions that are useful for research on behavior change, especially determinant studies (Peters and Crutzen 2024).

4 Intervention Mapping Steps

This section describes the IM steps. The emphasis is on the development phase (i.e., steps 1–4); therefore, in these steps, examples of public health interventions that use digital technology are provided, followed by a brief description of steps 5 and 6.

4.1 Step 1: A Logic Model of the Problem

The first step of IM involves a series of tasks that help to conduct a needs assessment of the health problem and to define the priority population. It is crucial to first understand the problem and what causes it before even thinking about what needs to change (step 2) and how to accommodate change (step 3).

4.1.1 Establish a Planning Group

The first task in step 1 is to compose a planning group that brings together important individuals with expertise, such as practitioners, policymakers, researchers, and members of the priority population. They are involved in all phases to collaboratively plan and co-create the intervention. This ensures that the intervention meets the needs of different stakeholders and maximizes the likelihood of developing something practical that relevant parties also use.

4.1.2 Conduct a Needs Assessment

A needs assessment is required to map factors contributing to the health problem. In this process, the PRECEDE Model (Green and Kreuter 2005) can be a useful framework because it helps to systematically organize the problem in a Logic Model (Bartholomew Eldredge et al. 2016). A Logic Model outlines the health problem, related behaviors and environmental conditions, and relevant determinants of those.

4.1.3 Define the Context

Defining the context of the intervention requires careful exploration of assets (i.e., opportunities that increase the potential effect and ensure adequate implementation). Examples of assets are persons (within specific organizations) that support the intervention, communication channels that allow for dissemination, or organizations that benefit the implementation.

4.1.4 State the Intervention Goal

Throughout the first IM step, new insights are constantly generated about the health problem and its causes. These findings have implications for the aim of the intervention and must be incorporated into the goal of the intervention.

> **An Example of Public Involvement Through an Advisory Board: The LETHE Project**
>
> Accumulating evidence demonstrates that modifiable factors risk factors contribute to the future risk for cognitive decline and dementia (Livingston et al. 2020; Jia et al. 2023). The LETHE project develops a comprehensive data collection platform and analysis system that allows individualized risk prediction and preventive lifestyle intervention for cognitive decline (Hanke et al. 2022; Rosenberg et al. 2024). The digital intervention is based on the successful FINGER protocol (Ngandu et al. 2015) and includes a smartphone application and smartwatch that encourage seniors to adopt positive lifestyle changes. For example, the app includes healthy habits that seniors can try, allows them to self-monitor physical activity and diet patterns, and offers brain training exercises.
>
> To develop the intervention, LETHE consists of a large European consortium that brings together various public and private organizations, including clinicians, researchers, and experts on information and communication technology. At the beginning of the project, an Advisory Board was set up, composing seven seniors living in Austria, Italy, Finland, and Sweden. Members of the Advisory Board are part of the priority population and include persons interested in the topic, at risk for developing dementia, or with mild dementia. They meet regularly with the project team and help to shape and inform the digital technology and research. Examples of the topics addressed during Advisory Board meetings are related to the use of technology by older persons, ethical issues, the protocol, materials for participants, and the recruitment strategy. To illustrate, the Advisory Board aided in designing a sub-study to explore usability aspects of additional interactive technology, including a robot and smart glasses. Specifically, they supported the decisional process in choosing what app functionalities could be delivered via the robot and smart glasses, and they critically revised a user manual to support participants while using these technologies. Their feedback helped the project team understand and anticipate the priority population's perspectives, preferences, and concerns.

4.2 Step 2: Outcomes and Objectives

In step 2 of IM, the focus shifts from the problem, and related behaviors and environmental conditions, toward the desired intervention outcomes.

4.2.1 State Expected Outcomes

Outcomes are formulated in terms of behaviors that reduce risk, promote health, or boost adherence of the priority population. Outcomes are also specified for agents at the relevant environmental levels (i.e., interpersonal, organizational, cultural, and political).

4.2.2 Specify Performance Objectives

The next step is to specify performance objectives for each outcome. Performance objectives define what sub-behaviors are needed to achieve the expected outcome.

4.2.3 Select Determinants

Subsequently, relevant behavioral determinants are selected to motivate individuals to achieve the performance objectives. It is vital to review existing research or conduct behavioral determinant research to identify important and changeable determinants.

4.2.4 Specify Change Objectives

The next task is to formulate the change objectives. In essence, change objectives state what aspects of the selected determinants need to change to achieve the performance objectives and thus reach the outcome.

Interesting Fact

Acyclic Behavior Change Diagrams (ABCDs) visually represent the assumptions regarding causal-structural chains that underlie putative active ingredients of behavior change interventions (Metz et al. 2022). Metz et al. (2023) illustrate how ABCDs can be used to investigate the intended use of a web-based sexual health intervention. A free web application to create ABCDs is available at: https://a-bc.eu/apps/abcd.

4.2.5 A Logic Model of Change

The Logic Model in step 1 contains a pathway of the problem. In step 2, a Logic Model of Change outlines the intended outcomes (at the level of health, related behaviors and environmental conditions, and determinants of those) after the intervention.

> **An Example to Illustrate Change Objectives: The SELFBACK app**
>
> Low Back Pain (LBP) is a major cause of disability and negatively impacts the quality of life. Every week, the SELFBACK app encourages its users to formulate self-management plans for physical activity training (Svendsen et al. 2022). Before the SELFBACK app was developed, the intervention outcomes were formulated in close collaboration with a planning group of physiotherapists, chiropractors, physicians, exercise physiologists, behavioral scientists, computer scientists, and app designers. Successively, for the outcomes, specific performance objectives were defined by departing from existing literature reviews and position papers and by exploring earlier intervention research. Table 1 exemplifies two performance objectives, their behavioral determinants, and specified change objectives as formulated by Svendsen et al. (2022). Subsequently, these objectives were linked to behavior change methods (in step 3) and translated into smartphone features (in step 4), such as functionalities to self-monitor steps, keep track of daily goals, do daily exercise activities, and read educational content. Additionally, an app feature was included to offer tips on managing back pain, such as relaxation techniques to alleviate stress.
>
> **Table 1** Matrix of change objectives (Svendsen et al. 2022)
>
> | **Behavioral outcome 1**: To increase the use of evidence-based self-management strategies | | | | | |
> |---|---|---|---|---|---|
> | Performance objectives | *Change objectives per personal determinant* | | | | |
> | | Knowledge | Skills | Fear-avoidance | Self-efficacy | Outcome expectations |
> | Make the decision to be physically active | Explain positive effects of physical activity on LBP | x | Recognize fearful thoughts and negative thinking in relation to physical activity | Express confidence in the ability to be physically active | Expect that physical activity will ease living with LBP |
> | Perform physical activities | List where and when physical activities can be performed | Demonstrate the ability to perform physical activities | Acknowledge that performing physical activities might result in a temporary increase in LBP | Express confidence in the ability to perform physical activities | Expect that performing physical activities will lead to a better, healthier life |
>
> Note. LBP = Low Back Pain

4.3 Step 3: Intervention Design

Where step 2 focuses on what to change, step 3 focuses on how to change it.

4.3.1 Generate Intervention Ideas, Components, Scope, and Sequence

Coming up with a suitable intervention idea is challenging. Involving the priority population can greatly help, for example, by brainstorming with the planning group members or organizing focus group discussions with the priority population. The involvement of the priority population also enhances the decisional process around the delivery of the intervention and its behavior change methods. For example, whether an intervention is delivered in an analog way, digitally, or a combination of both (i.e., blended).

4.3.2 Select Change Methods

Using appropriate behavior change methods will increase the likelihood that change in behavioral determinants is accomplished (Bartholomew Eldredge et al. 2016). Therefore, change methods are linked to the specified change objectives concerning a specific determinant. To illustrate, other behavior change methods are needed to change feelings of risk perception when aiming to enhance feelings of self-efficacy. Generally, it is accepted that behavior change methods can be used to address multiple change objectives across the specified performance objectives.

4.3.3 Account for Parameters of Use

When selecting behavior change methods, it is crucial to account for the parameters of use (i.e., conditions that determine if the method is effective or not). An often-used behavior change method to elicit risk perception is a fear appeal (e.g., health warnings on cigarette packages). Empirical evidence clearly shows that eliciting feelings of threat only works if individuals experience sufficient levels of self-efficacy to cope with the threat (Peters et al. 2013). Therefore, using fear appeals needs to be combined with a method that increases feelings of self-efficacy—otherwise, it might backfire.

4.3.4 Select and Design Appropriate Applications for Delivery

Once a set of behavior change methods has been selected, the next task involves determining the appropriate delivery methods for each one. In a sense, these practical applications are the vehicle to get the intervention messages (and its behavior change methods) across to the priority population and the environmental agents.

Digital technologies offer methods to deliver these change methods and account for use parameters, for example, via feedback notifications on a smartphone that are directly liked to lifestyle goals or by encouraging self-monitoring of steps and food intake. Consulting with the priority population can support selecting appropriate delivery applications for these efforts. To illustrate, the wide variety of digital delivery methods could range from webinar presentations to digital newsletters, infographics, app functionalities, websites, e-learnings, videos, or gamification elements.

Interesting Fact

Kok et al. (2016) developed a coding taxonomy of behavior change methods. In the supplementary materials, tables describe behavior change methods and their parameters for use. Additionally, these behavior change methods are linked to specific determinants of behavior, and examples are provided about their practical application.

An Example of Selecting Change Methods and Applications: Gaming Against Cyberbullying

Cyberbullying peaks in the seventh and eighth grades and has serious psychosocial consequences for victims (Hellfeldt et al. 2019). DeSmet et al. (2016) developed a story-driven game that focused on reducing bystander behavior to reduce cyberbullying.

Throughout step 3 of IM, DeSmet et al. (2016) selected behavior change methods based on extensive literature research and by conducting a meta-analysis on game design methodology (DeSmet et al. 2014). Earlier IM steps in this project revealed that attitudes and outcome expectations (i.e., behavioral determinants) were the strongest predictors of the bullying bystander effect. Therefore, the behavior change methods selected were specifically targeted at these determinants (Table 2).

Table 2 An example of behavior change methods and practical applications (DeSmet et al. 2016)

Performance objectives	Change objectives	Behavior change methods	Practical applications
1. Assess if a message is intended to hurt or is perceived as hurtful	1. Express confidence in recognizing a bully's intentions	Immediate feedback (*i.e., information about performance*) Contingent rewards (*i.e., rewards for behavior*) Modeling (*i.e., a model that shows desired behaviors*)	A serious game (including videos and cooperative learning) that is embedded in an educational curriculum
2. Never join or reinforce the bully	2. Express that assisting or laughing is just as bad as cyberbullying itself		

4.4 Step 4: Intervention Production

In step 4 of IM, the overall structure is defined, and successively the intervention materials are planned, produced, and pre-tested.

4.4.1 Refine Program Structure and Organization

The program structure provides an overview of the intervention organization. It describes the delivery by specifying who does what, when, and how. Additionally, it summarizes a time plan, the sequence, and the delivery of specific intervention components. For example, by outlining how analog and digital intervention components are combined in a blended intervention approach.

4.4.2 Plan to Produce Materials

Intervention materials are what participants see, read, hear, and feel. This includes various materials such as texts, slides, videos, guidelines, protocols, apps, websites, posters, etc. Each intervention material contains one or more behavior change methods and is delivered via a practical application, as specified in step 3. Carefully planning what, who, and when these materials are developed also allows organizers to plan the co-creation of these materials. This is essential to ensure they meet the needs of the priority population. A detailed description of co-creation is provided in "Participatory Approaches for Digital Public Health: Giving Voice to Values" chapter (Shrestha et al.) in this handbook.

4.4.3 Draft Messages, Materials, and Protocols

The intervention materials are developed, preferably following an iterative process of co-creation. This often includes using creative resources (e.g., photographers, web developers). It can be useful to pre-test early prototypes with the priority population and environmental agents, for example, via think-aloud sessions, individual interviews, or focus group interviews.

4.4.4 Pre-test, Refine, and Produce Materials

When drafts of the materials are prepared, it is critical to pre-test them before finalizing the content. A pre-test is a trial with implementers and intended participants before the intervention material is implemented. This helps to determine, for example, if the materials are engaging and understandable. A pre-test also helps to detect errors, bugs, and flaws. There is a wide variety of methods to pre-test, ranging from interviews to discuss materials, questionnaires about them, or running a brief pilot to explore feasibility aspects. It is generally accepted that using a variation of these methods helps to obtain more insight into directions for improvement.

> **An Example of the Production of an App and a Pre-test: the WhiteTeeth App**
>
> Adolescents who have fixed orthodontic appliances (e.g., brackets) have an increased risk of developing caries (Cruz and Edelstein 2016). Scheerman et al. (2018) developed the WhiteTeeth app that promotes oral hygiene among adolescents with orthodontic appliances.
>
> To develop the WhiteTeeth app (Scheerman et al. 2018), an iterative process—including a review, survey, and interviews—guided the selection of behavior change methods and practical applications. In step 4, a wireframe of the intervention was drafted and discussed with adolescents who studied at a university of applied science. Specifically, the students provided feedback on the intervention plan, app functionalities, and interface design. Subsequently, they presented their own directions to improve and optimize the intervention and its digital aspects. Based on this and intense discussion with the planning group, a 1.0 version of the WhiteTeeth app was developed. This version was first tested for bugs, which resulted in an improved 1.1 version that was pilot tested in a study with 28 adults with orthodontic appliances who used the WhiteTeeth app for 2 weeks. Afterward, they completed a survey that covered aspects of acceptability, ease of use, attractiveness, and usefulness of the app. The results were used to refine the app to a 1.2 version that was ready for implementation and future research.

4.5 Step 5: Planning Implementation

The impact of an intervention depends on the effect but also on its reach and implementation with completeness (i.e., whether everything is implemented) and fidelity (i.e., whether it is implemented in the right way) (Fernandez et al. 2019). Therefore, step 5 of IM focuses on planning the implementation. This step can also be used irrespective of the previous IM steps, for example, to scale up an existing intervention or use it in a different context (Bartholomew Eldredge et al. 2016).

4.5.1 Identify Stakeholders

When planning the implementation, the first task is to identify individuals who adopt (i.e., initiate use), implement (i.e., deliver), and maintain (i.e., continue) the intervention. Occasionally, different persons will be responsible for adoption, implementation, and maintenance. For example, managers are responsible for deciding to adopt a digital platform in a hospital setting, while clinicians implement it by using it in their daily work.

4.5.2 State Performance Objectives for Use

Quite similar to step 2 of IM, performance objectives are formulated that eventually lead to the adoption, implementation, and maintenance of the intervention. For example, (a) the manager takes part in an introduction meeting about a telemedicine platform, (b) the manager discusses the use of the platform with the board of directors, and (c) the manager signs an agreement to adopt the telemedicine platform in the hospital.

4.5.3 Design Implementation Interventions

The next task is to specify relevant determinants to achieve the performance objectives, formulate change objectives, and select methods to target these change objectives. Subsequently, the change objectives are translated into practical applications (similar to step 3 of IM) and, ultimately, material and other resources to support implementation (similar to step 4).

4.6 Step 6: Planning Evaluation

Step 6 of IM is about planning the evaluation of the intervention and its implementation. For a more comprehensive description of evaluation methodology see the "Evaluation of Digital Public Health Interventions" chapter, Lange et al. in this handbook.

4.6.1 Writing Evaluation Questions

Generally, the evaluation of interventions includes investigating the effect and the process. Research questions about the evaluation range from evaluating (a) the effect in outcomes and behaviors (IM steps 1 and 2), (b) the change in sub-behaviors and behavioral determinants (IM steps 2 and 3), the use of intervention applications and materials (IM steps 3 and 4), and the implementation and fidelity (IM steps 4 and 5).

4.6.2 Develop Measures and Specify the Design

Based on the research questions, an adequate set of outcome measurements is selected. For example, this can include quantitative scales to assess change in a user's quality of life, behavior and behavioral determinants, qualitative interviews based on acceptability and use of technology (Tamilmani et al. 2021), or the analysis of web statistics to examine the use of online intervention components (Metz et al. 2023).

Typically, evaluation studies are designed to investigate change after the intervention, as compared to before, and by comparing an intervention with a control group to ensure that changes can be attributed to exposure to the intervention.

4.6.3 Finalize the Evaluation Plan

After specifying the research questions, measurement instruments, and study design, the evaluation plan is finalized. It is recommendable to use reporting guidelines to carefully check if all important aspects are covered in the evaluation plan. An example of such a guideline is the CONSORT E-health (Consolidated Standards of Reporting Trials of Electronic and Mobile HEalth Applications and onLine TeleHealth) (Eysenbach and CONSORT-EHEALTH Group et al. 2011).

5 Closing Remarks

This chapter provides a crash course on Intervention Mapping, summarizing each step and its associated tasks. Overall, it provides an excellent beginning for readers interested in learning more about IM and its application in digital public health. By following the steps outlined in IM, intervention developers create a blueprint for their digital intervention, from design to implementation and evaluation. The examples used throughout the chapter showcase that IM is a versatile framework applicable to various health problems, settings, and contexts. Additionally, IM can be used to create new interventions or tailor existing ones for different priority populations and settings, as well as for scaling up interventions. This versatility allows for the applicability of IM in a wide range of projects, making it a valuable tool for intervention developers.

References

Bartholomew Eldredge LK, Markham CM, Ruiter RA, Fernández ME, Kok G, Parcel GS (2016) Planning health promotion programs: an intervention mapping approach, 4th edn. John Wiley & Sons, New York

Crutzen R, Peters GY (2023) A lean method for selecting determinants when developing behavior change interventions. Health Psychol Behav Med 11(1):2167719. https://doi.org/10.1080/21642850.2023.2167719

Cruz CL, Edelstein BL (2016) Linking orthodontic treatment and caries management for high-risk adolescents. Am J Orthod Dentofac Orthop 149(4):441–442. https://doi.org/10.1016/j.ajodo.2015.12.007

DeSmet A, Van Ryckeghem D, Compernolle S, Baranowski T, Thompson D, Crombez G et al (2014) A meta-analysis of serious digital games for healthy lifestyle promotion. Prev Med 69:95–107. https://doi.org/10.1016/j.ypmed.2014.08.026

DeSmet A, Van Cleemput K, Bastiaensens S, Poels K, Vandebosch H, Malliet S et al (2016) Bridging behavior science and gaming theory: using the intervention mapping protocol to design a serious game against cyberbullying. Comput Hum Behav 56:337–351. https://doi.org/10.1016/j.chb.2015.11.039

Eren H, Gauld C (2022) Smartphone use among young drivers: applying an extended theory of planned behaviour to predict young drivers' intention and engagement in concealed responding. Accid Anal Prev 164:106474. https://doi.org/10.1016/j.aap.2021.106474

Eysenbach G, CONSORT-EHEALTH Group (2011) CONSORT-EHEALTH: improving and standardizing evaluation reports of web-based and mobile health interventions. J Med Internet Res 13(4):e126. https://doi.org/10.2196/jmir.1923

Fernandez ME, Ten Hoor GA, van Lieshout S, Rodriguez SA, Beidas RS, Parcel G et al (2019) Implementation mapping: using intervention mapping to develop implementation strategies. Front Public Health 7:158. https://doi.org/10.3389/fpubh.2019.00158

Fishbein M, Ajzen I (2011) Predicting and changing behavior: the reasoned action approach. Taylor & Francis, New York

Garba RM, Gadanya MA (2017) The role of intervention mapping in designing disease prevention interventions: a systematic review of the literature. PLoS One 12(3):e0174438. https://doi.org/10.1371/journal.pone.0174438

Green LW, Kreuter MW (2005) Health promotion planning: an educational and ecological approach, 4th edn. McGraw-Hill Education, New York

Hanke S, Mangialasche F, Bödenler M, Neumayer B, Ngandu T, Mecocci P et al (2022) AI-based predictive modelling of the onset and progression of dementia. Smart Cities 5(2):700–714. https://doi.org/10.3390/smartcities5020036

Hazelzet E, Houkes I, Bosma H, de Rijk A (2022) How a steeper organisational hierarchy prevents change—adoption and implementation of a sustainable employability intervention for employees in low-skilled jobs: a qualitative study. BMC Public Health 22(1):2373. https://doi.org/10.1186/s12889-022-14754-w

Hellfeldt K, Lopez-Romero L, Andershed H (2019) Cyberbullying and psychological well-being in young adolescence: the potential protective mediation effects of social support from family, friends, and teachers. Int J Environ Res Public Health 17(1):45. https://doi.org/10.3390/ijerph17010045

Hilliard ME, Riekert KA, Ockene JK, Pbert L (2018) The handbook of health behavior change, 5th edn. Springer Publishing Company, New York

Jia J, Zhao T, Liu Z, Liang Y, Li F, Li Y et al (2023) Association between healthy lifestyle and memory decline in older adults: 10 year, population based, prospective cohort study. BMJ 380:e072691. https://doi.org/10.1136/bmj-2022-072691

Kok G, Gottlieb NH, Peters GJ, Mullen PD, Parcel GS, Ruiter RA et al (2016) A taxonomy of behaviour change methods: an intervention mapping approach. Health Psychol Rev 10(3):297–312. https://doi.org/10.1080/17437199.2015.1077155

Livingston G, Huntley J, Sommerlad A, Ames D, Ballard C, Banerjee S et al (2020) Dementia prevention, intervention, and care: 2020 report of the Lancet Commission. Lancet 396(10248):413–446. https://doi.org/10.1016/S0140-6736(20)30367-6

Metz G, Peters GY, Crutzen R (2022) Acyclic behavior change diagrams: a tool to report and analyze interventions. Health Psychol Behav Medi 10(1):1216–1228. https://doi.org/10.1080/21642850.2022.2149930

Metz G, Roosjen H, Zweers W, Crutzen R (2023) Evaluating use of web-based interventions: an example of a Dutch sexual health intervention. Health Promot Int 38:daab190. https://doi.org/10.1093/heapro/daab190

Moafa I (2022) Unravelling the effect of a dental public health intervention (ISAC): in the face of oral cancer early detection and prevention in the Jazan Region, Saudi Arabia. Doctoral thesis, Maastricht University. https://doi.org/10.26481/dis.20221024im

Ngandu T, Lehtisalo J, Solomon A, Levälahti E, Ahtiluoto S, Antikainen R et al (2015) A 2 year multidomain intervention of diet, exercise, cognitive training, and vascular risk monitoring versus control to prevent cognitive decline in at-risk elderly people (FINGER): a randomised controlled trial. Lancet 385(9984):2255–2263. https://doi.org/10.1016/s0140-6736(15)60461-5

O'Cathain A, Croot L, Sworn K, Duncan E, Rousseau N, Turner K et al (2019) Taxonomy of approaches to developing interventions to improve health: a systematic methods overview. Pilot Feasibility Stud 5:41. https://doi.org/10.1186/s40814-019-0425-6

Peters GJ, Crutzen R (2017) Pragmatic nihilism: how a theory of nothing can help health psychology progress. Health Psychol Rev 11(2):103–121. https://doi.org/10.1080/17437199.2017.1284015

Peters GJ, Crutzen R (2024) Knowing what we're talking about: facilitating decentralized, unequivocal publication of and reference to psychological construct definitions and instructions. Meta-Psychology, 8. https://doi.org/10.31234/osf.io/8tpcv

Peters GJ, Ruiter RA, Kok G (2013) Threatening communication: a critical re-analysis and a revised meta-analytic test of fear appeal theory. Health Psychol Rev 7(Suppl 1):S8–S31. https://doi.org/10.1080/17437199.2012.703527

Rosenberg A, Untersteiner H, Guazzarini AG, Bödenler M, Bruinsma J, Buchgraber-Schnalzer B. LETHE Consortium (2024) A digitally supported multimodal lifestyle program to promote brain health among older adults (the LETHE randomized controlled feasibility trial): study design, progress, and first results. Alzheimer's Res Ther 16(1): 252. https://doi.org/10.1186/s13195-024-01615-4

Ruiter RAC, Crutzen R (2020) Core processes: how to use evidence, theories, and research in planning behavior change interventions. Front Public Health 8:247. https://doi.org/10.3389/fpubh.2020.00247

Scheerman JFM, van Empelen P, van Loveren C, van Meijel B (2018) A mobile app (WhiteTeeth) to promote good oral health behavior among Dutch adolescents with fixed orthodontic appliances: intervention mapping approach. JMIR mHealth uHealth 6(8):e163. https://doi.org/10.2196/mhealth.9626

Strack F, Deutsch R (2004) Reflective and impulsive determinants of social behavior. Pers Soc Psychol Rev 8(3):220–247. https://doi.org/10.1207/s15327957pspr0803_1

Stutterheim SE, van der Kooij Y, Crutzen R, Ruiter RA, Bos A, Kok G (2025) Intervention mapping as a guide to developing, implementing, and evaluating stigma reduction interventions. Stigma Health 10(1):3–20. https://doi.org/10.1037/sah0000445

Svendsen MJ, Sandal LF, Kjaer P, Nicholl BI, Cooper K, Mair F et al (2022) Using intervention mapping to develop a decision support system-based smartphone app (selfBACK) to support self-management of nonspecific low back pain: development and usability study. J Med Internet Res 24(1):e26555. https://doi.org/10.2196/26555

Tamilmani K, Rana NP, Wamba SF, Dwivedi R (2021) The extended unified theory of acceptance and use of technology (UTAUT2): a systematic literature review and theory evaluation. Int J Inf Manage 57:102269. https://doi.org/10.1016/j.ijinfomgt.2020.102269

World Health Organization (1986) Ottawa charter for health promotion. WHO Regional Office for Europe, Copenhagen

Open Access This chapter is licensed under the terms of the Creative Commons Attribution 4.0 International License (http://creativecommons.org/licenses/by/4.0/), which permits use, sharing, adaptation, distribution and reproduction in any medium or format, as long as you give appropriate credit to the original author(s) and the source, provide a link to the Creative Commons license and indicate if changes were made.

The images or other third party material in this chapter are included in the chapter's Creative Commons license, unless indicated otherwise in a credit line to the material. If material is not included in the chapter's Creative Commons license and your intended use is not permitted by statutory regulation or exceeds the permitted use, you will need to obtain permission directly from the copyright holder.

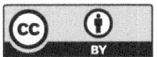

Evaluation of Digital Public Health Interventions

Oliver Lange, Paula Boskamp, Werner Brannath, Karina Karolina De Santis, Saskia Muellmann, Wolf Rogowski, and Heinz Rothgang

Abstract The evaluation of digital public health (DiPH) interventions is as necessary as the evaluation of any other medical or public health intervention. This chapter addresses the two important dimensions of evaluation: effectiveness and cost-effectiveness. In doing so, we ask (1) what is already known about the (cost-)effectiveness of DiPH interventions and (2) what factors should be considered when evaluating such interventions.

Although the body of literature is growing rapidly, the existing evidence is limited and often poor. So far, the effectiveness of DiPH interventions in terms of user outcomes was mainly assessed short-term (i.e., pre- vs. post-intervention) and compared to no intervention conditions. When assessing cost-effectiveness, it is important to distinguish between the perspectives of different types of decision makers (individuals, companies, healthcare payer, other public payers). In general, the estimated return on investment from a company perspective is positive in studies with a low quality of evidence, but negative in randomized controlled trials (RCTs) with a high quality of evidence.

O. Lange (✉) · W. Rogowski
Institute of Public Health and Nursing Research, Health Sciences, University of Bremen, Bremen, Germany

Leibniz Science Campus Digital Public Health Bremen, Bremen, Germany
e-mail: olange@uni-bremen.de

P. Boskamp · W. Brannath
Leibniz Science Campus Digital Public Health Bremen, Bremen, Germany

Competence Center for Clinical Trials Bremen, University of Bremen, Bremen, Germany

K. K. De Santis · S. Muellmann
Leibniz Science Campus Digital Public Health Bremen, Bremen, Germany

Leibniz Institute for Prevention Research and Epidemiology—BIPS, Bremen, Germany

H. Rothgang
Leibniz Science Campus Digital Public Health Bremen, Bremen, Germany

SOCIUM Research Center on Inequality and Social Policy, University of Bremen, Bremen, Germany

We argue that the evaluation of DiPH interventions requires alternative evaluation methods that, unlike the traditional methods (e.g., RCTs) could generate evidence faster and detect evidence gaps to be addressed in future studies.

Keywords Digital public health (DiPH) interventions · Evaluation · Effectiveness · Cost-effectiveness · Environmental impact · Evaluation methods

Abbreviations

CBA	Cost-benefit analysis
CEA	Cost-effectiveness analysis
CEEBIT	Continuous evaluation of evolving behavioral intervention technologies
CUA	Cost-utility analysis
DALY	Disability-adjusted life year
DiGA	Digitale Gesundheitsanwendung (digital health application)
DiPH	Digital public health
eHealth	Electronic health
EMA	Ecological momentary assessments
GHG	Greenhouse gas
HTA	Health technology assessment
ICER	Incremental cost-effectiveness ratio
JITAIs	Just-in-time adaptive interventions
LCA	Life-cycle assessment
mHealth	Mobile health
MOST	Multiphase optimization strategy
NICE	National Institute for Health and Care Excellence
QALY	Quality-adjusted life year
RCT	Randomized controlled trial
ROI	Return on investment
SMART	Sequential multiple assignment randomized trials
TAM	Technology acceptance model
UTAUT	Unified theory of acceptance and use of technology
WHP	Workplace health promotion
WTP	Willingness to pay

1 Introduction

The central concern of public health is to improve the benefits and efficiency of health-related interventions and to reduce health inequities while respecting the self-determination of individuals (Darmann-Finck et al. 2020). Within the world of evidence-based medicine, this implies that interventions to improve health should only be conducted if there is a proven net benefit for users. This requires a thorough evaluation of all new techniques and devices, such as those applied in the context of digital public health (DiPH). DiPH interventions (i.e., interventions supported by digital technologies), however, show features that might require an adaption of traditional evaluation frameworks and development of alternative methods before evaluation can be conducted. Therefore, in this chapter, we first explore what DiPH interventions are and what requirements are necessary for evaluation of such interventions. We subsequently discuss the effectiveness and efficiency of DiPH interventions. These discussions are centered around two questions: (1) What is the current evidence about the effectiveness, efficiency, and environmental impact of DiPH interventions and (2) What methods are available to evaluate DiPH interventions. We conclude by listing some points to consider for conducting evaluation of DiPH interventions.

2 Digital Public Health (DiPH) Interventions

While medicine focuses on individual-level health, public health always relates to the health of a population. Public health "comprises the entirety of all social, political and organizational efforts aimed at improving the health situation, reducing the likelihood of illness and death and increasing the life expectancy of groups [of individuals] or entire populations. Public health includes all organized, multidisciplinary and multi-professional approaches in disease prevention, health promotion, disease control, disease management, rehabilitation, and care" (Winslow 1920). DiPH can be considered as a comprehensive term for applying information and communication technologies to public health (Zeeb et al. 2020; see also Knöppler et al. 2016). While a consensus definition for DiPH is still lacking (Wienert et al. 2022), the term broadly refers to any electronic health (eHealth), mobile health (mHealth), and digital health tools and devices that could contribute to the improvement of a population's health. Furthermore, DiPH is relevant for any of the three levels of prevention (Wienert et al. 2022), including primary prevention (i.e., intervening before a health problem occurs), secondary prevention (i.e., reducing the impact of disease by medical treatment), and tertiary prevention (i.e., rehabilitation); see chapter "Public Health in the Digital Era: Digital Entry Points for Population Health" Why is it essential to address digital public health in an interdisciplinary way?, Maaß et al., in this handbook.

In the age of rapid technological development, the number of hardware- and software-based digital health technologies is increasing rapidly. For example, the number of mHealth apps available in the Apple App Store was more than 50,000 in the second quarter of 2022 (Ceci 2022). Besides software products, the number of devices, such as fitness trackers, smartwatches, and personal digital scales is also increasing. Beyond health apps, possible DiPH interventions also include digital software used by individuals for contact tracing (e.g., in the context of the COVID-19 pandemic) or by healthcare workers to notify health departments about new cases of a disease (Tom-Aba et al. 2020), digital platforms of health insurance providers to promote healthy behavior or to reimburse the costs of health services, and any interventions that use digitally linked devices (e.g., wearables or digitally linked accelerometers for physical activity promotion; Laranjo et al. 2021). Due to a wide variety of DiPH interventions, different requirements for the evaluation of such interventions are likely to exist (Tang et al. 2020).

Not all new devices may improve a population's health, highlighting the need for evaluation of such devices. However, the sheer speed of technological development generates new challenges for such evaluation. Thorough evaluations might require more time than the life cycle of specific products. Consequently, evaluation results might be available after the product is no longer available on the market. Hence the question of how evaluations should be conducted in this dynamically developing field of DiPH arises. This question is especially relevant because some digital health applications (the so-called *Digitale Gesundheitsanwendung* or DiGA) are already available on prescription in Germany.

3 Evaluation of DiPH Interventions

Different aspects of any intervention can be evaluated. For digital devices, *acceptance* is a prerequisite for successful implementation. Since the 1980s, extensive research has produced several Technology Acceptance Models (TAMs) (Davis 1985, 1989; Venkatesh and Davis 2000; Venkatesh and Bala 2008), which were later extended to the Unified Theory of Acceptance and Use of Technology (UTAUT model; Venkatesh et al. 2012). In this chapter we focus on effectiveness (with acceptance as a prerequisite) and efficiency as two important aspects of evaluation in a world characterized by limited resources. Additionally, we discuss the environmental impact of DiPH interventions, including carbon emissions, that is likely to gain more attention in the future.

Other aspects, such as ethics, need to be considered when evaluating DiPH interventions. These aspects are addressed in chapter "A Framework to Develop and Evaluate Digital Public Health Interventions", Pan et al., in this handbook, which describes a new framework to develop and evaluate DiPH interventions.

3.1 Evaluation of Effectiveness

From a public health point of view, it is crucial to disentangle potential financial gains for developers of technologies from any health benefits for technology users. Thus, evaluation of health benefits for users is crucial rather than the focus on mere technical development (De Santis et al. 2022a). The use of some technologies (e.g., health apps and wearables) could contribute to gains in at least two domains: (1) for individuals in terms of health promotion, disease prevention, monitoring, management, or health education, and (2) for healthcare policymakers by providing real-life, objective, self-tracked, and longitudinal data (Heidel and Hagist 2020). Evidence from both domains is required to decide which devices should be promoted and which should not.

3.1.1 What Is Known About the Effectiveness of DiPH Interventions?

The need to evaluate DiPH interventions has been extensively addressed in reviews with systematic methodology, such as systematic, scoping, or rapid reviews and overviews of reviews (De Santis et al. 2022a). Since the introduction of affordable internet on personal computers around the year 2000 and smartphone technology for personal use around the year 2010, the scientific literature on digital behavior change techniques primarily targets physical activity and healthy nutrition (Taj et al. 2019). DiPH interventions targeting healthy lifestyle may benefit various population groups, such as older adults (Muellmann et al. 2018). So far, however, the quality of existing evidence and reporting of effectiveness of DiPH interventions is poor (De Santis et al. 2022a; Eze et al. 2020).

It appears that DiPH interventions contribute to small health benefits for users under the following conditions: (1) in the short-term (i.e., when comparing user outcomes pre- vs. post-intervention), (2) relative to no intervention conditions (as opposed to other digital or non-digital intervention conditions), (3) for outcomes that can be measured objectively using digital devices (e.g., a number of steps per day measured by smartphones or activity trackers), and (4) if human support is provided (i.e., technical support or social network established with other study participants or study staff) (De Santis et al. 2022b; Muellmann et al. 2018). Although small health benefits may not be clinically meaningful, they could be sufficient to empower some populations, such as older people, to perform daily tasks required for independent living (De Santis et al. 2022b). However, it is unclear if DiPH interventions are superior to non-digital interventions. This is especially true in real-world conditions when DiPH interventions are delivered without human support. Furthermore, the long-term maintenance of any health benefits is unknown and the effectiveness for difficult-to-measure outcomes, such as well-being, is unclear (De Santis et al. 2022b; Muellmann et al. 2018).

Evaluation of DiPH interventions is not easy to accomplish for a number of reasons. First, it is unclear what methods should be used to evaluate the user outcomes of DiPH interventions. According to past reviews, the development of DiPH interventions is often guided by evaluation frameworks focusing on various aspects of behavior change theory (De Santis et al. 2022a). However, these reviews rarely addressed the theoretical underpinning of evaluation of user outcomes, indicating that this topic was either not mentioned in the primary studies or not coded by review authors (De Santis et al. 2022a). Complex or new methods may be required to adapt existing evaluation frameworks to evaluate user outcomes of digital health interventions (Hrynyschyn et al. 2022).

Second, evaluation of the effectiveness of any health intervention requires a standardized terminology that clearly defines the components and mode of delivery as well as the desired outcomes to be evaluated. Both requirements are, as yet, unfulfilled in the new field of DiPH interventions. For example, there was surprisingly little overlap in the primary studies included in the past reviews despite their focus on common intervention types (only digital) and health targets (only physical activity outcomes) (De Santis et al. 2022a). A lack of common terminology probably contributed to inclusion of different primary studies in such reviews and was also evident in incomplete reporting of DiPH intervention details and outcomes (De Santis et al. 2022a). Thus, standardization of terminology is required to evaluate the health outcomes of DiPH interventions.

Third, the effectiveness of DiPH interventions is affected by a complex set of factors. Similar to any health intervention, the evaluation of DiPH interventions should consider factors, such as a dose-response relationship (i.e., if higher doses contribute to larger benefits), the durability of any short-term effects in the absence of interventions, and the quality of adaptation towards the needs of the target population (e.g., children or older adults). Furthermore, user engagement needs to be considered when evaluating DiPH interventions (Saleem et al. 2021), especially if such interventions do not involve any human support. Finally, any add-on health benefits of DiPH interventions need to be investigated relative to traditional (non-digital) interventions (Muellmann et al. 2018).

The following section addresses some factors that could be considered when evaluating DiPH interventions. Hereby, we explain the adoption of evaluation frameworks, classic study designs usually used for evaluation of health interventions, alternative study designs for the digital environment, and digital data collection.

3.1.2 What Factors Should Be Considered When Evaluating DiPH Interventions?

Evaluation Frameworks

Frameworks that can be used to guide evaluation of DiPH interventions are still scarce. Most existing frameworks focus on evaluating digital health technologies without a focus on public health (Unsworth et al. 2021). To remedy this situation, members of the Leibniz ScienceCampus DiPH developed the DiPH framework (DigiPHrame, see chapter "A Framework to Develop and Evaluate Digital Public Health Interventions", Pan et al. in this handbook, and Jahnel et al. 2024). This framework was developed based on four steps: (1) scoping review of existing public health and digital health frameworks, (2) mapping of identified public health and digital health frameworks on the structure of the Health Technology Assessment (HTA) Core model, (3) consensus meeting with interdisciplinary experts from the Leibniz ScienceCampus DiPH, and (4) applying the framework on study cases. DigiPHrame consists of 182 questions structured in 12 domains, including health conditions and current public health interventions, technical aspects, usability, infrastructure and organization, implementation, intended and unintended health-related effects, social, cultural, and intersectional aspects, ethics, legal and regulatory, data security and data protection, cost and economics, and sustainability (Jahnel et al. 2024).

Study Designs for Evaluating DiPH Interventions

To assess the effectiveness of public health interventions, randomized controlled trials (RCTs) serve as a gold standard. However, due to the extended timeframe and rigidity of RCTs, these may not always be optimal for evaluating DiPH interventions. DiPH interventions depend on the rapid development of digital technologies and are complex concerning user needs and intervention components. Alternative study designs, which consider the characteristics of DiPH interventions to a certain extent, include the continuous evaluation of evolving behavioral intervention technologies (CEEBIT), multiphase optimization strategy (MOST), sequential multiple assignment randomized trials (SMART), micro-randomized trials, and N-of-1 trials (see Box 1).

> **Box 1 Alternative Study Designs for Evaluating Digital Health Interventions**
> Continuous evaluation of evolving behavioral intervention technologies (CEEBIT) (Mohr et al. 2013)
> Continuous evaluation concept, which compares different interventions included in one digital tool. New interventions can be added at any time. Interventions with inferior effects are terminated.
> **Multiphase optimization strategy (MOST)** (Collins et al. 2007)
> Multiphase concept for selecting and refining intervention components, followed by testing the overall intervention using an RCT.
> **Sequential multiple assignment randomized trials (SMART)** (Collins et al. 2007)
> Test concept for comparing multiple time-adaptive treatment strategies. Randomization to conditions at different time points, depending on the outcomes of the intervention up to that point. Data from multiple experimental groups are combined to test research questions of interest.
> **Micro-randomized trials** (Klasnja et al. 2015)
> Evaluation design for just-in-time adaptive interventions (JITAIs). Participants are randomized to different intervention conditions at critical time points. Short-time effects of different conditions are estimated and tested.
> **N-of-1 trials** (Kravitz et al. 2014)
> Trials with only one participant, who receives different interventions repeatedly in a randomized order. Individual intervention effects for the participant are estimated. Results of multiple N-of-1 trials can be combined.

Despite their existence, the alternative study designs are used less often than RCTs for evaluating digital health interventions (Pham et al. 2016). A recent scoping review (Hrynyschyn et al. 2022) identified only eight studies that used four alternative study designs (i.e., factorial designs, stepped-wedge designs, SMART, and micro-randomized controlled trials) to evaluate digital health interventions. The reasons for the infrequent use of alternative study designs are that they are considered to be more appropriate for intervention development (e.g., MOST, SMART, and micro-randomized trial) rather than for determining effectiveness (Gensorowsky et al. 2021) and that they are not considered as the gold standard. Therefore, some authors (e.g., Collins et al. 2007) recommend conducting an RCT after using any alternative study designs. Based on limited evidence so far, a general recommendation regarding the choice of a study design for evaluating DiPH interventions cannot be given as yet (Hrynyschyn et al. 2022).

Example of an Alternative Study Design: N-of-1 Trials

One example of an alternative evaluation method is the N-of-1 trial (Kravitz et al. 2014). In an N-of-1 trial, the effect of an intervention is evaluated for an individual participant. The participant receives the intervention or control for a predefined study duration, usually in a randomized order. The outcome is repeatedly recorded and compared between intervention and control periods. The effect of the intervention can be estimated and tested. If randomization is used, the bias due to time-depending confounders is minimized (Kravitz et al. 2014). Comparing different N-of-1 trials gives information about the heterogeneity of individual effects as opposed to RCTs that measure average effects (Kwasnicka et al. 2019). The average effects can also be investigated by combining the results of multiple N-of-1 trials (Kravitz et al. 2014).

N-of-1 trials can be used to evaluate DiPH interventions that are applied on an individual level. This approach allows investigation of interindividual differences in intervention effects, including which elements of the intervention are effective and for whom or whether there are different trajectories of change over time (Kwasnicka et al. 2019). Due to the cross-over type of evaluation, sample sizes are smaller than in RCTs. However, the N-of-1 trial cannot be applied in every situation. It requires a short-time intervention that can be randomized within a participant and an outcome that can be easily and repeatedly assessed. In one study (Sniehotta et al. 2012) the effect of goal-setting and self-monitoring of physical activity was tested in ten identical N-of-1 trials. While two participants each significantly benefited from goal-setting or self-monitoring, there were no significant effects for the other participants (Sniehotta et al. 2012).

Digital Data Collection

Digital and especially mobile technologies allow the collection of biological, behavioral, or environmental data (Kumar et al. 2013). This is done by the technology/application itself or via connected devices, like pedometers or smartwatches. Using digital data creates unique opportunities and challenges for evaluating digital health interventions.

Many digital technologies routinely and automatically collect primary data for technical reasons, such as for device functionality (e.g., apps used for monitoring of physical activity) or for personalizing content (e.g., apps sending reminders to complete sufficient physical activity per day). If these primary data are used for evaluation, this is considered a secondary data analysis (see chapter "Use of Secondary and Registry Data for Digital Public Health, Intemann et al. in this handbook). Automatically collected data can be used to investigate user involvement and engagement with digital health technologies (e.g., via data traffic, number of downloads, or use data). Additionally, effectiveness can be tested based on some user outcomes, such as physical activity. Possible outcomes for effectiveness include the number of steps, minutes in moderate-to-vigorous physical activity, or total physical activity in a chosen time period. The use of smartphones or some wearables also allows to include environmental covariates, like the weather or GPS location in evaluation models.

If data are repeatedly collected, this allows modeling of changes over time and time-depending covariates. It may be of interest under what conditions and for whom a DiPH intervention is effective. This is especially true for interventions targeting behavioral change that might be context-dependent. In psychology, such evaluation methods are called ecological momentary assessments (EMA) (Shiffman et al. 2008). The psychological state of participants in EMA is repeatedly assessed at strategically selected time intervals in real-world environments.

One advantage of digitally collected data is a lower effort since participants do not have to come to the research centers for measurements. As data are collected in daily life, this approach leads to a high external validity. Additionally, digital data collection may lead to a high density of data. Thus, with appropriate statistical methodology, higher statistical power can be achieved also with smaller sample sizes (Kumar et al. 2013). The examples of study designs that indeed rely on a high density of data over time are micro-randomized trials or N-of-1 trials.

However, some challenges must be considered in the context of digital data collection. Technical problems with digital devices may occur. For example, if participants' own devices are used, the digital intervention needs to work on different operating systems. Technical errors or connection issues may lead to missing data (Abdolkhani et al. 2020). Due to the real-life setting, the heterogeneity in the technology use by the participants may reduce the internal validity. For example, the assessment of physical activity depends on the participant carrying the smartphone or wearable at all times. Also, the digital literacy of the participants could influence their technology use. Combining these factors, missing values and high variability in collected data can be expected. To meet these challenges, a pilot study should be done to identify and fix technical errors and to test whether the instructions are clear and understandable for all participants. Technical support may also be required especially for participants with low digital literacy. Lastly, an appropriate evaluation strategy should be used to account for time series structure and missing data.

3.2 Evaluation of Cost-Effectiveness

DiPH technologies consume limited resources, so effectiveness and cost-effectiveness are relevant for their evaluation. As defined by Drummond et al. (2015), economic evaluation compares two or more interventions in terms of their cost and consequences. However, which costs and which consequences are to be investigated depends on the decision context.

In the following section, we distinguish between four decision contexts regarding the acquisition of DiPH technologies from limited resources: private decisions of individuals acquiring digital technologies on markets, coverage decisions taken by decision-makers in the public health and healthcare system, public decisions of policymakers with broader considerations than health alone and decisions by companies using DiPH interventions as investments into employee health. We briefly explain each context's essential characteristics, review the published evidence, and discuss methodological issues. Finally, we reflect on the possibilities of extending the economic evaluation perspective to a planetary perspective that does not only include the monetary costs.

Basic information on "What could be evaluated" in costs and economics has been presented as part of the DiPH framework (see chapter "A Framework to Develop and Evaluate Digital Public Health Interventions", Pan et al., in this handbook). To get more detailed information on the methodological particularities in the economic evaluation of DiPH, we refer to chapter "EPHO8: Assuring Sustainable Organizational Structures and Financing for Digital Public Health", Lange and Rogowski, in this handbook. Here, economic evaluation is introduced as a method to ensure sustainable financing of (digital) public health.

3.2.1 Informal Private Decisions About Acquiring DiPH Technologies

A central concept for economic evaluation linked to the decision context is the so-called "perspective", i.e., the question whose costs and benefits are considered. Unlike other public health interventions such as cancer screening, many potentially health-relevant digital technologies like pedometers or other wearable devices are bought on consumer markets. In terms of welfare economics, these applications can be regarded as *private goods and services*. In this case, it is up to the user to decide whether or not to download and use a digital health app based on their judgment of perceived costs and benefits. Only such private evaluation allows accounting for individual preferences.

On the other hand, such individual assessments of private, individual value can easily under-estimate the costs of data disclosure. Also, it is far from easy to evaluate the effectiveness of a digital tool in a realistic, unbiased manner (see above). Therefore, regulations like data safety laws are needed to ensure that digital goods do not incur harms that may not be perceived and thus are not included in the private evaluation of cost-effectiveness. Additionally, it might be of value to make information on the effectiveness and cost-effectiveness of available digital devices easily intelligible. This ensures well-informed private decisions about the acquisition of DiPH technologies. While it could be seen as a task of researchers to take this into account in their publication strategies, the provision of such information could also be left to the market or be organized in a non-profit way like the *Stiftung Warentest* in Germany.

3.2.2 Coverage Decisions Using Cost-Effectiveness and Cost-Utility Analysis

The need for publicly financed evaluations is more urgent if DiPH interventions are collectively funded by a national health service or a statutory health insurance system, thus turning these interventions into a public good. In this case, decision-makers need respective analyses to decide whether specific devices should be publicly reimbursed or not. Correspondingly, the standard context for which economic evaluation methods have been developed, and are applied, are coverage decisions made by healthcare and public health decision bodies. Respective bodies such as the English and Welsh National Institute for Health and Care Excellence (NICE) use cost-effectiveness analyses (CEA) and cost-utility analyses (CUA) as their standard tools.

CEA compares costs and a single health outcome.[1] Examples of CEA in the context of DiPH are analyses of costs per

- Kilogram weight loss (Little et al. 2017),
- Kilogram of fat loss (Chung et al. 2015; van Wier et al. 2012),
- Metabolic equivalent hours of walking and leisure activity per week (Maddison et al. 2015) or
- Quitter in smoking cessation interventions (Graham et al. 2013).

---

[1] In the US context, the term "CEA" is frequently used as a broader term encompassing CEA in the narrow sense as used here and CUA.

The (incremental) cost-effectiveness ratio (ICER) then summarizes how much additional money has to be spent on improving the respected endpoint by one (marginal) unit.

CUA compares costs to a generic measure of health gain, which can combine single or multiple effects. Possible outcomes of economic evaluation are costs per quality-adjusted life year (QALY) or costs per disability-adjusted life year (DALYs) gained. QALYs combine the health-related quality of life (0 corresponds with death and 1 with full quality of life) and life years. They allow for comparing very different and similar interventions with varying effects on health. Most importantly, they allow comparisons between health technologies aiming at indications (Drummond et al. 2015; Brazier et al. 2017). Among the 14 economic evaluations recently assessed by a systematic review of preventive Digital Public Health interventions (Lange 2023), twelve analyzed costs per QALY.

Economic evaluation can incorporate data from different sources. The three paradigm cases are economic evaluations based on (1) clinical trials (Ramsey et al. 2005), (2) observational data like routine data from sickness funds (Berger et al. 2012; Berger et al. 2009; Cox et al. 2009), and (3) decision-analytic models, which can incorporate all sorts of data and are typically based on data from literature reviews (Briggs et al. 2006). Even if observational studies appear highly relevant for evaluating DiPH interventions offered by sickness funds to their enrollees, own explorative searches conducted for this chapter mainly identified model- (see, e.g., the studies in Lange 2023) and trial-based (see, e.g., the studies in Law et al. 2022) health economic evaluations.

Though there are several CEA and CUA of digital health interventions (Lange 2023; Law et al. 2022), knowledge is scarce compared to the numerous DiPH technologies which could be applied. For example, more than 100,000 commercial physical activity apps are currently available in major app stores, but only a small number have undergone a formal cost-effectiveness analysis (Rondina et al. 2021). DiPH interventions, currently most frequently assessed by health economic evaluation, are web-based, text-message-based, and app-based to promote physical activity and weight loss, as well as interventions for smoking cessation (Lange 2023).

Lange (2023) reviewed economic evaluations that use decision-analytic modeling. While study-based economic evaluations are restricted to the short-term results of clinical trials, model-based analyses can more easily estimate costs and effects over longer time horizons. Accordingly, most model-based analyses have a medium or lifetime horizon, using various modeling approaches like Markov-, Multistate Life Table-, Discrete Event Simulation, or microsimulation models. Typically, the analyses estimated costs from the perspective of healthcare payers. Only two studies included societal costs in terms of productivity losses.

Regarding the final cost-effectiveness results, only two of the 14 studies Lange (2023) included reported that the expected costs of potentially avoided diseases exceed the intervention costs. Generally, the cost-effectiveness results are heterogeneous: the ICER of the included studies, which report cost per QALY, range between a min of −€3949 and a max of €114,211 (mean value of €20,955 per QALY). Thus, a general statement on DiPH interventions' cost-effectiveness is impossible. The cost-effectiveness ratio has to be determined separately for each DiPH intervention as it depends on various issues like the type of intervention, the setting, and the target population.

Other reviews report on the cost-effectiveness of overall digital application areas such as mHealth (Iribarren et al. 2017), eHealth (Sanyal et al. 2018), both mHealth and eHealth (de la Torre-Díez et al. 2015), or specific groups such as older people (Ghani et al. 2020) point towards the same direction.

3.2.3 Public Policy Decisions Using Cost-Benefit Analysis

DiPH interventions may also have consequences outside of healthcare, and decisions about their acquisition from scarce public budgets may be made by other than health and healthcare decision-makers. Moreover, digital interventions frequently have multiple benefits. Besides increasing health-related quality of life, for instance, an intervention that encourages commuting to work by bike rather than by private car can decrease presenteeism and absenteeism, and improve environmental impact or mental health and well-being.

Interventions which involve a diversity of benefits may be more susceptible to a cost-benefit analysis (CBA), which is not restricted to health-related endpoints but may include all kinds of consequences. To make them comparable, all outcomes of an intervention are expressed in monetary terms, thus allowing the integration of all effects into one figure. Moreover, recommendations follow immediately from this kind of analysis: As long as the monetary values of the consequences are higher than the monetary costs of an intervention, it should be pursued according to CBA. In CEA and CUA, an additional assessment is necessary to decide whether the ICER is regarded as satisfactory. To estimate the monetary value of outcomes, willingness to pay (WTP) analyses are performed.

This might appear as if CBA is generally superior to CEA or CUA. However, it must be kept in mind that the two methodological approaches lean towards quite different normative conceptions of what a desirable allocation of scarce resources looks like (Rogowski 2022). These conceptions are linked to the terms *welfarism* and *extra-welfarism* (Brouwer et al. 2008). Welfarists argue that the value of spending resources can only be determined by individuals and is best estimated by how much money individuals are willing to pay to receive this value. Extra-Welfarists argue that intersubjectively comparable measures of well-being, like capabilities rather than individual preferences, should guide economic analysis (Sen 1999). For a public health decision-maker whose primary concerns are health gains (and their distribution), CEA or CUA will likely be the more appropriate approach. In case a DiPH technology primarily provides other benefits than health gain, the acquisition of these technologies may better be left to the individuals' private valuation and market acquisition. CBA may be the more appropriate method for a policy maker outside the specific field of healthcare and public health, who has to account for very different dimensions of benefit.

Methods for estimating WTP are well established (MacIntosh 2010) and can also be applied to DiPH interventions. For example, WTP has been estimated as a weight loss maintenance intervention based on smart scales and text message support. The study revealed that the WTP per avoided percentage point of weight re-gain differed between £0.35 per month for users experienced with the intervention and £0.12 for the least experienced group. Also, highly educated and female respondents cared more about outcomes than costs (Mott et al. 2022). This stresses the importance of selecting adequate respondents for WTP surveys. Also, WTP is typically associated with income, so wealthier individuals' preferences bear a higher weight in WTP elicitation studies. This may be why a full CBA that compares benefits in terms of WTP with costs can rarely be identified for DiPH interventions. Further research would be necessary to provide better guidance on addressing these issues in the CBA of DiPH interventions.

The major challenges for conducting an economic evaluation of DiPH interventions do not lie in the cost side but somewhat in measuring effectiveness. Nevertheless, it is remarkable that economic evaluations, e.g., for prevention in older people (Huter et al. 2018), hardly account for the specific challenges the respective interventions raise for the measurement of effectiveness (see also: Lange 2023).

3.2.4 Company Decisions Using Return on Investment Analysis

A fourth decision context relevant to the economic evaluation of DiPH interventions is the decision of companies that use digital technologies as investments in workplace health promotion (WHP). Like for other investments, managers are interested in such interventions' return on investment (ROI) (an idea that could also be relevant for publicly financed healthcare systems).

There are several studies comparing costs and cost savings of digital WHP interventions, like weight management (Agrawal et al. 2021), physical activity promotion (Proper et al. 2004), stress management (Ebert et al. 2018), or combined programs (e.g., McKnight et al. 2018). Even if the analyses are sometimes labeled CBA, the benefits in these analyses typically consist of different types of direct and indirect costs like the costs of presenteeism, absenteeism, and saved medical expenditures due to avoided disease (Agrawal et al. 2021; Ebert et al. 2018). The latter are particularly relevant to public employers who co-fund their employees' healthcare.

It has to be noted that the considerations regarding assessing effectiveness above are also relevant for cost-effectiveness assessments: even if RCTs frequently lack external validity and suffer from overly shortened time horizons, there are high associations between study types and the outcomes of ROI analyses of WHP interventions. A systematic review of 51 ROI studies of WHP programs showed a clear inverse relation between ROI and study quality. While the mean ROI of all WHP studies was 1.38, the higher the study quality, the lower the ROI. RCTs even exhibited a negative mean ROI (Baxter et al. 2014).

3.2.5 Extending the Perspective to Include Environmental Benefits and Harms

A general recommendation for the economic evaluation of publicly funded interventions is that the analyses should use the *societal perspective*, i.e., considering all costs and benefits from all members of society (Drummond 2005).

However, DiPH may not only produce (un) intended monetary costs borne by others than the public healthcare payer. They also consume resources that are not easily susceptible to monetarization (for example, the use of the scarce absorption capacities of greenhouse gases (GHGs)). Since 2006 *health in all policies* has been a common demand, and there is now good reason to demand *climate in all policies* as well. Virtual services (e.g., telemedicine or virtual care) or DiPH interventions which encourage commuting by bike rather than by car could be assumed to avoid emissions. However, besides travel-related GHG emissions, these interventions also increase GHG emissions associated with the energy consumption of digital devices, servers, and networks, as well as indirect emissions related to the production of new devices.

Life-cycle assessment (LCA) is a well-developed methodology to analyze these emissions (DIN EN ISO 14040:2021–02 2021; DIN EN ISO 14044:2021–02 2021). LCA provides a standardized technique to assess the environmental impacts of a product throughout its life cycle, i.e., from the extraction of raw materials through its production and use phase until its final disposal. There are two approaches to conducting LCAs: process-based and cost-based LCA. Process-based LCA uses a bottom-up approach in which information about all environmentally relevant material and energy flows associated with a product system are collected, and their environmental impacts are estimated based on approved models (Matthews et al. 2018). Cost-based LCA pursues a top-down approach: using environmentally extended input-output tables, all environmental impacts of an economy (or different economies in multi-regional input-output models) are assigned to the economies' various industries. Using the *Leontief inverse*, emission factors per output for each industry can be calculated. By using the inverse, the whole supply chain is included. Using monetary values as units of calculation, these data allow for estimating the environmental impact per Euro spent for products from a certain industry (Minx et al. 2009; Huang et al. 2009).

There are different links between cost calculation in health economic evaluations and LCA. Following methodological standards of health economic evaluation, the analysis of costs should be based on the three steps of resource identification, measurement in physical units, and valuation (Drummond 2005). Since process-based LCA is based on data on resource consumption which are then valued (in terms of their environmental impacts, not their monetary values), there are theoretical similarities. Since bookkeeping data from cost-type-based accounts can also be used for cost-based LCA in healthcare (Zhang et al. 2022), the methodological link between LCA and cost assessment is even more visible (for further information on the methodology, see chapter "EPHO8: Assuring Sustainable Organizational Structures and Financing for Digital Public Health", Lange and Rogowski, in this handbook).

It should be noted that there are also links to the benefits side of economic evaluations. Generally, measuring effectiveness is a matter of balancing medical benefits and harms, and QALYs also allow aggregation of different positive and negative benefits. Likewise, methods could be found to include environmental advantages and disadvantages into the index of benefits in CUA, or they could be measured in terms of WTP in cost-benefit analysis. Further research is necessary on the appropriate integration of environmental concerns into economic evaluation.

Given the discussion about climate change, using LCA to estimate the GHG footprint of DiPH would be of particular interest. One recent systematic review assessed the evidence on the carbon footprint of virtual care and identified 23 studies that claimed to estimate a carbon footprint. However, the existing studies barely met the methodological standards set by the different guidelines. Therefore, even if many studies concluded that virtual care interventions are carbon-saving, these results must be handled with care. This is mainly because they replace individual travel with less carbon-intensive teleconsultation (Lange et al. 2022). More research on this important topic and its connection to health economic evaluation is necessary. Current evidence suggests that studies in this field still have a long way to go until the application of methodological standards, like in other fields of evidence-based medicine and public health, is a more widespread practice.

4 Conclusion

This chapter addressed two research questions: (1) What is already known about the (cost-)effectiveness of DiPH interventions and (2) What factors should be considered when evaluating such interventions. Although the body of literature on DiPH interventions is growing rapidly, the existing evidence is limited and often poor. Interestingly, the same is true for related areas, such as the effectiveness of digital nursing technologies (Huter et al. 2020; Krick et al. 2019). The potential of effectiveness analyses has yet to be fully explored and more extensively applied in this new and rapidly developing field of digital health technologies.

Evidence regarding the effectiveness of DiPH interventions in terms of user outcomes is limited. Further research is needed to evaluate the longer-term effects of such interventions, especially in the absence of the intervention. Furthermore, it is unclear if and under what conditions DiPH interventions are more effective than non-digital interventions when targeting the same health outcomes (e.g., physical activity promotion). Evaluation of effectiveness in terms of user outcomes may require a combination of RCTs (that are still considered the gold standard for evaluation, but are too slow for some purposes) with alternative study designs, such as CEEBIT, MOST, SMART, micro-randomized trials, and N-of-1 trials. As some of these study designs are relatively new, further research is needed to understand how these designs could contribute to evaluation of digital health technologies.

Reliable health economic evidence regarding DiPH interventions is also still scarce. A large share of decisions regarding DiPH interventions rests with market actors. Users base their decisions on individual preferences. Nevertheless, effectiveness and efficiency analyses could contribute to better-informed decision-making. If DiPH interventions are financed collectively, effectiveness and efficiency analyses from a societal perspective are even more urgently needed. Interestingly, ROI analyses show a negative correlation between the resulting ROI and the study's methodological quality. This relationship needs to be considered when methodological recommendations for economic evaluation are formulated. Similar to evaluation of user outcomes, a careful combination of methods may be required to evaluate the cost-effectiveness of DiPH interventions. Given the growing importance of environmental issues, their inclusion in evaluations seems inevitable. Thus, future studies should assess the environmental impact, such as the carbon footprint of DiPH interventions. Given the yet under-investigated link between the economic analysis and the environmental impact of DiPH interventions, this field will likely experience methodological development in the near future.

Note: An earlier version of this chapter was reproduced and made available within the doctoral thesis of Oliver Lange (2022).

References

Abdolkhani R, Gray K, Borda A, DeSouza R (2020) Quality assurance of health wearables data: participatory workshop on barriers, solutions, and expectations. JMIR mHealth uHealth 8(1):e15329. https://doi.org/10.2196/15329

Agrawal S, Wojtanowski AC, Tringali L, Foster GD, Finkelstein EA (2021) Financial implications of New York City's weight management initiative. PLoS One 16(2):e0246621. https://doi.org/10.1371/journal.pone.0246621

Baxter S, Sanderson K, Venn AJ, Blizzard CL, Palmer AJ (2014) The relationship between return on investment and quality of study methodology in workplace health promotion programs. Am J Health Promot 28(6):347–363. https://doi.org/10.4278/ajhp.130731-LIT-395

Berger ML, Mamdani M, Atkins D, Johnson ML (2009) Good research practices for comparative effectiveness research: defining, reporting and interpreting nonrandomized studies of treatment effects using secondary data sources: the ISPOR good research practices for retrospective database analysis task force report—Part I. Value Health 12(8):1044–1052. https://doi.org/10.1111/j.1524-4733.2009.00600.x

Berger ML, Dreyer N, Anderson F, Towse A, Sedrakyan A, Normand S-L (2012) Prospective observational studies to assess comparative effectiveness: the ISPOR good research practices task force report. Value Health 15(2):217–230. https://doi.org/10.1016/j.jval.2011.12.010

Brazier J, Ratcliffe J, Salomon JA, Tsuchiya A (2017) Measuring and valuing health benefits for economic evaluation, 2nd edn. Oxford University Press, Oxford. https://doi.org/10.1093/med/9780198725923.001.0001

Briggs A, Claxton K, Sculpher M (2006) Decision modelling for health economic evaluation. In: Handbooks in health economic evaluation series. Oxford University Press, Oxford

Brouwer WB, Culyer AJ, van Exel NJ, Rutten FF (2008) Welfarism vs. extra-welfarism. J Health Econ 27(2):325–338. https://doi.org/10.1016/j.jhealeco.2007.07.003

Ceci L (2022) Number of mHealth apps available in the Apple App Store from 1st quarter 2015 to 3rd quarter 2022. Statista. https://www.statista.com/statistics/779910/health-apps-available-ios-worldwide/. Accessed 16 Nov 2022

Chung LM, Law QP, Fong SS, Chung JW, Yuen PP (2015) A cost-effectiveness analysis of teledietetics in short-, intermediate-, and long-term weight reduction. J Telemed Telecare 21(5):268–275. https://doi.org/10.1177/1357633x15572200

Collins LM, Murphy SA, Strecher V (2007) The multiphase optimization strategy (MOST) and the sequential multiple assignment randomized trial (SMART): new methods for more potent eHealth interventions. Am J Prev Med 32(5 Suppl):S112–S118. https://doi.org/10.1016/j.amepre.2007.01.022

Cox E, Martin BC, Van Staa T, Garbe E, Siebert U, Johnson ML (2009) Good research practices for comparative effectiveness research: approaches to mitigate bias and confounding in the design of nonrandomized studies of treatment effects using secondary data sources: The International Society for Pharmacoeconomics and Outcomes Research Good Research Practices for retrospective database analysis task force report—Part II. Value Health 12(8):1053–1061. https://doi.org/10.1111/j.1524-4733.2009.00601.x

Darmann-Finck I, Rothgang H, Zeeb H (2020) Digitalisierung und Gesundheitswissenschaften—White Paper Digital Public Health. Gesundheitswesen 82(7):620–622. https://doi.org/10.1055/a-1191-4344

Davis FD (1985) A technology acceptance model for empirically testing new end-user information systems. Doctoral Thesis. Massachusetts Institute of Technology. https://dspace.mit.edu/handle/1721.1/15192. Accessed 30 Jun 2023

Davis FD (1989) Perceived usefulness, perceived ease of use, and user acceptance of information technology. MIS Q 13(3):319–339. https://doi.org/10.2307/249008

de la Torre-Díez I, López-Coronado M, Vaca C, Aguado JS, de Castro C (2015) Cost-utility and cost-effectiveness studies of telemedicine, electronic, and mobile health systems in the literature: a systematic review. Telemed J E Health 21(2):81–85. https://doi.org/10.1089/tmj.2014.0053

De Santis KK, Jahnel T, Matthias K, Mergenthal L, Al Khayyal H, Zeeb H (2022a) Evaluation of digital interventions for physical activity promotion: scoping review. JMIR Public Health Surveill 8(5):e37820. https://doi.org/10.2196/37820

De Santis KK, Mergenthal L, Christianson L, Zeeb H (2022b) Digital technologies for health promotion and disease prevention in older people: protocol for a scoping review. J Med Internet Res Res Protoc 11(7):e37729. https://doi.org/10.2196/37729

DIN EN ISO 14040:2021–02 (2021) Environmental management—Life cycle assessment—Principles and framework (ISO 14040:2006 + Amd 1:2020). https://www.iso.org/standard/76121.html. Accessed 30 Jun 2023

DIN EN ISO 14044:2021–02 (2021) Environmental management—Life cycle assessment—Requirements and guidelines (ISO 14044:2006 + Amd 1:2017 + Amd 2:2020). https://www.iso.org/standard/76122.html. Accessed 30 Jun 2023

Drummond MF, Sculpher MJ, Claxton K, Stoddart GL, Torrance GW (2015) Methods for the economic evaluation of health care programmes (Oxford medical publications), 4th edn. Oxford University Press, Oxford

Drummond ME, Sculpher MJ, Torrance GW, O'Brien BJ, Stoddart, GL (2005). Methods for the Economic Evaluation of Health Care Programmes (Oxford medical publications), 3th edn. Oxford University Press, Oxford

Ebert DD, Kählke F, Buntrock C, Berking M, Smit F, Heber E, Baumeister H, Funk B, Riper H, Lehr D (2018) A health economic outcome evaluation of an internet—based mobile-supported stress management intervention for employees. Scand J Work Environ Health 44(2):171–182. https://doi.org/10.5271/sjweh.3691

Eze ND, Mateus C, Cravo Oliveira Hashiguchi T (2020) Telemedicine in the OECD: an umbrella review of clinical and cost-effectiveness, patient experience and implementation. PLoS One 15(8):e0237585. https://doi.org/10.1371/journal.pone.0237585

Gensorowsky D, Lampe D, Hasemann L, Düvel J, Greiner W (2021) "Alternative study designs" for the evaluation of digital health applications—a real alternative? Z Evid Fortbild Qual Gesundhwes 161:33–41. https://doi.org/10.1016/j.zefq.2021.01.006

Ghani Z, Jarl J, Berglund JS, Andersson M, Anderberg P (2020) The cost-effectiveness of mobile health (mHealth) interventions for older adults: systematic review. Int J Environ Res Public Health 17(15):12. https://doi.org/10.3390/ijerph17155290

Graham AL, Chang Y, Fang Y, Cobb NK, Tinkelman DS, Niaura RS, Abrams DB, Mandelblatt JS (2013) Cost-effectiveness of internet and telephone treatment for smoking cessation: an economic evaluation of the iQUITT study. Tob Control 22(6):e11. https://doi.org/10.1136/tob accocontrol-2012-050465

Heidel A, Hagist C (2020) Potential benefits and risks resulting from the introduction of health apps and wearables into the German statutory health care system: scoping review. JMIR mHealth uHealth 8(9):e16444. https://doi.org/10.2196/16444

Hrynyschyn R, Prediger C, Stock C, Helmer SM (2022) Evaluation methods applied to digital health interventions: what is being used beyond randomised controlled trials? A scoping review. Int J Environ Res Public Health 19(9):5221. https://doi.org/10.3390/ijerph19095221

Huang YA, Lenzen M, Weber CL, Murray J, Matthews HS (2009) The role of input–output analysis for the screening of corporate carbon footprints. Econ Syst Res 21(3):217–242. https://doi.org/10.1080/09535310903541348

Huter K, Dubas-Jakóbczyk K, Kocot E, Kissimova-Skarbek K, Rothgang H (2018) Economic evaluation of health promotion interventions for older people: do applied economic studies meet the methodological challenges? Cost Effect Resour Alloc 16(1):14. https://doi.org/10.1186/s12962-018-0100-4

Huter K, Krick T, Domhoff D, Seibert K, Wolf-Ostermann K, Rothgang H (2020) Effectiveness of digital technologies to support nursing care: results of a scoping review. J Multidiscip Healthc 13:1905–1926. https://doi.org/10.2147/jmdh.S286193

Iribarren SJ, Cato K, Falzon L, Stone PW (2017) What is the economic evidence for mHealth? A systematic review of economic evaluations of mHealth solutions. PLoS One 12(2):e0170581. https://doi.org/10.1371/journal.pone.0170581

Jahnel T, Pan C, Pedros Barnils N, Muellmann S, Freye M, Dassow H, Lange O, Reinschluessel A, Rogowski W, Gerhardus A (2024) Developing and Evaluating Digital Public Health Interventions Using the Digital Public Health Framework DigiPHrame: A Framework Development Study J Med Internet Res 26:e54269. https://www.jmir.org/2024/1/e54269. https://doi.org/10.2196/54269

Klasnja P, Hekler EB, Shiffman S, Boruvka A, Almirall D, Tewari A, Murphy SA (2015) Microrandomized trials: an experimental design for developing just-in-time adaptive interventions. Health Psychol 34s(0):1220–1228. https://doi.org/10.1037/hea0000305

Knöppler K, Neisecke T, Nölke L (2016) Digital-Health-Anwendungen für Bürger: Kontext, Typologie und Relevanz aus Public-Health-Perspektive; Entwicklung und Erprobung eines Klassifikationsverfahrens. Bertelsmann Stiftung, Gütersloh. https://www.bertelsmann-stiftung.de/de/publikationen/publikation/did/digital-health-anwendungen-fuer-buerger/. Accessed 30 Jun 2023

Kravitz R, Duan N, The DEcIDE Methods Center N-of-1 Guidance Panel (2014) Design and implementation of N-of-1 trials: a user's guide. https://effectivehealthcare.ahrq.gov/sites/default/files/pdf/n-1-trials_research-2014-5.pdf. Accessed 30 Jun 2023

Krick T, Huter K, Domhoff D, Schmidt A, Rothgang H, Wolf-Ostermann K (2019) Digital technology and nursing care: a scoping review on acceptance, effectiveness and efficiency studies of informal and formal care technologies. BMC Health Serv Res 19(1):400. https://doi.org/10.1186/s12913-019-4238-3

Kumar S, Nilsen WJ, Abernethy A, Atienza A, Patrick K, Pavel M, Riley WT, Shar A, Spring B, Spruijt-Metz D, Hedeker D, Honavar V, Kravitz R, Lefebvre RC, Mohr DC, Murphy SA, Quinn C, Shusterman V, Swendeman D (2013) Mobile health technology evaluation: the mHealth evidence workshop. Am J Prev Med 45(2):228–236. https://doi.org/10.1016/j.amepre.2013.03.017

Kwasnicka D, Inauen J, Nieuwenboom W, Nurmi J, Schneider A, Short CE, Dekkers T, Williams AJ, Bierbauer W, Haukkala A, Picariello F, Naughton F (2019) Challenges and solutions for

N-of-1 design studies in health psychology. Health Psychol Rev 13(2):163–178. https://doi.org/10.1080/17437199.2018.1564627

Lange O (2022) Economic evaluation of digital public health. Dissertation, Fachbereich 11. Human—und Gesundheitswissenschaften der Universität Bremen, Bremen. https://doi.org/10.26092/elib/2187

Lange O (2023) Health economic evaluation of preventive digital public health interventions using decision-analytic modelling: a systematized review. BMC Health Serv Res 23:268. https://doi.org/10.1186/s12913-023-09280-3

Lange O, Plath J, Dziggel TF, Karpa DF, Keil M, Becker T, Rogowski WH (2022) A transparency checklist for carbon footprint calculations applied within a systematic review of virtual care interventions. Int J Environ Res Public Health 19(12):7474. https://doi.org/10.3390/ijerph19127474

Laranjo L, Ding D, Heleno B, Kocaballi B, Quiroz JC, Tong HL, Chahwan B, Neves AL, Gabarron E, Dao KP, Rodrigues D, Neves GC, Antunes ML, Coiera E, Bates DW (2021) Do smartphone applications and activity trackers increase physical activity in adults? Systematic review, meta-analysis and metaregression. Br J Sports Med 55(8):422–432. https://doi.org/10.1136/bjsports-2020-102892

Law L, Kelly JT, Savill H, Wallen MP, Hickman IJ, Erku D, Mayr HL (2022) Cost-effectiveness of telehealth-delivered diet and exercise interventions: a systematic review. J Telemed Telecare 30:420. https://doi.org/10.1177/1357633X211070721

Little P, Stuart B, Hobbs FR, Kelly J, Smith ER, Bradbury KJ, Hughes S, Smith PW, Moore MV, Lean ME, Margetts BM, Byrne CD, Griffin S, Davoudianfar M, Hooper J, Yao G, Zhu S, Raftery J, Yardley L (2017) Randomised controlled trial and economic analysis of an internet-based weight management programme: POWeR+ (positive online weight reduction). Health Technol Assess 21(4):1–62. https://doi.org/10.3310/hta21040

MacIntosh E (2010) Applied methods of cost-benefit analysis in health care. Oxford University Press, Oxford

Maddison R, Pfaeffli L, Whittaker R, Stewart R, Kerr A, Jiang Y, Kira G, Leung W, Dalleck L, Carter K, Rawstorn J (2015) A mobile phone intervention increases physical activity in people with cardiovascular disease: results from the HEART randomized controlled trial. Eur J Prev Cardiol 22(6):701–709. https://doi.org/10.1177/2047487314535076

Matthews HSH, Chris T, Matthews DH (2018) Life cycle assessment: quantitative approaches for decisions that matter. http://www.lcatextbook.com/. Accessed 30 Jun 2023

McKnight T, Demuth JR, Wilson N, Leider JP, Knudson A (2018) Assessing effectiveness and cost-benefit of the trinity hospital twin city fit for life program for weight loss and diabetes prevention in a rural midwestern town. Prev Chronic Dis 15:E98. https://doi.org/10.5888/pcd15.170479

Minx JC, Wiedmann T, Wood R, Peters GP, Lenzen M, Owen A, Scott K, Barrett J, Hubacek K, Baiocchi G (2009) Input–output analysis and carbon footprinting: an overview of applications. Econ Syst Res 21(3):187–216. https://doi.org/10.1080/09535310903541298

Mohr DC, Cheung K, Schueller SM, Hendricks Brown C, Duan N (2013) Continuous evaluation of evolving behavioral intervention technologies. Am J Prev Med 45(4):517–523. https://doi.org/10.1016/j.amepre.2013.06.006

Mott DJ, Ternent L, Vale L (2022) Do preferences differ based on respondent experience of a health issue and its treatment? A case study using a public health intervention. Eur J Health Econ 24(3):413–423. https://doi.org/10.1007/s10198-022-01482-6

Muellmann S, Forberger S, Möllers T, Bröring E, Zeeb H, Pischke CR (2018) Effectiveness of eHealth interventions for the promotion of physical activity in older adults: a systematic review. Prev Med 108:93–110. https://doi.org/10.1016/j.ypmed.2017.12.026

Pham Q, Wiljer D, Cafazzo JA (2016) Beyond the randomized controlled trial: a review of alternatives in mHealth clinical trial methods. JMIR mHealth uHealth 4(3):e107. https://doi.org/10.2196/mhealth.5720

Proper KI, de Bruyne MC, Hildebrandt VH, van der Beek AJ, Meerding WJ, van Mechelen W (2004) Costs, benefits and effectiveness of worksite physical activity counseling from the employer's perspective. Scand J Work Environ Health 30(1):36–46. https://doi.org/10.5271/sjweh.763

Ramsey S, Willke R, Briggs A, Brown R, Buxton M, Chawla A, Cook J, Glick H, Liljas B, Petitti D, Reed S (2005) Good research practices for cost-effectiveness analysis alongside clinical trials: the ISPOR RCT-CEA task force report. Value Health 8(5):521–533. https://doi.org/10.1111/j.1524-4733.2005.00045.x

Rogowski W (2022) Ideale ohne Ideologie in der Ökonomik. Evidenzbasierte Verbindung positiver und normativer Ökonomik als Mittel der Ideologiekritik (ideals sans ideology in economics. Evidence-based conjunction of positive and normative economics for preventing ideology). Zeitschrift für Wirtschafts—und Unternehmensethik 23(1):57–92. https://doi.org/10.5771/1439-880X-2022-1

Rondina R, Hong M, Sarma S, Mitchell M (2021) Is it worth it? Cost-effectiveness analysis of a commercial physical activity app. BMC Public Health 21(1):1950. https://doi.org/10.1186/s12889-021-11988-y

Saleem M, Kühne L, De Santis KK, Christianson L, Brand T, Busse H (2021) Understanding engagement strategies in digital interventions for mental health promotion: scoping review. JMIR Ment Health 8(12):e30000. https://doi.org/10.2196/30000

Sanyal C, Stolee P, Juzwishin D, Husereau D (2018) Economic evaluations of eHealth technologies: a systematic review. PLoS One 13(6):e0198112. https://doi.org/10.1371/journal.pone.0198112

Sen A (1999) The possibility of social choice. Am Econ Rev 89(3):349–378. https://doi.org/10.1257/aer.89.3.349

Shiffman S, Stone AA, Hufford MR (2008) Ecological momentary assessment. Annu Rev Clin Psychol 4:1–32. https://doi.org/10.1146/annurev.clinpsy.3.022806.091415

Sniehotta FF, Presseau J, Hobbs N, Araújo-Soares V (2012) Testing self-regulation interventions to increase walking using factorial randomized N-of-1 trials. Health Psychol 31(6):733–737. https://doi.org/10.1037/a0027337

Taj F, Klein MCA, van Halteren A (2019) Digital health behavior change technology: bibliometric and scoping review of two decades of research. JMIR mHealth uHealth 7(12):e13311. https://doi.org/10.2196/13311

Tang MSS, Moore K, McGavigan A, Clark RA, Ganesan AN (2020) Effectiveness of wearable trackers on physical activity in healthy adults: systematic review and meta-analysis of randomized controlled trials. JMIR mHealth uHealth 8(7):e15576. https://doi.org/10.2196/15576

Tom-Aba D, Silenou BC, Doerrbecker J, Fourie C, Leitner C, Wahnschaffe M, Strysewske M, Arinze CC, Krause G (2020) The surveillance outbreak response management and analysis system (SORMAS): digital health global goods maturity assessment. JMIR Public Health Surveill 6(2):e15860. https://doi.org/10.2196/15860

Unsworth H, Dillon B, Collinson L, Powell H, Salmon M, Oladapo T, Ayiku L, Shield G, Holden J, Patel N, Campbell M, Greaves F, Joshi I, Powell J, Tonnel A (2021) The NICE evidence standards framework for digital health and care technologies—developing and maintaining an innovative evidence framework with global impact. Digit Health 7:20552076211018617. https://doi.org/10.1177/20552076211018617

van Wier MF, Dekkers JC, Bosmans JE, Heymans MW, Hendriksen IJ, Pronk NP, van Mechelen W, van Tulder MW (2012) Economic evaluation of a weight control program with e-mail and telephone counseling among overweight employees: a randomized controlled trial. Int J Behav Nutr Phys Act 9:112. https://doi.org/10.1186/1479-5868-9-112

Venkatesh V, Bala H (2008) Technology acceptance model 3 and a research agenda on interventions. Decis Sci 39(2):273–315. https://doi.org/10.1111/j.1540-5915.2008.00192.x

Venkatesh V, Davis FD (2000) A theoretical extension of the technology acceptance model: four longitudinal field studies. Manage Sci 46(2):186–204. https://doi.org/10.1287/mnsc.46.2.186.11926

Venkatesh V, Thong J, Xu X (2012) Consumer acceptance and use of information technology: extending the unified theory of acceptance and use of technology. MIS Q 36(1):157–178. https://doi.org/10.2307/41410412

Wienert J, Jahnel T, Maaß L (2022) What are digital public health interventions? First steps toward a definition and an intervention classification framework. J Med Internet Res 24(6):e31921. https://doi.org/10.2196/31921

Winslow CE (1920) The untilled fields of public health. Science 51(1306):23–33. https://doi.org/10.1126/science.51.1306.23

Zeeb H, Pigeot I, Schuz B (2020) Digital public health—An overview. Bundesgesundheitsblatt Gesundheitsforschung Gesundheitsschutz 63(2):137–144. https://doi.org/10.1007/s00103-019-03078-7

Zhang X, Albrecht K, Herget-Rosenthal S, Rogowski W (2022) Estimation of carbon footprints for hospital care based on routine G-DRG accounting data in Germany: an application to acute decompensated heart failure. J Indus Ecol 26:1528–1542. https://doi.org/10.1111/jiec.13294

Open Access This chapter is licensed under the terms of the Creative Commons Attribution 4.0 International License (http://creativecommons.org/licenses/by/4.0/), which permits use, sharing, adaptation, distribution and reproduction in any medium or format, as long as you give appropriate credit to the original author(s) and the source, provide a link to the Creative Commons license and indicate if changes were made.

The images or other third party material in this chapter are included in the chapter's Creative Commons license, unless indicated otherwise in a credit line to the material. If material is not included in the chapter's Creative Commons license and your intended use is not permitted by statutory regulation or exceeds the permitted use, you will need to obtain permission directly from the copyright holder.

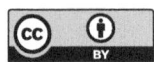

Challenges for Digital Public Health

Cyberspaces: Modifying the Digital Environment for Health Promotion and Prevention

A. L. Stark-Blomeier, J. Albrecht, and C. Dockweiler

Abstract Digital transformation is creating new digital spheres of experience and venues for everyday interaction. New cyberspaces are emerging that have the potential to fundamentally change the way we live and communicate. The conceptual understanding of spaces, places, and environments is changing. This has implications for understanding health-promoting settings. The questions arise whether the common understanding of settings and the setting approach of the World Health Organization is still appropriate today and what challenges and opportunities for health promotion and prevention arise with the expansion of settings to digital spaces, places, and environments.

Keywords Space · Place · Settings-based · Health promotion · Prevention · Virtual · Social context

Abbreviations

ICT   Information and communication technologies
JMD   Jugendmigrationsdienst
VR   Virtual reality
WHO   World Health Organization

A. L. Stark-Blomeier and J. Albrecht shared authority.

A. L. Stark-Blomeier (✉) · J. Albrecht · C. Dockweiler
Chair of Digital Public Health, Department of Social Sciences, Faculty of Arts and Humanities, University of Siegen, Siegen, Germany
e-mail: lea.stark-blomeier@uni-siegen.de

© The Author(s) 2025
H. Zeeb et al. (eds.), *Digital Public Health*, Springer Series on Epidemiology and Public Health, https://doi.org/10.1007/978-3-031-90154-6_9

1 Introduction

The concept of cyberspace and its impact on health promotion and prevention is becoming increasingly relevant due to the ongoing digitalization of our everyday lives. Cyberspaces are virtual spaces on the internet that offer new opportunities and challenges for the dissemination of health information and the promotion of health-conscious behavior. So far, it is debatable whether cyberspaces can be understood as a setting for health promotion and prevention. The World Health Organization (WHO 1998) defines settings as a "[…] place or social context in which people engage in daily activities in which environmental, organizational and personal factors interact to affect health and wellbeing" (ibid.). Based on this understanding of the setting, the question arises to what extent the term "cyberspace" is compatible with the setting approach and definition of the WHO. Accordingly, this chapter aims to highlight the importance of cyberspaces for settings-based health promotion and prevention. For this purpose, the connections between the terms "cyberspaces" and the functional and conceptual meanings of "space," "place," and "social environment" will be presented. Subsequently, the suitability of cyberspaces as settings for health promotion and prevention will be discussed along the WHO approach. Furthermore, different approaches to settings-based health promotion and prevention in cyberspaces will be outlined to derive implications for the future design of settings-based health promotion and prevention.

2 Methods

This chapter is based on the one hand on systematic literature analyses conducted by the authors as part of a research project on digital settings-based health promotion and prevention. The project "Lebensweltbezogene Gesundheitsförderung und Prävention im Zeitalter der Digitalisierung" was funded from November 2019 to January 2022 by the "Verband der Privaten Krankenversicherung e.V.." On the other hand, a recent exploratory literature analysis was conducted on the topic of cyberspace.

As part of the research project, the current state of research on digital health promotion and prevention in settings was investigated through various literature searches. First, a scoping review was conducted that aimed to "assess the range of scientific literature focusing on digital health promotion and primary prevention in settings" (Stark et al. 2022). The search was conducted in the databases MEDLINE, SocINDEX, PsycINFO, PSYNDEX, IEEE Xplore, BASE, and Web of Science. Search terms like "health promotion," "prevention," "living environment," "setting," "technology," and "digital" were used. Literature between 2010 and January 2020 was included, while reviews were excluded. The review was based on a broad understanding of settings, which also included less formalized settings such as neighborhoods and households. The findings were subsequently updated and supplemented in a Horizon Scan, where the setting approach of the WHO with a narrower definition of settings as formal organizations, was used for this in-depth search. In the Horizon Scan, future predictions were made, and the research results on the current state of research and practice were updated by conducting study, project, and social media searches, telephone interviews with experts, and an online Delphi survey. Study and project searches were conducted in March 2021 via PubMed, Google Scholar, at www.clinicaltrials.gov, in technical journals, in project databases, and on health promotion/science websites. Social media research was conducted on YouTube and Twitter in October 2021. The telephone interviews (March–April 2021) with six experts in the science and practice of digital and settings-based prevention and health promotion were conducted as semi-structured guided interviews based on Meuser and Nagel (1991) and analyzed according to Kuckartz (2018). The online-based Delphi survey (September to November 2021) was implemented in two stages via the software "Unipark" with experts in science and practice (Stark et al. 2023b). Open questions were evaluated using qualitative content analysis according to Kuckartz (2018). Closed questions were evaluated using descriptive quantitative analyses and the Mann-Whitney U test to determine group differences using SPSS.

The explorative literature search was conducted in March 2023 in the scientific databases PsycInfo, PSYNDEX, MEDLINE, Social Science Open Access Repository, and the grey literature search engines Google Scholar and Google. To get a first overview and a rough classification of the main topic, the keywords "place," "space," "context," and "environment" in combination with the terms "definition," "term," "word," "concept," "origin," "background," and "etymology" were searched. The terms "functional" and "conceptual" were added to identify the meanings and relationships of terms. The terms "prevention," "health promotion," and "setting-based" were complimented. Only publications in German and English were selected, and no time limit was set.

3   Cyberspaces: On the Transformation of the Conceptual and Functional Understanding of Place, Space, and Environment in the Course of Digitalization

To understand the evolution and meaning of the term "cyberspace," the following subchapters will focus on the terms "space," "place," "environment," and "cyberspace" and explain their functional and conceptual meanings.

3.1   *Spaces*

Everyday life occurs through living, interacting, and moving across and within spaces and involves spatial behaviors and relationships (Dodge and Kitchin 2001). The term "space" means "denoting time or duration" or "the amount of time contained in a specified period." Another understanding is "physical extent or area, extent in two or three dimensions" (Oxford University Press 2023a, n. p.).

Furthermore, space can be specified contextually as "physical space," "geographic space," and "social space" (Bourdieu 2018). The difference is that physical space refers to the actual, tangible space that exists in the physical world, including the objects and structures within it. It is often defined by dimensions such as length, width, and height. Geographical space refers to the physical space on the Earth's surface and in the atmosphere. It includes features such as landforms, bodies of water, climate, and vegetation (Mazur and Urbnek 1983). Social space refers to the space in which social interactions take place. It is defined by the relationships between people and groups and by the norms, values, and cultural practices that shape those relationships. Social space is often less tangible than physical or geographical space; it cannot exist without them, but it can influence how people interact and communicate (Bourdieu 2018; Tække 2002; Adams and Warf 1997). Examples of social space include public spaces such as parks and streets and online spaces such as social media platforms and discussion forums.

The sociologist Bourdieu shows that physical space influences the way people interact in social space and that physical conditions define social space. In this regard, architecture and design play a significant role in shaping physical space and how this can impact social dynamics, as social interactions and relationships are influenced by the way spaces are organized and designed (Bourdieu 2018; Qvortrup 2002). Similarly, Bourdieu highlights the importance of social space concerning identity and group membership, as well as the impact of technology on how physical space is experienced and how social interactions occur (Bourdieu 2018). Spiegel (2000) also argues that the importance of space in social sciences is significant, as it plays an important role in the analysis of social processes and the connection between space and society. The term "space" is used to analyze the impact of social, political, and economic processes on spatial structures and vice versa. It is important to consider the different dimensions of "space" (physical and geographic vs. social, cultural, and political) to conduct a complete social process analysis (Spiegel 2000).

Accordingly, if in the broader sense, "space" is understood as "social space," then it encompasses more than just a geographical or physical space based solely on the restriction to 3D spatial properties and underlying physical laws (Bourdieu 2018; Ferreira and Vale 2021; Spiegel 2000; Tække 2002). Thus, "spaces are produced and given meaning through social practices that create places" (Dodge and Kitchin 2001).

3.2 Places

The word "place" comes from the Greek term "plateia (hodos)" which means "broad (way)" and from the Latin terms "placea" and "platea," meaning "courtyard, open space, or avenue" (Maslovskaya 2019; Qazimi 2014). In general language, we use the word "place" for settlements, cities, neighborhoods, or well-known public spaces (e.g., a square or castle) or refer to a restaurant or café as our favorite place (Cresswell 2008).

In geography, the phrase "place" has been understood primarily as locations defined as objective, definable points in space since the 1970s. Over time, various psychologists and philosophers took up the concept and discussed, in particular, the meaning of places for people, defining places as meaningful locations (Cresswell 2008; Qazimi 2014). The philosopher Martin Heidegger connects "place" with the concept of "dwelling." Thus, the meaning of places "elaborated into 'a place – to dwell' – the process of making a place a home" (Qazimi 2014). Accordingly, dwelling in places allows us to establish an identity, grant us meaning, and find a place of belonging (Malpas 2014). In this understanding, a place is not only a location but has a physical landscape or structure and a "sense of place." The sense of place relates to the above-mentioned meaning that is associated with a place, both individual and shared (Cresswell 2008). With the advent of humanistic geography, people's subjective experience in places became the focus, and the researchers analyzed the relationship between people and places and how people make their environments into places. As an opposing approach, inspired by Marxism, it was argued that places are not only about a positive sense of connectedness but are associated with power. Thus, places are social constructs reflecting the society and social processes that created them. As another research branch, critical cultural geographers in the 1990s examined the influence of places and their meanings on social exclusion. Therefore, the interaction of place and its meanings, practices, and identities leads to normative constructions of a place. Things, practices, and people can be labeled as "in place" or "out of place" according to place-based norms (ibid.).

In summary, a place does not only refer to a spatial location but also to its meanings constructed by culture and society (Anthamatten 2022), referring to the physical and social dimensions of a place. Here, the distinction from "spaces" becomes clear: "with 'space' becoming 'place' as it gains psychological or symbolic meaning" (Altman and Zube 1989). Places can be further characterized. Ardoin et al. (2012) distinguish four dimensions: biophysical, socio-cultural, political-economic, and psychological. The biophysical characteristics of a place include the landscape as well as the plants and animals. The socio-cultural characteristics comprise the cultural practices and demographic conditions within the place, the psychological characteristics include the person's internal features and relationship to the place, and lastly, the political-economic characteristics refer to job opportunities, financial considerations, and political boundaries in a place (ibid.).

3.3 (Social) Environments

The term "environment" means "the action of circumnavigating, encompassing, or surrounding something; the state of being encompassed or surrounded" (Oxford University Press 2023b). The environment "is defined as all external forces and factors to which an organism or aggregate of organisms is actually or potentially responsive" (Jeong 1997) and consists of at least three components: the natural, the human-made, and the social environment (ibid.). The environment is an essential component of geography that aims at learning about people, places, environments, and their interaction (RGS 2008, as cited in Demeritt 2009). Other disciplines, such as public health, use the concept by analyzing the effects of the environment on peoples' life or health. In different models, researchers systematize the environment or its determinants relevant to their research field. For example, the socio-ecological model by Bronfenbrenner states that health is affected by the interplay of the individual, community, and environment and distinguishes between physical, social, and political environmental factors (Kilanowski 2017).

The social environment encompasses "socio-economic factors (e.g., employment, education), physical surroundings (e.g., neighborhood and work conditions), social relations (e.g., within a community or workplace) and power arrangements (e.g., political empowerment, individual and community control and influence)" (Lillie-Blanton and Laveist 1996) within which people function and interact. The term "social context" is partly used synonymously with social environment (Biamino 2011). Others define social contexts with being "in the presence of another person" (Rolison et al. 2018) or being a member in a social group (Langner et al. 2013).

Compared to "places" and "spaces," the meaning of environments differs. While the environment comprises all surroundings of a person or object of interest, a space refers more to a physical or geographic location on Earth that can influence social interactions and relationships through its design and architecture. Further, one can refer to a social space in which people interact and build relationships, and space can become a place when it produces and provides social meanings.

3.4 Cyberspaces

With the development of the internet and the expansion of investment in information and communication technologies (ICTs) as transformative technologies, society has changed in many ways. The construction of a virtual world, alongside the physical world, created changes in social, cultural, political, institutional, and economic life through "cyberspace" (Ferreira and Vale 2021). However, the understanding of "cyberspace" has evolved in recent years. Compared to space and place, "cyberspace" is described as a concept with various forms of definitions that are based on technological, social, and cultural perspectives. In this context, "cyberspace" is considered to be a "space of virtual reality, the notional environment within which electronic communication (esp. via the internet) occurs" (Oxford University Press 2023a, b, c).

Since the 1980s, the term "cyberspace" has already been used to describe, on a technical level, the virtual world of computer networks or artificial reality (Ferreira and Vale 2021; Kitchin 1998). Ottis and Lorents (2010) consider "cyberspace" from a purely technological perspective, defining it as "a global domain within the information environment consisting of the interdependent network of information technology infrastructures, including the Internet, telecommunications networks, computer systems, and embedded processors and controllers" (ibid.).

Furthermore, Dodge and Kitchin (2001) emphasize that "cyberspace" is a space created through the interaction of computers and users that contains digital and virtual elements (ibid.). From a communication studies perspective, Riva and Galimberti (1997) agree, describing "cyberspace" as a virtual space where people communicate with each other through technology. This digital interactive communication leads to a new construction of subjectivity based on three psychosocial roots: (1) networked reality, (2) virtual conversation, and (3) identity construction. Accordingly, cyberspaces construct identities where individuals can establish a new sense of self and control through interaction. The authors describe "cyberspace" as a space that provides a convincing simulation of the physical presence of others while maintaining anonymity. Thus, communication technologies can be seen as transparent interfaces that enable communication in a virtual space between interlocutors (ibid.). Considering "cyberspace" as a conceptual digital information space within ICTs means that it does not consist of a single homogeneous space but rather of a multitude of cyberspaces, each offering a different form of digital interaction and communication and creating new forms of social relationships and identities that are different from analog spaces and places (Dodge and Kitchin 2001).

From the perspective of humanistic geography, the consideration of cyberspaces initially focused on physical locations. Since "cyberspace" can only come into being through physical elements (e.g., hardware, software, Internet routers, and computers), the connection to the physical world cannot be dismissed. Compared to physical space, which exists unconditionally, "cyberspace" thus differs by the dependence on the existence of physical space (Bryant 2001). Despite the dependence on physical space, Kwan (2001) points out that the creation of a virtual space removes geographic landmarks and information about distances and directions (ibid.).

Cyberspace enables new forms of communication and interaction that change the way we interact with each other, and these social interactions and relationships are influenced by the way cyberspaces are organized and designed (Ferreira and Vale 2021). According to this, various scholars argue that the understanding of "cyberspace" should not be limited to technical aspects but should include cultural and social components (Dodge and Kitchin 2001; Ferreira and Vale 2021; Kalay and Marx 2006; Strate 1999; Tække 2002). Furthermore, some scholars have increasingly come to recognize some virtual spaces as places because cyberspaces should be considered as meaningful locations constructed by culture and society, or in other words, as places (Kalay and Marx 2006; Relph 2007). In doing so, some authors argue for understanding and designing cyberspaces as "web places" rather than "web pages" or as "places" rather than "spaces" (Kalay and Marx 2006; Kitchin and Dodge 2015). Their rationale is that "cyberspace" is a stage for everyday economic, cultural, and other human activities. As a result, there is an opportunity to design it in line with place-like principles. In this context, designing "cyberspace" as a place means not only enabling social interaction but also, like physical places, embodying and expressing cultural values (Kalay and Marx 2006; Strate 1999). On that basis, "cyberspace" can be understood as an abstract construct in which, with social and technological development parallel to physical reality, a space emerges that does not conform to the physical definition of geographic space (Tække 2002). However, "cyberspace" cannot be considered independent of the physical or real world either, as its existence depends on it (Ferreira and Vale 2021). Instead, from this perspective, "cyberspace" becomes a meaningful place constructed by culture and society (Kalay and Marx 2006).

Cyberspace can be further characterized. Accordingly, it "is not a stable space that is already there. It is an ongoing and highly performative process constituted by temporary assemblages of data, people, devices, infrastructure and space" (Ferreira and Vale 2021). This perspective is also shared by Strate (1999), who emphasizes that "cyberspace" is not a single, unified entity but rather a collection of different spaces that are interconnected and interdependent (ibid.). As mentioned before, cyberspace does not consist of a single homogeneous space but rather a multitude of cyberspaces, each offering a different form of digital interaction and communication. These spaces can generally be divided into the domains of conventional telecommunications (such as the telephone), virtual reality (VR), and internet technologies, with new hybrid spaces emerging continuously due to the rapid convergence of technologies (Kalay and Marx 2006). For example, social media platforms as internet technologies increasingly provide new opportunities for digital interaction (Lupton 2015). However, the boundaries between different forms of "cyberspace" are often fuzzy and blurred, and the physical and virtual elements influence each other (Strate 1999). Approaches to systematically classify and map "cyberspace" are proving challenging, as they must capture the unimaginable complexity of cyberspaces systems (Jiang and Ormeling 1997, 2000; Strate 1999).

4 Cyberspaces in Settings-Based Health Promotion and Prevention

The emergence and continuous development of cyberspaces imply changes in all spheres of life and society. This may change our understanding of settings for health promotion and prevention and bring new directions for health promotion. In the following, the WHO's setting definition and approach will be presented with regard to the concepts mentioned above, and the meaning of cyberspaces as settings will be discussed.

4.1 Setting Definition and Setting Approach

The setting approach is a key strategy in health promotion that emphasizes the connections between people, places, and environments. Accordingly, effective health promotion requires interventions in the places, environments, and contexts we live in (Dooris et al. 2022a). Settings have long been used as a means (and place) for health promotion. However, the setting approach extends beyond this, as it considers that places, environments, and contexts impact health and seeks "to embed health within the culture, ethos and core business of settings" (Dooris et al. 2022b).

Considering the historical development of the setting approach, it becomes apparent that various disciplines, e.g., sociology and geography, have contributed to it (Dooris et al. 2022b; Green et al. 2000). Beginning in the 1980s, the WHO developed the "Health for All by the Year 2000" program that recognized the social, economic, physical, and political determinants of health. In 1986, the WHO launched the "Ottawa Charter for Health Promotion" (Dooris et al. 2022b). Here, the term "setting" was initially mentioned as a relevant determinant of health: "Health is created and lived by people within the settings of their everyday life; where they learn, work, play and love. Health is created by caring for oneself and others, by being able to take decisions and have control over one's life circumstances, and by ensuring that the society one lives in creates conditions that allow the attainment of health by all its members" (WHO 1986). With this conceptual definition, the WHO shifted the focus from the pathogenetic model of disease to health potentials, considering the above-mentioned sense of place and sense of self. In that context, the WHO's "Healthy Cities" program was the first to aim at developing healthy settings—understood as complex and holistic systems (Dooris et al. 2022b).

In the 1990s, the Healthy Cities program was expanded to countries of the Global North, other area-based settings (e.g., Healthy Villages, Islands, Regions), and organizational settings (e.g., Healthy Schools, Hospitals, Workplaces) (ibid.). The setting approach was consolidated in 1998 with the WHO's "Health Promotion Glossary," defining settings as a "place or social context in which people engage in daily activities in which environmental, organizational, and personal factors interact to affect health and wellbeing [...]. A setting is also where people actively use and shape the environment and thus create or solve problems relating to health. Settings can normally be identified as having physical boundaries, a range of people with defined roles, and an organizational structure" (WHO 1998). Thus, the setting approach focuses on structures, people, and places and understands settings not only as a medium to reach a target group but also as a context that influences health and involves a commitment to integrate health into a setting's cultures, structures, and routines (Dooris et al. 2022a). Further, it focuses on organizations as the setting approach demands actions in the form of organizational development and changes to the physical environment, organizational structures, administration, and management (WHO 1998).

In the 2000s, the setting approach was further strengthened by various policy papers by the WHO that focused on the development of healthy settings. The approach was applied to new settings, like villages or residential care. By the end of the twentieth century, the setting approach was well-established internationally. This development continues today, and the setting approach is continuously reflected, and new emerging settings, such as social media or digital settings, are being discussed (Dooris et al. 2022b). However, it is important to mention that until today there is still an unclear theoretical foundation and implementation practice of the setting approach. The current discussion continues to be characterized by a lack of a generally accepted definition of the term "setting" and related terms such as "living or social environment" (Dadaczynski 2019).

4.2 Cyberspaces as Settings

Previously, we defined the term "setting" as places or social contexts where peoples' everyday activities take place and health is affected. To answer whether cyberspaces can be understood as settings, it is thus necessary to examine whether cyberspaces are places or social contexts. We have postulated that cyberspaces are understood as digital/virtual spaces that emerge through the interaction of people using ICTs. As shown, it is currently not certain whether cyberspaces can be understood as places. Some scientists argue in favor of this because cyberspaces enable everyday human activities and can display social values. Thus, cyberspaces as places contain meanings constructed by society. There is a need for further research on what characterizes a place. The term "social context" is used synonymously with "social environment" and differentiates in its meaning of places; thus, its meaning should be distinguished from that of places. Environments are one's surroundings, in terms of social environment, the social relations one engages with, and social circumstances under which one lives (e.g., power constellations). "Cyberspace" is partly defined as the technological, virtual, or notional environment of people communicating via information and communication technologies. Further, scientists support the thesis that "cyberspace" has a social dimension and "has created a virtual social environment in which people can meet, negotiate, collaborate, and exchange goods and information" (Barak 2008).

As mentioned before, "cyberspace" can be differentiated into various forms, each offering a different way of digital interaction. These include different applications of internet technologies or virtual reality. Especially with the development of Web 2.0, which is synonymous with the "social web," new opportunities for digital interaction have emerged through social media platforms such as Twitter or Instagram (Lupton 2015). Regarding the definition of settings, it must be considered if the different cyberspaces, respective forms of digital interaction that are part of peoples' everyday life, have an impact on their health. Research is still in its infancy, but initial studies show, for example, that the use of social media or VR can, under certain conditions, damage or promote health (see also Social Media in Digital Public Health, Sina et al. in this handbook; Alonzo et al. 2021; Ghahramani et al. 2022; Healy et al. 2022; Nichols and Patel 2002).

According to the WHO's setting approach, a setting also comprises organizational structures. Organizational structures determine how organizations try to control behavior and complete tasks, for example, through specialization and formalization (Quigg et al. 2016). On the one hand, traditional organizations increasingly use cyberspaces, e.g., social media platforms, to communicate with target groups or stakeholders. An example is the application Second Life, a "fantasy

Web world where users create and act out life through avatars [...]. More than 80 major brands have created (and paid for) a virtual presence in Second Life in order to reach the site's more than 13 million visitors" (Hallahan 2020). On the other hand, digital organizations with digital business models and electronic value creation processes, e.g., e-commerce, are located directly in "cyberspace" (Hallahan 2020; Stark et al. 2023a). The question remains whether the different forms of cyberspaces, such as social media platforms or VR gatherings, can be understood as organizations. Companies operating a social media platform consist of employers and employees—organizations with formal structures. When considering social media platforms as a medium for digital communication, the focus is more on informal social communities, which cannot necessarily be defined as an organization with formal structures. Thus, the classification of social media as organizations is less evident (Stark et al. 2023a).

In summary, neither the concept of "cyberspace" nor "setting" are uniformly defined and understood in the scientific community. Although specific forms of "cyberspace" can be understood as settings, if a certain definition and interpretation of the terms are applied, it is not possible to make a final and universally valid judgment. In the following section, we will look at how other scientists evaluate "cyberspace" in terms of the WHO's setting approach.

As one example, Loss et al. (2014) theoretically discuss whether social media platforms can constitute novel settings for health promotion. For this purpose, they analyze whether characteristics of settings/the setting approach are applicable. First, they support a realignment of the setting definition: "As many of our daily activities have shifted to cyberspace, we argue that online social interaction may gain more importance than geographic closeness for defining a 'setting'" (ibid.). In favor of social media platforms as settings for health promotion, they argue that these offer social interaction, are part of everyday life, allow the pursuit of professional/leisure time activities, and display organizational structures (e.g., terms of use, common technical features that structure interaction, i.e., users profiles, options for posting/feedback). According to the authors, however, there are other setting characteristics for which it remains unclear whether an application to social media platforms is possible. Discussions are needed regarding whether social media platforms are based on shared values, norms, and sanctions, influence the users´ health, and are permanent/consistent. Regarding the setting approach, social media platforms offer the possibility to address individuals in the setting, to build upon their capacities/skills, and partly to seek the participation of setting members and empower them (for further information about participation, see also Participatory approaches for digital public health—giving voice to values, Shrestha et al. in this handbook). It remains unclear if changes to the environment and organizational structures (e.g., technical applications that influence health behavior) and building partnerships within the setting or with other settings are possible on social media platforms (ibid.).

Also, Levin-Zamir et al. (2022) state that the expansion of social media and virtual environments "has reshaped the traditional definition of health-promoting settings" (ibid.). They discuss social media and virtual worlds as examples of new settings for health promotion. First, the authors present the benefits of social media platforms in terms of health promotion, including their everyday use by many people, the high reach, the reach of "hard to reach" groups, and the possibility of social mobilization and social support. They refer to the article of Loss et al. and conclude that the definition of social media as a setting remains unclear. Next, the authors describe social virtual worlds as online 3D multiuser virtual environments where people interact through an avatar as their virtual selves. In their article, the authors highlight the value of these "places" for maintaining health. Thus, they present that staying in the virtual environment, which reacts to the user's interactions, and the associated immersion and social presence of virtual worlds can influence the user's feelings and perceptions (e.g., feelings of belonging or a sense of place identity) and accordingly, the user's health. They conclude that social virtual worlds provide "engaging immersive avatar-based health promotion settings where health interventions can be implemented, as well as giving access to peer-led social support and education" (ibid.).

4.3 Approaches of Health Promotion and Prevention in Cyberspaces

The various forms of digital interaction and communication in cyberspaces and their influence on social relationships and behavior have opened new opportunities for health promotion and prevention. Networking or campaigns on social media platforms or interventions via ICTs are some of the approaches that can be used in cyberspaces to promote health and prevent diseases (see also Social Media in Digital Public Health, Sina et al. in this handbook; Levin-Zamir et al. 2022; Lupton 2015; McElhinney et al. 2018). Following the subdivision of cyberspaces according to Kalay and Marx (2006), two exemplary approaches to settings-based health promotion and prevention in internet technologies as well as virtual reality will be discussed.

With the development of digital street work, the model project "JMD Digital"[1] of the "Jugendmigrationsdienst"[2] (JMD) is one example of possibilities of settings-based health promotion and prevention in cyberspace. The concept of digital street work is based on a settings-based approach and comprises outreach psychosocial and health-related services for people who are not or are no longer reached by the established care system (Gusy 2020; Institut für E-Beratung der Technischen Hochschule Nürnberg Georg Simon Ohm 2022). It includes outreach work (non-content based) and the generation of original content on the respective profile page of the JMD (content-based). The outreach work is carried out defensively (systematic placement of postings on social media to draw attention to consulting offers),

---

[1] Further information: www.jugendmigrationsdienste.de/jmd-digital
[2] Institution in the field of youth migration service in Germany.

indirectly (mouth-to-mouth advertising by peers of the target group), or directly (targeted contact and announcement of the role and function via chat). As part of the project, the new virtual counseling approach, "digital street work" was tested on the social media platforms Facebook and Instagram and supplemented by further counseling structures via the online counseling platform "JMD4You." In this way, young people from rural areas seeking advice can be supported and advised in the sense of setting-oriented work in their familiar online environment on Facebook and Instagram.

The platform "JMD4You" uses different communication channels (chat or direct messages with counselors, forums on various topics), which are supposed to reproduce the structures of the traditional analog counseling context. The digital street work is based on approaches in analog street work and means the outreach work of socio-pedagogical specialists in the familiar online environment to reach young people at a low threshold who have not yet taken advantage of any services offered by the JMD. The goal of the digital street workers is to point out misinformation on social media platforms, depending on the focus of the topic (e.g., opportunities for social participation), to correct this by disseminating verified information in a targeted manner, and to point people to local offers of help if questions remain. Digital street work acts as a bridge between analog and digital work by providing targeted information about services offered by local youth migration services and other sources of help. The third component of the project is the provision of a virtual world, which for the time being, however, only relates to topics of professional integration. Here, the virtual world is to be understood as a virtual simulation, which means immersion in a comic story via an app. The goal of this story is for the user to virtually go through job application processes in Germany and playfully experience a simulation of a job interview. It is also designed to assist in writing cover letters and resumes using various digital explanations and checklists. Users may even make direct contact with a JMD employee on-site.

Through a physical infrastructure (servers, routers, and cables for communication via computers), the project creates cyberspace via internet technologies, including a virtual reality through which and in which people can interact. Through the exchange of personal information, as well as in the context of one's identity and contact with others, both the online counseling service platform and the virtual experience via the app can become a place where the users gather personal experiences, connect social meanings, and are influenced in their behavior and interactions. However, the social meanings attributed to the online counseling service platform, as well as the virtual experience via the app, may change over time, for example, as the platform evolves or as user behavior changes. Accordingly, counseling situations on various (health) topics can also be understood as social contexts, as they are an environment in which people interact and exchange ideas.

With the increasing use of virtual reality technology in various fields, there has been a growing interest in exploring its potential in promoting health and preventing diseases (Galliers et al. 2017; Gilbert et al. 2013; Gorini et al. 2008; Levin-Zamir et al. 2022). VR technology provides an immersive and interactive experience that can simulate different environments and situations, making it a potentially effective tool for health promotion and disease prevention. In behavioral health promotion, for example, applications are used to simulate exposure to smoking or alcohol and help people make healthier choices. A concrete example of a settings-based approach to health promotion and prevention in cyberspaces in virtual reality is the Second Life project.[3] As mentioned before, Second Life is a social virtual world in which multiuser virtual environments are created by allowing different users to interact, communicate, trade, and even build new virtual spaces in the form of avatars. These interactions occur in a virtual space generated by computers and can be explored by users through their avatars. While Second Life's space is dependent on a physical space where physical infrastructure (servers) enables virtual interaction, it provides users with an experiential environment in which they can move and act virtually within a given social context. Second Life users can create and design their own identities and spaces, making their virtual space a place for self-realization and self-development. By replicating physical structures, users can engage in activities and build relationships in Second Life that are similar in some respects to those in the physical world. In this sense, Second Life can be seen as a place that is shaped and given social meaning by users through their interactions and creativity. At the same time, Second Life is also a virtual place shaped by its digital design and technical characteristics.

Suomi et al. (2014) examined health-related resources in Second Life and identified two ways in which it has an impact on users' health. Firstly, people with disabilities and illnesses can be supported in building social interactions and connections using Second Life, which, in turn, contributes to their social participation and promotes health. Accordingly, virtual worlds offer the potential to foster a more democratic society by creating opportunities for individuals who encounter challenges in their real-life circumstances (ibid.). Furthermore, users can utilize health-related resources in Second Life, such as information or virtual worlds where health-related activities can be performed. This includes, for example, entering virtual operating theaters for educational purposes or accessing consultation rooms to obtain health-related information or support (Beard et al. 2009; Suomi et al. 2014). The development of such health-related resources in Second Life is oriented toward user groups. As a relatively high proportion of users in Second Life have a disability, a relatively large number of health-related resources associated with consultation rooms related to disability-related issues can be found in Second Life. However, according to Suomi et al. (2014), these resources are underutilized, and activity in health-related resources is relatively low. It should be emphasized that it is the responsibility of Second Life operators and those responsible for health-related resources within the virtual world to manage these resources. This means that these resources are made available sustainably or, alternatively, deactivated based on high or low usage patterns of these resources (ibid.). This demonstrates a high level of control over the range of use and, thus, the structures of Second Life on the part of the operators and health promotion stakeholders.

---

[3] Further information: www.secondlife.com

The establishment of long-term and consistent relationships in virtual reality worlds is, however, difficult, as the identity of avatars does not necessarily correspond to their real identity and therefore does not necessarily represent the reality or values and norms of the users (ibid.). However, behaviors from virtual worlds may well have an impact on the real world. For example, users in Second Life engage in a range of health-related activities that may or may not consciously affect behavior in real life. The extent to which spending time in virtual realities such as Second Life impact health remains an open question. Conscious effects might include, for example, actively seeking out health services after virtual counseling. Unconscious effects could occur, for example, when the virtual identity does not match the real identity.

5 Implications for Settings-Based Health Promotion and Prevention

Cyberspaces, such as social media platforms or virtual reality, influence health and are increasingly used as spaces to implement health promotion and prevention measures. However, it cannot be conclusively clarified whether cyberspaces can be defined as a setting according to the WHO criteria. To use the potential of cyberspaces for health promotion and prevention and overcome the real and potential challenges in implementation, clarification of the specific WHO criteria for cyberspaces is necessary. This clarification should include an official statement on the definition of cyberspaces, such as social media platforms or VR gatherings as settings, and roles for health promotion and prevention. Based on this, some cyberspaces could be included in the healthy setting program.

Further research is needed for this. For example, there is a scientific debate about whether cyberspaces can be understood as conceptual digital places within information and communication technologies (including platforms or virtual realities) and designed accordingly to promote health. At the same time, it has been highlighted that as the digital transformation progresses, physical boundaries are dissolving and are replaced or extended by digital boundaries. For example, these digital boundaries can be understood as limits in digitally mediated social interaction (e.g., asynchronous/synchronous, text-based/video-based), which need to be further defined and systematized in future research.

Following the recommendation of Loss et al. (2014) as well as Levin-Zamir et al. (2022), the question remains as to how structural elements of cyberspaces affect users in terms of health and to what extent users can influence structural elements of cyberspaces (Loss et al. 2014). In addition to the systematization of cyberspaces, it is also advisable to review a possible classification of the different forms of cyberspaces regarding their structure. Such a classification or systematization can provide an orientation framework for actors in health promotion and prevention to identify structures of cyberspaces and to consider the possible effects of cyberspaces on health. This, in turn, can support the planning, implementation, and evaluation of interventions in cyberspaces or in the development of health-promoting cyberspaces.

Regardless of whether cyberspaces are officially or consensually defined as settings, cyberspaces should be understood as stages for everyday activities with an impact on the health of users and should thus receive more attention as potential subjects for health promotion and prevention. So far, cyberspaces, like social media platforms, are mainly used to reach the target groups with behavioral interventions and unidirectional digital health information (Levin-Zamir et al. 2022; Stark et al. 2022). In the sense of holistic health promotion according to the setting approach, however, the context of the setting or the technical, social, organizational, and environmental conditions should also be examined. Only in this way can cyberspaces be used effectively for health promotion in the future and can be changed to become healthy spaces, environments, places, or settings.

References

Adams PC, Warf B (1997) Introduction: cyberspace and geographical space. Geogr Rev 87:139–145. https://doi.org/10.1111/j.1931-0846.1997.tb00067.x

Alonzo R, Hussain J, Stranges S, Anderson KK (2021) Interplay between social media use, sleep quality, and mental health in youth: a systematic review. Sleep Med Rev 56:101414. https://doi.org/10.1016/j.smrv.2020.101414

Altman I, Zube EH (1989) Public places and spaces. Human Behavior and Environment, Springer US, Boston, MA

Anthamatten P (2022) Geography and health. In: Naidoo J, Wills J (eds) Health studies: an introduction, 4th edn. Palgrave Macmillan, Singapore, pp 125–155

Ardoin NM, Schuh JS, Gould RK (2012) Exploring the dimensions of place: a confirmatory factor analysis of data from three ecoregional sites. Environ Educ Res 18:583–607. https://doi.org/10.1080/13504622.2011.640930

Barak A (2008) Psychological aspects of cyberspace: theory, research, applications. Cambridge University Press, Cambridge, New York

Beard L, Wilson K, Morra D, Keelan J (2009) A survey of health-related activities on second life. J Med Internet Res 11:e17. https://doi.org/10.2196/jmir.1192

Biamino G (2011) Modeling social contexts for pervasive computing environments. In: 2011 IEEE international conference on pervasive computing and communications workshops (PERCOM Workshops). IEEE, Seattle

Bourdieu P (2018) Social space and the genesis of appropriated physical space. Int J Urban Reg Res 42:106–114. https://doi.org/10.1111/1468-2427.12534

Bryant R (2001) What kind of space is cyberspace? Minerva 5:138–155

Cresswell T (2008) Place: encountering geography as philosophy. Geography 93:132–139. https://doi.org/10.1080/00167487.2008.12094234

Dadaczynski K (2019) Prävention und Gesundheitsförderung in Settings und Lebenswelten. In: Haring R (ed) Gesundheitswissenschaften. Springer, Berlin, Heidelberg, pp 403–412

Demeritt D (2009) From externality to inputs and interference: framing environmental research in geography. Trans Inst Br Geogr 34:3–11. https://doi.org/10.1111/j.1475-5661.2008.00333.x

Dodge M, Kitchin R (2001) Mapping cyberspace. Routledge, London, New York

Dooris M, Kokko S, Leeuw E d (2022a) Evolution of the settings-based approach. In: Kokko S, Baybutt M (eds) Handbook of settings-based health promotion. Springer, Cham, pp 3–22

Dooris M, Kokko S, Baybutt M (2022b) Theoretical grounds and practical principles of the settings-based approach. In: Kokko S, Baybutt M (eds) Handbook of settings-based health promotion. Springer, Cham, pp 23–44

Ferreira D, Vale M (2021) From cyberspace to cyberspatialities? Fennia 199(1). https://doi.org/10.11143/fennia.100343

Galliers J, Wilson S, Marshall J, Talbot R, Devane N, Booth T, Woolf C, Greenwood H (2017) Experiencing EVA Park, a multi-user virtual world for people with aphasia. ACM Transact Access Comput 10:1–24. https://doi.org/10.1145/3134227

Ghahramani A, de Courten M, Prokofieva M (2022) The potential of social media in health promotion beyond creating awareness: an integrative review. BMC Public Health 22:2402. https://doi.org/10.1186/s12889-022-14885-0

Gilbert RL, Murphy NA, Krueger AB, Ludwig AR, Efron TY (2013) Psychological benefits of participation in three-dimensional virtual worlds for individuals with real-world disabilities. Int J Disabil Dev Educ 60:208–224. https://doi.org/10.1080/1034912X.2013.812189

Gorini A, Gaggioli A, Vigna C, Riva G (2008) A second life for eHealth: prospects for the use of 3-D virtual worlds in clinical psychology. J Med Internet Res 10:e21. https://doi.org/10.2196/jmir.1029

Green LW, Poland BD, Rootman I (2000) The settings approach to health promotion. In: Poland BD, Green LW, Rootman I (eds) Settings for health promotion: linking theory and practice. Sage, Thousand Oaks, CA, pp 1–43

Gusy B, (2020) Streetwork/Aufsuchende soziale Arbeit, https://doi.org/10.17623/BZGA:Q4-i117-3.0

Hallahan K (2020) Crises and risk in cyberspace. In: Heath RL, O'Hair D (eds) Handbook of risk and crisis communication. Routledge, London, pp 412–445

Healy D, Flynn A, Conlan O, McSharry J, Walsh J (2022) Older adults' experiences and perceptions of immersive virtual reality: systematic review and thematic synthesis. JMIR Serious Games 10:e35802. https://doi.org/10.2196/35802

Institut für E-Beratung der Technischen Hochschule Nürnberg Georg Simon Ohm (2022) Aufsuchende digitale Beratungsmethoden: Handlungsleitfaden der wissenschaftlichen Begleitforschung des Projektes JMD DIGITAL—Virtuelle Beratungsstrukturen für ländliche Räume. https://www.jugendmigrationsdienste.de/fileadmin/media/jmddigital/Leitf%C3%A4den/IEB_Leitfaden_Aufsuchende_digitale_Beratungsmethoden.pdf. Accessed 28 Mar 2023

Jeong D-Y (1997) A sociological implication of environment in social development. Korea J Popul Dev 26:1–13

Jiang B, Ormeling F (1997) Cybermap: the Map for Cyberspace. The Cartographic Journal 34(2):111–116. https://doi.org/10.1179/caj.1997.34.2.111

Jiang B, Ormeling F (2000) Mapping Cyberspace: Visualizing Analysing and Exploring Virtual Worlds. The Cartographic Journal 37(2), 117–122. https://doi.org/10.1179/0008704.37.2.p117

Kalay YE, Marx J (2006) Architecture and the internet: designing places in cyberspace. First Monday. https://doi.org/10.5210/fm.v0i0.1563

Kilanowski JF (2017) Breadth of the socio-ecological model. J Agromedicine 22:295–297. https://doi.org/10.1080/1059924X.2017.1358971

Kitchin RM (1998) Towards geographies of cyberspace. Progr Hum Geogr 22:385–406. https://doi.org/10.1191/030913298668331585

Kitchin R, Dodge M (2015) 'Placing' cyberspace: geography, community and identity. Inf Technol Educ Soc 16:23–43. https://doi.org/10.7459/ites/16.1.03

Kuckartz U (2018) Qualitative Inhaltsanalyse: Methoden, Praxis, Computerunterstützung, 4th edn. Grundlagentexte Methoden, Beltz Juventa, Weinheim, Basel

Kwan M-P (2001) Cyberspatial cognition and individual access to information: the behavioral foundation of cybergeography. Environ Plann B Plann Des 28:21–37. https://doi.org/10.1068/b2560

Langner S, Hennigs N, Wiedmann K-P (2013) Social persuasion: targeting social identities through social influencers. J Consum Market 30:31–49. https://doi.org/10.1108/07363761311290821

Levin-Zamir D, Bertschi IC, McElhinney E, Rowlands G (2022) Digital environment and social media as settings for health promotion. In: Kokko S, Baybutt M (eds) Handbook of settings-based health promotion. Springer International Publishing, Cham, pp 205–224

Lillie-Blanton M, Laveist T (1996) Race/ethnicity, the social environment, and health. Soc Sci Med 43:83–91. https://doi.org/10.1016/0277-9536(95)00337-1

Loss J, Lindacher V, Curbach J (2014) Online social networking sites-a novel setting for health promotion? Health Place 26:161–170. https://doi.org/10.1016/j.healthplace.2013.12.012

Lupton D (2015) Health promotion in the digital era: a critical commentary. Health Promot Int 30:174–183. https://doi.org/10.1093/heapro/dau091

Malpas J (2014) Rethinking dwelling: Heidegger and the question of place. https://jeffmalpas.com/wp-content/uploads/Rethinking-Dwelling-Heidegger-and-the-Questi.pdf. Accessed 28 Mar 2023

Maslovskaya O (2019) The role of urban squares in the spatial concept of being. IOP Conf Ser Earth Environ Sci 272:32242. https://doi.org/10.1088/1755-1315/272/3/032242

Mazur E, Urbnek J (1983) Space in geography. GeoJournal 7(2). https://doi.org/10.1007/BF00185159

McElhinney E, Kidd L, Cheater FM (2018) Health literacy practices in social virtual worlds and the influence on health behaviour. Glob Health Promot 25:34–47. https://doi.org/10.1177/1757975918793334

Meuser M, Nagel U (1991) ExpertInneninterviews — vielfach erprobt, wenig bedacht. In: Garz D, Kraimer K (eds) Qualitativ-empirische Sozialforschung. VS Verlag für Sozialwissenschaften, Wiesbaden, pp 441–471

Nichols S, Patel H (2002) Health and safety implications of virtual reality: a review of empirical evidence. Appl Ergon 33:251–271. https://doi.org/10.1016/s0003-6870(02)00020-0

Ottis R, Lorents P (2010) Cyberspace: definition and implications. In: Armistead L (ed) Proceedings of the 5th International Conference on Information Warfare and Security: the Air Force Institute of Technology. Academic Conferences Limited, Dayton, OH, pp 267–270

Oxford University Press (2023a) Oxford English Dictionary: Space. https://www.oed.com/view/Entry/185414?rskey=uvHsZC&result=1&isAdvanced=false#eid. Accessed 28 Mar 2023

Oxford University Press (2023b) Oxford English Dictionary: Environment. https://www.oed.com/view/Entry/63089?. Accessed 17 Mar 2023

Oxford University Press (2023c) Oxford English Dictionary: Cyberspace. https://www.oed.com/view/Entry/250879?rskey=z2ycaC&result=2#eid. Accessed 28 Mar 2023

Qazimi S (2014) Sense of place and place identity. Eur J Soc Sci Educ Res 1:306. https://doi.org/10.26417/ejser.v1i1.p306-310

Quigg M, Lopez J, Rice M, Grimaila M, Ramsey B (2016) Cyberspace and organizational structure: an analysis of the critical infrastructure environment. In: Rice M, Shenoi S (eds) Critical infrastructure protection x. Springer, Cham, pp 3–25

Qvortrup L (2002) Cyberspace as representation of space experience: in defence of a phenomenological approach. In: Qvortrup L, Jensen JF, Kjems E, Lehmann N, Madsen C (eds) Virtual space. Springer, London, pp 5–24

Relph E (2007) Spirit of place and sense of place in virtual realities. Techné 10:17–25. https://doi.org/10.5840/techne20071039

Riva G, Galimberti C (1997) The psychology of cyberspace: a socio-cognitive framework to computer-mediated communication. New Ideas Psychol 15:141–158. https://doi.org/10.1016/S0732-118X(97)00015-9

Rolison MJ, Naples AJ, Rutherford HJV, McPartland JC (2018) Modulation of reward in a live social context as revealed through interactive social neuroscience. Soc Neurosci 13:416–428. https://doi.org/10.1080/17470919.2017.1339635

Spiegel SL (2000) Traditional space vs. cyberspace: the changing role of geography in current international politics. Geopolitics 5:114–125. https://doi.org/10.1080/14650040008407694

Stark AL, Geukes C, Albrecht J, Dockweiler C (2022) Digitale Anwendungen in der Planung und Umsetzung von verhältnisorientierter Gesundheitsförderung und Prävention in settings: Ergebnisse eines scoping reviews (digital applications in the planning and implementation of structural health promotion and prevention settings: results of a scoping review). Gesundheitswesen. https://doi.org/10.1055/a-1757-9264

Stark AL, Albrecht J, Dockweiler C (2023a) Digitale Transformation in Settings—Entwicklung eines neuen Begriffsverständnisses digitalisierter Settings entlang des Settingansatzes. In: Dockweiler C, Stark AM, Albrecht J (eds) Settingbezogene Gesundheitsförderung und Prävention in der digitalen Transformation: Transdisziplinäre Perspektiven, 1st edn. Nomos, Baden-Baden, pp 19–52

Stark AL, Albrecht J, Dongas E, Choroschun K, Dockweiler C (2023b) Zukunftstrends und Einsatzmöglichkeiten digitaler Technologien in der settingbezogenen Prävention und Gesundheitsförderung—Eine Delphi-Befragung (future trends and possible applications of digital technologies in setting-based prevention and health promotion-a Delphi survey). Bundesgesundheitsblatt Gesundheitsforschung Gesundheitsschutz 66:320–329. https://doi.org/10.1007/s00103-023-03669-5

Strate L (1999) The varieties of cyberspace: problems in definition and delimitation. West J Commun 63:382–412. https://doi.org/10.1080/10570319909374648

Suomi R, Mäntymäki M, Söderlund S (2014) Promoting health in virtual worlds: lessons from second life. J Med Internet Res 16:e229. https://doi.org/10.2196/jmir.3177

Tække J (2002) Cyberspace as a space parallel to geographical space. In: Qvortrup L, Jensen JF, Kjems E, Lehmann N, Madsen C (eds) Virtual space. Springer, London, pp 25–46

World Health Organization (1986) Ottawa charter for health promotion. World Health Organization, Ottawa, ON. Accessed 28 Mar 2023

World Health Organization (1998) Health promotion glossary. World Health Organization, Geneva. Accessed 28 Mar 2023

Open Access This chapter is licensed under the terms of the Creative Commons Attribution 4.0 International License (http://creativecommons.org/licenses/by/4.0/), which permits use, sharing, adaptation, distribution and reproduction in any medium or format, as long as you give appropriate credit to the original author(s) and the source, provide a link to the Creative Commons license and indicate if changes were made.

The images or other third party material in this chapter are included in the chapter's Creative Commons license, unless indicated otherwise in a credit line to the material. If material is not included in the chapter's Creative Commons license and your intended use is not permitted by statutory regulation or exceeds the permitted use, you will need to obtain permission directly from the copyright holder.

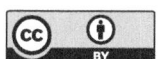

Digital Public Health in Europe: Was the COVID-19 Pandemic an Enabler for Healthcare Digitalization?

Laura Maaß, Brian Li Han Wong, Rok Hrzic, Ave Põld, Juan José Rachadell, Marine Delgrange, Robin van Kessel, and Stefan Buttigieg

Abstract Digital public health has influenced how healthcare is delivered and how health data is used for research and the monitoring of infectious diseases. The COVID-19 pandemic prompted a broader adoption of digital health interventions for public health purposes in several European countries. The European Union passed regulations to ensure data security and developed data hubs for international health data exchange to improve healthcare and public health research in the region.

Laura Maaß and Brian Li Han Wong have contributed equally to this work.

L. Maaß (✉)
SOCIUM Research Center on Inequality and Social Policy, University of Bremen, Bremen, Germany

Leibniz Science Campus Digital Public Health Bremen, Bremen, Germany

Digital Health and Artificial Intelligence Section, European Public Health Association, Utrecht, The Netherlands

Digital Public Health Taskforce, Association of Schools of Public Health in the European Region (ASPHER), Brussels, Belgium
e-mail: laura.maass@uni-bremen.de

B. L. H. Wong
Digital Health and Artificial Intelligence Section, European Public Health Association, Utrecht, The Netherlands

Department of International Health, Care and Public Health Research Institute—CAPHRI, Maastricht University, Maastricht, The Netherlands

Digital Public Health Taskforce, Association of Schools of Public Health in the European Region (ASPHER), Brussels, Belgium

R. Hrzic
Department of International Health, Care and Public Health Research Institute—CAPHRI, Maastricht University, Maastricht, The Netherlands

Digital Public Health Taskforce, Association of Schools of Public Health in the European Region (ASPHER), Brussels, Belgium

A. Põld
Institute of Family Medicine and Public Health, University of Tartu, Tartu, Estonia

J. J. Rachadell
Digital Health and Artificial Intelligence Section, European Public Health Association, Utrecht, The Netherlands

Institute for Evidence Based Health—ISBE, Lisbon, Portugal

M. Delgrange
Guy's and St Thomas' NHS Foundation Trust, Westminster, UK

NHS Leadership Academy, Leeds, UK

R. van Kessel
Department of International Health, Care and Public Health Research Institute—CAPHRI, Maastricht University, Maastricht, The Netherlands

Digital Public Health Taskforce, Association of Schools of Public Health in the European Region (ASPHER), Brussels, Belgium

LSE Health, Department of Health Policy, London School of Economics and Political Science, London, UK

S. Buttigieg
Digital Health and Artificial Intelligence Section, European Public Health Association, Utrecht, The Netherlands

Digital Public Health Taskforce, Association of Schools of Public Health in the European Region (ASPHER), Brussels, Belgium

Ministry for Health, Valletta, Malta

University of Malta, Msida, Malta

This chapter will present the essential European digital health and digital public health regulations (e.g., the General Data Protection Regulation). It will discuss the European Health Data Space and the importance of equitable access to digital public health interventions. This chapter will then analyze selected national perspectives through seven country case studies. These applied digital public health in various settings: through educational websites, patient portals, telemedicine, medical apps on prescription, infectious disease surveillance systems, and many more. By ensuring equitable access to these interventions and balancing investment in digital public health between populations with high levels of access and those with limited access, Europe can create a future where everyone can access quality health services, regardless of location or socioeconomic status.

Keywords Europe · General Data Protection Regulation · European Health Data Space · Healthcare systems

Abbreviations

AI	Artificial Intelligence
CPIAS	Support Centers for the Prevention of Nosocomial Infections
CRPD	Central Registry of Patient Data
DHSC	Department of Health and Social Care

DiGA	Digital Health Applications
DiPA	Digital Care Applications
DiPH	Digital Public Health
EHDS	European Health Data Space
eHDSI	Health Digital Service Infrastructure
EHIS	Estonian National Health Information System
eHealth	Electronic Health
EHR	Electronic Health Records
ePrescription	Electronic Prescription
eReferral	Electronic Referral
EU	European Union
GDHM	Global Digital Health Monitor
GDPR	General Data Protection Regulation
GP	General practitioner
mHealth	Mobile Health
NHS	National Health Service
OECD	Organisation for Economic Co-operation and Development
RCT	Randomized Controlled Trials
SINAVE	National Epidemiologic Surveillance System
UK	United Kingdom

1 Introduction

Digital public health (DiPH) refers to using digital technologies, such as mobile applications, Electronic Health Records (EHR), and wearable devices, to improve population health outcomes and support achieving public health goals Maaß et al., (2024). The complexity is explained more in detail in Chapter "Why Is It Essential to Address Digital Public Health in an Interdisciplinary Way?" in this handbook. The main goal of DiPH is to leverage technology to create more effective, efficient, and sustainable healthcare systems. This involves harnessing data, digitizing processes, and creating digital solutions that can help to identify and address public health challenges, improve (access to) health services, support health decision-making for health promotion, and improve patient outcomes (Barros et al. 2019; van Kessel et al. 2022a; World Health Organization 2021a).

Health systems globally undergo various digital transformations as technology and data increasingly play a crucial role in monitoring, understanding, and addressing public health challenges (Kraus et al. 2021). Digital technologies in public health have become increasingly widespread in recent years as countries aim to improve health outcomes, increase efficiency, and enhance the quality of health services (Odone et al. 2019). These digital transformations have been driven by various factors, including the need to reduce healthcare costs, improve patient outcomes, and increase the efficiency of healthcare systems (Barros et al. 2019). As a result of technological advancements, health and social care providers are increasingly relying on digital tools and platforms to improve the quality of care and make it more accessible to patients (Cordeiro 2021). At the same time, the proliferation of digital technologies in societies at large have given rise to a myriad of health challenges that stem from the digital world, such as problematic internet use, dark commercial patterns, and misinformation (van Kessel et al. 2025).

According to the European Observatory on Health Systems and Policies, the COVID-19 pandemic response in Europe accelerated the adoption and implementation of digital health tools that influenced healthcare delivery and public health activities. Primarily, countries invested in communication and information systems, monitoring and surveillance, supporting the provision of health services, and vaccination programs supported through digital tools. However, European countries were positioned quite differently at the start of the pandemic, with only some having good digital health integration in their healthcare systems. In contrast, others had either an incomplete development in that area (such as having the technical infrastructure but with relatively restrictive regulations) or no integration at all (Fahy et al. 2021).

Even after the crisis portion of the pandemic was officially declared over in 2023, DiPH is being considered a critical strategy for addressing Europe's challenges, including aging populations, chronic diseases, and limited healthcare resources (Wong et al. 2022). Many European countries have made substantial investments in digital technologies to improve the delivery of healthcare services, several of which are at the forefront of digital public health and digital transformation of health (Barros et al. 2019; Digital Europe 2022). In recent years, telemedicine and EHRs have been two of the most commonly implemented interventions in European healthcare systems. Telemedicine refers to using technology, such as video conferencing and remote monitoring, to provide healthcare services to patients who cannot access care in person. This has proven particularly useful during the COVID-19 pandemic, in rural or underserved areas, and with patients with mobility issues, as it allows them to receive care remotely (Butzner and Cuffee 2021). EHRs, on the other hand, are digital versions of a patient's medical history, which healthcare providers can access to help them make more informed patient care decisions. EHRs have been shown to improve patient safety and diagnosis accuracy and reduce the time spent on administrative tasks (Manca 2015; Menachemi and Collum 2011). Other digital technologies are also being used to transform European healthcare systems; these include Artificial Intelligence (AI) to analyze and monitor medical, demographic, behavioral, and environmental data (Panteli et al. 2025), generate content and communicate risks (Mahl et al. 2025). Additionally, digital technologies for public health are used as wearable devices and mobile apps that allow healthcare providers and patients to monitor their (patients') health and wellness (Butryn et al. 2021; Zia et al. 2022).

Digital technologies generate vast amounts of data, which can be applied to monitoring individual health-related parameters, identifying risk factors, and evaluating the effectiveness of public health interventions. This data can also be used to develop personalized health plans and support evidence-based decision-making by public health officials. Algorithms and Machine earning can help healthcare providers and epidemiologists identify patterns and trends in the health data of patients or populations, enabling them to predict and prevent potential health issues or conduct surveillance on ommunicable and non-communicable diseases (Fahy et al. 2021).

Another essential goal of DiPH in Europe is to improve the accessibility of healthcare services, particularly in rural and underserved areas, as the internet and, by extension, digital (public) health is not currently equally accessible to everyone (van Kessel et al. 2022b; World Health Organization 2022). Digital technologies can connect patients with healthcare providers, allowing for remote consultations and care management. This can significantly reduce barriers to care, such as long distances and transportation difficulties, and helps ensure all individuals have access to high-quality healthcare services. In addition to improving access to care and leveraging data and analytics, DiPH in Europe also focuses on empowering individuals to manage their health. This can be achieved through mobile health (mHealth) applications and wearable devices, which can provide individuals with access to real-time health information and support them in making healthier lifestyle choices (Lavallee et al. 2020). Besides using digital technologies to improve diagnosis and treatment, European countries also started to apply DiPH in health promotion and prevention settings. These interventions fit best under "technology-supported lifestyle behavioral interventions" as defined by Parati et al. (2019). Such projects range from remote blood pressure measurement to behavior monitoring, health education, motivational support, reduction of isolation, and prolonged independent living (Parati et al. 2019; De Santis et al. 2023). However, so far, there is no substantial extension towards setting-based health promotion, tackling structural and upstream health determinants.

However, digital transformation in the public health sector has challenges, especially from a governance and data security point of view: digitally vulnerable groups are at greater risk of being on the wrong side of the digital divide and, therefore, should be placed at the center of digital transformations and developments in health across the region (van Kessel et al. 2022a, c; Organisation for Economic Co-operation and Development 2022a). As more and more sensitive health information is collected and stored digitally, it is essential to have robust security measures in place to protect this data from unauthorized access and misuse. Additionally, there are concerns about the potential for digital technologies to create new inequalities as a result of haphazard implementation or suboptimal regulatory and reimbursement frameworks (van Kessel et al. 2022b, d; Holly et al. 2023).

This chapter will explore the current state of DiPH in Europe and examine the key trends, challenges, and opportunities in this rapidly evolving field. We will highlight essential European regulations and initiatives influencing DiPH, such as the General Data Protection Regulation (GDPR) or the European Health Data Space (EHDS). Through country case studies, we aim to offer a deeper understanding of the role of digital technologies and healthcare systems' transformations in shaping the future of public health in Europe.

2 The Digital Public Health Playing Field in Europe

2.1 The General Data Protection Regulation: An Enabler or a Barrier to Digital Public Health?

Personal health data flows play a central role in the development of DiPH. The cornerstone of the European Union's (EU) data governance framework is the GDPR (European Union 2016a). The GDPR harmonized data protection across the EU and sought to balance the increased protection and empowerment of data subjects with enhancing the circulation of personal data. In pursuing these objectives, it conferred new rights (e.g., the "right to be forgotten"), highlighted the responsibility and accountability of data controllers and processors throughout the data lifecycle, and set the conditions for the processing of sensitive personal data, including health data (Marelli and Testa 2018). Of particular interest to public health is the secondary processing of health data, where the GDPR requires either the acquisition of explicit (expanded) consent or arguing that the processing is performed in the public interest for the production of statistics while adhering to the principle of data minimization (e.g., pseudonymization), or for scientific research (European Union 2016b).

However, the scope of the GDPR may be insufficient to protect against potentially harmful practices emerging in developing digital infrastructures and products for welfare and healthcare (Kostkova 2018; Kuntsman et al. 2019; van Zoonen 2020). This challenge is exemplified by four tensions (Marelli et al. 2020):

1. data minimization versus Big Data, where the data requirements for training predictive algorithms are at odds with the principles of purpose limitation and data minimization enshrined in the GDPR;
2. sensitive versus non-sensitive data, where the linkage of datasets unrelated to health (e.g., lifestyle data) or pseudonymized datasets (e.g., genetic data) afford the ability to infer health status or the identity of a data subject;
3. active, informed consent versus passive acquiescence, where the data subjects provide consent without much thought after being presented with complex terms of service or faced with steep social costs for non-consent and non-use of a digital platform; and
4. the promise versus the peril of predictive analytics, where the GDPR provides little recourse against algorithmic bias.

In this case, the GDPR is "a stepping stone, pointing towards the need to evolve data protection beyond the old paradigm, yet not fully committed to doing so" (Mayer-Schönberger and Padova 2016). In particular, the GDPR seems unable to contend with the rapid expansion of the digital (public) health ecosystem. Nowadays, this includes large transnational corporations with the ability to collect a broad range of datasets and use them to construct powerful (if not always beneficent) digital tools (Marelli et al. 2020). Suggestions for a remedy range from a fundamental reconsideration of the value of greater precision in service provision (Prainsack 2020) through a greater empowering of the data subject, i.e., patient, consumer, or citizen, through emphasizing co-creation (Muller et al. 2021) and decentralizing data stewardship (Janssen et al. 2020), to a more rigorous treatment of predictive analytics in future regulation (Buiten 2019; Mühlhoff 2021).

2.2 Regulations on Mobile Medical Devices in the European Union

Health data collected via personal medical devices can be exempted from GDPR in the case of public health and scientific research interest. Yet, the rules for such data collection and processing are not harmonized among the EU member states (Minssen 2022). To support member states in improving health data quality, discoverability, and regulation, the European Medicines Agency and the Heads of Medicines Agencies Big Data Task Force recommend establishing a cross-EU platform for accessing and analyzing health care data in a decentralized manner: The Data Analysis and Real World Interrogation Network (Grundy et al. 2019; Mulder 2019). This platform could also help to improve the legislation supporting the collection and processing of health data, as well as review systems and processes related to medical devices in EU countries (Minssen 2022).

Another problematic area related to health data handling can be seen across most mHealth apps in the EU, which neither provide users with privacy policy information nor enable them to withdraw consent and delete their health data (European Union 2016c). As a potential solution, app stores, which are currently not regulated under the GDPR, could conduct a form of self-regulation by translating GDPR privacy provisions into pre-approval requirements for app developers (European Union Agency For Network and Information Security 2018; Fong 2017). The project *Label2Enable*, funded through Europe Horizon by the EU, developed a health app quality assessment framework in the form of an International Organization for Standardization certificate. App developers can assess their products individually among the criteria of *healthy and safe*, *easy to use*, *secure data*, and *robust build* (Hoogendoorn 2023). However, the integration of this framework in the design process of health apps is currently not enforced, meaning it is up to the developers to choose whether to use it.

In October 2020, Germany was the first to regulate digital health applications (DiGA) as mobile medical devices. Since 2021, digital care applications (DiPA) have been available in the German healthcare market, though the uptake of DiGAs in clinical practices has arguably been lackluster (Schmidt et al. 2024a). Following a preliminary registration phase of usually one year, during which they can already be marketed, these medical apps must prove their effectiveness through randomized controlled trials (RCT) to be prescribed by physicians and reimbursed by health insurance. Further, applying developers need to provide robust data protection frameworks in their applications to secure user data (Federal Institute for Drugs and Medical Devices Germany 2023a). Nevertheless, discussions in the scientific community arise about whether RCTs' tightly framed study design is suitable for the fast-changing digital environment (Guo et al. 2020). By allowing healthcare providers to prescribe medical apps, patients can be directed to specific, clinically-validated apps that have been shown to improve outcomes for particular conditions. This can help ensure that patients use safe, effective, and appropriate apps for their needs. The regulation of medical apps such as DiGA and DiPA can serve as quality labels in addition to the *Label2Enable* (Maaß et al. 2022). The reimbursement of DiGA and DiPA can further reduce the financial burden for patients who might otherwise struggle to afford digital health solutions. This can improve access to digital health offers for vulnerable populations and help to ensure that everyone can benefit from the potential advantages of digitalization (Wangler and Jansky 2022). However, whether these potentials materialize is unclear, given the small number of DiGA and DiPA and the limited coverage of health topics. Since 2020, regulating medical apps as medical devices was also implemented in France (Della Vecchia et al. 2022).

2.3 Towards the European Health Data Space

In 2011, the EU passed the *Cross-Border Healthcare Directive* (2011/24/EU) to promote cooperation on healthcare between member states and facilitate access to safe and high-quality cross-border healthcare. Of particular relevance to DiPH, the directive aimed to create an EU-wide network of national authorities responsible for electronic health (eHealth) to facilitate the voluntary exchange of health information among member states, including patient summaries (European Union 2011). In combination, these efforts led to the creation of the eHealth Digital Service Infrastructure (eHDSI), also known as the *MyHealth@EU* platform, enabling cross-country exchange of patient summaries and electronic prescriptions (ePrescriptions) since 2019 (European Court of Auditors 2019). However, the voluntary nature of participation in the data exchange platform, combined with weak demand, has led to the involvement of only ten member states by the end of 2022 (Marcus et al. 2022).

In 2025, the Regulation on the EHDS was ratified, which provides a new framework for sharing and using health data across the EU (European Commission 2025). Spurred by the COVID-19 pandemic and the data challenges faced, this regulation was the culmination of a significant political movement as part of the European Strategy of Data (European Commission 2025b), one of which was health. Once fully implemented, the EHDS Regulation will help EU member states to:

1. Support individuals to take control of their health data
2. Support the use of health data for better healthcare delivery, better research, innovation, and policy-making
3. Enable the EU to make full use of the potential offered by a safe and secure exchange, including the use and reuse of health data (European Commission 2025a).

The EHDS regulation builds on existing EU legislation, such as the Data Act and the Data Governance Act, which provide the legal framework for collecting, processing, and sharing personal data. The AI Act also plays a role alongside the EHDS regulation. It provides a regulatory framework within which AI can be used ethically in the EU, including for the purpose of healthcare (Schmidt et al. 2024b). The interplay between these different pieces of legislation are crucial in ensuring that the EHDS can effectively facilitate the sharing of health data and are actively being worked on during the writing of this chapter.

2.4   Equitable Access to Digital Public Health in Europe

The COVID-19 pandemic has demonstrated the transformative potential of DiPH to revolutionize healthcare by leveraging technology for the mass-scale collection, analysis, and dissemination of health data and provision of health services, irrespective of geographic location (Murray et al. 2020). However, it also highlighted some novel threats to human health (Catalani et al. 2023, van Kessel et al. 2025). As it stands, the benefits of DiPH are not equally distributed among Europe, and there remain substantial challenges for public health policy and practice to ensure that all European populations have equitable access to DiPH and can meaningfully harness its benefits (Wong et al. 2022; World Health Organization 2022). Various drivers, such as patterns in access, use, and engagement with digital technologies, vary across populations, regions, and countries (van Kessel et al. 2023a, b), while being important determinants for accessing data and digital technologies (van Kessel et al. 2023c). For instance, digital health technologies are generally more widely used in urban areas, while they are less used by those from ethnic minorities and those facing language barriers (World Health Organization 2022). As such, it will be crucial to balance investment in empowering populations with high levels of access to DiPH with allocating resources to people with limited access to level the playing field. Additionally, digital health literacy is another important issue that needs attention. This is further discussed in Chapter "Digital Health Literacy", Zeeb and Dratva in this handbook.

Among the populations with high levels of access to and use of technologies and internet connectivity, investment in digital infrastructure and capacity can enable them to benefit from improved health outcomes and reduced healthcare costs (Asian Development Bank 2018; van Kessel et al. 2022b). For example, telemedicine can help people with chronic conditions manage their health more effectively (Corbett et al. 2020; Ma et al. 2022), while remote monitoring can help patients with chronic diseases avoid hospitalization (National Health Service England 2023; Peyroteo et al. 2021; Taylor et al. 2021). Digital health technologies can also help improve women's empowerment and gender equality by facilitating skills acquisition, health education, and social interaction, while allowing cost-effective health services (Borges do Nascimento et al. 2025). Additionally, investment in DiPH can help support the development of new and innovative health technologies, which can be scaled and applied in different contexts to benefit other populations (Labrique et al. 2018).

Creating equitable DiPH systems requires a balanced allocation of resources. While increasing investment for high-access populations can improve health outcomes and reduce costs, achieving social justice in Europe hinges on ensuring DiPH access for all. To ensure that no one is left behind in the digital era, it is crucial to bridge divides to avoid creating DiPH systems that exacerbate existing healthcare inequalities (Ibrahim et al. 2021). Therefore, pursuing health equity should guide the design of digital health ecosystems to prevent the deepening of existing health inequalities (van Kessel et al. 2022c).

Nevertheless, many European populations, particularly those in rural and remote areas, still lack sufficient access to technology and the Internet (Gomes & Dias 2024). Resources must be allocated to building digital infrastructure, enhancing digital literacy, and training health workers to address this digital divide. For example, investment in digital infrastructure can extend healthcare services to remote and rural areas where traditional health services are limited or non-existent. Building digital literacy can help ensure all populations have the skills and knowledge to use DiPH effectively. Training health workers can help them deliver quality care through DiPH. The case studies in the subsequent section will shed light on the current state of DiPH in different European countries.

3 Examples of Digital Public Health in Europe by Country

This section will highlight selected DiPH initiatives before and during the COVID-19 pandemic for seven European countries and provide future perspectives for DiPH in these countries (see Fig. 1). The selected countries represent Europe's big and small states as well as those with higher and lower gross domestic products per capita. Additionally, the comparison includes countries from the west to the east of the European continent, but also representatives from the EU (every country but the United Kingdom) or Organisation for Economic Co-operation and Development (OECD) member states (every country but Malta).

According to the Global Digital Health Monitor (GDHM), all selected countries are on the fourth to fifth overall digital health phase (Global Digital Health Monitor 2023). The GDHM is an interactive digital resource that tracks, monitors, and evaluates the use of digital technology for health across countries. It scores countries based on 23 indicators through seven domains:

1. Leadership and governance
2. Strategy and investment
3. Legislation, policy and compliance
4. Workforce
5. Standards and interoperability
6. Infrastructure
7. Services and applications

It then classifies countries (overall and in each domain) into phases of development (phase 5 being the most advanced). However, only the first three categories and the overall rating provided data for the majority of the selected countries and are displayed in Table 1.

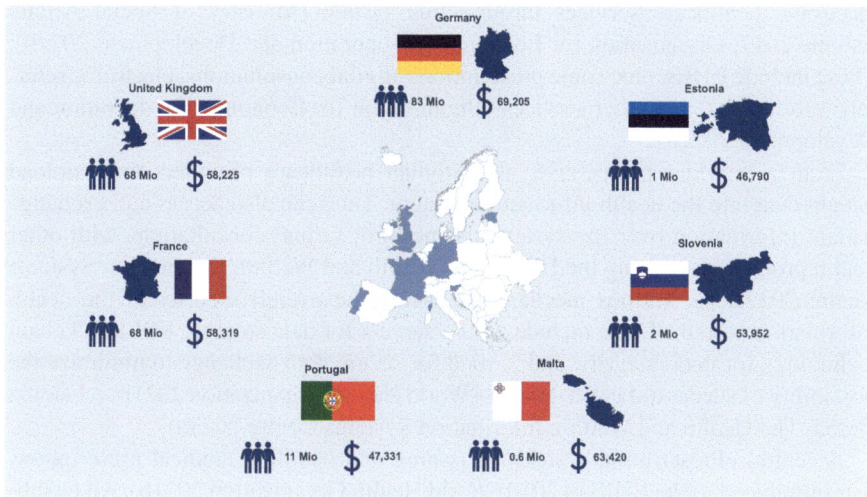

Fig. 1 Included countries with population and 2023 gross domestic product per capita as purchasing power parity in US$. (Source: own figure based on World Bank 2023)

Table 1 Included countries' rating according to the Global Digital Health Monitor (2023)

Country	Score			
	Overall	Legislation, policy and compliance	Infrastructure	Leadership and Governance
Estonia	Phase 5	Phase 5	Phase 4	Phase 5
France	Phase 5	Phase 5	Phase 5	Phase 5
Germany	Phase 5	Phase 5	Phase 5	Phase 5
Malta	Phase 4	Phase 4	Phase 4	Phase 4
Portugal	Phase 5	Phase 5	Phase 5	Phase 5
Slovenia	Phase 5	Phase 5	Phase 4	Phase 4
United Kingdom	Phase 5	Phase 4	Phase 5	Phase 5

(Source: own figure using data from the Global Digital Health Monitor (2023))

3.1 Estonia

The Estonian National Health Information System (EHIS) was launched in 2008 (The Health and Welfare Information Systems Centre 2023a). One part of EHIS, the Patient Portal, enables patients to access their health records, book medical appointments, use digital referrals, sign declarations of intent, and more (Merimaa and Vanker 2020; The Health and Welfare Information Systems Centre 2023a, b). Estonians can access this portal through the well-established ID-card-based infrastructure. More than 96% of all Estonians can securely access various electronic healthcare services through this system (Ministry of Social Affairs Estonia 2017; Organisation for Economic Co-operation and Development 2022b). These include EHRs, electronic prescriptions, digital consultations, electronic referrals (eReferrals), and other services (Organisation for Economic Co-operation and Development 2022a).

From a provider perspective, all Estonian healthcare providers must upload patient data into the health information system. They can also access and exchange patient information over the system and perform virtual consultations with other health professionals using the EHIS (The Health and Welfare Information Systems Centre 2023a, b). Various mechanisms ensure the overall security of the health information system. These include secure servers for data storage, KSI Blockchain technology for data integrity, and X-road for secure data exchange to minimize the possibility of successful cyber-attacks (World Health Organization 2021b; e-Estonia 2025a; The Health and Welfare Information Systems Centre 2023a).

A central ePrescription system for issuing and handling medical prescriptions was introduced to the EHIS in 2010 (World Health Organization 2021b). All healthcare providers and pharmacies are connected to this system. It is designed to be user-friendly, automatically accounts for reimbursements, and enables users to see prescription histories and issue repeat prescriptions in just a few clicks (World Health Organization 2021b; e-Estonia 2025b).

The existing digital infrastructure in Estonia enabled a timely response to the COVID-19 pandemic. At the pandemic's start, Estonia started allowing ePrescriptions to be issued via phone calls between doctors and patients. It quickly increased the range of digital consultations leading to 46% of Estonians reporting teleconsultations during the COVID-19 pandemic, compared with a 39% EU average (World Health Organization 2021b; Organisation for Economic Co-operation and Development and European Observatory on Health Systems and Policies 2021). Estonia was also among the first countries to issue the EU digital COVID-19 passport (Schengenvisa 2021).

On a European level, Estonia strongly collaborates with other countries to enable Europeans to obtain prescription medication anywhere in Europe. Since 2019, the ePrescription system has allowed Estonian and Finnish patients to retrieve electronically prescribed medicine from pharmacies in the respective neighboring country (European Commission 2022). The system has since expanded through collaboration with Croatia, Portugal, Poland, Spain, Greece, Lithuania, Latvia, and the Czech Republic, with additional EU countries expected to join in the near future (Estonian Health Insurance 2025). In addition to the ePrescription services, Estonia actively contributes to the cross-EU eHDSI. The country has a reciprocal patient health data exchange system with Portugal and a one-way agreement where doctors from France and Luxembourg can consult the health data of Estonians. The aim is to roll out electronic cross-border health services in 25 EU countries by 2025 (European Commission 2023; Kivi 2023). Additionally, in October 2020, Estonia and the World Health Organization announced they are working together on various DiPH projects related to vaccination cards, ePrescriptions, electronic dispensing systems, and the *European Roadmap for the Digitalization of National Healthcare Systems* (World Health Organization 2020).

The future development goals for eHealth in Estonia entail multiple targets linked to primary prevention and technological development. An important focus area is personalized medicine, supported by digital public health research with genetic data from the Estonian biobank. The aim is to improve primary disease prevention via population risk screening combining genetic and electronic health data for identifying individuals with high genetic risk for conditions such as breast cancer or cardiovascular disease (Viigimaa et al. 2022; Estonian Health Insurance News 2024; University of Tartu 2023). Estonia is also focused on further improving the security aspects of exchanging health data, establishing legal frameworks to support health data used for public health research, improving data collection quality, and decreasing healthcare inequities (European Union 2015; Foresight Centre 2020). The launch of the updated Health Portal in November 2023 represents a major step forward- laying the foundation for a future where every Estonian citizen can seamlessly engage with their health data and benefit from more equitable, data-driven care (Estonian Health Insurance 2024).

3.2 France

In France, digital health governance is shared across several administrative bodies, such as the *Digital Health Delegation* and the *Digital Health Agency* (Ministry of Health and Prevention France 2022a, b, 2023a, b). The *Digital Health Delegation*, an entity attached to the Ministry of Health, has created a comprehensive roadmap to develop and implement digital health solutions and projects across the national healthcare landscape (Ministry of Health and Prevention France 2022b).

The *Ségur du Numérique en Santé* program, funded by a two billion EUR investment from the European Recovery and Resilience Fund, aims to promote flexible and secure health data sharing between health professionals and patients for improved prevention and treatment (Ministry of Health and Prevention France 2023c). This program is being implemented through the roll-out of the national digital health platform *Mon Espace Santé* (Mon espace santé 2021). *Mon Espace Santé* offers patients a secure online portal for accessing their health records, including lab results, imaging, and ePrescriptions, as well as direct communication with healthcare professionals via the secure messaging service *MSSanté* (Mailiz 2023). So far, however, many challenges have hindered the platform's wide adoption, including a reluctance among clinicians to use the platform due to its time-consuming nature, lack of compatibility with existing patient record systems, and data privacy and security concerns among patients.

However, France has made notable progress in collecting and analyzing health data at a national level. Implementing a National Health ID (Identifiant National de Santé) for all patients in 2021 has enabled healthcare professionals and organizations to exchange health data more easily. Additionally, a single platform, *Pro Santé Connect*, was established to identify registered healthcare professionals and allows them to access all national digital health services, such as patient records, enhancing the security and efficiency of access to patient data (Ministry of Health and Prevention France 2023b). The country has also established a *Health Data Hub*, a centralized infrastructure to collect and make health data accessible for clinical and medical research purposes. The hub provides public health authorities with a comprehensive view of the population's health status, identifying emerging health trends and facilitating effective responses to public health threats (Health Data Hub 2023). Building upon its advancements in those domains, France contributed to the progress of the EHDS initiative during the country's presidency of the European Council. This included the national adoption of the *Systematized Nomenclature of Medicine - Clinical Terms* framework and the harmonization of European evaluation criteria for assessing digital medical devices (Ministerial Delegation for Digital Health France 2022).

During the COVID-19 pandemic, the implementation of the *Système d'information national de suivi du dépistage COVID-19* laid down the foundations of a more robust digital surveillance system (Clinisys 2023). Since 2021, genomic surveillance systems of COVID-19 variants, vaccination tracking, and database pairings have helped improve epidemic monitoring and serve as a model for future surveillance efforts (Santé Publique France 2022a). To further support oversight, France developed *Géodes,* an online platform that aggregates and visualizes various indicators collected by *Santé Publique France* through surveys and surveillance systems. It presents the data in an accessible format, including interactive maps, tables, and graphs (Santé Publique France 2023).

Additionally, France has leveraged digital tools to monitor and manage infections and epidemics through the *e-Sin* application (Santé Publique France 2021a). The app streamlines internal reporting processes and transmits data on outbreaks of antibiotic-resistant bacteria to the regional Support Centers for the Prevention of Nosocomial Infections (CPIAS) and regional health agencies. The CPIAS provide expertise to the facilities and to the regional health agencies, allowing for rapid implementation of measures to prevent further spread. The data submitted through the platform is also compiled and analyzed nationally by *Santé Publique France*. It may trigger national alerts and be shared with the national research centers as part of a nationwide alert system (Santé Publique France 2021a).

Finally, *Santé Publique France* leverages digital technology and the internet to communicate health promotion and prevention messages. The agency disseminates information on healthy behaviors and health risks through online platforms. In line with the national health strategy, the agency sets specific prevention and health promotion aims for each life stage and uses national data to monitor progress against those objectives. In 2021, for example, the agency launched the digital campaign *en parler, c'est déjà se soigner* to address mental health among young people. The campaign provides various digital tools, including a website, phone line, and online chat to facilitate access to mental health resources and foster community among individuals facing similar challenges (Santé Publique France 2021b).

3.3 Germany

The healthcare system in Germany is complex and decentralized, with different levels of government and various stakeholders involved. An example of this problem was the initiation of the organization *gematik* which should have supposedly formed the digital infrastructure since 2004. The organization was owned by the major stakeholders of the German healthcare system, all with different interests and agendas. This resulted in postponed deadlines for implementing the infrastructure for digital healthcare services (Schmitz 2019). In 2019, the federal government took over the *gematik* (§291a Sozialgesetzbuch 5 2022). The government decision to expand the *gematik* to the national digital agency for health from 2024 is currently on hold as the Digital-Agency-for-Health-Act did not pass the final vote before re-elections in 2025.

The national health portal (*gesund.bund.de*) started in 2020. It was an evidence-based open-access website run by governmental health institutes. The portal intended to inform citizens on various health- and disease-related topics and informs users about digital health tools in Germany, like EHRs, DiGA, and telemedicine. The aim was to empower patients to actively engage in their treatment, improve patient health literacy and competencies and foster patient sovereignty (gesund.bund.de 2023). However with only 12 million estimated visitors per year, it remains debatable whether or not the portal has any impact on the health of the German population.

The introduction of DiGA put Germany back on the international digital health playing field. These apps could benefit the healthcare system as treatment alternatives and support. By allowing healthcare providers to prescribe medical apps, patients can be directed to specific, clinically-validated apps that have been shown to potentially improve outcomes for particular conditions (Maaß et al. 2022). Since their introduction in 2020 and until 31 December 2024, 861 thousand app prescriptions have been used (with nearly 400 thousand in 2024 alone). This corresponds to the activation of 81% of all app codes prescribed in total during the same timespan. Even in 2025, there has been no single DiPA approved for reimbursement. One third each of all used DiGA referred to mental health and metabolic diseases which also represent the areas with the most available DiGA. Over 70% of all app users are female and between 30-50 years old (National Association of Statutory Health Insurance Funds 2025). From a prescriber's perspective, however, until the end of 2023, 44% of all healthcare professionals (including physicians and therapists) had never prescribed a DiGA and only 26% had prescribed at least 6 DiGA in the last 12 months (Grobe et al. 2024). A study published in 2022 presented concerns among primary physicians in regards to data protection (61%) and doubts regarding the effectivity (59%). However, physicians also named doubts in patient motivation to use the apps, unavailability of testing options for the practitioners, high bureaucratic and organizational burdens, insufficient information material, and technical problems as barriers to the deployment of DiGA (Obermann 2022). The low support for DiGA from the side of healthcare professionals could limit the effect these apps could have on the German healthcare system.

EHRs have been available in Germany since 2021 (Ministry of Health Germany 2019). Since the implementation of an opt-out-procedure in January 2025, the health insurances must offer an EHR to all insured persons who have not objected (Ministry of Health Germany 2025). Theoretically, citizens shall be able to use their EHR for all healthcare provided in hospitals or by ambulatory practicing physicians as well as pharmacies. As of April 2025, this was possible for one quarter of all healthcare providers and 50 million EHRs had been opened by mid-May 2025 (Gematik 2025). An EHR data donation, as decided by each record owner, for public health research will potentially be available from 2026 (Techniker Health Insurance 2025).

The *Health Data Lab*, founded in 2019, grants researchers access to secondary data based on health insurance claims data of all people with statutory health insurance in Germany for public health research in 2025. This includes data on diagnoses, prescribes medication, and information on inpatient hospital stays among other data. Additionally, data from the EHRs will be added in 2026. The lab assesses the re-identification risk and the intended scientific benefit of each research application before granting access to the data. The goal is to provide data for the long-term evaluation of health conditions and the healthcare system and improve treatment (Federal Institute for Drugs and Medical Devices Germany 2025).

3.4 Malta

The initial wave of digital transformation in healthcare in Malta between 2003 and 2007 was punctuated by the creation of Malta's Integrated Health Information System (IHIS), culminating in a strategic plan established in 2003. Unfortunately, after a lengthy evaluation procedure, the tender for the IHIS had to be discontinued in 2007. Consequently, the government's focus shifted to procuring critical IT systems and services for Mater Dei Hospital. The most crucial among these were the radiology information system, picture archiving and communication system, integrated laboratory information system, order communications system, and a health level 7 interface engine (Muscat et al. 2019).

Mater Dei Hospital's IT systems, which went live concurrently with the launch of the hospital in late 2007, were initially exclusive to Mater Dei Hospital. However, due to the structure of Malta's public health service, these systems needed to be extended to other government hospitals and health centers to enable the health service to function as well as possible. This extension took several years but ultimately established a nationwide health IT network. Consequently, the period from the late 2000s was characterized by the need to narrow the information gap between the public and private health sectors (Mongin-Bulewski 2008). In response, the Maltese government introduced the *myHealth* portal, providing patients and doctors with access to specific medical records (Malta Information Technology Agency 2023).

The first version of *myHealth*, launched in 2012, offered access to case summaries, lab test results, and medical imaging reports, among other data. The uptake of this service was initially limited due to security constraints requiring national e-ID credentials. However, with the overhaul of the national e-ID system in 2014–2015 and the issuance of new national ID cards, the uptake of the *myHealth* service began to increase. This was further boosted by releasing a new, mobile-friendly version of *myHealth* in 2017, including additional data sources such as vaccinations. By September 2018, 50,000 patients had connected with doctors through *myHealth*, marking it as one of the government's most successful online services (Agius 2018).

In 2016, the Ministry for Health initiated work on a suite of national eHealth services to further its digital healthcare ambitions. These services were incorporated into the government's *Connected eGovernment* project to unite multiple IT service applications under one umbrella. This project, co-financed by the European Regional Development Fund, included initiatives like National Electronic Health Records, Electronic Patient Records for Primary Health Care, Health Data Exchange, Patient Registries, Patient Data Consent Management System, and the Pharmaceutical Affairs System (Malta Information Technology Agency 2017).

In parallel to these national developments, Malta also engaged in cross-border eHealth initiatives. After successful participation in the second phase of the *Smart Open Services for European Patients* project from 2011–2014 (European Commission 2017), the Ministry for Health secured funds from the *Connecting Europe Facility* for implementing and deploying cross-border patient summary services. These services targeted to support EU citizens needing unscheduled health care while traveling in EU countries and went live in December 2019 and has been followed by the EU-funded mheme project in April 2025 to facilitate healthcare for citizens traveling abroad or living in Malta (Government of Malta 2025).

The COVID-19 Pandemic in Malta proved to be a catalyst and empowered the implementation of the COVID-19 Public Health Response Team in the early days of the pandemic. Through this expertise, Malta was one of four out of 27 EU member states to have implemented all four main pillars of the EU Digital response to COVID-19 (European Court of Auditors 2023):

1. a contact tracing app called "COVID Alert Malta" supported by a contact-tracing gateway,
2. a national EU digital passenger locator form,
3. the EU Digital COVID Certificate, and
4. the exchange of international passenger locator forms.

Despite facing the resourcing challenges of a small island state, Malta managed multiple DiPH initiatives. These put open data, data flows, and data automation in the center of the interventions as the COVID-19 operations had to be effectively scaled up and down through numerous national and political events (Ministry of Health Malta 2023a). Eventually, a COVID-19 result submission portal was implemented. It was supported by federal legislation and linked to the official COVID-19 Test, Track and Trace System supported by cloud-based customer relationship management systems (Ministry of Health Malta 2020).

Social media related to federal health authorities and the Ministry for Health also significantly boosted, reaching more than 116,000 followers over two years (Ministry of Health Malta 2023b). The community played an intrinsic role in developing health services throughout the COVID-19 pandemic. A national Telemedicine Centre was set up, supported by *Primary HealthCare*, and centralized all healthcare-related communications directed towards primary care. This center also had a critical role in overseeing the health of thousands of COVID-19 patients, with more than 200,000 online consultations in two years (Calleja 2021).

The future of digitalization in Malta looks bright with the recent launch of the *Malta National Healthcare Systems Strategy 2023–2030*. The strategy strongly emphasizes digitalization supported with a planned concrete deliverable and governance through developing a multi-sectorial digital health steering committee.

The utilization of digital health services in Malta, particularly the national patient portal, myHealth, saw a significant surge during the COVID-19 pandemic. The portal, which gives citizens and patients secure online access to their health data, experienced a threefold increase in usage. This surge reflects the growing desire among the Maltese population for increased online engagement with health services. Indeed, research indicates a widespread wish to evolve *myHealth* into a singular, comprehensive, patient-centric portal for all online interactions with healthcare providers (Ministry of Health Malta 2022).

3.5 Portugal

Portugal's health sector has been considered one of the national digital transformation agenda priorities during the last decade. Gradually, a process of healthcare digitalization made digital prescriptions the norm for medication and diagnostic tests (clinicians must provide a specific justification if they intend to print a prescription on paper). Other examples of digitalization included the migration from a paper-based system of epidemiological surveillance to EHRs and digital systems (Rachadell 2021).

However, different degrees of digital transformation must be noted. In some areas, digitalization was limited to directly transferring a paper-based system to a digital strategy, as with the national epidemiologic surveillance system (SINAVE). The original version of the system was based on paper forms that had to be physically sent through a sequential hierarchy of health authorities. In contrast, the digital version consisted of the same process but with digital documents, which conferred some advantages in accountability, data analysis capabilities, and overall system speed. In other areas, the digital transformation has included the digitalization of existing processes and the use of new technologies to reinvent and improve old procedures, as is the case with the implementation of EHRs in Portugal. Though the initial process was a direct transfer from a paper-based health records system to an EHR system, the new design showed advantages in information availability and accessibility. For instance, all the patient's information was now centralized in the same online repository, which can be accessed by healthcare professionals, including medical doctors, nurses, and public health authorities. However, subsequent system iterations have changed how patient information is managed. Presently, citizens can log in to their national healthcare system account and control access to their health information. They can decide which healthcare professionals should be granted access and if they want to be notified when their information is accessed (Diáro Da República Eletrónico 2009, 2013, 2014; Ministry of Health Portugal 2023).

The COVID-19 pandemic accelerated the digital health transformation already underway in Portugal. The need for large-scale contact tracing capabilities in epidemiologic surveillance exposed some limitations in the previous digital SINAVE. This led to the development of a new system geared explicitly towards COVID-19 control (TraceCOVID-19). The most recent iteration of the system changed several processes that had not been altered during the implementation of the first digital version. The latest system automatically connected numerous healthcare databases, including laboratory results for COVID-19 tests. Further, it allowed for the automatic issuance of health declarations by public health authorities. Lastly, it encouraged the participation of citizens in their surveillance through a COVID-19 telemonitoring system based on auto-reported symptoms. This last feature changed the process of epidemiologic surveillance in Portugal. It is no longer a unidirectional path through a hierarchy of public health authorities but an interactive process incorporating citizens' feedback. For instance, TraceCOVID-19 would notify medical doctors if patients report specific symptoms (Serviços Partilhados do Ministério da Saúde 2021). As this system was used specifically for the pandemic response, it is no longer in widespread use. Instead, Portugal went back to using SINAVE as its main system for epidemiological surveillance.

Portugal continues to prioritize the digital transformation of its healthcare system, most recently through the National Ecosystem of Health Information Strategy. The strategy delineates a shared vision for the Portuguese healthcare system, including the national healthcare system and all healthcare stakeholders (Serviços Partilhados do Ministério da Saúde 2019).

3.6 Slovenia

Digitalization of the Slovene healthcare system began in the mid-2000s with the publication of the *eHealth 2010* strategic document (Ministry of Health of the Republic of Slovenia 2005). However, it was not until 2016 that the digitalization process gained significant momentum (Stanimirović and Matetić 2020). This coincides with adopting the *Resolution on the National Health Care Plan 2016–2025* (Official Gazette of the Republic of Slovenia 2016) and the conclusion of the pilot phase of the eHealth project (Ministry of Health Slovenia 2021). These developments resulted in a unified health data infrastructure that links various health databases and telemedicine services. The system includes the Central Registry of Patient

Data (CRPD), ePrescriptions, electronic appointments and eReferrals, electronic triage, teleradiology, and monitoring for stroke patients (National Institute of Public Health of the Republic of Slovenia 2023).

There was a significant level of digitalization in healthcare and public health in Slovenia even before the COVID-19 pandemic. More than 90% of all prescriptions and referrals were created using the eHealth infrastructure in 2019, while the number of documents stored in the CRPD increased fivefold since 2016 to encompass specialist reports, microbiology reports, discharge letters, ambulatory exam reports, vaccinations, and other patient records (Stanimirović and Matetić 2020). A governmental analysis indicates that digitalization was associated with approximately 40 million EUR in savings from 2016 to 2018 (Ministry of Public Administration of the Republic of Slovenia 2019).

The built-up eHealth capacity proved to be critical in enabling continuity of care during the pandemic (European Observatory on Health Systems and Policies 2021), with more than 60% of the population consulting their physician or receiving a prescription online or by telephone (Organisation for Economic Co-operation and Development and European Observatory on Health Systems and Policies 2021). The national patient portal (zVEM) played a central role by creating a one-stop shop for health services and information (European Observatory on Health Systems and Policies 2021). This was also enabled by the changes in the reimbursement rules of the national health insurance institute during the pandemic that allowed the reimbursement of teleconsultations (Health Insurance Institute of Slovenia 2021). In addition, most complementary insurance schemes began to offer video call applications allowing patients to connect with a general practitioner (Generali 2022).

Crucial for public health and health research, the current health data infrastructure links various national databases, including national cancer and central population registries. However, gaps remain in the health information system. For example, data from long-term healthcare services are inadequately captured, and there is currently no scope for linkage between health and other sectors like employment (European Observatory on Health Systems and Policies 2021).

The short-term future of digital health in Slovenia will be shaped by the new healthcare digitalization strategy for 2022–27, which the government presented in November 2022 (Ministry of Health of the Republic of Slovenia 2023; Ministry of Health of the Republic of Slovenia and European Commission 2022). Its key objectives include streamlining the governance of eHealth services, infrastructures, and health data, implementing a standardized electronic patient record supporting medical imaging, and creating a national framework for telemedicine. The strategy also aims to enable the secondary use of health data in preparation for participating in the EHDS. Finally, the strategy also foresees greater use of health data to support policy and public health decision-making.

3.7 The United Kingdom

Advancing digital transformation in healthcare has long been a key objective in England. In 2019, the five-year framework for reforming general practitioner (GP) contracts emphasized enabling practices to adopt a digital-first approach through access to medical records and digital prescription services (British Medical Association and National Health Service England 2019). Concurrently, the National Health Service's (NHS) Long-Term Plan, published in the same year, established a target for clinicians to access patient records and granted all patients the right to online GP consultations by 2024 (National Health Service England 2022). Recognizing the necessity for digital transformation beyond the health sector, the United Kingdom (UK) government's white paper on adult social care reform, issued in 2021, allocated £150 million over three years to support digital investment in social care. The document recognized the imperative of enhancing data collection and quality, integrating with NHS systems, and improving internet connectivity in care homes (Department of Health and Social Care United Kingdom 2022).

The COVID-19 pandemic accentuated the need for digital public health, as the NHS track and trace app was swiftly implemented nationwide. The app, which used Bluetooth technology to notify individuals who had come into contact with COVID-19-positive individuals, is estimated to have prevented around one million cases, 44,000 hospitalizations, and 9600 deaths during its first year alone (Kendall et al. 2023). Although integrating digital technologies to advance public health may take longer, it is also an integral part of the national strategy. The 2022 *digital health and social care plan* outlines the rollout of public health digital tools from March 2024–2025 (National Health Service England 2022).

The NHS is a pioneer in collecting health data at the national level. One such example is the *Compendium*, which comprises a collection of indicators that offer a comprehensive understanding of population health at national, regional, and local levels. These indicators are used to compare local areas, understand population health challenges, and examine the impact of factors such as unemployment and education on health inequalities (National Health Service England 2017). A range of other studies have been undertaken nationwide, such as the *National Study of Health and Well-being*, which tracks the mental health and emotional well-being of parents and children over time (National Health Service England 2021), as well as the *What About Youth* survey, which was launched to enhance the health of young people (Ipsos 2015). The nature of the healthcare system facilitates data collection at the national level since all publicly available health services are provided by the NHS trusts, which are overseen by NHS England, a non-departmental body of the Department of Health and Social Care (DHSC).

Health Education England, another body of the DHSC, provides national leadership for the education and training of health and public health professionals in

England. The *e-Learning for Healthcare* platform offers over 150 standardized and quality-assured programs to increase the accessibility and integration of population health information into healthcare practice ((National Health Service Health Education England 2023a). It contains a *Population Well-being Portal*, which covers a wide range of topics from sexual health to tobacco dependence (National Health Service Health Education England 2023b). Interactive learning sessions were developed around *All Our Health*, an evidence framework to guide healthcare professionals in promoting health and preventing illness (Office for Health Improvement and Disparities England 2015). Lastly, the toolkit *Embedding public health into clinical services* aims to support leaders and service managers in redesigning services to prioritize prevention (National Health Service Health Education England 2021).

4 Conclusion

The pandemic response caused the rapid development and scaling of some DiPH solutions. These days, DiPH plays a significant role in determining the health of Europe's population. Digital technologies and AI offer the potential to create new tools and systems to support and improve public health efforts and outcomes across the region. By leveraging these technologies, public health practitioners and policymakers can collect and analyze vast amounts of data, understand public health trends and patterns, and target public health interventions more effectively.

Overall, the case studies discussed in this chapter demonstrate the potential for digital public health to play a transformative role in improving public health outcomes in Europe. For example, Estonia has established a comprehensive national EHR system, while England leveraged digital technologies to enhance public health research efforts. France has taken a comprehensive approach to digital health, focusing on creating a seamless and integrated healthcare system, and Germany was the first country to use medical apps on prescriptions for healthcare. At the same time, Malta has utilized telemedicine to improve access to healthcare for its citizens. Portugal has applied digital technologies to improve its mental health services, while Slovenia has used digital tools to enhance its disease surveillance efforts. So far, all countries have mainly focused on increasing the application of DiPH in healthcare and surveillance. However, more developments in digital health solutions for primary prevention and health promotion are necessary to improve public health across Europe. By continuing to build on these efforts and addressing the challenges and opportunities presented by DiPH, Europe can continue to lead the way in developing innovative and effective public health solutions for the benefit of its citizens.

Despite all these advancements, questions still remain regarding the long-term impact of DiPH tools and interventions in Europe after the COVID-19-related upsurge. Firstly, many digital tools used to support healthcare delivery and public health activities were either completely new or existing solutions that were scaled for the first time in an emergency context. Thus there are still significant gaps in evidence on their impact, efficacy, and cost-effectiveness. Better evidence must be developed to inform future policymakers on digital health tools' added value and implementation. Secondly, although some countries already had a regulatory framework to enable digital health tools, in many cases, the tensions between existing regulations and the need for a quick pandemic response were solved with temporary adaptations. It is yet unknown if digital health tools implemented based on interim legal measures will be restricted once again when the COVID-19 pandemic no longer poses a significant threat. Securing permanent advancements for European - and indeed global - DiPH will require a supportive policy environment that removes barriers to implementation and actively fosters the adoption and expansion of digital health solutions.

References

§291a Sozialgesetzbuch 5 (2022) Elektronische Gesundheitskarte als Versicherungsnachweis und Mittel zur Abrechnung (Electronic health card as proof of insurance and means of billing). BGBl 1, S. 2793. https://dejure.org/gesetze/SGB_V/291a.html

Agius M (2018) Family doctors to get access to patients' hospital records online. Maltatoday. https://www.maltatoday.com.mt/lifestyle/health/89308/new_services_on_myhealth_website_to_make_life_easier_for_doctors_and_patients. Accessed 29 May 2025

Asian Development Bank (2018) Guidance for investing in digital health. In: ADB sustainable development working paper series. Asian Development Bank, Mandaluyong City. https://doi.org/10.22617/WPS179150-2

Borges do Nascimento et al. (2025) https://www.thelancet.com/journals/landig/article/PIIS2589-7500(25)00022-6/fulltext

Barros PP, Bourek A, Brouwer W, Lehtonen L, Barry M, Murauskiene M, Riccardi W, Siciliani L, Wild C, Koch S, Saranto K, European Commission (2019) Assessing the impact of digital transformation of health services. In: Report of the Expert Panel on effective ways of investing in Health (EXPH). Publications Office of the European Union, Luxembourg. https://doi.org/10.2875/644722

British Medical Association, National Health Service England (2019) Investment and evolution: a five-year framework for GP contract reform to implement. The NHS long term plan. NHS England, London

Buiten MC (2019) Towards intelligent regulation of artificial intelligence. Eur J Risk Regul 10(1):41–59. https://doi.org/10.1017/err.2019.8

Butryn B, Chomiak-Orsa I, Hauke K, Pondel M, Siennicka A (2021) Application of machine learning in medical data analysis illustrated with an example of association rules. Procedia Comput Sci 192:3134–3143. https://doi.org/10.1016/j.procs.2021.09.086

Butzner M, Cuffee Y (2021) Telehealth interventions and outcomes across rural communities in the United States: narrative review. J Med Internet Res 23(8):e29575. https://doi.org/10.2196/29575

Calleja C (2021) Doctors hold more than 200,000 online consultations during pandemic. 24/7 Telemedicine service for digital visits with doctors proves popular. Times Malta. https://timesofmalta.com/articles/view/doctors-hold-more-than-200000-online-consultations-during-pandemic.919243. Accessed 29 May 2025

Catalani V, Townshend HD, Prilutskaya M, Roman-Urrestarazu A, van Kessel R, Chilcott RP, Banayoti H, McSweeney T, Corazza O (2023) Profiling the vendors of COVID-19 related product on the Darknet: an observational study. Emerg Trends Drugs Addict Health 3:100051. https://doi.org/10.1016/j.etdah.2023.100051

Clinisys (2023) The IT heart of SI-DEP—France's national Covid-19 screening platform. https://www.clinisys.com/at/en/case-studies/sidep-project-en/. Accessed 29 May 2025

Corbett JA, Opladen JM, Bisognano JD (2020) Telemedicine can revolutionize the treatment of chronic disease. Int J Cardiol Hypertens 7:100051. https://doi.org/10.1016/j.ijchy.2020.100051

Cordeiro JV (2021) Digital technologies and data science as health enablers: an outline of appealing promises and compelling ethical, legal, and social challenges. Front Med 8:647897. https://doi.org/10.3389/fmed.2021.647897

De Santis KK, Mergenthal L, Christianson L, Busskamp A, Vonstein C, Zeeb H (2023) Digital technologies for health promotion and disease prevention in older people: scoping review. J Med Internet Res 25:e43542. https://doi.org/10.2196/43542

Della Vecchia C, Leroy T, Bauquier C, Pannard M, Sarradon-Eck A, Darmon D, Dufour J-C, Preau M (2022) Willingness of French general practitioners to prescribe mHealth apps and devices: quantitative study. JMIR Mhealth Uhealth 10(2):e28372. https://doi.org/10.2196/28372

Department of Health and Social Care United Kingdom (2022) Policy paper. People at the heart of care: adult social care reform white paper. https://www.gov.uk/government/publications/people-at-the-heart-of-care-adult-social-care-reform-white-paper. Accessed 29 May 2025

Diáro Da República Eletrónico (2009) Assembleia da República Lei n.º 81/2009 de 21 de Agosto (Assembly of the Republic Law no. 81/2009 of August 21). https://files.dre.pt/1s/2009/08/16200/0549105495.pdf. Accessed 29 May 2025

Diáro Da República Eletrónico (2013) No. 248/2013, Series 1 of 2013-08-05. https://dre.pt/dre/en/detail/order/248-2013-499034. Accessed 29 May 2025

Diáro Da República Eletrónico (2014) No. 5855/2014, Series 2 of 2014-05-05. https://dre.pt/dre/en/detail/tipo/5855-2014-25688419. Accessed 29 May 2025

DigitalEurope (2022) A digital health decade: driving innovation in Europe. Digital Europe, Brussels

e-Estonia (2025a) Digital healthcare. e-Estonia. https://e-estonia.com/programme/digital-healthcare/. Accessed 29 May 2025

e-Estonia (2025b) e-Prescription. https://e-estonia.com/solutions/e-health-2/e-prescription/. Accessed 29 May 2025

Estonian Health Insurance (2024). Health Portal. Available online: https://tervisekassa.ee/en/organisation/e-health-products/healthportal. Accessed on May 28, 2025

Estonian Health Insurance News (2024). Eestis on kanda kinnitamas uued sõeluuringud. Available online. https://www.tervisekassa.ee/uudised/eestis-kanda-kinnitamas-uued-soeluuringud. Accessed on May 28, 2025.

Estonian Health Insurance (2025). Digital prescription. Available online. https://tervisekassa.ee/en/people/pharmaceuticals/digitalprescription. Accessed on May 28, 2025.

European Commission (2017) Smart Open Services - Open eHealth Initiative for a European Large Scale Pilot of Patient Summary and Electronic Prescription. European Commission. https://cordis.europa.eu/project/id/224991. Accessed 29 May 2025

European Commission (2022) Digital public administration factsheet 2022. European Commission, Brussels

European Commission (2025a) European health data space. https://health.ec.europa.eu/ehealth-digital-health-and-care/european-health-data-space_en. Accessed 29 May 2025

European Commission (2025b) A European strategy for data. European Commission. https://digital-strategy.ec.europa.eu/en/policies/strategy-data. Accessed 29 May 2025

European Commission (2023) Electronic cross-border health services. https://health.ec.europa.eu/ehealth-digital-health-and-care/electronic-cross-border-health-services_en. Accessed 29 May 2025

European Commission (2025) https://eur-lex.europa.eu/eli/reg/2025/327/oj/eng

European Court of Auditors (2019) EU actions for cross-border healthcare: significant ambitions but improved management required. European Union, Brussels. https://doi.org/10.2865/280048

European Court of Auditors (2023) Tools facilitating travel within the EU during the COVID-19 pandemic. In: Relevant initiatives with impact ranging from success to limited use. Publications Office of the European Union, Luxembourg. https://doi.org/10.2865/62115

European Observatory on Health Systems and Policies, Albecht T, Polin K, Brinovec RP, Kuhar M, Poldrugovac M, Rehberger PO, Rupel VP, Vracko P (2021) Slovenia: Health system review. World Health Organization, Regional Office for Europe, Copenhagen

European Union (2011) Directive 2011/24/EU of the European Parliament and of the Council of 9 March 2011 on the application of patients' rights in cross-border healthcare. https://eur-lex.europa.eu/legal-content/EN/TXT/?uri=CELEX:02011L0024-20140101. Accessed 29 May 2025

European Union (2015) E-tervise visioon 2025. E-tervise strateegiline arenguplaan 2020. (eHealth Vision 2025. eHealth Strategic Development Plan 2020). EU, Brussels

European Union (2016a) Regulation (EU) 2016/679 of the European Parliament and of the Council of 27 April 2016 on the protection of natural persons with regard to the processing of personal data and on the free movement of such data, and repealing Directive 95/46/EC (General Data Protection Regulation). https://eur-lex.europa.eu/eli/reg/2016/679/oj. Accessed 29 May 2025

European Union (2016b) Art. 89 GDPR. Safeguards and derogations relating to processing for archiving purposes in the public interest, scientific or historical research purposes or statistical purposes. https://gdpr.eu/article-89-processing-for-archiving-purposes-scientific-or-historical-research-purposes-or-statistical-purposes/. Accessed 29 May 2025

European Union (2016c) Directive (EU) 2016/1148 of the European Parliament and of the council of 6 July 2016 concerning measures for a high common level of security of network and information systems across the union. https://eur-lex.europa.eu/eli/dir/2016/1148/oj. Accessed 29 May 2025

European Union Agency For Network and Information Security (2018) Privacy and data protection in mobile applications. A study on the app development ecosystem and the technical implementation of GDPR. ENISA, Heraklion. https://doi.org/10.2824/114584

Fahy N, Williams GA, Habicht T, Köhler K, Jormanainen V, Satokangas M, Tynkkynen L-K, Lantzsch H, Winklemann J, Cascini F, AGd B, Morsella A, Poscia A, Ricciardi W, Silenzi A, Farcasanu D, Scintee SG, Vladescu C, Delgado EB, Pueyo EA, Romero FE (2021) Use of digital health tools in Europe: before, during and after COVID-19. Policy brief, no. 42. European Observatory on Health Systems and Policies, Copenhagen

Federal Institute for Drugs and Medical Devices Germany (2023a) DiGA. Digital health applications. https://www.bfarm.de/EN/Medical-devices/Tasks/DiGA-and-DiPA/Digital-Health-Applications/_node.html;jsessionid=9081513AEC138A926675EB0E7D1C4DFD.internet272. Accessed 29 May 2025

Federal Institute for Drugs and Medical Devices Germany (2025) Health data lab. https://www.healthdatalab.de/about/. Accessed 29 May 2025

Fong A (2017) The role of app intermediaries in protecting data privacy. Int J Law Inf Technol 25(2):85–114. https://doi.org/10.1093/ijlit/eax002

Foresight Centre (2020) The future of healthcare in Estonia. Scenarios up to 2035. Foresight Centre, Tallinn.

Gematik (2025) Aktuelles | Die Zahlen steigen: Die ePA-Nutzung steigt deutschlandweit (News | The numbers show: EHR use is increasing throughout Germany). https://www.gematik.de/newsroom/news-detail/epa-nutzung-steigt Accessed 29 May 2025

Generali (2022) Halo doktor. Ko je zdravnik samo en klik stran (Halo doktor. Remote doctor. Also at weekends and on public holidays). https://halodoktor.si/generali/. Accessed 29 May 2025

gesund.bund.de (2023) Your source of information on health issues. Ministry of Health, Germany. https://gesund.bund.de/en. Accessed 29 May 2025

Global Digital Health Monitor (2023) Global digital health index. Country profile portugal. https://monitor.digitalhealthmonitor.org/country_list. Accessed 29 May 2025

Government of Malta (2025) Mheme EU project. https://health.gov.mt/eu-projects/mheme-eu-project/. Accessed 29 May 2025

Gomes & Dias (2024) https://link.springer.com/article/10.1007/s11205-024-03452-2

Grobe TG, Weller L, Braun A, Szecsenyi J (2024) Schriftreihe zur Gesundheitsanalyse—Band 45. Barmer Arztreport 2024. Digitale Gesundheitsanwendungen—DiGA (Publication series on health analysis, vol 45. Barmer physician report. Digital health applications—DiGA). Barmer, Berlin. https://www.bifg.de/media/dl/Reporte/Arztreporte/2024/barmer-arztreport-2024.pdf

Grundy Q, Chiu K, Held F, Continella A, Bero L, Holz R (2019) Data sharing practices of medicines related apps and the mobile ecosystem: traffic, content, and network analysis. Br Med J 364:l920. https://doi.org/10.1136/bmj.l920

Guo C, Ashrafian H, Ghafur S, Fontana G, Gardner C, Prime M (2020) Challenges for the evaluation of digital health solutions—a call for innovative evidence generation approaches. NPJ Digit Med 3(1):110. https://doi.org/10.1038/s41746-020-00314-2

Health Data Hub (2023) Health data hub. https://www.health-data-hub.fr/. Accessed 29 May 2025

Health Insurance Institute of Slovenia (2021) Izvajalcem zdravstvenih storitev. Navodilo o beleženju in obračunavanju zdravstenih storitev in izdanih materialov (Instruction on recording and reimbursing healthcare services and materials). https://api.zzzs.si/ZZZS/info/egradiva.nsf/0/c82bdb0f7a50f864c125867f00436abe/$FILE/OKR_ZAE_3-21_P.pdf. Accessed 29 May 2025

Holly L, Wong BLH, van Kessel R, Awah I, Agrawal A, Ndili N (2023) Optimising adolescent wellbeing in a digital age. Br Med J 380:e068279. https://doi.org/10.1136/bmj-2021-068279

Hoogendoorn P (2023) Label2Enable. About CEN-ISO/TS 82304–2. https://label2enable.eu/about-cen-iso-ts-82304-2. Accessed 29 May 2025

Ibrahim H, Liu X, Zariffa N, Morris AD, Denniston AK (2021) Health data poverty: an assailable barrier to equitable digital health care. Lancet Digit Health 3(4):e260–e265. https://doi.org/10.1016/s2589-7500(20)30317-4

Ipsos MORI (2015) Health and wellbeing of 15 year olds in England: findings from the What About YOUth? survey 2014. NHS Digital, London

Janssen H, Cobbe J, Singh J (2020) Personal information management systems: a user-centric privacy utopia? Internet Policy Rev 9(4):1–25. https://doi.org/10.14763/2020.4.1536

Kendall M, Tsallis D, Wymant C, Di Francia A, Balogun Y, Didelot X, Ferretti L, Fraser C (2023) Epidemiological impacts of the NHS COVID-19 app in England and Wales throughout its first year. Nat Commun 14(1):858. https://doi.org/10.1038/s41467-023-36495-z

Kivi G (2023) Eestlaste terviseandmed muutuvad Euroopa arstidele kättesaadavaks ja vastupidi (Estonians' health data becomes available to European doctors and vice versa). The Health and Welfare Information Systems Centre (TEHIK). https://www.tehik.ee/uudis/eestlaste-terviseandmed-muutuvad-euroopa-arstidele-kattesaadavaks-ja-vastupidi. Accessed 29 May 2025

Kostkova P (2018) Disease surveillance data sharing for public health: the next ethical frontiers. Life Sci Soc Policy 14(1):16. https://doi.org/10.1186/s40504-018-0078-x

Kraus S, Schiavone F, Pluzhnikova A, Invernizzi AC (2021) Digital transformation in healthcare: analyzing the current state-of-research. J Bus Res 123:557–567. https://doi.org/10.1016/j.jbusres.2020.10.030

Kuntsman A, Miyake E, Martin S (2019) Re-thinking digital health: data, appication and the (im)possibility of 'opting out'. Digital Health 5:2055207619880671. https://doi.org/10.1177/2055207619880671

Labrique AB, Wadhwani C, Williams KA, Lamptey P, Hesp C, Luk R, Aerts A (2018) Best practices in scaling digital health in low and middle income countries. Global Health 14(1):103. https://doi.org/10.1186/s12992-018-0424-z

Lavallee DC, Lee JR, Austin E, Bloch R, Lawrence SO, McCall D, Munson SA, Nery-Hurwit MB, Amtmann D (2020) mHealth and patient generated health data: stakeholder perspectives on opportunities and barriers for transforming healthcare. Mhealth 6:8. https://doi.org/10.21037/mhealth.2019.09.17

Ma Y, Zhao C, Zhao Y, Lu J, Jiang H, Cao Y, Xu Y (2022) Telemedicine application in patients with chronic disease: a systematic review and meta-analysis. BMC Med Inform Decis Mak 22(1):105. https://doi.org/10.1186/s12911-022-01845-2

Maaß L, Freye M, Pan C-C, Dassow H-H, Niess J, Jahnel T (2022) The definitions of health apps and medical apps from the perspective of public health and law: qualitative analysis of an interdisciplinary literature overview. JMIR mHealth uHealth 10(10):e37980. https://doi.org/10.2196/37980

Maaß et al. (2024): https://www.nature.com/articles/s41746-024-01078-9

Mahl et al. (2025) https://gh.bmj.com/content/10/5/e018545

Mailiz (2023) m@ailiz. La messagerie sécurisée proposée par les Ordres de sante (The secure messaging system proposed by the health orders). https://mailiz.mssante.fr/. Accessed 29 May 2025

Malta Information Technology Agency (2017) CONvErGE: €40 million investment in ICT. Mita. https://procurement.mita.gov.mt/events/converge-40-million-investment-in-ict/. Accessed 29 May 2025

Malta Information Technology Agency (2023) myHealth. Mita. https://myhealth.gov.mt/. Accessed 29 May 2025

Manca DP (2015) Do electronic medical records improve quality of care? Yes. Can Fam Phys 61(10):846–847

Marcus JS, Martens B, Carugati C, Bucher A, Godlovitch I (2022) The european health data space. European Parliament, Brussels. https://doi.org/10.2139/ssrn.4300393

Marelli L, Testa G (2018) Scrutinizing the EU General Data Protection Regulation. Science 360(6388):496–498. https://doi.org/10.1126/science.aar5419

Marelli L, Lievevrouw E, Van Hoyweghen I (2020) Fit for purpose? The GDPR and the governance of European digital health. Policy Stud 41(5):447–467. https://doi.org/10.1080/01442872.2020.1724929

Mayer-Schönberger V, Padova Y (2016) Regime change? Enabling big data through Europe's new data protection regulation. Sci Technol Law Rev 17(2). https://doi.org/10.7916/stlr.v17i2.4007

Menachemi N, Collum TH (2011) Benefits and drawbacks of electronic health record systems. Risk Manage Healthc Policy 4:47–55. https://doi.org/10.2147/rmhp.S12985

Merimaa K, Vanker E (2020) Terviseportaal. In: Eelanalüüs (Health portal. Preliminary analysis). Ministry of Social Affairs, Tallinn

Ministerial Delegation for Digital Health France (2022) Digital Health actions and initiatives under the French Presidency of the Council of the European Union during the first semester of 2022. Ministry of Health and Prevention France, Paris

Ministry of Health and Prevention France (2022a) Organisation de la délégation ministérielle au numérique en santé (Organization of the ministerial delegation for digital health). Ministry of Health and Prevention France. https://sante.gouv.fr/ministere/organisation/organisation-des-directions-et-services/article/organisation-de-la-delegation-ministerielle-au-numerique-en-sante. Accessed 29 May 2025

Ministry of Health and Prevention France (2022b) Study on digital health implementation in the EU. Final report. EY Consulting property. https://esante.gouv.fr/sites/default/files/media_entity/documents/dns-pfue_final-report_digital-health-vf.pdf. Accessed 29 May 2025

Ministry of Health and Prevention France (2023a) Le Ségur du numérique en santé (Ségur of digital health). Ministry of Health and Prevention France. https://esante.gouv.fr/segur. Accessed 29 May 2025

Ministry of Health and Prevention France (2023b) La transformation numérique de notre système de santé commence ici, pour vous et avec vous! (The digital transformation of our health system starts here, for you and with you!). Ministry of Health and Prevention France. https://esante.gouv.fr/. Accessed 29 May 2025

Ministry of Health and Prevention France (2023c) Comprendre le ségur du numérique en santé. Présentation, objectifs et périmètre (Understanding the segur of digital health. Presentation, objectives and scope). Ministry of Health and Prevention France, Paris

Ministry of Health Germany (2019) Schnellere Termine, mehr Sprechstunden, bessere Angebote für gesetzlich Versicherte. Terminservice- und Versorgungsgesetz (Faster appointments, more consultation hours, better services for people with statutory health insurance. Appointment Service and Care Act). https://www.bundesgesundheitsministerium.de/terminservice-und-versorgungsgesetz.html. Accessed 29 May 2025

Ministry of Health Malta (2020) Covid result submission malta. https://covidresultsubmission.gov.mt/. Accessed 29 May 2025

Ministry of Health Malta (2022) A national health systems strategy for Malta 2023–2030. Investing successfully for a healthy future. Ministry of Health Malta, Valletta

Ministry of Health Malta (2023a) COVID19-Malta. COVID19-Data. Github. https://github.com/COVID19-Malta/COVID19-Data. Accessed 29 May 2025

Ministry of Health Malta (2023b) saħħa. Facebook. https://www.facebook.com/sahhagovmt. Accessed 29 May 2025

Ministry of Health Germany (2025) Die elektronische Patientenakte (ePA) für alle (The electronic health record (EHR) for everyone). https://www.bundesgesundheitsministerium.de/themen/digitalisierung/elektronische-patientenakte/epa-fuer-alle.html. Accessed 29 May 2025

Ministry of Health of the Republic of Slovenia (2005) eHealth 2010. Strategy for informatization of the Slovenian health care system 2005–2010. Ministry of Health of Slovenia, Ljubljana

Ministry of Health of the Republic of Slovenia (2023) Digitalisation is the key step to a modern health system. https://www.gov.si/en/news/2023-01-13-digitalisation-is-the-key-step-to-a-modern-health-system/. Accessed 29 May 2025

Ministry of Health of the Republic of Slovenia, European Commission (2022) Slovenija – e-zdravje za bolj zdravo družbo. REFORM/SC2021/061 (Slovenia - eHealth for a healthier society). Ministry of Health of the Republic of Slovenia, Ljubljana

Ministry of Health Portugal (2023) SINAVE. National epidemiological surveillance system. https://www.spms.min-saude.pt/2020/07/sinave-2/#googtrans(pt%7Cen). Accessed 29 May 2025

Ministry of Health Slovenia (2021) [eHealth]. Ministry of Health Slovenia. https://www.gov.si/zbirke/projekti-in-programi/ezdravje/. Accessed 29 May 2025

Ministry of Social Affairs Estonia (2017) Factsheet. In: E-health in Estonia. Republic of Estonia, Tallinn

Minssen T (2022) European regulation of medical devices: introduction. In: Cohen I, Minssen T, Price WN II, Robertson C, Shachar C (eds) The Future of Medical Device Regulation: Innovation and Protection. Cambridge University Press, Cambridge, pp 47–114

Mon espace santé (2021) Le service public pour gérer sa santé. Vous avez la main sur votre santé (The public service to manage your health. You have control over your health). https://www.monespacesante.fr/. Accessed 29 May 2025

Mongin-Bulewski C (2008) The Mater Dei Hospital project: a quantum leap for healthcare in Malta. Hospital Healthcare Europe. https://hospitalhealthcare.com/news/the-mater-dei-hospital-project-a-quantum-leap-for-healthcare-in-malta/. Accessed 29 May 2025

Mühlhoff R (2021) Predictive privacy: towards an applied ethics of data analytics. Ethics Inf Technol 23(4):675–690. https://doi.org/10.1007/s10676-021-09606-x

Mulder T (2019) Health Apps, their Privacy Policies and the GDPR. Eur J Law Technol 1(1)

Muller SHA, Kalkman S, van Thiel GJMW, Mostert M, van Delden JJM (2021) The social licence for data-intensive health research: towards co-creation, public value and trust. BMC Med Ethics 22(1):110. https://doi.org/10.1186/s12910-021-00677-5

Murray CJL, Alamro NMS, Hwang H, Lee U (2020) Digital public health and COVID-19. Lancet Public Health 5(9):e469–e470. https://doi.org/10.1016/s2468-2667(20)30187-0

Muscat HA, Pace J, Buttigieg S (2019) Digital Health in Malta. In: Muscat NA, Melillo T, Cauchi D (eds) Public health in malta. 1999-2019. The story of public health in malta, vol 20th Anniversary Edition. Malta Association of Public Health Medicine, Valletta, pp 25–28

National Association of Statutory Health Insurance Funds (2025) DiGA-Bericht des GKV-Spitzenverbandes 2024. Bericht über die Inanspruchnahme und Entwicklung der Versorgung mit Digitalen Gesundheitsanwendungen. Berichtszeitraum: 01.09.2020–31.12.2024 (DiGA Report of the National Association of Statutory Health Insurance Funds 2024. Report on the utilization and development of care with digital health applications. Reporting period: 01.09.2020–31.12.2024). Berlin: National Association of Statutory Health Insurance Funds

National Health Service England (2017) Compendium–Public health indicators. NHS England. https://digital.nhs.uk/data-and-information/publications/statistical/compendium-public-health/current. Accessed 29 May 2025

National Health Service England (2021) National study of health and wellbeing: children and young people. NHS England. https://digital.nhs.uk/data-and-information/areas-of-interest/public-health/national-study-of-health-and-wellbeing-children-and-young-people. Accessed 29 June 2025

National Health Service England (2022) Policy paper. A plan for digital health and social care NHS England. https://www.gov.uk/government/publications/a-plan-for-digital-health-and-social-care/a-plan-for-digital-health-and-social-care. Accessed 29 May 2025

National Health Service England (2023) Remote monitoring for patients with chronic conditions in the Midlands. NHS England. https://transform.england.nhs.uk/covid-19-response/technology-nhs/remote-monitoring-for-patients-with-chronic-conditions-in-the-midlands/. Accessed 29 May 2025

National Health Service Health Education England (2021) Embedding public health in to clinical services toolkit-workbook. NHS England, London

National Health Service Health Education England (2023a) elfh. elearning for healthcare. https://portal.e-lfh.org.uk/. Accessed 29 May 2025

National Health Service Health Education England (2023b) elfh. elearning for healthcare. Population wellbeing portal. https://www.e-lfh.org.uk/programmes/population-wellbeing-portal/. Accessed 29 May 2025

National Institute of Public Health of the Republic of Slovenia (2023) Slovenian eHealth solutions at a glance. https://ezdrav.si/jezik-anglesko/. Accessed 29 May 2025

Obermann K (2022) Digital health applications (DiGA) in practice: Findings and experiences. In: Doctors in the future market of health 2022. A representative Germany-wide survey of service providers by Stiftung Gesundheit in cooperation with the information company DiGA Info. Stiftung Gesundheit, Hamburg

Odone A, Buttigieg S, Ricciardi W, Azzopardi-Muscat N, Staines A (2019) Public health digitalization in Europe: EUPHA vision, action and role in digital public health. Eur J Public Health 29(Supplement_3):28–35. https://doi.org/10.1093/eurpub/ckz161

Office for Health Improvement and Disparities England (2015) All our health: personalised care and population health. A framework of evidence to guide healthcare professionals in preventing illness. Protecting health and promoting wellbeing. https://www.gov.uk/government/collections/all-our-health-personalised-care-and-population-health. Accessed 29 May 2025

Official Gazette of the Republic of Slovenia (2016) Resolucijo. O nacionalnem planu zdravstvenega varstva 2016–2025 »Skupaj za družbo zdravja« (ReNPZV16–25)(Resolution on the national health care plan 2016–2025 "Together for a healthy society"). Official Gazette of the Republic of Slovenia, Ljubljana.

Organisation for Economic Co-operation and Development (2022a) Health data governance for the digital age. OECD, Paris. https://doi.org/10.1787/68b60796-en

Organisation for Economic Co-operation and Development (2022b) The development of the Estonian health system performance assessment framework. Situational analysis report. OECD, Paris

Organisation for Economic Co-operation and Development, European Observatory on Health Systems and Policies (2021) State of Health in the EU. In: Estonia Country Health Profile 2021. OECD, Paris. https://doi.org/10.1787/1313047c-en

Panteli et al. (2025) https://www.thelancet.com/journals/lanpub/article/PIIS2468-2667(25)00036-2/fulltext

Parati G, Pellegrini D, Torlasco C (2019) How digital health can be applied for preventing and managing hypertension. Curr Hypertens Rep 21(5):40. https://doi.org/10.1007/s11906-019-0940-0

Pärna K, Snieder H, Läll K, Fischer K, Nolte I (2020) Validating the doubly weighted genetic risk score for the prediction of type 2 diabetes in the Lifelines and Estonian Biobank cohorts. Genet Epidemiol 44(6):589–600. https://doi.org/10.1002/gepi.22327

Petrone J (2022) From Tallinn to Lisbon: ePrescription is now accessible in more European countries. e-Estonia. https://eestonia.com/from-tallinn-to-lisbon-eprescription-is-now-accessible-in-more-european-countries/. Accessed 29 May 2025

Peyroteo M, Ferreira IA, Elvas LB, Ferreira JC, Lapão LV (2021) Remote monitoring systems for patients with chronic diseases in primary health care: systematic review. JMIR Mhealth Uhealth 9(12):e28285. https://doi.org/10.2196/28285

Prainsack B (2020) The political economy of digital data: introduction to the special issue. Policy Stud 41(5):439–446. https://doi.org/10.1080/01442872.2020.1723519

Rachadell J (2021) 9.C. Round table: digital innovation to fight the pandemic, what is here to stay? Eur J Public Health 31(Supplement_3). https://doi.org/10.1093/eurpub/ckab164.625

Santé Publique France (2021a) E-sin: signalement externe des infections nosocomiales (E-sin: external reporting of nosocomial infections). https://www.santepubliquefrance.fr/maladies-et-traumatismes/infections-associees-aux-soins-et-resistance-aux-antibiotiques/infections-associees-aux-soins/articles/e-sin-signalement-externe-des-infections-nosocomiales. Accessed 29 May 2025

Santé Publique France (2021b) La santé mentale au temps de la COVID-19: en parler, c'est déjà se soigner (Mental health at the time of COVID-19: talking about it is already taking care of itself). https://www.santepubliquefrance.fr/presse/2021/la-sante-mentale-au-temps-de-la-covid-19-en-parler-c-est-deja-se-soigner. Accessed 29 May 2025

Santé Publique France (2022a) La recherche au cœur du plan de surveillance génomique du territoire français de variants du Sars-Cov-2 (Research at the heart of the genomic surveillance plan for the French territory of Sars-Cov-2 variants). https://www.santepubliquefrance.fr/presse/2022/la-recherche-au-caeur-du-plan-de-surveillance-genomique-du-territoire-francais-de-variants-du-sars-cov-2. Accessed 29 May 2025

Santé Publique France (2022b) La santé à tout âge (Health at any age). https://www.santepubliquefrance.fr/la-sante-a-tout-age/la-sante-a-tout-age. Accessed 29 May 2025

Santé Publique France (2023) Géodes: Géo Données en santé publique (Géodes: geo data in public health). https://geodes.santepubliquefrance.fr/#c=home. Accessed 29 May 2025

Schengenvisa (2021) Estonia becomes one of the first countries to join EU Digital COVID-19 passport. https://www.schengenvisainfo.com/news/estonia-becomes-one-of-the-first-countries-to-join-eu-digital-covid-19-passport/. Accessed 29 May 2025

Schmitz S (2019) Entwicklung der elektronischen Gesundheitskarte—BMG übernimmt Kommando (Development of the electronic health card—BMG takes over command). Best Pract Onkol 14(5):157. https://doi.org/10.1007/s11654-019-0146-6

Schmidt et al. (2024a) https://www.nature.com/articles/s41746-024-01137-1

Schmidt et al. (2024b) https://doi.org/10.1038/s41746-024-01221-6

Serviços Partilhados do Ministério da Saúde (2019) Enesis 20–22. Estratégia nacional para o ecossisteme de informação de saúde. Versão Preliminar para Consulta Pública (Enesis 20–22. National Strategy for the Health Information Ecosystem. Preliminary Version for Public Consultation). SPMS, Lisbon

Serviços Partilhados do Ministério da Saúde (2021) Trace COVID-19. In: Gestão de vigilâncias. Manual de utilizador 2022 (Trace COVID-19. Surveillance management. User's manual 2022). SPMS, Lisbon

Stanimirović D, Matetić V (2020) Can the COVID-19 pandemic boost the global adoption and usage of eHealth solutions? J Glob Health 10(2):0203101. https://doi.org/10.7189/jogh.10.0203101

Taylor ML, Thomas EE, Snoswell CL, Smith AC, Caffery LJ (2021) Does remote patient monitoring reduce acute care use? A systematic review. BMJ Open 11(3):e040232. https://doi.org/10.1136/bmjopen-2020-040232

Techniker Health Insurance (2025) Forschungsdatenspende in der elektronischen Patientenakte (ePA) (Research data donation in the electronic patient record (EHR)). https://www.tk.de/techniker/leistungen-und-mitgliedschaft/online-servicesversicherte/elektronische-patientenakte-tk-safe/elektronische-patientenakte-forschungsdatenspende-2190328. Accessed 29 May 2025

The Health and Welfare Information Systems Centre (2023a) Health information system. https://www.tehik.ee/en/health-information-system. Accessed 29 May 2025

The Health and Welfare Information Systems Centre (2023b) Digital referral. https://tehik.ee/en/digital-referral. Accessed 29 May 2025

Transform Health (2023) Health data governance principles. https://healthdatagovernance.org/principles/. Accessed 29 May 2025

University of Tartu (2023) University of Tartu received €30 million to develop a centre of excellence for personalised medicine. https://genomics.ut.ee/en/University-of-Tartu-received-30-million-to-develop-a-centre-of-excellence-for-personalised-medicine. Accessed 29 May 2025

van Kessel R, Wong BLH, Forman R, Gabrani J, Mossialos E (2022a) The European Health Data Space fails to bridge digital divides. BMJ 378:e071913. https://doi.org/10.1136/bmj-2022-071913

van Kessel R, Wong BLH, Rubinić I, O'Nuallain E, Czabanowska K (2022b) Is Europe prepared to go digital? Making the case for developing digital capacity: an exploratory analysis of Eurostat survey data. PLoS Digit Health 1(2):e0000013. https://doi.org/10.1371/journal.pdig.0000013

van Kessel R, Hrzic R, O'Nuallain E, Weir E, Wong BLH, Anderson M, Baron-Cohen S, Mossialos E (2022c) Digital health paradox: international policy perspectives to address increased health inequalities for people living with disabilities. J Med Internet Res 24(2):e33819. https://doi.org/10.2196/33819

van Kessel R, Wong BLH, Clemens T, Brand H (2022d) Digital health literacy as a super determinant of health: more than simply the sum of its parts. Internet Interv 27:100500. https://doi.org/10.1016/j.invent.2022.100500

van Kessel R, Kyriopoulos I, Wong BLH, Mossialos E (2023a) The effect of the COVID-19 pandemic on digital health–seeking behavior: big data interrupted time-series analysis of google trends. J Med Internet Res 25:e42401. https://doi.org/10.2196/42401

van Kessel R, Kyriopoulos I, Mastylak A, Mossialos E (2023b) Changes in digital healthcare search behavior during the early months of the COVID-19 pandemic: a study of six English-speaking countries. PLoS Digit Health 2(5):e0000241. https://doi.org/10.1371/journal.pdig.0000241

van Kessel et al. (2023c) https://www.ncbi.nlm.nih.gov/pmc/articles/PMC11774227/, https://www.sciencedirect.com/science/article/pii/S138650562400176X

van Kessel et al. (2025) https://www.ncbi.nlm.nih.gov/pmc/articles/PMC11774227/

van Zoonen L (2020) Data governance and citizen participation in the digital welfare state. Data Policy 2:e10. https://doi.org/10.1017/dap.2020.10

Viigimaa M, Jürisson M, Pisarev H, Kalda R, Alavere H, Irs A, Saar A, Fischer K, Läll K, Kruuv-Käo K, Mars N, Widen E, Ripatti S, Metspalu A (2022) Effectiveness and feasibility of cardiovascular disease personalized prevention on high polygenic risk score subjects: a randomized controlled pilot study. Eur Heart J Open 2(6):oeac079. https://doi.org/10.1093/ehjopen/oeac079

Wangler J, Jansky M (2022) Welche Potenziale und Mehrwerte bieten DiGA für die hausärztliche Versorgung? – Ergebnisse einer Befragung von Hausärzt*innen in Deutschland (What potential and added value do DiGA offer for primary care? Results of a survey of general practitioners in Germany). Bundesgesundheitsblatt, Gesundheitsforschung, Gesundheitsschutz 65(12):1334–1343. https://doi.org/10.1007/s00103-022-03608-w

Wong BLH, Maaß L, Vodden A, van Kessel R, Sorbello S, Buttigieg S, Odone A (2022) The dawn of digital public health in Europe: implications for public health policy and practice. Lancet Reg Health 14:100316. https://doi.org/10.1016/j.lanepe.2022.100316

World Bank (2025) GDP per capita, PPP (current international $). World Bank. https://data.worldbank.org/indicator/NY.GDP.PCAP.PP.CD?name_desc=true. Accessed 26 Jun 2023

World Health Organization (2020) Estonia and WHO to work together on digital health and innovation. WHO. https://www.who.int/europe/news/item/07-10-2020-estonia-and-who-to-work-together-on-digital-health-and-innovation. Accessed 29 May 2025

World Health Organization (2021a) Global strategy on digital health 2020–2025. WHO, Geneva

World Health Organization (2021b) Estonia: digital technologies ensuring continuity in access to essential medicines during the COVID-19 pandemic. WHO, Copenhagen

World Health Organization (2022) Equity within digital health technology within the WHO European region: a scoping review. WHO, Copenhagen

Zia A, Aziz M, Popa I, Khan SA, Hamedani AF, Asif AR (2022) Artificial intelligence-based medical data mining. J Pers Med 12(9):1359. https://doi.org/10.3390/jpm12091359

Open Access This chapter is licensed under the terms of the Creative Commons Attribution 4.0 International License (http://creativecommons.org/licenses/by/4.0/), which permits use, sharing, adaptation, distribution and reproduction in any medium or format, as long as you give appropriate credit to the original author(s) and the source, provide a link to the Creative Commons license and indicate if changes were made.

The images or other third party material in this chapter are included in the chapter's Creative Commons license, unless indicated otherwise in a credit line to the material. If material is not included in the chapter's Creative Commons license and your intended use is not permitted by statutory regulation or exceeds the permitted use, you will need to obtain permission directly from the copyright holder.

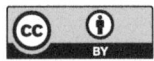

Global Perspectives on Digital Public Health: A Framework

Luís Velez Lapão

Abstract This chapter addresses the evolution from global health to public health and back to global public health, as well as delving into the establishment of digital public health, where globalization has played a critical role.

We examine a set of examples of global application of digital public health from both Europe and Africa (Angola, Cape Verde, and São Tomé and Principe) contexts. This includes case studies of collaborations comprising several institutions leveraging their different skills and expertise, fully encompassing the concept of global public health.

Design science is presented as a relevant scientific approach to support the implementation of digital public health, and a specific framework is provided to relate concrete public health functions with digital public health development opportunities. This can also be used as an agenda for research in global digital public health.

In conclusion, a set of global digital public health challenges are summarised. It is argued that capacity building will play a role as public health professionals need to understand how to leverage digital health to bridge the gap with other areas of health. Digital public health could establish a new global and environmental health paradigm within the next ten years, paving the way to digital planetary health.

Keywords Digital health · Global health · Global digital public health · Sustainable development goals · Universal health coverage · Digital transformation

L. V. Lapão (✉)
WHO Collaborating Center for Health Workforce Policy and Planning, and Digital & Smart Healthcare Laboratory UNIDEMI, Universidade Nova de Lisboa, Lisbon, Portugal

Intelligent Systems Associate Laboratory (LASI), Guimarães, Portugal

WHO Technical Advisory Group on Health Emergency Preparedness, Response and Resilience (Preparedness 2.0), Geneva, Switzerland
e-mail: luis.lapao@nms.unl.pt

Abbreviations

EHR	Electronic health records
HRMS	Health Remote Monitoring Systems
HUG	Geneva University Hospitals
ICT	Information and communication technologies
LMIC	Low-and-middle-income countries
MoH	Ministry of Health
NASA	National Aeronautics and Space Administration
PHC	Primary Health Care
STP	Sao Tome and Principe
UHC	Universal Health Coverage
UNL	Universidade Nova de Lisboa

1 Introduction

Europe and the world are facing three major structural changes: (a) the climate crisis, having a significant impact on public health; (b) the digitalization of the low-growth economy, which could play a significant role in mitigating climate change and its impacts on public health; and (c) demographic change, which is associated with the increase in multi-morbidities that lead to a growing demand for more health services. The COVID-19 pandemic has affected our lives in many ways, including how people see public health and climate change. It has created the conditions for the almost exponential growth in telemedicine and digitalization in healthcare. This was an opportunity for digital public health (Silva et al. 2022).

We need to underline that the world is facing an increasing level of innovation and integration of digital technologies to address public health and environmental problems due to the digitalization of working processes and the "uberization" of many health services. Furthermore, the UN Secretary-General and the Director-General of the World Health Organization have both recently declared that we are currently fighting a climate "pandemic" in the same way we are fighting COVID-19. Responding to public health, animal health, and environmental challenges and risks is increasingly high on the agenda of policymakers. With the support of Germany, WHO is establishing a pandemic intelligence hub in Berlin, recognizing the need to put emphasis on establishing practices that provide more real-time insights to inform policy-making for preparedness and response to health emergencies and strengthening health systems. The aim is to transform global health into planetary health.

1.1 Globalization of Health

Global health is now an established concept. However, through the evolution of concepts like international and diplomatic health, the need to integrate the global interlinks of health was firmly established. The recent pandemic has shown the implications of global health and the need for both better frameworks and shared design of policies. Naturally, the WHO has a role in this, and it has promoted a shared responsibility among international players under the framework of sustainable development goals (Koplan et al. 2009).

Another significant trend is the advance of the implementation science after many years of documented health intervention failures (Theobald et al. 2018). Even more important are the newly identified global health challenges, like fast sharing of quality information, sustainable cooperation, and equity. Global health is indeed a process in the making, possibly towards a more comprehensive and sustainable "planetary health" approach (Whitmee et al. 2015). This process started many years ago when health started to receive extensive international attention and had several important stages. The adoption of Universal Health Coverage (UHC) in 1978 at the WHO assembly in Alma-Ata (Kazakhstan), the Millennium Declaration by the United Nations General Assembly in 2000, and the renewed commitment to Universal Health Coverage in December 2012 were decisive events. More recently, in 2020, the COVID-19 pandemic also underlined the importance and relevance of a global health perspective and the best framework for action.

The process of globalization in healthcare presented clear clues, such as:

- Impacts of global health social determinants on modern societies.
- Shifts in demand from childhood care to elderly care.
- People's near-limitless ability to move around the world and transport pathogenic microorganisms quicker than ever.
- Exasperating economics of environmental exploitation, loss of wildlife diversity, and the terrible consequences for the health of populations.

The deterioration of the working conditions, occurring both in agriculture and in factories, and the emergence of digital platform workers contribute to an epidemic of mental health problems across societies globally. The increasing role of the food industry (and its conglomerates) and the logistics thereof must be considered, especially considering the two significant "lost contests" of tobacco and sugar—despite the WHO pushing for more stringent rules, regulations on both industries remain weak. All these factors represent substantial threats to global health.

Today, it is clear that the globalization of health is an important phenomenon. There are numerous relevant aspects, such as:

- The speed of disease spread and transmission due to the increased mobility (and detrimental behavior) of people acting as disease vectors.

GLOBAL DIGITAL PUBLIC HEALTH

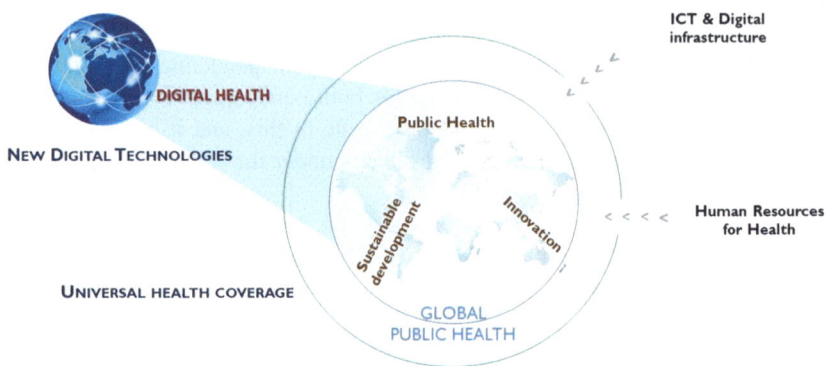

Fig. 1 Global digital public health context. (Source: own figure, adapted from Maia et al. 2015, reprinted with permission from the authors)

- The economic impact of the persistence of some communicable diseases like malaria or yellow fever in poorer areas (mostly in Africa);
- The emergence of global health initiatives supported by international technical and financial agencies (both public and private) that often bring as much distress (and some disruption to health services) as attempts to mitigate disease impact.

All these activities have led to the emergence of a global market for health services and professionals (qualified human resources). However, the proliferation of new information and digital technologies (e.g., telemedicine, mobile health) and the perception that social and economic inequities cannot be resolved without improving health levels (and universal health coverage) in all countries is calling for a new paradigm. The digitalization of healthcare and public health leads to global digital public health (Fig. 1).

1.2 The Dawn of Global Health: From the Navigators to the Second Millennium

In a time when we start rethinking globalization, it is important to go back to understand its dawn. Global health is very much related to human migrations and traveling, and history has plenty to display. One may argue that "viable economic and cultural" globalization started with the European navigations to Africa, America, and Asia. At the lowermost corner of Europe, at the crossroad between the Atlantic Ocean and the Mediterranean Sea, Portuguese and Spanish navigators had an immense impact on the globalization of commerce across the world. The discovery of new lands led to new commercial exchanges (from pepper to new materials and knowledge) but also new diseases (e.g., influenza and malaria). But before these health threats started to decimate populations, there was a disease that killed many of the sailors on their voyages, scurvy, known since the times of Hippocrates (Walter 1979). The Portuguese navigators soon discovered a remedy to mitigate scurvy while on the open sea for a long time, as the caravels (ships with triangular sales) began to range farther and farther away. As these travelers went around the Cape of Good Hope, they almost immediately discovered the value of oranges and lemons, already abundant in Iberia. In fact, lemons are especially abundant sources of vitamin C, which prevents scurvy.

The voyage of Vasco da Gama towards India (1498) was heavily affected by scurvy. The sailors were involuntarily saved when they traded with some Arabian ships loaded with oranges before landing at Mombasa (now in Kenya) (Martini 2003). On the return journey from India, the sailors managed to bring some oranges with some effect on scurvy survival, as was registered by the fleet reporter.

Oranges were one of the "healthy" secrets revealed by the Portuguese to enable long sailing trips. The astrolabe (used to calculate astronomical positions and latitude with precision) and gunpowder were some of the other essential technologies to enable mercantilism, European colonialism, and the first stage of globalization. It wasn't until much later that the Royal Navy physician James Lind advanced the knowledge of scurvy prevention and treatment. However, it took almost another half century until his insights became broadly accepted (Baron 2009).

Renaissance and later medicine further improved the knowledge about symptoms and later combined it with the knowledge of anatomy and physiology. But a huge event was about to change public health forever. In August of 1854, a suburb of London was severely hit by a terrible outbreak of cholera. John Snow took this opportunity to test an idea about the existence of a specific source of the disease (McLeod 2000).

The mapping (dot by dot) of the infected patients enabled him to identify a water pump as the potential origin of the disease, indicating that contaminated water was the key source of the epidemic. With this exercise, the fundamental principle of public health was established. Mapping and tracing infected persons became part of the new public health information system and laid the groundwork for today's data-rich health information systems.

Today, many recognize that globalization and technology have created a "flat" world (Friedman 2006). Recent advances in information and communication technologies (ICTs) have also contributed towards "condensing" the world to almost resemble a village. The latest progresses in ICTs, like smart networks or mobile 5G and soon 6G, have shown incredible promises in addressing significant challenges in healthcare coverage, including more preventive approaches, in several regions of the world. Nowadays, telemedicine services ensure the provision of accessible, cost-effective, and often specialized care to distant areas (Maia et al. 2019).

According to the World Health Organization (WHO), telemedicine pertains to the delivery of healthcare using different approaches embedded in the health ICT network (nowadays, largely supported by digital telecommunication services), with a secure and private sharing of data based on ISO 27001 standards. It aims to advance healthcare, ranging from individual to population levels, by allowing the exchange of "real-time" patient information for diagnosis and management of health problems, primary healthcare and prevention, and education of physicians or other health workers via distance learning (Masic et al. 2009). Telemedicine, or more generally "digital health," is now a new and accepted paradigm as a comprehensive channel for healthcare services delivery, enabling opportunities to strengthen patients' active participation (Peyroteo et al. 2021; Ryu et al. 2017). The digital "revolution" will enable more active and participative patients to assume responsibility for managing their health.

The earliest known mention of the telemedicine notion can be traced back to 1879, to a text in *The Lancet*, which described the effective diagnosis of a child over the phone and the 1905 long-distance transfer of electrocardiograms by a Dutch physician (Ryu 2010). It became common for the wealthier to call their doctors by telephone; these were often the first citizens to install a phone in their towns so they could be reached. In April 1924, Radio News magazine allegedly introduced another notion of telemedicine by using the term "radio doctor" to describe the potential for remote communication between a patient and a physician through the radio (Waqas et al. 2020).

The use of telegraph technology was already common during the American Civil War for both transfers of mortality data and remote delivery of medical care (i.e., treatment guidance). New telecommunication infrastructures that accompanied the deployment of train lines even improved reach to remote regions. However, the first modern example of telemedicine was seen when, in 1969, the National Aeronautics and Space Administration (NASA) used radio telecommunications to monitor the astronauts' well-being during the Apollo 11 mission to the moon.

The contemporary form of telemedicine, however, appeared more recently with the advent and evolution of the internet, which supported the use of web-based videoconferencing, high-quality and secure data transfer, and web-based distance learning platforms operating at a much lower cost (and, thus, easier to use). The potential of telemedicine in strengthening global health systems was also recognized by the WHO, leading to the establishment of the Global Observatory for eHealth in 2005 (WHO 2006).

In 2009, the telemedicine unit of the Global Observatory for eHealth registered the development of telemedicine in four main specialties of medicine (telepathology, teleradiology, telepsychology, and teledermatology) in the WHO member states. This report pointed out an impressive development that had been made in providing radiology services at a distance, implemented in 33% of WHO member states. 20% of the countries reported conducting a national review or evaluation of telemedicine, and 50% reported that they had created institutions dedicated to the development of telemedicine solutions (WHO 2006).

The globalization of health is very much linked with digitalization and improving access to care. A recent WHO report emphasized the role of eHealth in achieving universal health coverage, aligned with the 1978's message from Alma Ata WHO General Assembly (WHO 2015).

Telemedicine services around the world established in the most recent decade are considered central in accomplishing the health-focused sustainable development goal #3, to "ensure healthy lives and promote well-being for all at all ages," and more specifically #3.8, to "achieve universal health coverage." From 2010 to 2016, the speed of the evolution of telemedicine was considered the highest ever since. By 2016, at least 83% of the countries had reported a mobile health (mHealth) initiative, the scale-up of teleradiology services (from 33% to 77%), telepathology or teledermatology services (in about 50% of countries), and telepsychiatry (in 33% of countries) (WHO 2006).

Very importantly, eLearning initiatives were reported from about 84% of countries, while the development of national electronic health records (EHR) was mentioned by only 47% of the member states, with very different levels of implementation accomplished. Telemedicine platforms for education purposes are more advanced than the implementation of EHR. A critical factor is the development of appropriate legal regulations. Acknowledging the role of regulations, about 78% of the countries have created legislation ensuring the privacy of EHR data.

Nevertheless, very few countries had correctly assessed the mHealth programs under development, limiting our knowledge of the proper use of mobile health, its barriers and facilitators, and which elements could be considered to be good practices (WHO 2006). While these data were reported before the COVID-19 pandemic and indicate significant development steps in the field of telemedicine before, one must be aware that this information was provided by government organizations (often overly optimistic) and was heavily focused on government-run telehealth initiatives.

COVID-19 was a game changer, an opportunity to make a difference while leveraging the digital technologies available to tackle a set of new challenges and improve the health systems' resilience to the pandemic. A recent study looked at the use of telemedicine in primary healthcare (PHC) during COVID-19 and identified 44 studies showing just how important it was (Silva et al. 2022). The results showed both the positive and negative impacts on the quality of PHC and the inability to take advantage of the potential of technologies during the pandemic. It also pointed out that PHC must improve planning, response capabilities, training, embrace a more extensive use of ICT, and manage challenges like services deployment, making appropriate use of scientific evidence since digital health provides important development options and must be integrated into health and public services (Maia et al. 2019).

2 Global Health and the Rise of Telemedicine

Information and communication technologies (ICT) have been used for a long time to support healthcare systems innovation, especially in higher-income countries. But low and middle-income countries (LMIC) have also participated in proof of concept pilots and more extensive digital health programs, often as a significant contribution towards attaining universal health coverage (UHC) (Seneviratne and Peiris 2019; Goncalves et al. 2021).

2.1 Global Health and the Establishment of Telemedicine

Telemedicine could be used to connect healthcare services in different countries, even on different continents (WHO 2017). Regardless of the promising potential of telemedicine to address global health problems, especially in low-and-middle-income countries (LMIC), its scale-up has been unsatisfactory, and many telemedicine services fail to sustain their implementation shortly after initial funding or a pilot phase. Capacity building is another challenge, and the telemedicine technique shortage threatens the full deployment of telemedicine services. Therefore, it is essential to identify successful models of telemedicine implementation in LMIC to recognize commonalities and extract experiences that would be useful for implementers, policymakers, and future researchers (Kim and Zuckerman 2019; Maia et al. 2019).

In sub-Saharan Africa, and more specifically in the Portuguese-speaking countries context, telemedicine has already been successfully implemented in programs that could be leveraged further (Goncalves et al. 2021; Correia et al. 2018; Correia et al. 2017).

One example of specialized collaborative care in global health is in Sao Tome and Principe (STP), a lower-income, developing, and small archipelago state with a weak economy. STP's national health system is fragile and lacks fundamental infrastructure, technology facilities, and human resources to meet basic population health demands. Portugal is the leading destination for severely ill patients from STP, with about 200 evacuations per year. The Valle Flor Foundation provides the technology and management between the two health systems. Several times a year, a group of surgeons visits STP to deliver basic surgery procedures previously selected via digital consultation between the surgeons in Portugal and the physicians at STP. Likewise, another example of global health procedures linking the Portuguese HNS with STP is the use of telemedicine to triage patients for medical evacuations. These evacuations play a key role as the last level of care and still constitute a significant financial and social challenge for evacuated patients (Goncalves et al. 2021). In STP, the potential for leveraging telemedicine to deliver essential global healthcare services in LMIC supported by the international community is evident.

However, in most LMIC countries, there is the potential for telemedicine to be used to reduce healthcare costs, improve access, and advance health outcomes. It is, therefore, essential to move beyond the WHO stance: it is vital to implement telemedicine services as a crucial tool contributing to the quality of healthcare from a global health perspective (Maia et al. 2019).

Another example comes from Angola. The Angolan Ministry of Health (MoH) is promoting the "municipalization" of health as a strategy to improve healthcare coverage, which means prioritizing the strengthening of the national health system at the district level.

To attain this aim, the MoH decided to support the strategy with a national telemedicine network. To build up this network, a partnership was created with the

Geneva University Hospitals (HUG) and the Portuguese Universidade Nova de Lisboa (UNL). Telemedicine units were built in strategic locations to enable distance education and tele-expertise activities, using software and hardware developed by HUG adapted to local specifications and conditions. Designated physicians in each hospital were trained to use the telemedicine platform. Two technical groups were constituted to analyze the problems and identify appropriate solutions. Seven telemedicine platforms were installed, and by 2022, more than 100 health professionals were trained to use the platform.

One of the aims was to provide distance education activities. For this purpose, a set of 70 courses was prepared, recorded, and webcast. The courses were very well received (96% of participants were very satisfied). However, the use of tele-expertise second opinion connections was limited. This was largely explained by limited computer literacy, restricted availability of computers, and low motivation among the physicians to contact other colleagues for support. Global health is a team effort made possible by digitalization, and this message needs to be promoted. Other significant aspects were the legislative and regulatory framework fragilities and the limitations to internet access in most hospital facilities. The scale-up process to include other sites was interrupted due to financial (and strategic) constraints. These obstacles highlight that a clear strategy, more and better technology investment, and proper capacity when building activities are needed to include other sites and address a growing population demand (Correia et al. 2018).

Correia et al. (2018) provide some evidence of how important global telemedicine services truly are in order to cope with both the geography and the shortage of medical specialties in a remote place like Cape Verde. Here, global telemedicine services support the cardiological monitoring and evacuation procedures from Cape Verde to Portugal, aiming at improving quality and reducing cost (Correia et al. 2017). The monitoring of post-evacuation patients has the potential to save significant resources by avoiding additional evacuations. Moreover, this example of global telemedicine collaborative service—including collaborations with India and Brazil—could even avoid more evacuations as many cases could be treated and followed locally with remote technical specialist support, thus contributing to a more balanced and resilient health system and supporting an overall public health goal.

The impressive success in responding to pediatric cardiologic situations highlighted the importance of telemedicine as another tier of the Cape Verde health system. Other areas (like ophthalmology, dermatology, etc.) can also benefit from global digital health, given the high demand for these specialized services. It is important to realize that the country has neither the technical level nor the number of patients in some areas to justify the existence of some specialties. Also relevant is the growing demand due to the epidemiologic transition towards non-communicable diseases and the geographical dispersion of populations and services. Global digital health seems to be the only solution for which first experiences are now available and where tangible results, both nationally and internationally, can provide insights (Lapão 2012).

As global digital health grows in offering a larger set of services, it needs to consider both business and organizational issues. For that purpose, the MOMENTUM approach can be used to identify priorities. Global digital services provide some clinical advantages, such as second-opinion support, better use of sophisticated equipment, and improved learning. However, the patients reap the most significant benefits. The advantages—if the approach is fully implemented—include quicker diagnostics, less time on waiting lists, cost reduction, and access to teleconsultation from the nearest health facility (Correia et al. 2018).

3 Global Digital Public Health

3.1 Digital Public Health

Public health has gained overall appreciation in recent years. From Ebola outbreaks to the COVID-19 pandemic, the role of public health action has been present in the media and our lives in recent years. For instance, to tackle COVID-19, several measures were adopted, aiming at reducing patient travel to healthcare facilities to prevent the spread of the SARS-CoV-2 virus. Indeed, numerous digital tools have been developed, and existing ones have been improved since 2020. Digital health also means a more efficient way of using medical resources, either by introducing easy ways of accessing care or smart decision support systems like Artificial Intelligence. In this way, digital health has evolved as a priority worldwide and has also changed public health (Lapão 2012).

Digital interventions have been deployed in different settings, from primary health care to specific disease contexts (e.g., diabetes epidemics), to digitally trace infected patients and provide capacity building of public health information. However, it is important to reflect on the implementation process and its delays in the healthcare sector and digital public health with its heavy base in ICT infrastructure and capacities. The implementation of digital information systems in healthcare presents various challenges and obstacles. While the technology itself is important, the organizational side of the digitalization process (i.e., clearly identifying the clinical and other processes required) and the service delivery processes (e.g., interaction with patients, like teleconsultations or the monitoring of vital signs) are equally, if not more crucial to implementation (Wong et al. 2022).

3.2 From Primary Healthcare to Universal Access

Primary health care is the first line of care and the first line of global health. Digital primary healthcare (PHC), supported by new types of digital sensors, the Internet of Things, and the emergence of sophisticated Big Data tools, has opened new opportunities for improving the delivery of PHC services and providing additional and relevant data to public health surveillance. Remote monitoring systems play an important role and help improve patient access globally (Peyroteo et al. 2021). The flexibility of these digital systems has been visibly demonstrated during the COVID-19 pandemic.

The so-called health remote monitoring systems (HRMS) offer benefits such as quicker response to PHC patients' demands, allowing for reduced waiting times at both hospital emergency rooms and PHC centers (Kim and Zuckerman 2019; Lapão 2012). The HRMS mainly targets patients with chronic diseases, often older adults, or COVID-19-infected patients who experience less severe symptoms.

A recent systematic review of the literature on HRMS identified 26 studies with chronic patients in the PHC setting, showing interesting aspects of the progress of digitalizing PHC processes, as well as some relevant limitations. The review predominantly documented cases of patients with diabetes and cardiovascular diseases (representing 62% of all cases). Regarding the implementation of these digital interventions, the greatest difficulties were the integration with existing PHC information systems and the changing working practises of healthcare professionals.

The PHC context now has global reach, as digital services allow mobile patients to interact with their family medicine teams (Wang 2016). Digital PHC integrates multidisciplinary PHC teams and patients, often with complex, chronic pathologies at risk of imbalances in their health status. The chronic care model provides a useful theoretical framework to organize digital care delivery and the involvement of both patients and care teams in the design and implementation processes (Yeoh et al. 2018). The globalization of PHC requires improved digital platforms where matching technology with PHC practices in interventions using sensors and wearables for remote monitoring is critical as a source of information for chronic disease management. A mature digitalization of PHC will imply proper access to real-time information via digital platforms encompassing sensor networks. These networks will provide a significant amount of data that will allow not only a better response to patients but also crucial information to be used in public health, both for surveillance and planning.

A critical area of application for digital technologies globally is diabetes prevention and care. Diabetes increasingly spreads around the globe and can be seen as associated with globalization. Digital health interventions have the potential to help the health systems overcome several diabetes-specific challenges, including an insufficient supply of medicines and materials, poor adherence to guidelines by healthcare professionals, poor adherence to treatment by patients, a lack of access to information or data, and the frequent loss of patients to follow-up. Combined with proper decision support systems, digital public health can help by providing protocol checklists, giving prompts and alerts as per protocols, enhancing communication between healthcare providers and patients, and compiling the schedules of healthcare providers. This can also aid in routine public health data collection by increasing the secondary use of electronic medical records and health management information systems (Correia et al. 2021).

3.3 Digital Contact Tracing

Contact tracing is an excellent example of a public health intervention when combined with other actions like physical distancing, testing, and proper vaccination. It was one of the first measures installed to prevent and guide people's behavior during the COVID-19 pandemic in many European countries. Some digital solutions have been deployed around the world to improve the contact tracing process, motivated mainly by the limited availability of adequately trained public health surveillance experts. A systematic review has been investigating the impact of digital contact tracing on patients infected with COVID-19 (Unim et al. 2022).

Among 27 studies, sixteen were modeling methods, and only eleven were actual population-based studies. Several technologies have been used, including GPS, Bluetooth-based, and manual tracing, amongst others. Unfortunately, the usage approval rate of digital contact tracing apps in the population varied significantly, from 19% to almost 100%. During the COVID-19 pandemic, digital contact tracing was usually combined with other actions (like lockdowns or masks).

The studies generally characterize digital contact tracing as a digital public health tool. Security and privacy were seen as essential constraints but were addressed by only about a third of the situations studied.

Besides the limited knowledge about contact tracing, there are a couple of studies that have shown that digital contact tracing has indeed contributed to reducing further COVID-19 transmission, especially where a sufficiently large population adopted the applications and where there was a combined approach with other public health actions (Correia et al. 2021). Nevertheless, it is important to recognize that inadequate communication strategies and security and privacy constraints might have limited the success of contact tracing apps. These limitations need to be addressed so that digital contact tracing will become an important and effective public health tool, hopefully in time for the next pandemic.

3.4 European School on Health Information

Health information skills inequalities have been recognized as a barrier to the proper development of digital public and global health. Limitations in the COVID-19 pandemic response with respect to digital public health solutions in many European countries confirm this. A global health response requires well-trained public health experts. The InfAct Joint Action on Health Information project (https://www.inf-act.eu/) aims to increase health information capacities across European member states. The previously identified inequalities led to the design and inauguration of the first European School on Health Information. It took place online in 2020, reaching participants from 17 different countries in Europe.

The course topics were selected, aiming to contribute to global health preparedness and the convergence of European HI standard methods and fundamentals, including innovative inputs from the InfAct experts (Lapao et al. 2021). Now, this platform is part of the European Health Information Portal, providing relevant information within the training section (https://www.healthinformationportal.eu/).

3.5 Promoting Global Digital Public Health

3.5.1 From Telemedicine to Pandemics

There is a global interest in promoting global digital public health, with the WHO leading this effort. There are still some challenges, but the main concepts of digital health are already a mainstream issue. However, there are still challenges and obstacles with respect to digital public health implementation. Global digital public health was substantially expanded during the COVID-19 Pandemic. The perception of the use of digital tools in health generally improved (Lapao et al, 2021a), and a clearer vision of the biggest challenges to be faced in the coming years (digital health experts, infrastructure, data protection, privacy, ethics) emerged.

The process of digitalizing public health has already shown the value of tools that were critical in the management of the COVID-19 pandemic (contact tracing, geographical information systems, and decision-supporting systems). However, implementation is still a complex procedure, and it is clear that more evidence-based methodologies need to be used. Digitalization encompasses the combination of technology and healthcare expertise. As such, sharing and communication are essential to reach the full potential that this area can bring us.

Digital solutions have been implemented to address COVID-19, which may, with respect to the major global health issue of climate change, help reduce CO_2 emissions and help improve quality of life. Digital systems, including Artificial Intelligence, robots, and drones, are now changing the paradigm of public health and environment management. These new technologies, both supporting individuals and institutional systems, are thought to offer possible solutions to several global problems. However, bolder steps are warranted to fully address these complex problems with the digitalization of healthcare and public health. We need a more audacious approach to contribute to a significant change in access to public health and to deliver relevant and more-real time insights for public health and policymaking.

3.5.2 Global Digital Public Health Framework

To leverage the full impact of global public health in the coming decades, global digital public health, supported by new digital technologies like information systems, mobile health, sensors, Artificial Intelligence, etc., is an important concept.

Global digital public health components are based on the functions of global health and can be conceived under a systems lens that focusses on:

- Governance and leadership;
- Public health data collection and management;
- Analytics and decision-making;
- Policy dialogue and engaging with populations.

This global digital public health framework implies that a public health function should be supported by digital technology adoption while considering the following two aspects: (i) implementation research to understand what works under which conditions, and (ii) feedback into the health system, emergency response, and public health programs for a leaner and more flexible decision-making and policy management process (Oderkirk et al. 2021; Lapao et al. 2023).

Digital technologies should also be implemented and assessed with consideration to additional principles and aims:

- Establish a framework to promote a proper design of global public health digital services and to enable the establishment of a research agenda;
- Evaluation of health impact for nimble course corrections in global public health programming;
- Focus on addressing the inequalities (health and digital) and the needs of vulnerable populations;
- Proper management of risk, bias, and unintended harm (i.e., digital transparency);
- Include human- and community-centeredness in design, as well as the implementation and evaluation of best practices;
- Emphasis on building community resilience (through participatory practices, engagement, literacy, social media, etc.);
- Consideration of the use of integrated epidemiological and social science analytics;
- Generation and sharing of evidence on what works and what doesn't by using open science and new partnerships to build better systems, interventions, and practices.

4 Conclusion: Challenges Ahead

Due to the complex nature of the global health information ecosystem our societies and communities live in, a global digital public health approach can be applied to guide investment with the highest global health impact, to reduce harm to health at the individual, community, and population health levels, and to support social cohesion and trust in emergency response and interventions dealing with crises such as epidemics, climate change, and food chain disruptions.

The proposed framework encompasses a set of challenges requiring attention from global health institutions:

- First and foremost, the need for a digitally well-prepared health workforce for digital leadership, process improvement, and clinical quality;
- The need for institutions to define a long-term strategic roadmap to tackle the change in the health services delivery process (i.e., deploying new digital public health channels);
- A solid regulatory framework for digital public health;
- The development of essential strategies and partnerships to combat the tricky procurement of new digital;
- Last but not least, a close collaboration with the academia to both leverage new knowledge and provide information on lessons learned;

Digital public health could establish a new paradigm and practice in global and environmental health within the next 10 years, paving the way to planetary health. Public health professionals urgently need to understand how to leverage digital health in order to bridge gaps with other areas of healthcare and across the world. A global digital public health framework could contribute to enabling a change in the role of patients in the global health value chain. For Europe, the new European Health Data Space strategy combined with the European Green Deal may provide an inspiring way forward in this crucial area.

Acknowledgments The author would like to acknowledge the contributions from the discussions with Prof. Hajo Zeeb, Prof. Mélanie Maia, and Dr. Tina Purnat (WHO); and also the Fundação para a Ciência e a Tecnologia (FCT—MCTES) for its financial support via the project UIDB/00667/2020 (UNIDEMI).

References

Baron JH (2009) Sailors' scurvy before and after James Lind—a reassessment. Nutr Rev 67(6):315–332
Correia A, Azevedo V, Lapão LV (2017) A Implementação da Telemedicina em Cabo Verde: Factores Influenciadores. Acta Med Port 30(4):255–262
Correia J, Lapão LV, Mingas RF, Augusto HA, Balo MB, Maia MR, Geissbuhler A (2018) Implementation of a telemedicine network in Angola: challenges and opportunities. J Health Inf Dev Countries 12(1):1–14
Correia JC, Meraj H, Teoh SH, Waqas A, Ahmad M, Lapão LV, Pataky Z, Golay A (2021) Telemedicine to deliver diabetes care in low-and middle-income countries: a systematic review and meta-analysis. Bull World Health Organ 99(3):209
Friedman TL (2006) The world is flat [updated and expanded]: a brief history of the twenty-first century. Macmillan, New York
Goncalves C, da Mata A, Lapão LV (2021) Leveraging technology to reach global health: the case of telemedicine in São Tomé and Príncipe health system. Health Policy Technol 10(3):100548
Kim T, Zuckerman JE (2019) Realizing the potential of telemedicine in global health. J Glob Health 9(2):020307

Koplan JFB et al (2009) Towards a common definition of global health. Lancet 373:1993–1995

Lapão LV (2012) Cape Verde's Santiago Island health system review. WHO, Geneva

Lapao L, Peyroteo M, Paulo M (2021) European school on health information: strengthening public health information workforce in Europe. Eur J Public Health 31(Supplement_3):64–403

Lapão LV, Peyroteo M, Maia M, Seixas J, Gregório J, Da Silva MM, Heleno B, Correia JC (2021a) Implementation of digital monitoring services during the COVID-19 pandemic for patients with chronic diseases: design science approach. J Med Internet Res 23(8):e24181

Lapao LV, Correia JC, Jevtic M (2023) Public health framework for smart cities within the comprehensive approach to sustainability in Europe: case study of diabetes. Sustainability 15(5):4269

Maia MR, Correia AJ, Lapão LV (2015) Policy Paper Telemedicina-Um meio para a saúde global. Um caminho para o acesso universal à saúde. Global Health and Tropical Medicine Instituto de Higiene e Medicina Tropical Universidade Nova de Saúde. https://www.ihmt.unl.pt/policy-paper-telemedicina-um-meio-para-a-saude-global-um-caminho-para-o-acesso-universal-a-saude/. Accessed Jul 2023

Maia MR, Castela E, Pires A, Lapão LV (2019) How to develop a sustainable telemedicine service? A pediatric telecardiology service 20 years on-an exploratory study. BMC Health Serv Res 19(1):1–16

Martini E (2003) How did Vasco da Gama sail for 16 weeks without developing scurvy? Lancet 361(9367):1480

Masic I, Pandza H, Kulasin I, Masic Z, Valjevac S (2009) Tele-education as method of medical education. Med Arch 63(6):350

McLeod KS (2000) Our sense of snow: the myth of John snow in medical geography. Soc Sci Med 50(7–8):923–935

Oderkirk J, Tomlinson N, Elgar K (2021) Case study: digital transformation of public health systems. In: Development co-operation report. Shaping a just digital transformation. OECD, Paris. https://doi.org/10.1787/3a83c9cc-en. Accessed Apr 2023

Peyroteo M, Ferreira IA, Elvas LB, Ferreira JC, Lapão LV (2021) Remote monitoring systems for patients with chronic diseases in primary health care: systematic review. JMIR Mhealth Uhealth 9(12):e28285

Ryu S (2010) History of telemedicine: evolution, context, and transformation. Healthc Inf Res 16(1):65

Ryu B, Kim N, Heo E, Yoo S, Lee K, Hwang H et al (2017) Impact of an electronic health record-integrated personal health record on patient participation in health care: development and randomized controlled trial of MyHealthKeeper. J Med Internet Res 19(12):e8867

Seneviratne M, Peiris D (2019) Digital health in low-and middle-income countries. In: Revolutionizing tropical medicine: point-of-care tests, new imaging technologies and digital health, pp 566–583 https://doi.org/10.1002/9781119282686.ch32

Silva CRDV, Lopes RH, de Goes Bay O Jr, Martiniano CS, Fuentealba-Torres M, Arcêncio RA, Lapão LV, Uchoa SADC (2022) Digital health opportunities to improve primary health care in the context of COVID-19: scoping review. JMIR Hum Factors 9(2):e35380

Theobald S, Brandes N, Gyapong M, El-Saharty S, Proctor E, Diaz T, Wanji S, Elloker S, Raven J, Elsey H, Bharal S (2018) Implementation research: new imperatives and opportunities in global health. Lancet 392(10160):2214–2228

Unim B, Zile-Velika I, Misins J, Pavlovska Z, Lapão L, Peyroteo M, Palmieri L (2022) Systematic review on digitals tools used for contact tracing of COVID-19 patients: Interim results. Eur J Public Health 32(Supplement_3). https://doi.org/10.1093/eurpub/ckac129.063

Walter JF (1979) Scurvy resulting from a self-imposed diet. West J Med 130(2):177

Wang W (2016) The global reach of family medicine and community health. Fam Med Commun Health 4(3):2–3

Waqas A, Teoh SH, Lapão LV, Messina LA, Correia JC (2020) Harnessing telemedicine for the provision of health care: Bibliometric and scientometric analysis. J Med Internet Res 22(10):e18835

Whitmee S, Haines A, Beyrer C, Boltz F, Capon AG, de Souza Dias BF, Yach D et al (2015) Safeguarding human health in the anthropocene epoch: report of The Rockefeller Foundation—Lancet Commission on planetary health. Lancet 386(10007):1973–2028.

Wong BLH, Maaß L, Vodden A, van Kessel R, Sorbello S, Buttigieg S, European Public Health Association (2022) The dawn of digital public health in Europe: implications for public health policy and practice. Lancet Reg Health 14:100316

World Health Organization (2006) Building foundations for eHealth: progress of member states: report of the WHO Global Observatory for eHealth. https://apps.who.int/iris/handle/10665/43599. Accessed Jul 2023

World Health Organization (2015) Atlas of eHealth country profiles: the use of eHealth in support of universal health coverage: based on the findings of the third global survey on eHealth, vol 3. WHO, Geneva. https://www.who.int/publications/i/item/9789241565219. Accessed Jul 2023

World Health Organization (2017) Global diffusion of eHealth: Making universal health coverage achievable: report of the third global survey on eHealth. WHO, Geneva. https://apps.who.int/iris/handle/10665/252529. Accessed Jul 2023

Yeoh EK, Wong MC, Wong EL, Yam C, Poon CM, Chung RY, Chong M, Fang Y, Wang HH, Liang M, Cheung WW (2018) Benefits and limitations of implementing chronic care model (CCM) in primary care programs: a systematic review. Int J Cardiol 258:279–288

Open Access This chapter is licensed under the terms of the Creative Commons Attribution 4.0 International License (http://creativecommons.org/licenses/by/4.0/), which permits use, sharing, adaptation, distribution and reproduction in any medium or format, as long as you give appropriate credit to the original author(s) and the source, provide a link to the Creative Commons license and indicate if changes were made.

The images or other third party material in this chapter are included in the chapter's Creative Commons license, unless indicated otherwise in a credit line to the material. If material is not included in the chapter's Creative Commons license and your intended use is not permitted by statutory regulation or exceeds the permitted use, you will need to obtain permission directly from the copyright holder.

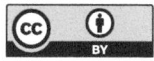

Digital Health Inequality

T. Brand, P. S. Herrera-Espejel, and H. Busse

Abstract Unequal health outcomes across population groups as defined by, for example, socio-economic status, gender, minority status, or sexual orientation are a major public health concern. Health interventions may unintentionally add to these health inequalities through differences in access, usage, and effectiveness (intervention-generated inequalities). Since access and usage of digital tools are known to be socially patterned, digital public health interventions are at a high risk of generating inequality effects ("the digital divide"). In this chapter, we collate evidence on digital divides and their implications for health inequalities and discuss potential solutions for minimizing the risk of intervention-generated inequalities. We argue that the involvement of diverse population groups in the development process of digital public health interventions is a central element for achieving equitable outcomes.

Keywords Health inequality · Health inequity · Digital divide · Digital public health interventions · Intervention-generated inequalities

1 Introduction

Health inequalities, or more precisely health inequities, are differences in health outcomes between individuals or groups of individuals that originate from their unequal access to scarce societal resources—e.g., financial resources, political power, knowledge, beneficial social relationships—and that are considered unfair (Kawachi et al. 2002; Phelan et al. 2010). Public health research has investigated the influence of these social determinants on various health outcomes for many decades, and the aim of reducing inequalities in health has found its way into many national and international policy agendas (Bundesregierung der Bundesrepublik Deutschland 2015; Marmot and Bell 2018; World Health Organization 2013). Over the last two

---

T. Brand (✉) · P. S. Herrera-Espejel · H. Busse
Leibniz Institute for Prevention Research and Epidemiology—BIPS, Bremen, Germany
e-mail: brand@leibniz-bips.de

decades, the question of whether certain types of public health interventions increase or decrease health inequalities has gained attention (Lorenc et al. 2013).

With the rise of digital ubiquity and the expansion of digital health interventions, the question of whether digital population-based health interventions exacerbate or mitigate existing health inequities has gained particular attention (Wirtz, Logie, and Mbuagbaw 2022). Among the positive attributes of digital health interventions are accessibility, reach, personalization, and program flexibility. Additionally, they offer opportunities to engage with users at any time and in any environment, and are generally inexpensive. These attributes are used to explain their potential and increased popularity in health promotion and prevention (Bert et al. 2014). Aside digital interventions at the individual level, digital transformations at the community and organizational levels for better health and well-being are ongoing. However, digitalization also provides entry points for health inequalities. As suggested by Jahnel and colleagues in their "Digital Rainbow Model" (with reference to the socio-ecological model of health by Dahlgren and Whitehead), digitalization permeates all levels of determinants of health inequities (Jahnel et al. 2022). This highlights that despite the potential benefits of digitalization, there is a risk of maintaining or even exacerbating existing inequalities in health, which underlines the importance of investigating potential differential effects of digital interventions and transformations.

Our aim in this chapter is to collate evidence and reflections on health interventions using digital tools from an equity-in-health perspective. Here, the critical question is whether digital health interventions use their potential to diversify information and services and tailor them to the needs of different population groups or whether they merely replicate or amplify real-world inequalities, leaving already disadvantaged population groups even further behind.

2 Dimensions of the Digital Divide

Since access and usage of digital tools are known to be socially patterned, digital public health interventions are at a high risk of generating inequality effects ("the digital divide"). Current literature suggests that the dynamics of the digital divide can be observed and analyzed along three vertical lines: access, usage, and effectiveness (van Deursen and van Dijk 2018; Vassilakopoulou and Hustad 2023).

The first-order divide, access, addresses differences between individuals, groups, geographic areas, and socio-economic levels in terms of how they are able to access internet services, mobile devices, computing hardware, or other connected devices (OECD 2001; Pick and Sarkar 2016; Rivera et al. 2023). Inequalities in access are commonly measured with macro-level variables reflecting accessibility patterns to information and communication technology software and infrastructure connectivity (Ragnedda 2019). Further dimensions of an access divide include differences in the capacity to "maintain use of the internet over time" (e.g., software subscriptions) and access "peripheral equipment (e.g. printers or screens) [...] that make the use of the internet more convenient" (van Deursen and van Dijk 2019).

If access is established, the second-order divide, usage, relates to different patterns of technology use. Empirical contributions examine adoption patterns and frequency of use of internet users (Hargittai 2002), as well as how people locate content online and their search and networking preferences. Research on second-order inequalities explores how cognitive and technical competencies for finding, understanding, evaluating, and creatively using digital tools and information among different demographics can lead to a continuing digital divide (Mubarak and Suomi 2022).

Of equal importance, the term digital exclusion describes the situation when established internet users are unable to meaningfully benefit from the use of online content available to them (Honeyman et al. 2020). This is referred to as the third-order divide, or "empowerment divide", and is defined by differences in the effective outcomes from digital content among different internet user populations. In their majority, studies addressing digital exclusion focus on specific usability issues or biases in design and user research, which disadvantage groups with different digital dexterities. Assessments of the effectiveness of digital interventions center on how exposure to the same intervention content result in differential outcomes depending on participants' personal, cultural, or socio-economic resources (Ragnedda and Ruiu 2017; van Deursen and Helsper 2015).

In addition to these three orders, a fourth order may also be considered in terms of inequalities to privacy preservation and meaningful consent to share personal data. On this subject, Hamoud Alhazmi et al. (2022) suggest that "a new type of digital divide [may be] related to information privacy." Referred to as a "digital privacy divide," the term is used in connection to an individual's power to informedly fulfill their general data protection rights (e.g., General Data Protection Regulation (GDPR) in Europe, state-level data privacy law compliance in the USA, etc.) in light of modern information and communication technology networks, cloud computing, and storage services. Although still emerging, literature on the digital privacy divide puts forward inequalities between groups with diverse socio-economic and digital literacy levels concerning algorithm awareness, privacy and security risk perceptions, and trust in the institutions processing one's data (Honeyman et al. 2020). Awareness is not the only issue here. The third-order divide also links to back inequality in financial resources to, for example, buy safer devices or program licenses that reduce the amount of data tracking and advertisement exposure compared to "free" program versions. Overall, the causes and mechanisms underlying the three levels of the digital divide are multifaceted, encompassing personal, social, community, and societal determinants. Additionally, they are related to technical developments and interventions (Max et al. 2025).

3 Public Health Interventions and the Digital Divide

Digital public health interventions refer to the integration of various types of digital technologies to enhance essential public health operations, such as health promotion, surveillance, population-wide prevention campaigns, and epidemiological research (Iyamu et al. 2022). Commonly used digital technologies include websites (eHealth interventions), text messages, email feedback or prompts, or mobile applications (mHealth interventions). Further uses of digital technologies may involve sensors or other virtual assistive technologies to promote physical activity and reduce the risk of falling in older adults (Pech et al. 2021). Digital divides are reinforced when integrating digital technologies in public health interventions either impedes or favors certain population groups' access, use, and/or effective participation with their personal or health-related data.

3.1 Evidence for Digital Health Inequality

Reviews on the equity effects of digital interventions have indeed highlighted stark inequalities among target populations. For example, a review by Western et al. (2021), including 19 randomized controlled trials in the area of physical activity promotion, found digital interventions to be only effective for those in a high socio-economic position and not effective for changing physical activity in those in a low socio-economic position. Similarly, another systematic review by Szinay et al. (2022), distinguishing between uptake, engagement with, and effectiveness of digital interventions for weight-related behaviors, found differences across inequality indicators concerning the engagement and effectiveness of included interventions. Other reviews on the topic reported mixed or inconclusive findings, highlighting the lack of and, at times, complexity around interpreting available data on inequality domains (Birch et al. 2022; Czwikla et al. 2021). As a result, there is a limited amount of evidence on how digital health interventions impact health equity (Reiners et al. 2019), and the available evidence tends to be varied on the more specific aspects related to equity.

Our own overview of several literature reviews on the topic suggests that the majority of studies on digital public health interventions fail to adequately consider all dimensions of digital inequities and divides as part of their research design and methodology. In their scoping review, Iyamu and colleagues (Iyamu et al. 2022) found that most literature on the digital divide in the domain of digital public health only covers the first two divide orders, focusing either on unequal access to digital technologies or the use of adjacent services (Iyamu et al. 2022). In another instance, Schroeer and colleagues (Schroeer et al. 2021) found that only one study out of the eleven addressed the digital divide as a limitation. In either case, the literature studying the interdependence of digital health literacy and health outcomes of particular at-risk populations is limited (Choukou et al. 2022). Considerations on the "empowerment divide" or privacy preservation rights are seldom addressed or even recognized as such.

3.2 Access to Participation and Misrepresentation

From the outset, unequal access to digital technologies excludes the most deprived communities and geographic areas both from using digital health tools and participating in digital intervention studies. For example, Honeyman et al. (2020) found that aging residents in the UK are less likely to own a mobile phone or have internet connectivity. In another case, they also found that impoverished communities were also less likely to access mobile technology from their homes on a regular basis, meaning that although some groups own mobile devices, they may not use similar mobile phone data plans allowing them to access web-based content equally. Reiners et al. (2019) stress the importance of not only identifying social factors that make a difference in access across the whole population but also in population subgroups (e.g., older migrant women). However, there is a lack of research on technology access in specific communities around the world. As such, the understanding of the intersectionality of groups within groups is lacking, and consequently, there is a failure to tailor interventions and extrapolate results.

For researchers looking to understand and mitigate first-order digital divides, the lack of diversity in research presents a challenge for equitable and inclusive design, as discrepancies in one context do not always hold true in another. For example, Mubarak and Suomi (2022) and Shi and colleagues (Zhen et al. 2024) found that older adults have a higher degree of digital literacy in contexts where they receive immediate support from family members and other social support structures when using the internet and electronic devices.

3.3 Digital Literacy and Generalizability Issues in Evaluation of Interventions

Digital literacy refers to the "confidence and ability of an individual to use a variety of digital technologies" (Choukou et al. 2022). Beyond access to the technology itself, differing skill levels affect the ability to find and retrieve the content of the digital intervention, interact and communicate with the digital tool, or create self-made content, leading to different outcomes among target groups. It is crucial for researchers considering the use of specific digital tools or applications for public health intervention to identify differences in digital literacy among population subgroups to reduce disparities.

At the point of delivery, even though some groups can equally access software or specific devices, this does not guarantee equal use of the available functionalities.

Different uses, although subtle, may impede participants from being able to equally contribute to or benefit from the intervention. In their review, Reiners et al. (2019) conclude that most digital interventions using self-management approaches for chronic diseases, which requires a certain degree of agency and technical competencies, did not consider differences between socio-demographic characteristics of the participants and their digital skills. The studies featured a high risk of non-response bias, which decreased the generalizability of their results. As such, conclusions of most studies may only reliably be extrapolated to participants who owned a smartphone, had continuous access to an internet connection, and had specific language and literacy skills.

Digital health literacy levels vary widely between and within countries and are unequally distributed, as, for instance, in Germany (De Santis et al. 2021). Response differences due to unquantified bias from different literacy levels can cause a lack of internal validity or incorrect assessments in further evaluation stages. For example, the unequal data losses in evaluation and follow-up procedures will affect the interpretation of results between different subgroups and lead to incomplete conclusions. In their review, Schroeer et al. (2021) find that data collected from digital interventions in social media forums are hard to interpret due to possible variability in the tone or intention of different individuals. As a consequence, participatory digital formats are prone to selection bias, where the vast majority of participants are skewed toward higher socio-economic backgrounds.

3.4 Lack of User-Centeredness and Intervention Effectiveness

Although the term digital divide implies a dichotomy, the term is, in fact, used to describe a wide array of individuals from different communities who have different usage conditions, skills, and needs, which evolve over time, as suggested by Reiners et al. (2019). For researchers, it is necessary to facilitate as much equivalent effectiveness as possible among different subsets throughout the delivery stages and beyond.

On this topic, Jarke (2021) explains that an underlying reason for the low uptake of digital services is that participants from different socio-demographic backgrounds may not respond equally "well to the life worlds, use contexts and use practices" of different digital interventions. As for other types of interventions in other domains, if the users "are not satisfied with the system, they will not use it, or will not use it correctly and efficiently." As exemplified in a past systematic review (Clare 2021), despite the proven potential of mobile health applications to improve individual health in several preventative domains, at an aggregate level, such interventions are not equally used or effective for different population subgroups.

3.5 Digital Privacy Preservation and Informed Consent

In addition to issues of access, use, and effectiveness, interventions using digital health components raise ethical challenges related to informed consent and other digital privacy rights. Failure to consider the ethical and privacy values of different groups may lead to designing interventions that do not truly provide equitable, informed consent conditions for participants. Furthermore, it is insufficient to merely require consent over direct data use in the intervention, as concerns about device safety and data confidentiality might still prevail. In terms of study quality, these concerns might affect the accuracy of self-reported data or raise the risk of attrition during delivery phases.

Although research is lacking in this field, Honeyman et al. (2020) assert that perceptions of privacy constitute an essential element in deciding whether or not to use digital health technologies in one way or another. One of the few papers mentioning privacy in their scoping review, from Mackert et al. (2016), explored how perceptions of privacy and trust impacted the adoption of digital health technology in the USA. The study found that lower levels of digital health literacy are associated with lower trust in services provided by public authorities and health technology vendors.

4 Solutions to Digital Divides in Digital Public Health Interventions

There are many ways in which researchers and practitioners can address all aspects of the digital divide in the design, implementation, delivery, and/or evaluation stages of a health intervention (see Fig. 1).

Digital Divide Dimension	Risks & Challenges	Potential Solutions
1st dimension Reach & Access	• No or slow internet connection • No or out-dated devices • Lack of software subscriptions • Low storage and data volume	• Enable intervention on different devices • Use preferred platforms or apps in target group • Provide appropriate devices and data volume • Provide non-digital alternatives
2nd dimension Usage & Engagement	• Differential attrition • Participants cannot operate the system • Content is not understandable • Content is not meaningful	• Involve target groups in content creation • Provide content in easy-to-understand language • Use audio-visual material along written formats • Provide digital literacy trainings
3rd Dimension Effectiveness & Empowerment	• Differential effectiveness • Participants cannot translate information into behavior change	• Adopt "phygital" and hybrid approaches • Combine with higher-level intervention elements (e.g. policy or organizational level)
4th Dimension Data Privacy Preservation	• Disparities in meaningful consent • Gaps in algorithm awareness • Different privacy and security risk perceptions	• Conduct preliminary pilot studies on consent literacy • Plan for formative research to identify motivations for consent among populations subgroups • Hold data management workshops with selected members of communities

Fig. 1 Risks for inequality and potential solutions across the different domains of the development and implementation of a digital health intervention. (Source: own figure)

4.1 Supporting Accessibility to Digital Public Health Interventions

Creating hybrid solutions will enable communities with limited access to digital devices and applications to participate in the intervention. Providing "phygital" solutions, a combination of in-person and online elements to an intervention, may reduce inequalities in reach and access. When designing an intervention with digital and physical tools, Clare (2021) suggests that researchers can be better informed by listening to the experiences of individuals in the target communities of study.

Regarding accessibility, Reiners et al. (2019) also suggest that digital material should be designed to be mobile-friendly and available offline as a standard. The availability of multiple platforms avoids disparities as it considers the different preferences or motivations of different subsets to use digital content. For example, the literature provides evidence that older age groups prefer computers over mobile phones. As stated above, digital interventions should also be optimized for assistive technology such as screen readers, large or simplified text, text-to-speech, and keyboard or commands.

4.2 Supporting Digital Literacy to Ensure Equitable Use Opportunities

Digital health literacy depends on both the users and the system deploying health services or interventions (Jenkins et al. 2022). As such, support, training, and tailored outreach strategies that consider disparities in digital health literacy are as important as designing the intervention itself to be as understandable and usable as possible. It is also essential to ensure that the support is equally distributed or provided among different vulnerable communities (Choukou et al. 2022).

Jenkins et al. (2022) stress that interventions should focus on groups with low digital health literacy levels on both the individual and systemic levels. As an option, researchers may consider offering training workshops to prepare participants to correctly use technology during the delivery stages, identify specific needs, and design interventions accordingly (Choukou et al. 2022). Moreover, frameworks such as the eHealth literacy framework by Norgaard et al. (2015) are useful methodological tools to inform interventions designed before their implementation and delivery. These frameworks help researchers to identify the level of digital health literacy of sampled populations and adapt digital content and materials to reduce barriers among groups with lower levels of digital health literacy. It is, however, important to note that literacy is not always the main barrier. Other factors in everyday life, such as other demands or time restrictions, may be of equal or higher importance for the use of digital health tools.

4.3 Involving the Target Group to Enable Effectiveness

Literature on the co-creation of digital technology indicates that addressing user expectations is a critical step to ensure the adoption and effective use of information systems (Freimuth and Quinn 2004; Jarke 2021). To optimize effectiveness and quality, the identified needs of the target population should be incorporated into all aspects of an intervention from the beginning of the development process. In this regard, adopting co-design, community-based, and participatory approaches during the design stages helps to identify specific mechanisms to improve uptake and engagement with digital tasks required in the interventions.

Moreover, directly engaging with members of the communities during the development process of the interventions has been recommended. Armaou et al. (2020) argue that to tackle community health inequalities, interventions should show cultural sensitivity in their methodology. They suggest using sampling procedures that represent targeted communities' characteristics. For instance, through co-designing and collaborative methods, researchers can identify population language and socio-cultural characteristics and explore "individual literacy, numeracy skill level and psychomotor capabilities" (Armaou et al. 2020).

4.4 Addressing Data Privacy Rights and Consent

Considerations of the appropriate communication of legal and ethical documentation are key to ensuring equal preservation of rights among participants from all population subsets. From the perspective of Nebecker and colleagues (2019), one solution to preserve privacy and obtain meaningful consent is to conduct preliminary pilot studies and plan for formative research aimed at identifying the specific barriers and motivations of culturally diverse individuals to participate in interventions. One key theme is addressing the doubts or worries that participants may have regarding technical functionalities and the safety of digital tools. Along with pilot studies, workshops with selected members of target communities may also be helpful to inform participants on planned data management practices and enable researchers to amend privacy practices to meet socio-cultural needs and preferences.

5 Further Considerations

Broadly speaking, when looking at the type of digital interventions currently tried, tested, and evaluated for health promotion and prevention, reviews have identified what can be described as individual-level, behavior-change interventions (Rose et al. 2017). Due to the focus of individual-level interventions on characteristics such as attitudes, intentions, ability, and individual agency (Adams et al. 2016), there is a risk that these types of more "downstream" interventions will maintain or possibly increase existing inequalities (Lorenc et al. 2013). In contrast, "upstream" interventions, focusing on social, community-level, or policy-level factors (and thus tackling the more structural and environmental determinants of health), are postulated to have more potential to decrease existing inequalities with a potential to lead to co-benefits, such as wider sustainability outcomes (Lorenc et al. 2013).

While individual-level approaches have been a common focus, the broad term "digital health" may also refer to technologies such as those included in health informatics, health systems, and further digital health transformations. When considering these with regard to health promotion and prevention, a range of further uses of digital technologies thus become apparent. One example might be using digital approaches to train intervention staff, lay health workers, or others involved at an organizational level. This is supported by one of the strategies suggested in the World Health Organization guideline on "recommendations on digital interventions for health system strengthening," which is based on evidence from provider-to-provider telemedicine and serves to provide health services at a distance while linking less skilled workers with more specialist ones. So long as access to technology is granted and possible personnel expenses are considered, provider-to-provider telemedicine is regarded as an equitable digital intervention in remote settings (World Health Organization 2019). Similarly, digital health worker decision supports, digital tracking of participant's health status, and digital provision of training and educational content to health workers are regarded as helpful digital means, particularly in rural communities, despite further considerations around network availability, access to electricity, lower levels of training and literacy with technologies, and possible limited access to mobile devices (World Health Organization 2019).

The existing evidence base has predominantly focused on digital technologies for individual-level interventions in public health. Therefore, it is of immense importance that a range of further options for digitalization for health promotion and prevention, going beyond the individual level, should be considered, trialed, and investigated concerning equity effects (Donatella Rita et al. 2024). More "upstream" digital interventions, such as the digitalization of settings, communities, and structures, in particular, warrant further attention and considerations, given their potential to impact existing inequalities positively (Lorenc et al. 2013).

5.1 Combining Digital Components with In-Person Components: The Role of Intervention Modality

A further complication in determining the equity effects of digital interventions is the finding that, contrary to the name, many digital interventions often incorporate at least some in-person components and/or face-to-face contact (Western et al. 2021). As a typical example, the 'HEYMAN' health lifestyle program for young men incorporated a total of seven components, including a responsive website, a wearable physical activity tracker, as well as weekly face-to-face sessions at a university (Ashton et al. 2017). To further illustrate this point, in the systematic review of Szinay et al. (2022) (focused on digital interventions for the promotion of weight-related behaviors), the third most common reason for excluding a study in the screening process was because the intervention was not purely digital. This makes disentangling potential differential or negative effects stemming from the digital nature of the intervention difficult as it carries the question of whether potential inequalities arise because of the overall intervention design or because of the digital elements of the intervention.

Thus, the majority of digital intervention studies inherently include some in-person contact. While this makes it harder to accumulate evidence on the potential differential effects of digital technologies, in many cases, there might be valid reasons for in-person contact. In-person contact at the start of the research study might include recruiting participants into the study or setting up and explaining the technologies (e.g., wearables, online portals, etc.) used in the study. This might provide benefits for actively supporting the user in the use of technology, enhancing the user's digital health literacy and thus limiting access barriers or dropout later on in the study or process (Santarossa et al. 2018). Face-to-face components may also be used as a means to increase the adoption of digital interventions amongst disadvantaged groups. In such cases, appropriately trained facilitators might be present to connect digital services to those user groups. In the mental health field, a review of digital interventions for children and adolescents found that interventions that included an in-person element with a professional, peer, or parent were associated with greater effectiveness, adherence, and lower dropout than fully automatized or self-administered interventions (Lehtimaki et al. 2021).

Next to in-person contact, any face-to-face contact (either in-person or virtual) or additional communication elements might enhance the intervention experience and effectiveness. Guidance through e-coaching has been found to be a common feature and engagement strategy in digital mental health promotion interventions (Saleem et al. 2021), and other research studies generally indicate the benefit that human support can play in the effectiveness or adherence to online interventions (Mohr et al. 2011). A review on internet-based interventions for health behavior change also highlighted how additional methods of communication, such as through text messages, can enhance the effectiveness of digital interventions (Webb et al. 2010). Face-to-face intervention components offer a great chance to overcome barriers to access and use of digital interventions as this contact can be used to train the participants in using the digital intervention, to assure that a certain level of technology use is present, or to strengthen the digital health literacy of the user, allowing for better engagement with the digital technology at hand.

However, with regard to more sensitive or stigmatized topics, digital-only interventions, without in-person contact, might be advantageous. For example, a review in the area of sexual health promotion concluded that digital technologies are effective tools for learning about sexual health and perform better than face-to-face interventions at improving sexual health knowledge (Bailey et al. 2010). Another study found text messages to be a feasible, acceptable, and sensitive way to screen women for postpartum depression (Lawson et al. 2019). Moreover, a review of studies on problem gambling showed that digital interventions might be promising, as these might reduce barriers in accessing professional help (Van Der Maas et al. 2019).

5.2 Are Targeted Approaches the Solution?

As pinpointed by Armaou et al. (2020) in their umbrella review, only a handful of studies deal specifically with inequities affecting the representation of indigenous, LGBTQIA+, and certain culturally and linguistically diverse communities. The authors found that most studies on the digital divide in public health focus on systematically underserved populations from urban areas in the USA, while fewer studies focus on other underserved populations residing outside the USA (Armaou et al. 2020). If the needs of the disadvantaged group are unknown or neglected, developing digital interventions that target said group can be an effective option to counteract inequalities. The targeted approach can support positive identification in groups with shared backgrounds and common issues. It can also help gather data about the preferences and needs of population groups that would otherwise be discriminated against by algorithms. However, in most other cases, diversification of universal approaches, i.e., adapting an intervention to the needs and preferences of different population groups, is preferable for a couple of reasons: targeted approaches can be stigmatizing in the sense that they assume that disadvantaged population groups are somewhat different and problematic; they can essentialize social categories by ignoring the within-groups heterogeneity and reinforce existing stereotypes about the behavior and preferences of people from these groups; and lastly, it is certainly not possible to develop and maintain specific digital interventions for a large number of disadvantaged groups. The politics of prioritizing the needs of one disadvantaged group over the other may be influenced by the level of their political organization and advocacy and can be unfair.

5.3 Real-World Applications

Judgment on the long-term use and potential implementation of digital interventions in the real world remains difficult. As the effects of digital interventions are typically measured short-term, and engagement in digital interventions has been found to be limited and reducing over time, transferring findings from research into the real world and to broader user groups becomes problematic (Romeo et al. 2019). For example, one review in the area of mental health apps reported that intervention completion rates were as low as 2.8% in the real world, which differed substantially from trials on the same program (completion rates of 22.5%), showing that research data might not be transferable and that implementation might differ from reported trials (Fleming et al. 2018).

With the progress of digital transformation, as noted by Brown and colleagues (Brown et al. 2022), the potential of adopting digital public health interventions depends on the technology being intentionally developed with a focus on diversity, equity, and inclusion from its inception, rather than those elements being incorporated retroactively. This highlights the need to consider equity effects, among others, right from the start of intervention development or evaluations. While most digital interventions reported on in this chapter were developed in research settings, the research-practice gap and lack of knowledge about implementing digital interventions into real life—also in terms of potential inequalities—need to be acknowledged.

5.4 Urgent Need for Better Research and Data

Across the studies and reviews in the field of digital technologies and health promotion and prevention, one consistent finding is that there is still a scarcity of data on the differential effects of digital interventions (Brown et al. 2022; Love et al. 2017). This is similar to the literature on equity effects of non-digital interventions (Attwood et al. 2016), highlighting the urgent need for more research and data to assess possible unequal effects of existing interventions.

In order to expand the much-needed evidence on potential differential effects of interventions, it is crucial that studies on digital technologies are powered accordingly and be conducted with adequate sample sizes so analyses on equity subgroups or interaction effects can be undertaken (Czwikla et al. 2021). The PROGRESS-Plus dimensions of place of residence, race/ethnicity, occupation, gender, religion, education, socio-economic status (SES), and social capital, as well as age, disability, and sexual orientation, may be used as potential starting points to assess dimensions of inequality for stratified analyses (O'Neill et al. 2014). The available literature also raises a need for better reporting of equity effects. A Cochrane review investigating how equity impacts are reported across systematic reviews highlights the need for improvement in reporting, such as by providing definitions of health equity, providing more details about analytical approaches used, and transparent reporting of judgments made by review authors (Welch et al. 2022).

Given the available evidence on the potential for digital interventions to maintain or increase existing inequalities in health, it is vital to consider unintended effects of digital public health interventions. As alluded to by Schuez and Urban (2020), possible negative side effects of digital interventions can occur at the individual level (e.g., false health recommendations based on unreliable data; reiterations of existing stereotypes; personal data leakages), level of social relationships (e.g., increases in stigmatization) or at the health services level (e.g., unequal access to and use of technologies). One way to consider potential unintended consequences may be by actively establishing "dark" logic models for digital public health interventions (Bonell et al. 2015). Making potential negative outcomes explicit might help in the early identification of crucial aspects and components in a study that might help avoid unequal effects in access, update, or use of a given digital technology. Moreover, it might help identify suitable measurements for adverse effects or outcomes (e.g., differential uptake of intervention, differential drop-out).

Besides looking at primary studies and synthesis for evidence of the digital divide, available real-world data can be used to assess equity impacts and potential mechanisms of eHealth or mHealth interventions. Several digital technology providers make their data available and allow access to larger data sets, thus offering further potential for investigating inequalities within secondary data analyses. For instance, the social network platform Twitter® provides free access to data, having shown in the past how attitudes toward COVID-19 vaccines varied by region (Liu and Liu 2021) or how physical activity in urban green space varied by season (Roberts et al. 2017), and Facebook® has made data collected through the COVID-19 symptom survey and movement range maps available, located approximately at the county and regional levels. Fitbit®, a popular company for activity and health tracking, includes a data dictionary and recommendations for researchers (https://healthsolutions.fitbit.com/researchers/faqs/) In addition, it is crucial to consider study design decisions that might unintentionally enhance inequities across research stages by, for instance, minimizing study eligibility criteria and carefully designing the screening process into the study (Rebecca et al. 2024). The importance of selecting valid tools and measurements, as well as ensuring that digital health interventions keep abreast of constantly evolving technological innovations, is also important (Max et al. 2025).

5.5 Towards a Deeper Understanding of Inequality

From the perspective of diffusion of innovation theory, inequality in the uptake of a new digital health intervention is to be expected (Rogers 2003). There will always be "early adopters" and "laggards." Similarly, Whitehead (1992) argued that differences between population groups should not be regarded as unfair as long as the disadvantaged group is enabled with the means to catch up soon. So, is it simply a matter of time until differences in the uptake of new digital health interventions between population groups disappear? Given the structural barriers, the different levels of health literacy, and the misrepresentation of disadvantaged groups in the development process, a "wait and see" approach is certainly not the best solution. However, this perspective also reminds us not to judge the equity impact of a new intervention too soon. For example, during the COVID-19 pandemic, many older adults substantially increased their digital competencies, which may reduce the age gap in digital health interventions. Stopping the development of a set of new health interventions at an early stage due to their potential inequality effects would slow down the dynamics of innovation in the field and thus also all the potential beneficial effects. However, even if inequality in uptake is a temporary phenomenon, it becomes harmful when a new digital tool replaces an older non-digital alternative. For example, more and more health services provide online tools for booking an appointment. If appointments can only be booked online, it would exclude all those who do not have access to the internet or have the skills to operate the system.

In many cases, it is quite challenging to determine the threshold when inequalities are harmful. If a digital health intervention is effective among persons with high SES but not among those with a low SES, a negative equity effect is clearly identifiable (Western et al. 2021). There may, however, be other scenarios where this is less clear-cut. Assume a digital health promotion program is effective across all SES groups, but the most substantial effects are found in the highest SES group. Should we discontinue this program due to its differential effectiveness, although it has beneficial effects in all groups? If we elaborate on this scenario further, it becomes clear that we have to consider the alternatives to the (set of) digital interventions under study and other potential uses of the relevant resources. Thus, for a comprehensive assessment, we would need to know how the digital intervention performs across SES strata compared to a non-digital alternative. It could be the case that the magnitude of the inequality effect is equal across both alternatives or even smaller in the digital intervention. This would indicate that introducing the digital intervention in question would not widen existing inequalities. Assuming that we have enough data, we could also evaluate the equity effects of this intervention with regard to other inequality factors, such as gender, minority status, or sexual orientation—plus the intersection of these factors. The more factors we analyze, the more likely it is that we find some inequality effects. From an inequality-sensitive perspective, we would welcome more and more complex analyses of the equity effect. Still, we also see the need for a broader discussion on how to interpret and evaluate the findings. This pertains, for example, to questions on how to judge (1) the relevance of differential access in comparison to differential effectiveness, (2) no effectiveness versus lower effectiveness in disadvantaged groups, (3) inequality in digital interventions in comparison to non-digital interventions, (4) inequality in a small number of subgroups when there is a large number of subgroups in the analysis.

One crucial category for a comprehensive evaluation of inequality effects is what Lorenc and Oliver (2014) called "opportunity cost harms." These are defined by authors as "the potential benefits which may be foregone as a result of committing resources to ineffective or less effective interventions, or to less serious public health problems" and are argued to outweigh any other category of harms (Lorenc and Oliver 2014). For an adequate judgment on whether digital interventions are effective or ineffective, and for whom, we have to consider if investment in other (e.g., non-digital or upstream) interventions would entail a more substantial contribution to health equity.

6 Conclusion

Future research needs to better understand how and why different digital public health interventions influence health inequalities, particularly in the sphere of digital interventions; in the case of those with likely potential for "opportunity cost harms," better reporting of and attention to equity effects is urgently required. In this chapter, we discuss some potential solutions for digital health inequalities. A greater number of more substantial studies are needed to provide evidence of whether such measures positively impact health inequalities. Wrapping up the evidence so far, we would argue that the meaningful involvement of diverse population groups throughout the different phases of development and research on new digital public health interventions is key to reducing the risk of differential access, usage, and effectiveness.

References

Adams J, Mytton O, White M, Monsivais P (2016) Why are some population interventions for diet and obesity more equitable and effective than others? The role of individual agency. PLoS Med 13:e1001990
Alhazmi H, Imran A, Alsheikh MA (2022) How do socio-demographic patterns define digital privacy divide? IEEE Access 10:11296–11307
Andrea L, Wirtz Carmen H, Logie Lawrence, Mbuagbaw (2022) Addressing Health Inequities in Digital Clinical Trials: A Review of Challenges and Solutions From the Field of HIV Research Abstract Epidemiologic Reviews 44(1) 87–109 https://doi.org/10.1093/epirev/mxac008
Armaou M, Araviaki E, Musikanski L (2020) eHealth and mHealth interventions for ethnic minority and historically underserved populations in developed countries: an umbrella review. Int J Commun Well Being 3:193–221
Ashton LM, Morgan PJ, Hutchesson MJ, Rollo ME, Collins CE (2017) Feasibility and preliminary efficacy of the 'HEYMAN' HEALTHY lifestyle program for young men: a pilot randomised controlled trial. Nutr J 16:1–17
Attwood S, Van Sluijs E, Sutton S (2016) Exploring equity in primary-care-based physical activity interventions using PROGRESS-plus: a systematic review and evidence synthesis. Int J Behav Nutr Phys Act 13:60
Bailey JV et al (2010) Interactive computer-based interventions for sexual health promotion. Cochrane Database Syst Rev (9):CD006483
Bert F, Giacometti M, Gualano MR, Siliquini R (2014) Smartphones and health promotion: a review of the evidence. J Med Syst 38:1–11
Bianca D., Rivera Claire, Nurse Vivek, Shah Chastidy, Roldan Adiebonye E., Jumbo Mohammad, Faysel Steven R., Levine David, Kaufman Aimee, Afable (2023) Do digital health interventions hold promise for stroke prevention and care in Black and Latinx populations in the United States? A scoping review Abstract BMC Public Health 23(1) https://doi.org/10.1186/s12889-023-17255-6
Birch JM et al (2022) A systematic review of inequalities in the uptake of, adherence to, and effectiveness of behavioral weight management interventions in adults. Obes Rev 23:e13438
Bonell C, Jamal F, Melendez-Torres G, Cummins S (2015) 'Dark logic': Theorising the harmful consequences of public health interventions. J Epidemiol Community Health 69:95–98
Brown S-A et al (2022) The pursuit of health equity in digital transformation, health informatics, and the cardiovascular learning healthcare system. Am Heart J Plus Cardiol Res Pract 17:100160
Bundesregierung der Bundesrepublik Deutschland (2015) Gesetz zur Stärkung der Gesundheitsförderung und der Prävention (Präventionsgesetz—PrävG). Bundesgesetzblatt, Bonn, pp 1368–1379
Choukou M-A, Sanchez-Ramirez DC, Pol M, Uddin M, Monnin C, Syed-Abdul S (2022) COVID-19 infodemic and digital health literacy in vulnerable populations: a scoping review. Digit Health 8:20552076221076927

Clare CA (2021) Telehealth and the digital divide as a social determinant of health during the COVID-19 pandemic. Netw Model Anal Health Inf Bioinform 10:26

Czwikla G et al (2021) Equity-specific effects of interventions to promote physical activity among middle-aged and older adults: results from applying a novel equity-specific re-analysis strategy. Int J Behav Nutr Phys Act 18:65

De Santis KK, Jahnel T, Sina E, Wienert J, Zeeb H (2021) Digitization and health in Germany: cross-sectional nationwide survey. JMIR Public Health Surveill 7:e32951

Donatella Rita, Petretto Gian Pietro, Carrogu Luca, Gaviano Roberta, Berti Martina, Pinna Andrea Domenico, Petretto Roberto, Pili (2024) Digital determinants of health as a way to address multilevel complex causal model in the promotion of Digital health equity and the prevention of digital health inequities: A scoping review Journal of Public Health Research 13(1) https://doi.org/10.1177/22799036231220352

Fleming T, Bavin L, Lucassen M, Stasiak K, Hopkins S, Merry S (2018) Beyond the trial: systematic review of real-world uptake and engagement with digital self-help interventions for depression, low mood, or anxiety. J Med Internet Res 20:e9275

Freimuth VS, Quinn SC (2004) The contributions of health communication to eliminating health disparities. Am J Public Health 94:2053–2055

Hargittai E (2002) Second-level digital divide: differences in people's online skills. First Monday 7. https://doi.org/10.5210/fm.v7i4.942

Honeyman M, Maguire D, Evans H, Davies A (2020) Digital technology and health inequalities: a scoping review. Public Health Wales NHS Trust, Cardiff

Iyamu I et al (2022) Challenges in the development of digital public health interventions and mapped solutions: findings from a scoping review. Digit Health 8:20552076221102255

Jahnel T, Dassow H-H, Gerhardus A, Schüz B (2022) The digital rainbow: digital determinants of health inequities. Digit Health 8:1–10

Jarke J (2021) Co-creating digital public services for an ageing society: evidence for user-centric design. Springer, Berlin

Jenkins CL et al (2022) Digital health intervention design and deployment for engaging demographic groups likely to be affected by the digital divide: protocol for a systematic scoping review. JMIR Res Protoc 11:e32538

Kawachi I, Subramanian S, Almeida-Filho N (2002) A glossary for health inequalities. J Epidemiol Community Health 56:647–652

Lawson A, Dalfen A, Murphy KE, Milligan N, Lancee W (2019) Use of text messaging for postpartum depression screening and information provision. Psychiatr Serv 70:389–395

Lehtimaki S, Martic J, Wahl B, Foster KT, Schwalbe N (2021) Evidence on digital mental health interventions for adolescents and young people: systematic overview. JMIR Ment Health 8:e25847

Liu S, Liu J (2021) Public attitudes toward COVID-19 vaccines on English-language twitter: a sentiment analysis. Vaccine 39:5499–5505

Lorenc T, Oliver K (2014) Adverse effects of public health interventions: a conceptual framework. J Epidemiol Commun Health 68:288–290

Lorenc T, Petticrew M, Welch V, Tugwell P (2013) What types of interventions generate inequalities? Evidence from systematic reviews. J Epidemiol Community Health 67:190–193

Love RE, Adams J, van Sluijs EMF (2017) Equity effects of children's physical activity interventions: a systematic scoping review. Int J Behav Nutr Phys Act 14:134

Mackert M, Mabry-Flynn A, Champlin S, Donovan EE, Pounders K (2016) Health literacy and health information technology adoption: the potential for a new digital divide. J Med Internet Res 18:e6349

Marmot M, Bell R (2018) The sustainable development goals and health equity. Epidemiology 29:5–7

Max J, Western Eline S, Smit Thomas, Gültzow Efrat, Neter Falko F, Sniehotta Olivia S, Malkowski Charlene, Wright Heide, Busse Carmen, Peuters Lucia, Rehackova Angelo, Gabriel Oteșanu Ben, Ainsworth Christopher M, Jones Michael, Kilb Angela M, Rodrigues Olga, Perski Alison, Wright Laura M, König (2025) Bridging the digital health divide: a narrative review of the causes implications and solutions for digital health inequalities Health Psychology and Behavioral Medicine 13(1). https://doi.org/10.1080/21642850.2025.2493139

Mohr D, Cuijpers P, Lehman K (2011) Supportive accountability: a model for providing human support to enhance adherence to eHealth interventions. J Med Internet Res 13:e1602

Mubarak F, Suomi R (2022) Elderly forgotten? Digital exclusion in the information age and the rising Grey digital divide. Inquiry 59:00469580221096272

Nebeker C, Torous J, Bartlett Ellis RJ (2019) Building the case for actionable ethics in digital health research supported by artificial intelligence. BMC Med 17:137

Norgaard O et al (2015) The e-health literacy framework: a conceptual framework for characterizing e-health users and their interaction with e-health systems. Knowl Manage E-Learn 7:522–540

OECD (2001) Understanding the digital divide. https://www.oecd-ilibrary.org/content/paper/236405667766

O'Neill J et al (2014) Applying an equity lens to interventions: using PROGRESS ensures consideration of socially stratifying factors to illuminate inequities in health. J Clin Epidemiol 67:56–64

Pech M, Sauzeon H, Yebda T, Benois-Pineau J, Amieva H (2021) Falls detection and prevention systems in home care for older adults: myth or reality? J Med Internet Res Aging 4:e29744

Phelan JC, Link BG, Tehranifar P (2010) Social conditions as fundamental causes of health inequalities: theory, evidence, and policy implications. J Health Soc Behav 51(Suppl):S28–S40

Pick J, Sarkar A (2016) Theories of the digital divide: critical comparison. In: 49th Hawaii International Conference on System Sciences (HICSS), Hawaii, 5–8 Jan. 2016, pp 3888–3897

Ragnedda M (2019) Conceptualising the digital divide. In: Bruce M, Massimo R (eds) Mapping the digital divide in Africa. Amsterdam University Press, Amsterdam, pp 27–44

Ragnedda M, Ruiu ML (2017) Social capital and the three levels of digital divide. In: Ragnedda M, Muschert G (eds) Theorizing digital divides. Routledge, London, pp 21–34

Rebecca A, Krukowski Kathryn M, Ross Max J, Western Rosie, Cooper Heide, Busse Cynthia, Forbes Emmanuel, Kuntsche Anila, Allmeta Anabelle Macedo, Silva Yetunde O, John-Akinola Laura M, König (2024) Digital health interventions for all? Examining inclusivity across all stages of the digital health intervention research process Abstract Trials 25(1) https://doi.org/10.1186/s13063-024-07937-w

Reiners F, Sturm J, Bouw LJ, Wouters EJ (2019) Sociodemographic factors influencing the use of eHealth in people with chronic diseases. Int J Environ Res Public Health 16:645

Roberts H, Sadler J, Chapman L (2017) Using twitter to investigate seasonal variation in physical activity in urban green space. GEO 4:e00041

Rogers EM (2003) Diffusion of innovations. Free Press, New York

Romeo A et al (2019) Can smartphone apps increase physical activity? Systematic review and meta-analysis. J Med Internet Res 21:e12053

Rose T et al (2017) A systematic review of digital interventions for improving the diet and physical activity behaviors of adolescents. J Adolesc Health 61:669–677

Saleem M, Kühne L, De Santis KK, Christianson L, Brand T, Busse H (2021) Understanding engagement strategies in digital interventions for mental health promotion: scoping review. JMIR Ment Health 8:e30000

Santarossa S, Kane D, Senn CY, Woodruff SJ (2018) Exploring the role of in-person components for online health behavior change interventions: can a digital person-to-person component suffice? J Med Internet Res 20:e8480

Schroeer C, Voss S, Jung-Sievers C, Coenen M (2021) Digital formats for community participation in health promotion and prevention activities: a scoping review. Front Public Health 9:713159

Schuez B, Urban M (2020) Unintended consequences and side effects of digital health technology: a public health perspective. Bundesgesundheitsblatt Gesundheitsforschung Gesundheitsschutz 63:192–198

Szinay D, Forbes C, Busse H, DeSmet A, Smit ES, König LM (2022) Is the uptake, engagement and effectiveness of mobile interventions for the promotion of weight-related behaviours equal for all? A systematic review. Obes Rev 24(3):e13542

Van Der Maas M et al (2019) Internet-based interventions for problem gambling: scoping review. JMIR Ment Health 6:e9419

van Deursen AJAM, Helsper EJ (2015) The third-level digital divide: Who benefits most from being online? In: Communication and information technologies annual, vol 10. Emerald Group, pp 29–52

van Deursen AJAM, van Dijk JAGM (2018) The first-level digital divide shifts from inequalities in physical access to inequalities in material access. New Media Soc 21:354–375

van Deursen AJ, van Dijk JA (2019) The first-level digital divide shifts from inequalities in physical access to inequalities in material access. New Media Soc 21:354–375

Vassilakopoulou P, Hustad E (2023) Bridging digital divides: a literature review and research agenda for information systems research. Inf Syst Front 25:955–969

Webb T, Joseph J, Yardley L, Michie S (2010) Using the internet to promote health behavior change: a systematic review and meta-analysis of the impact of theoretical basis, use of behavior change techniques, and mode of delivery on efficacy. J Med Internet Res 12:e1376

Welch V et al (2022) How effects on health equity are assessed in systematic reviews of interventions. Cochrane Database Syst Rev 1(1):MR000028

Western MJ, Armstrong MEG, Islam I, Morgan K, Jones UF, Kelson MJ (2021) The effectiveness of digital interventions for increasing physical activity in individuals of low socioeconomic status: a systematic review and meta-analysis. Int J Behav Nutr Phys Act 18:148

Whitehead M (1992) The concepts and principles of equity and health. Int J Health Serv 22:429–445

World Health Organization (2013) Health 2020. A European policy framework and strategy for the 21st century. WHO Regional Office for Europe, Copenhagen

World Health Organization (2019) WHO guideline: Recommendations on digital interventions for health system strengthening. World Health Organization, Geneva

Zhen, Shi Xixi, Du Juan, Li Rongting, Hou Jingxuan, Sun Thammarat, Marohabutr (2024) Factors influencing digital health literacy among older adults: a scoping review Frontiers in Public Health 12 https://doi.org/10.3389/fpubh.2024.1447747

Open Access This chapter is licensed under the terms of the Creative Commons Attribution 4.0 International License (http://creativecommons.org/licenses/by/4.0/), which permits use, sharing, adaptation, distribution and reproduction in any medium or format, as long as you give appropriate credit to the original author(s) and the source, provide a link to the Creative Commons license and indicate if changes were made.

The images or other third party material in this chapter are included in the chapter's Creative Commons license, unless indicated otherwise in a credit line to the material. If material is not included in the chapter's Creative Commons license and your intended use is not permitted by statutory regulation or exceeds the permitted use, you will need to obtain permission directly from the copyright holder.

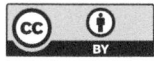

Digital Health Literacy

Hajo Zeeb and Julia Dratva

Abstract Digital health literacy (DiHL) is a new and evolving concept. Given the ongoing digitalization of health, social and other systems, and the shift of health-related information and communication exchange into the digital space, it is becoming an increasingly important qualification for citizens, but also for health workers. The DiHL concept has recently begun to move away from being solely an issue for individuals or patients to an issue for populations and health providers. Privacy and ethical issues associated with digital technology use and data sharing are also closely related to digital health literacy.

The chapter provides an overview of the field, moving from definitions and the evolution of the underlying concept to an overview of core instruments for the assessment of digital health literacy, with selected results on empirical findings from various populations. After discussing critical aspects of current concepts and available knowledge on digital health literacy levels, we provide an outlook that goes beyond enhancing not only individual capacities but also organizational digital health literacy.

Keywords Digital health literacy · Digital transformation · eHealth · eHEALS · Measurement

Abbreviations

DiHL   Digital Health Literacy
DHLI   Digital Health Literacy Instrument

H. Zeeb (✉)
Leibniz Science Campus Digital Public Health, Leibniz Institute for Prevention Research and Epidemiology—BIPS, Bremen, Germany
e-mail: zeeb@leibniz-bips.de

J. Dratva
Institute of Public Health, ZHAW Zurich University of Applied Sciences, Winterthur, Switzerland

Medical Faculty, University of Basel, Basel, Switzerland

© The Authors(s) 2025
H. Zeeb et al. (eds.), *Digital Public Health*, Springer Series on Epidemiology and Public Health, https://doi.org/10.1007/978-3-031-90154-6_13

DHTL-AQ	Digital Health Technology Literacy Assessment Questionnaire
eHEALS	eHealth Literacy Scale
eHLS	eHealth Literacy Scale (Hsu et al. 2014)
eHLQ	eHealth Literacy Questionnaire
HLS19	Health Literacy Survey 2019
PB-mHL	Problem-Based mHealth Literacy Scale
PRE-HIT	Patient Readiness to Engage in Health Internet Technology

1 Introduction

Smartphones and tablets are ubiquitous, and the demands on users of digital information and communication technologies in terms of skills and knowledge are already very high. The digital transformation of the entire healthcare system will further increase these requirements in the future, and the complexity of the applications will continue to rise. As a result, being able to use, understand and apply digital technology and online information is becoming a key qualification for empowered, digitally confident citizens and patients.

This development was substantially accelerated in many countries during the COVID-19 pandemic, as personal contacts had to be limited, and numerous digital offers to sustain the functioning of health and social systems were introduced at previously unencountered speed and breadth. Such offers and developments included video consultations; extensive digital information on the course of the pandemic (and all aspects associated with it); and a social media avalanche of information, misinformation, and discussions (see Box 1 for an example).

Box 1 Insights into Digital Transformation During the COVID-19 Pandemic: Primary Care in Australia (Source: Own Figure)
COVID-19: transformation of primary care in Australia

How did informatics and digital health strategies support the primary care response to COVID-19 in Australia? In a rapid scoping review based on 29 eligible papers, the authors (Jonnagaddala et al. 2021) found that telehealth was the central digital health response. Mobile applications and telephone (national) hotlines were increasingly relevant to support primary care delivery and public health, e.g., through information provision to healthcare professionals and support for child health and nutrition counselling. Adapted funding arrangements for a "digital-first" response to COVID-19 strengthened this development. Telephonic consultations, however, were much more important than video consultations. Among the main inhibitors were knowledge and capacity gaps among care providers as well as access to affordable technology, and unclear funding, along with ethical and privacy concerns. Validated applications and suitable technology, trained staff, and good communication between healthcare professionals were some of the facilitating factors reported.

For many citizens, these developments represented an unforeseen challenge. With access to analog offers and contact with others limited or even prohibited, rapid adaptation of technology became a necessity, even for those who had yet to contemplate going digital for their health needs. On the other hand, the more digitally prone were faced with a rapidly accelerated evolution of health information and health care offers requiring more enhanced skills and additional motivation to test new functions and systems. Notably, the use of technology for health, including digital health information sharing, is socially patterned. In Australia, an online consumer preference survey clearly showed that willingness to use technologies for health was associated with educational attainment (Lee et al. 2022), a finding that has been replicated in other countries as well (Makowsky et al. 2021; Doyle et al. 2021).

Digital health literacy is a central component of any digitally transformed health system as DiHL, addressing important individual and structural aspects that are key to an appropriate and equitable modern (public) health system. Offering technologies that are not accepted, trusted, or used skillfully by the public, patients, and providers alike will be fruitless from a systems perspective. Thus, tackling barriers like technology access, low levels of digital communication skills of providers, and limited trust in privacy, among others, will be an important challenge for modern health and social systems, and different perspectives and developments will need to be considered. From a user perspective, digital technology and digitally conveyed health information may well be overwhelming and be seen to be driven by technical opportunities rather than by user needs. The user needs approach will promote digital health literacy through the necessary interactions and the development of user-centered cases. Sufficient ability to critically engage with the digital transformation of the health system, including shared decision-making, may already be a core component of citizen digital empowerment (Bittlingmayer et al. 2020). For example, as digital technologies (including Artificial Intelligence applications) are increasingly becoming a larger part of the personal, health care, and public health spheres, the understanding of and critical engagement with the technology, its potential, and limitations, becomes crucial for the workforce and public alike.

In addition, the question of which role institutions and organizations take on in the quest to advance digital health literacy has become a matter of discussion as the DiHL concept moves away from being solely an issue for individuals or patients to an issue for populations and health providers. DiHL is also a pivotal capacity in order to advance discussions around privacy and ethical issues associated with digital technology use and data sharing (as discussed in Chapter "Open Data for DiPH Research vs. Data Protection", Buchner et al. in this handbook).

This chapter aims to provide a comprehensive overview of the evolving concept of digital health literacy. We review digital health literacy definitions, empirical methods, and data on digital health literacy in different countries. We also offer a critical assessment of the status and the developments regarding digital health literacy assessments in various populations, highlighting knowledge gaps, potential biases, and future directions of research and assessment.

2 Definitions of Digital Health Literacy

Digital Health Literacy is considered a central precondition to ensure a successful digital transformation of health systems and health communication and to maximize the impact of the digital transformation regarding the population's empowerment and health management competencies. At the same time, what exactly constitutes digital health literacy is still under much debate. This lack of a clear definition is related to the similar lack of a clear definition of eHealth, today more often referred to as digital health: In 2005, Oh et al. stated "eHealth…has become an accepted neologism despite the lack of an agreed-upon clear or precise definition" (Oh et al. 2005). It is reasonable to assume that the discussion on the definition of digital health literacy as an interactive and dynamic concept needs to be ongoing, given the constant development of new technologies and their continuous implementation into everyday life and the health system.

2.1 Relationship Between Health and Digital Literacy

Digital health literacy has its roots in "health literacy." Initially, the concept of health literacy consisted of basic literacy skills needed to understand prescriptions, physician's recommendations, or health bills. It was further developed to include communication and critical literacy (Nutbeam 2000) to obtain, process, and understand basic health information and "services needed to make appropriate health decisions" (Ratzan and Parker 2000). The current health literacy definition adopted by the WHO (Nutbeam and Muscat 2021) underlines the mediating role and responsibility of society, health stakeholders, and health services to enable health literacy (Box 2). It is understood as a complex and life-long social construct, which includes social practices, social and material interactions, and social norms (Bauer 2019).

> **Box 2 Definitions (Source: Own Figure Using Definitions from Nutbeam and Muscat 2021; Oh et al. 2005; Norman and Skinner 2006a; Griebel et al. 2018)**
> **Health Literacy** (Health promotion glossary, Nutbeam and Muscat 2021)
> Health literacy represents the personal knowledge and competencies accumulated through daily activities, social interactions, and across generations. Personal knowledge and competencies are mediated by the organizational structures and availability of resources that enable people to access, understand, appraise, and use information and services in ways that promote and maintain good health and well-being for themselves and those around them.
> **eHealth** (Oh et al. 2005)
> "e-health is an emerging field in the intersection of medical informatics, public health and business, referring to health services and information

Digital Health Literacy

> delivered or enhanced through the Internet and related technologies." (based on (Eysenbach 2001).
> **eHealth Literacy** (Norman and Skinner 2006a)
> "...the ability to seek, find, understand, and appraise health information from electronic sources and apply the knowledge gained to addressing or solving a health problem."
> **Digital Health Literacy** (Griebel et al. 2018)
> "...a dynamic and context specific set of individual and social factors, as well as consideration of technological constraints in the use of digital technologies to search, acquire, comprehend, appraise, communicate, apply and create health information in all contexts of health care with the goal of maintaining of improving the quality of life throughout the lifespan."

The term eHealth literacy surfaced during the first years of the twenty-first century. Numerous definitions with different nuances circulated, but a common understanding was that eHealth was "the use of electronic technologies in health, health care and public health." eHealth literacy was not only about technical developments, but "a state-of-mind, a way of thinking, an attitude, and a commitment for networked, global thinking, to improve health care locally, regionally, and worldwide by using information and communication technology" (Eysenbach 2001). In fact, eHealth was considered to be less about the health of the people or population health but more about health services delivery (health care, health system, health sector, or health industry). eHealth literacy, later called digital literacy, accordingly addressed the question of which skills or competencies were needed by the public to participate and make use of these new services, communication technologies, and systems.

3 Digital Health Literacy: Challenges in Conceptualizing and Measuring an Evolving Concept

Digital health literacy is a multi-literacy concept, illustrated by the Lily model (Fig. 1) (Norman and Skinner 2006a). The model comprises a set of six core skills needed for eHealth literacy.

Two of these are non-specific to digital health literacy (1) traditional literacy (functional literacy, basic education) and (2) information literacy (ability to manage and appraise information). The other four contain specific aspects regarding digital health literacy: (3) media literacy (ability to deal with media and information gained from media), (4) computer literacy (ability to use computers), (5) science literacy (ability to understand and interpret scientific findings), and (6) health literacy (ability to interact with the health system for one's own health).

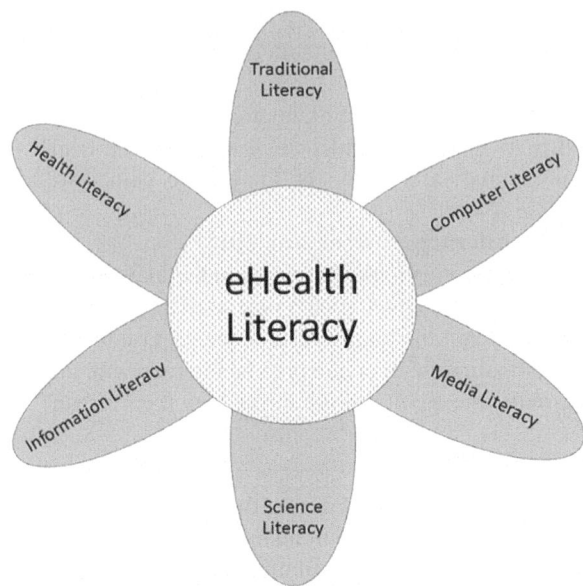

Fig. 1 Lily model of eHealth literacy. (Source: based on Norman and Skinner 2006a)

Various changes have been suggested and partly implemented since the concept was first published: Norman himself pointed out that eHealth literacy evolves according to technological and societal changes and that a subscale on social media or mobile internet use was needed (Norman 2011). Van der Vaart and Drossaert (2017), among others, underlined the need to adapt the definition to the current technological and digital media (web 2.0) and developed an instrument incorporating respective skills (see Table 1). Next to critique regarding the limited focus on skills and competencies assessed by eHEALS, researchers pointed out that the motivation (Kayser et al. 2018) and the readiness (Koopman et al. 2014) to apply literacies is key for digital health literacy to have the intended impact on health. The skills alone will not improve health.

The discussion about further modifications to the Lily model of eHealth includes several aspects that we summarize in the following paragraphs:

- New modes of information-seeking behavior need to be considered

Information literacy—one core component of digital health literacy—has evolved to include new forms of information provision and seeking behavior. Individuals no longer only seek information from experts provided for the population or a specific target group in print and novel media. The public provides and co-creates content. Sharing information with others (prosuming) is increasingly common, while passive information seeking (consuming) is also very common as information is provided abundantly on social media and the internet.

Table 1 eHealth and digital literacy measurement instruments (adapted and extended from Bittlingmayer et al. 2020)

Name/ Reference	Scope	Dimensions	Items	Psychometric analyses	Development/ validation sample	Language
eHEALS (Norman and Skinner 2006b)	General digital health literacy	6 Dimensions: (1) traditional literacy, (2) information literacy, (3) media literacy, (4) computer literacy, (5) science literacy, and (6) health literacy (Lily model)	8 Items, 5-point Likert scale	Factor analyses, item-scale correlations, test-retest reliability 6 months from baseline	Development: USA 13–17 years; validation: different adult populations	Original English, translated in numerous languages
eHLS (Hsu et al. 2014)	Functional, interactive, and critical eHealth literacy in relation to individual health behavior	3 dimensions: (1) functional, (2) interactive, (3) critical evaluation	12 Items, 5-point Likert scale	Fit indices	Development: Taiwan, college students	Taiwanese
eHLQ (Kayser et al. 2018)	eHealth Literacy Framework (eHLF)	7 dimensions: (1) using technology to process health information, (2) understanding of health concepts and language, (3) ability to actively engage with digital services, (4) feel safe and in control, (5) motivated to engage with digital services, (6) access to digital services that work, and (7) digital services that suit individual needs	35 Items	Confirmatory factor analyses	Development: >18 years	Danish, English

(continued)

Table 1 (continued)

Name/Reference	Scope	Dimensions	Items	Psychometric analyses	Development/validation sample	Language
DHLI (van der Vaart and Drossaert 2017)	Complete spectrum of Health 1.0 and Health 2.0 skills, including actual competencies	6 Dimensions: (1) PC/smartphone operational skills, (2) web navigation skills, (3) information searching skills, (4) evaluating reliability (5) determining relevance to oneself, (6) adding self-generated content, (7) protecting and respecting privacy	21 Items, 4-point Likert scale	Internal consistencies, Total scale explained variance, test-retest analysis	>18 years	Danish, English
PRE-HIT (Koopman et al. 2014)	Readiness to use internet resources to access health, and chronic patients	8 Dimensions: (1) health information need, (2) computer/internet experience, (3) computer anxiety, (4) preferred mode of interaction, (5) relationship with doctor, (6) cellphone expertise, (7) internet privacy, and (8) no news is good news	28 Items sorted into 8 factors, four-point Likert scale	Cronbach's alpha, test/retest-reliability (3 months)	Development: Patients with chronic conditions: diabetes, hypertension, heart failure, coronary artery disease	English
DHTL-AQ (Yoon et al. 2022)	Ability to use digital health technology, services, and data	2 dimensions: (1) digital functional, (2) digital critical literacy	34 Items, 4 categories	Cronbach's alpha, model fit analyses, correlation with task ability assessment, eHEALS, Newest Vital Sign	Development: Korea, >18 years	Korean, English
PB-mHL (Zhang and Li 2022)	mHealth (mobile) literacy, problem-based approach	8 Dimensions: (1) mHealth desire, (2) mobile phone operational skills, (3) acquiring mHealth information, (4) acquiring mHealth services, (5) understanding of medical terms, (6) mobile-based patient–doctor communication, (7) evaluating mHealth information, (8) mHealth decision-making	33 Self-reported items, 8 domains	Cumulatively explained variance, Cronbach's alpha, factor loadings, composite reliability values, average variance extracted values, second order model fit indices	Development: China, 30–60 years	Chinese

Name/Reference	Scope	Dimensions	Items	Psychometric analyses	Development/validation sample	Language
HLS19-DIGI (HLS$_{19}$ Consortium 2022)	General health literacy, accompanied by two instruments on interaction with digital resources (DIGI-INT, 2 items) and frequency of use of digital devices (DIGI-DD, 6 items)	1 Dimension: dealing with digital information	8 Items	Cronbach's alpha, confirmatory factor analyses, Rasch Partial Credit Models, and content, discriminatory, and predictive validity	13 European countries, >18 years	13 European languages

eHEALS eHealth Literacy Scale, *PRE-HIT* Patient Readiness to Engage in Health Internet Technology, *eHLQ* eHealth Literacy Questionnaire, *eHLS* eHealth Literacy Scale, *DHLI* Digital Health Literacy Instrument, *HLS19* Health Literacy Survey 2019

- Media literacy extends to a large variety of media

Media ranges from traditional media (newspapers, journals, TV, and radio) to internet websites, blogs, or social media. While some of the content is the same as in traditional media, just provided in a digital format such as digitalized newspapers or books, other content is only available via new media where the origin or validity of the information is sometimes less transparent. Media competency has thus become more challenging, and critical appraisal of available content an essential skill.

- Computer literacy has been replaced by digital device literacy

The devices that allow access to digital health information have evolved from desk computers to tablets or mobile phones and will evolve further. The complexity extends to digital devices that provide not only health information by others but of one's own health through collecting individual health data (mobile applications). Computer literacy thus extends to the skill in using more devices in parallel, new applications, and digital modes of interacting with health services or health providers, such as online appointment tools, telehealth, or sharing mobile health data.

- Science literacy is insufficient in the age of data

While until recently, scientific evidence was provided with explanations and interpretations by scientists, policymakers, or scientific journalists, more and more evidence is provided without an expert interpretation but as mere data points or graphs. Thus, data literacy describes the skills needed to understand and interpret science better than science literacy. Data literacy covers the competencies to access, appraise, and interpret scientific and health data. It further includes the ability to understand and apply basic data security, such as self-protection and the critical appraisal of consequences. Data literacy is becoming an increasingly important skill.

- Organizational and societal digital health literacy needs to be included

As health literacy incorporates societal and organizational responsibility to enable the health literacy of the public, digital health literacy must follow suit. The empowerment of patients or the public to interact with digital health systems must be accompanied by digitally health-literate organizations and institutions.

Given the complexity and different skills, it is intuitive that digital health literacy is more than the addition of different literacy skills or two literacy concepts, namely health literacy and digital literacy (Kickbusch et al. 2021; Paige et al. 2018; van Kessel et al. 2022). There is an interaction between the two, respectively the different skills, that is further modified by individual and societal characteristics. It is these interactions and modifiers that provide both public health opportunities and risks to strengthen or weaken digital health literacy.

4 Measuring Digital Health Literacy

Since the very first digital health literacy instrument, eHEALS, developed by (Norman and Skinner 2006b), various instruments have been developed and published. Most have been tested for their psychometric properties, and some have been validated in different populations.

The most investigated among all remains eHEALS. An important critique relates to the lack of incorporation of skills needed in the era of social media (Lee et al. 2021). Another critique often voiced is the fact that eHEALS was developed in youths, who are assumed to be more experienced in digital technologies. Further, as it has been validated in different populations and age groups, and although in some cases different factor structures depending on the studied population have been reported ranging from a one-factor to a three-factor structure, a single-factor structure is the most consistent finding. Indeed, a benefit of eHEALS is the availability in numerous languages and of comparable data due to its frequent use.

While most instruments build on eHEALS, which is a general population health literacy scale, the newer ones add additional aspects, such as Web 2.0 skills (van der Vaart and Drossaert 2017), mobile technologies (Yoon et al. 2022), or they target specific groups. The PRE-Hit instrument, for example, addresses the health literacy of patients (Koopman et al. 2014), while the eHealth Literacy Scale (eHLS) was used to investigate college students (Hsu et al. 2014). A more recent instrument aimed to improve the main limitation of self-report type instruments, the subjectivity of the response, by adding problem-based questions (Zhang and Li 2022). The new WHO Action Network M-POHL instrument is an 8-item questionnaire for adult populations, with additional questionnaires to measure interaction with digital devices and the frequency of digital resource use (The HLS_{19}-Consortium of the WHO Action Network M-POHL 2022).

The development of new instruments is a reaction to the constantly changing required skills and technological developments, as well as an improved understanding of mediating factors of digital health literacy and health outcomes.

Table 1 presents major published instruments and provides essential characteristics (name, background, validation studies, language, construction (items, factors), psychometric properties).

4.1 Digital Health Literacy Levels in Different Populations

DiHL has been assessed internationally in the general population and select population groups in recent years, applying diverse instruments and using a multitude of concepts and tools. However, due to this heterogeneity of instruments, the comparability of quantitative results is limited. We provide a broad overview of study results in different populations indicating the approaches used in the respective studies.

General population surveys aiming to assess DiHL, e.g., in Germany and Greece, have been conducted, applying various measurement approaches. (Xesfingi and Vozikis 2016) used the eHEALS questionnaire to measure digital health literacy among a convenience sample of Greeks aged 15 years and above, showing that 48.6% had low or fair DiHL, and almost 10% categorized as having high DiHL. Age and education were the strongest correlates of digital health literacy in the sample, but general computer and information literacy were also strongly associated with DiHL (or eHealth as termed by the authors). In Germany, Schaeffer and colleagues (Schaeffer et al. 2021) measured DiHL shortly before and during the COVID-19 pandemic, using a new tool with some relationship to the DHLI instrument (van der Vaart and Drossaert 2017). Digital health literacy labeled as problematic or inadequate was most common in those with low education and among participants above age 65. Overall, the proportion of participants with problematic or inadequate DiHL was 75.8% before the Corona pandemic, while this proportion decreased to 70.5% in the survey conducted in mid-2020. The group with inadequate DiHL decreased from 66.4 to 57.5%, indicating substantial DiHL gains during the pandemic, where health information and health care strongly shifted into the digital space. In an even larger representative German survey conducted online in 2020, Kolpatzik et al. (2020) found limited DiHL (measured by DHLI) reported by 52.4%. Older persons in this survey also showed lower DiHL but less pronounced than in the Schaeffer et al. survey. Migrant status was not associated with DiHL level, but education level showed associations similar to those reported elsewhere. A 2014 survey in Israel used translated versions of the eHEALS tool and showed relatively high levels of eHealth literacy (3.37–3.6 on the 0–4 scale) across three ethnically different participant groups. As group differences were marked when comparing general health literacy, the authors interpreted this high DiHL level as an empowering advantage conferred by internet-based health information offers (Neter et al. 2021). An overview of digital health literacy findings from 13 national surveys using the HLS_{19}-instrument that was also applied in (Schaeffer et al. 2021) indicated that mean scores varied substantially between countries (range 42–79 on a 0–100 scale), with the highest values observed in Norway and lowest in Germany. In the entire sample of more than 29,000 respondents, lower mean scores were found for vulnerable populations, including those with bad self-perceived health, financial deprivation, and low educational attainment (Levin-Zamir et al. 2021). Digital health literacy scores were correlated with general health literacy ($r = 0.53$) as well as other specific literacies.

DiHL is being studied increasingly in select patient populations, often with linkage to specific digital therapeutic approaches (Griffith and Monkman 2017) or health information seeking (Jia et al. 2021) for which DiHL plays a role. There was an increase in studies of this type during the COVID-19 pandemic as therapeutic concepts had to be shifted to reduce personal contact between healthcare providers and patients.

Populations include cancer patients and their caregivers (Verma et al. 2022), patients with spinal cord injury (Singh et al. 2022), and many other patient groups, e.g., (Ramstad et al. 2022; Han et al. 2018). Public health studies investigate digital health literacy among healthy older adults (Berkowsky 2021), parents (Jaks et al. 2019; Juvalta et al. 2020), students (Lotto et al. 2021), and refugee and migrant populations (Wangdahl et al. 2021), to name a few.

An overall picture similar to findings for general health literacy emerges, whereby DiHL is socially patterned and differs between the age groups, with elderly persons often displaying lower levels of DiHL across measurement tools used and groups studied. There is some evidence that persons with low self-rated health have lower digital health literacy levels. While there are few common implications of the numerous and different studies on DiHL, they indicate a strong research interest in the topic fueled by the digital transformation of the health system and the ongoing shift of health information (exchanges) into the digital space. The COVID-19 pandemic seems to have instigated improvements in DiHL, and it will be interesting to see whether these gains persist in the future.

5 Critical Interpretation of Digital Health Literacy Definitions and Data

It has been noted that current definitions of digital health literacy have moved beyond the early understanding and now have a stronger focus on empowerment and self-determination in the context of seeking and working with digital health information. This development clearly reflects the fact that the limited focus on the ability to appropriately handle electronic health information is now broadened to include different sources of health information (such as apps, tracking devices, etc.) and a wide set of sub-competencies that, in sum, support the user or patient as sovereign and competent actor and manager of the digital health information flow. The downside of the strongly contextualized newer definitions of digital health literacy is their increasing complexity and fuzziness, which can lead to problems of demarcation, clarity, and applicability. There is a clear risk of overburdening the concept with multidimensional challenges arising from the rapid and dynamic evolution of the digital health and social landscape. At the same time, achieving a high level of digital health literacy and, thus, digital self-determination is becoming ever more challenging in the light of increasing data and information availability and data use by public and private actors in the health field and beyond. Thus, specific results of digital health literacy studies that indicate particular problems in evaluating and applying digital health information should not come as a surprise, as objectively, the difficulties to obtain a coherent, digitally supported insight into health issues and their determinants or concomitant features becomes increasingly difficult. Nevertheless, it is interesting to see the conceptual links of modern digital health literacy to foundational public health documents such as the Ottawa Charter on health promotion with its broad approach, including individual as well as societal and environmental factors and actions. An integrated digital health literacy concept may hence gain increasing importance for modern public health and its foundations in socio-ecological models (as discussed in Chapter "Public Health in the Digital Era—Digital Entry Points for Population Health", Jahnel et al. in this handbook).

Regarding the measures of digital health literacy, we already pointed to some of the limitations of the current instruments: subjectivity, incomparability, changing demands, and technologies. Many instruments used in health and public health research rely on subjective data. It is the norm to test instruments' psychometric properties and validate them against objective data, comparable instruments, or by means of qualitative data. While some studies try to somewhat objectively measure digital health literacy with problem-based approaches, proficiency, or knowledge tests, the correlation of subjective and objective evaluation of health literacy skills has not been investigated, neither in labs nor real life and the external validation against health endpoints is lacking for all currently published health literacy instruments. Further, an improved understanding of the associated factors of digital health literacy is needed to be sure of its internal validity. The incomparability can be surmounted with studies either applying different instruments simultaneously or the same instrument across studies, age groups and continents, as well as time. Comparability across time is challenging as further technological developments emerge, and the implementation of digital health applications, as well as the public use of digital technologies, is still on the rise. The COVID-19 pandemic has accelerated digital health service provision, which might lead to increasing competition between digital and traditional health services. Citizens and patients are faced with increasingly complex demands in order to benefit from these developments fully.

A lack of representativeness of many DiHL surveys must be noted, however, and with respect to distinct subgroups such as elderly persons or persons with direct or parental migration experience, selective participation in studies remains an issue. Nevertheless, results from existing DiHL surveys mostly show a strong socio-economic and age-related gradient. Empirical data thus underline a digital divide, and (Sieck et al. 2021) have pointed out that DiHL and internet connectivity can be seen as "super social determinants of health" as they have implications for all other social determinants of health. Thus, there is a strong case for digitally inclusive health and social systems, with clear strategic development of technology access and digital health literacy in the population. Participatory approaches supporting self-determination and the appropriateness of technological solutions for diverse socio-economic groups are especially important. If it is true that DiHL—whatever its exact definition—has already become a core factor in health services use and public health advancement, then more intense DiHL monitoring in the population will be needed in order to identify old and new gaps and provide the evidence base for targeted interventions and improvements. Such developments will need to be linked to the overall digital transformation and the evolution of digital public health (Wong et al. 2022).

Finally, we note that an overall implication of individual-centered DiHL testing is that potentially identified deficits can be subject to training and individual capacity gain. However, the case can be made that more attention should be paid to improving bad designs, simplifying access, and reducing unnecessary technological complexity of digital health technologies. In this vein, standardized instruments that measure the (un-) suitability of digital technology offers for health purposes might be an essential addition to the digital health evaluation instrument suite.

6 Outlook

Overall, digital health literacy continues to be a new and still evolving concept. What becomes clear is that digital health literacy can no longer be seen as an individual competency that can be "learned" and then subsequently applied, irrespective of context. Bittlingmayer (Bittlingmayer et al. 2020) talks of digital health literacy as a social practice but critically notes that there is as yet no assessment instrument available that allows the assessment of digital health literacy under this social practice perspective. Moreover, linking digital health literacy to self-determination and increased well-being remains a challenge for measurement strategies and approaches. Interdisciplinary methods beyond (relatively) simple quantitative approaches may be needed to further advance the understanding of this concept.

Given the relative novelty of the concept and the fast transformation of the digital health landscape, it is not surprising that major research gaps exist. While, fortunately, there are European initiatives that use harmonized instruments to measure digital health literacy in different countries, there is still a substantial dearth of information on population-wide and subgroup digital health literacy levels and requirements for improvement and change. Instrument validation and further methods development, as pointed out earlier, remains on the agenda, and conceptual work on approaches to more thoroughly investigate links between health and socio-economic status and digital health literacy is needed, as well as implementation research on best and sustainable ways to advance population and system digital health literacy.

What is currently known regarding the characteristics of digital health literacy in diverse populations nevertheless indicates that actions to strengthen various digital health literacy domains seem strongly required. Such efforts should not, or not exclusively, focus on individuals and their competencies and skills but also take a systems perspective in order to identify structural leverage points supporting digital health literacy. Co-creation of massive online courses (Perestelo-Perez et al. 2020) may be one way to develop and apply learning materials that not only enhance digital health literacy but also strengthen shared decision-making regarding health matters. It is currently unclear whether demographic changes with increasing proportions of "digital natives" and the ongoing digital transformation of societies worldwide will inadvertently lead to higher digital health literacy in the future, but is it clear that a potential for an increasing digital divide exists that is likely also to affect digital health literacy, and consequently health. Equity-oriented digital public health needs to counteract this potential and systematically strengthen digital health literacy in and for all population groups.

References

Bauer U (2019) The social embeddedness of health literacy. In: Okan O, Bauer U, Levin-Zamir D, Pinheiro P, Sørensen K (eds) International handbook of health literacy research, practice and policy across the lifespan. Policy Press, Bristol

Berkowsky RW (2021) Exploring predictors of eHealth literacy among older adults: findings from the 2020 CALSPEAKS survey. Gerontol Geriatr Med 7:23337214211064227. https://doi.org/10.1177/23337214211064227

Bittlingmayer UH, Dadaczynski K, Sahrai D, van den Broucke S, Okan O (2020) Digital health literacy-conceptual contextualization, measurement, and promotion. Bundesgesundheitsblatt, Gesundheitsforschung, Gesundheitsschutz 63(2):176–184. https://doi.org/10.1007/s00103-019-03087-6

Doyle AM, Bandason T, Dauya E, McHugh G, Grundy C, Dringus S, Dziva Chikwari C, Ferrand RA (2021) Mobile phone access and implications for digital health interventions among adolescents and young adults in Zimbabwe: cross-sectional survey. JMIR mHealth uHealth 9(1):e21244. https://doi.org/10.2196/21244

Eysenbach G (2001) What is e-health? J Med Internet Res 3(2):e20. https://doi.org/10.2196/jmir.3.2.e20

Griebel L, Enwald H, Gilstad H, Pohl A-L, Moreland J, Sedlmayr M (2018) eHealth literacy research—Quo vadis? Inform Health Soc Care 43(4):427–442. https://doi.org/10.1080/17538157.2017.1364247

Griffith J, Monkman H (2017) Usability and eHealth literacy evaluation of a mobile health application prototype to track diagnostic imaging examinations. Stud Health Technol Inform 234:150–155

Han HR, Hong H, Starbird LE, Ge S, Ford AD, Renda S, Sanchez M, Stewart J (2018) eHealth literacy in people living with HIV: systematic review. JMIR Public Health Surveill 4(3):e64. https://doi.org/10.2196/publichealth.9687

Hsu W, Chiang C, Yang S (2014) The effect of individual factors on health behaviors among college students: the mediating effects of eHealth literacy. J Med Internet Res 16(12):e287. https://doi.org/10.2196/jmir.3542

Jaks R, Baumann I, Juvalta S, Dratva J (2019) Parental digital health information seeking behavior in Switzerland: a cross-sectional study. BMC Public Health 19(1):225. https://doi.org/10.1186/s12889-019-6524-8

Jia X, Pang Y, Liu LS (2021) Online health information seeking behavior: a systematic review. Healthcare 9(12):1740. https://doi.org/10.3390/healthcare9121740

Jonnagaddala J, Godinho MA, Liaw ST (2021) From telehealth to virtual primary care in Australia? A rapid scoping review. Int J Med Inform 151:104470. https://doi.org/10.1016/j.ijmedinf.2021.104470

Juvalta S, Kerry MJ, Jaks R, Baumann I, Dratva J (2020) Electronic health literacy in Swiss-German parents: cross-sectional study of eHealth literacy scale unidimensionality. J Med Internet Res 22(3):e14492. https://doi.org/10.2196/14492

Kayser L, Karnoe A, Furstrand D, Batterham R, Christensen KB, Elsworth G, Osborne RH (2018) A multidimensional tool based on the eHealth literacy framework: development and initial validity testing of the eHealth literacy questionnaire (eHLQ). J Med Internet Res 20(2):e36. https://doi.org/10.2196/jmir.8371

Kickbusch I, Piselli D, Agrawal A, Balicer R, Banner O, Adelhardt M, Capobianco E, Fabian C, Singh Gill A, Lupton D, Medhora RP, Ndili N, Ryś A, Sambuli N, Settle D, Swaminathan S, Morales JV, Wolpert M, Wyckoff AW, Xue L, Bytyqi A, Franz C, Gray W, Holly L, Neumann M, Panda L, Smith RD, Georges Stevens EA, Wong BLH (2021) The lancet and financial times commission on governing health futures 2030: growing up in a digital world. Lancet 398(10312):1727–1776. https://doi.org/10.1016/S0140-6736(21)01824-9

Kolpatzik K, Mohrmann M, Zeeb H (2020) Digitale Gesundheitskompetenz in Deutschland. KomPart, Berlin

Koopman RJ, Petroski GF, Canfield SM, Stuppy JA, Mehr DR (2014) Development of the PRE-HIT instrument: patient readiness to engage in health information technology. BMC Fam Pract 15(1):18. https://doi.org/10.1186/1471-2296-15-18

Lee J, Lee EH, Chae D (2021) eHealth literacy instruments: systematic review of measurement properties. J Med Internet Res 23(11):e30644. https://doi.org/10.2196/30644

Lee CMY, Thomas E, Norman R, Wells L, Shaw T, Nesbitt J, Frean I, Baxby L, Bennett S, Robinson S (2022) Educational attainment and willingness to use technology for health and to share health information—the reimagining healthcare survey. Int J Med Inform 164:104803. https://doi.org/10.1016/j.ijmedinf.2022.104803

Levin-Zamir DV, Pelikan J, Biro E, Boggild H, Bruton L, De Gani SM, Gibney S, Griebler R, Griese L, Klochanova Z, Kucera Z, Thomas L, Mancin J, Miksova D, Pettersen KS, Le C, Finbraten HS, Guttersrud O, Schaeffer D, Ribeiro da Silva C, Sorensen K, Straßmayr C, Telo de Arriaga M, Vrdela M, for the HLS-19 Consortium of the WHO Action Network M-POHL (2021) Digital health literacy. In: The HLS19 Consortium of the WHO Action Network M-POHL (ed) International report on the methodology, results, and recommendations of the European Health Literacy Population Survey 2019–2021 (HLS19) of M-POHL. Austrian National Public Health Institute, Vienna

Lotto M, Maschio KF, Silva KK, Ayala Aguirre PE, Cruvinel A, Cruvinel T (2021) eHEALS as a predictive factor of digital health information seeking behavior among Brazilian undergraduate students. Health Promot Int 38:daab182. https://doi.org/10.1093/heapro/daab182

Makowsky MJ, Jones CA, Davachi S (2021) Prevalence and predictors of health-related internet and digital device use in a sample of south Asian adults in Edmonton, Alberta, Canada: results from a 2014 community-based survey. JMIR Public Health Surveill 7(1):e20671. https://doi.org/10.2196/20671

Neter E, Brainin E, Baron-Epel O (2021) Group differences in health literacy are ameliorated in ehealth literacy. Health Psychol Behav Med 9(1):480–497. https://doi.org/10.1080/21642850.2021.1926256

Norman C (2011) eHealth literacy 2.0: problems and opportunities with an evolving concept. J Med Internet Res 13(4):e125. https://doi.org/10.2196/jmir.2035

Norman C, Skinner H (2006a) eHealth literacy: essential skills for consumer health in a networked world. J Med Internet Res 8(2):e9. https://doi.org/10.2196/jmir.8.2.e9

Norman CD, Skinner HA (2006b) eHEALS: the eHealth literacy scale. J Med Internet Res 8(4):e27. https://doi.org/10.2196/jmir.8.4.e27

Nutbeam D (2000) Health literacy as a public health goal: a challenge for contemporary health education and communication strategies into the 21st century. Health Promot Int 15(3):259–267

Nutbeam D, Muscat DM (2021) Health promotion glossary 2021. Health Promot Int 36(6):1578–1598. https://doi.org/10.1093/heapro/daaa157

Oh H, Rizo C, Enkin M, Jadad A (2005) What is eHealth (3): a systematic review of published definitions. J Med Internet Res 7(1):e1. https://doi.org/10.2196/jmir.7.1.e1

Paige SR, Stellefson M, Krieger JL, Anderson-Lewis C, Cheong J, Stopka C (2018) Proposing a transactional model of eHealth literacy: concept analysis. J Med Internet Res 20(10):e10175. https://doi.org/10.2196/10175

Perestelo-Perez L, Torres-Castano A, Gonzalez-Gonzalez C, Alvarez-Perez Y, Toledo-Chavarri A, Wagner A, Perello M, Van der Broucke S, Diaz-Meneses G, Piccini B, Rivero-Santana A, Serrano-Aguilar P (2020) IC-Health Project: development of MOOCs to promote digital health literacy: first results and future challenges. Sustainability 12(16):6642

Ramstad KJ, Brors G, Pettersen TR, Deaton C, Palm P, Rotevatn S, Wentzel-Larsen T, Norekval TM (2022) eHealth technology use and eHealth literacy after percutaneous coronary intervention. Eur J Cardiovasc Nurs 22:472–481. https://doi.org/10.1093/eurjcn/zvac087

Ratzan SC, Parker RM (2000) Introduction. In: Selden CR, Zorn M, Ratzan SC, Parker RM (eds) National library of medicine current bibliographies in medicine: health literacy. NLM pub. no. CBM 2000–1. National Institutes of Health, U.S. Department of Health and Human Services, Bethesda, MD

Schaeffer D, Gille S, Berens EM, Griese L, Klinger J, Vogt D, Hurrelmann K (2021) Digital health literacy of the population in Germany: results of the HLS-GER 2. Gesundheitswesen 85:323–331. https://doi.org/10.1055/a-1670-7636

Sieck CJ, Sheon A, Ancker JS, Castek J, Callahan B, Siefer A (2021) Digital inclusion as a social determinant of health. NPJ Digit Med 4(1):52. https://doi.org/10.1038/s41746-021-00413-8

Singh G, Sawatzky B, Nimmon L, Mortenson WB (2022) Perceived eHealth literacy and health literacy among people with spinal cord injury: a cross-sectional study. J Spinal Cord Med 46:118–125. https://doi.org/10.1080/10790268.2021.1963140

The HLS19-Consortium of the WHO Action Network M-POHL (2022) The HLS_{19}-DIGI instrument to measure digital health literacy. Factsheet. Austrian National Public Health Institute, Vienna

van der Vaart R, Drossaert C (2017) Development of the digital health literacy instrument: measuring a broad spectrum of health 1.0 and health 2.0 skills. J Med Internet Res 19(1):e27. https://doi.org/10.2196/jmir.6709

van Kessel R, Wong BLH, Clemens T, Brand H (2022) Digital health literacy as a super determinant of health: more than simply the sum of its parts. Internet Interv 27:100500. https://doi.org/10.1016/j.invent.2022.100500

Verma R, Saldanha C, Ellis U, Sattar S, Haase KR (2022) eHealth literacy among older adults living with cancer and their caregivers: a scoping review. J Geriatr Oncol 13(5):555–562. https://doi.org/10.1016/j.jgo.2021.11.008

Wangdahl J, Dahlberg K, Jaensson M, Nilsson U (2021) Arabic version of the electronic health literacy scale in Arabic-speaking individuals in Sweden: prospective psychometric evaluation study. J Med Internet Res 23(3):e24466. https://doi.org/10.2196/24466

Wong BLH, Maaß L, Vodden A, van Kessel R, Sorbello S, Buttigieg S, Odone A (2022) The dawn of digital public health in Europe: implications for public health policy and practice. Lancet Reg Health 14:100316. https://doi.org/10.1016/j.lanepe.2022.100316

Xesfingi S, Vozikis A (2016) eHealth literacy: in the quest of the contributing factors. Interact J Med Res 5(2):e16. https://doi.org/10.2196/ijmr.4749

Yoon J, Lee M, Ahn JS, Oh D, Shin S-Y, Chang YJ, Cho J (2022) Development and validation of digital health technology literacy assessment questionnaire. J Med Syst 46(2):13. https://doi.org/10.1007/s10916-022-01800-8

Zhang L, Li P (2022) Problem-based mHealth literacy scale (PB-mHLS): development and validation. JMIR mHealth uHealth 10(4):e31459. https://doi.org/10.2196/31459

Open Access This chapter is licensed under the terms of the Creative Commons Attribution 4.0 International License (http://creativecommons.org/licenses/by/4.0/), which permits use, sharing, adaptation, distribution and reproduction in any medium or format, as long as you give appropriate credit to the original author(s) and the source, provide a link to the Creative Commons license and indicate if changes were made.

The images or other third party material in this chapter are included in the chapter's Creative Commons license, unless indicated otherwise in a credit line to the material. If material is not included in the chapter's Creative Commons license and your intended use is not permitted by statutory regulation or exceeds the permitted use, you will need to obtain permission directly from the copyright holder.

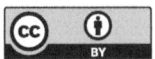

Public Health Goes Digital—Or Not? Ethical Considerations Concerning Limits and Necessary Alternatives

Dagmar Borchers and Regina Müller

Abstract Digitalization is making significant advancements in public health, but does it lead to good healthcare for everyone? Our analysis presents the accomplishments of digitalization in the field of public health and explores their ethical implications, for example, regarding access to healthcare. The analysis focuses on the ethical obligation of society to provide alternatives to digital public health services for those who cannot or do not wish to participate in digital healthcare. In the present transitional period, we suggest that such an obligation (still) exists. We draw our analysis on the principles of public health ethics, including the well-being and health of the population as a value, societal responsibility, justice and equality, and health as a fundamental element of a good life. Different challenges are identified for various groups due to age-related physical and mental limitations, illness, disabilities, and marginalized social categories. We highlight the distinct needs and claims of these groups based on ethical values in public health ethics. Society bears the responsibility of providing alternative solutions for those who are physically incapable of participating in digital processes. Similarly, for individuals and groups who desire inclusion but face inadequate representation, societal efforts must be made to integrate them into digital public health initiatives. However, we face a more complex ethical question regarding the societal obligation to support individuals who willingly abstain from digitalization. Overall, the analysis emphasizes the importance of considering ethical obligations in the context of digital public health, encompassing both the provision of alternatives for those unable to engage and the inclusion of those currently excluded from digital processes.

Keywords Public health ethics · Digital ethics · Justice · Responsibility · Discrimination

D. Borchers (✉) · R. Müller
Applied Philosophy, Department of Philosophy, University of Bremen, Bremen, Germany
e-mail: borchers@uni-bremen.de; regina.mueller@uni-bremen.de

1 Introduction

Digitalization seems to be a matter of course today—within the domain of public health as well as in other sections of contemporary societies. Public health publications discuss how it works, how it proceeds, and what more needs to be done. There are still gaps and deficiencies, but it seems to be a consensus that digital progress should proceed as quickly as possible. However, is this the best path to provide good healthcare for everyone?

There might be some doubts. In the following chapter, we will first highlight some of the successes of digitalization in public health and then offer some considerations against unlimited digitalization within public health. We will ask where problems and limits lie—not to recommend overcoming them, but to look for alternative options. It will be a plea for limits, for maintaining alternatives for those with problems participating in a digitalized world.

For some, this might seem a strange argumentation: shouldn't it be clear that digitalization is a process that cannot and should not be stopped or hindered? Digital tools are an essential part of almost everyone's daily life. Most people look at their smartphone or laptop most of the time, at least several times a day (and night). People live in a digitalized world. And supposing the goal is to provide good healthcare (including prevention and health promotion), it is well-advised to develop services, technologies, and programs that will be part of this world—otherwise, they would not successfully reach people. In addition, digitalization in the healthcare sector has already brought numerous advantages, such as enhanced efficiency and improved access to information (for an overview of opportunities and risks of Artificial Intelligence (AI) and digitalization in the healthcare sector, see, for example, Glauner et al. (2022)).

However, considerations arise regarding those who may become lost, experience significant difficulties in participating, or face exclusion. The underlying questions are whether everyone should be integrated into the digitalized world as much as possible or whether some should be allowed to stay outside if they don't want to or can't participate, for example, because of a disease. We will consider the following fundamental question: do we as a society have an ethical obligation to provide alternatives to digital healthcare for people who cannot and/or do not want to go digital? We assume that at least in a transition period like today, we (still) have this obligation.

2 Not Radically Negative: The Success Stories

2.1 *The Digital Landscape in Public Health Continues to Evolve*

In today's digital age, people are increasingly connected online; smartphone and app use have increased rapidly, and most spend much of their time online (Holst 2020; Pew Research Center 2021a, b). To effectively reach and support people, we must meet them where they are—in the digitalized world. In the meantime, a plethora of digital health applications, tools, and services have emerged to meet a wide range of needs and preferences. These digital technologies offer, for example, resources, including information, preventative measures, and specialized support for people with diseases.

The digital landscape is also evolving in the field of public health. Although there is no uniform definition of what digitalization in public health actually means (Nievas Soriano et al. 2019; Public Health England 2017; Dadaczynski and Tolks 2018), in our understanding, digitalization in the field of public health refers to digital innovations, technologies, and data focusing on the (promotion of) health and well-being of populations, through the prevention of disease and injury, especially including considerations of health inequalities (Zeeb et al. 2020). Digitalization in public health encompasses various technologies, including, for example, applications that collect data from internet platforms and social media to monitor diseases, assess population health, and determine health risks. Further, the analysis of large amounts of data generated by public health systems using data analytics methods and AI-based techniques can help, for example, to identify disease patterns, predict epidemics, develop prevention strategies, and optimize resource utilization (Aiello et al. 2020; Hamilton and Hopkins 2019; Li et al. 2021). Another example is Electronic Health Records (EHRs) (see also Chap. "Surveillance of Population Health and Well-being (EPHO1)", Ahrens and Pigeot, in this handbook). EHRs are digital patient information records, including the patients' medical histories, diagnoses, treatment plans, and medication data. In the ideal case, EHRs enable seamless communication and information exchange between patients, physicians, different healthcare facilities, and providers. Other examples are telecommunications technologies (telemedicine), mobile apps (mHealth), and wearables for disease prevention and health promotion. For example, users can 'track' their health through apps—in turn, the app supports self-care, provides health information, and promotes healthy behavior. There is an immense number of apps on the market (with varying quality) with which users can track their fitness, manage medications, or receive health tips, for example (Kao and Liebovitz 2017; Marcolino et al. 2018). These are just a few examples and do not cover the broad range of technologies that (will) come into play in digital public health.

2.2 *Advantages of Digitalization in Public Health*

The advantages of digitalization in public health are—at least in part—remarkable, with various contributing factors. One of these factors is the diversity of available technologies, which serve multiple purposes, functions, and aim at different target groups. Though we cannot give an overview here, we generally believe that the diversity of digital technologies enables people to engage in health issues in ways that align with their different needs and preferences. There is an app for every imaginable health need these days. And through the use of algorithms and AI, digital health applications can provide personalized information and recommendations. The broad range of offerings may enable a digital engagement with health and illness that addresses specific needs and situations.

Furthermore, digitalization in public health may strengthen the autonomy and empowerment of the users. Through access to information and resources, users can make informed decisions about their health, seamlessly communicate with their healthcare providers, and actively participate in their own treatment. In this respect, digital health solutions might enable individuals to take more responsibility for their health.

In addition, digitalization in public health may improve access to healthcare. Technologies, such as apps, can enable remote care and help receive timely and convenient healthcare services. By providing remote services and overcoming geographical barriers, digital solutions might bridge the gap between individuals and healthcare providers and may improve access to healthcare, particularly for individuals in rural areas or with limited mobility.

Digitalization in public health thus might offer a promising future through the broad range of technologies, personalized services, and empowerment of users. In addition, digitalization may improve access to healthcare services and ensure that more people receive the care they need, regardless of their geographical location or physical limitations.

3 Nor Radically Positive: A Discussion of Limits

3.1 Asking Critical Questions for Ethical Reasons

In addition to these successes, increasingly critical voices can be heard calling for a thorough and systematic examination of the risks regarding digitalization processes in public health (Chauvin and Lomazzi 2017; Lupton 2018; Wong et al. 2022). What is of particular interest to us are the ethical aspects, especially the ethical aspects of public health (Mastroianni et al. 2019; Peckham and Hann 2009; Kass et al. 2015). Public health ethics finds its roots in various ethical theories, particularly consequentialism and deontology (Siegel and Merritt 2019). It also draws inspiration from ethical concepts, such as social justice and human rights (Siegel and Merritt 2019), civic virtue (Jennings 2007), ethical aspects of care (Roberts and Reich 2002), or relational dimensions (Kenny et al. 2010). Despite different understandings of the normative basis for public health ethics, we see commonalities: public health ethics considers the *well-being and health of the population as a value*. The focus is on achieving the best outcome for the health and well-being of communities, not for individuals. Added to this, public health ethics emphasizes the *responsibility of societies and their institutions* to care for the health of their population. This includes, for example, governments, healthcare facilities, healthcare professionals, and society as a whole as subjects of responsibility. Often, there is a special emphasis on *justice and equality*. Considerations and recommendations regarding actions aim to reduce health disparities and to increase equal opportunities for everyone to lead a healthy life. Throughout this section, we will concentrate on aspects of societal and institutional responsibility and justice, basically understood as an equal chance for everybody to have access to quality healthcare.

3.2 Different Challenges for Different Groups

Who is being addressed here? There are people who, due to *age-related physical and mental limitations,* are not or are no longer able to operate digital devices. It can become difficult for them, for example, to use their smartphones or laptops in a successful way to find suitable health apps, digital health services, or just the relevant health information on the internet. A large group of non-users (8.5 million in Germany over the age of 60 in 2021/22) is already at risk of not being included should healthcare be offered (solely) digitally (Kurz and Richter-Kuhlmann 2023). At present, this group presumably includes all those who have not yet or are not sufficiently engaged with digital technologies, primarily because digital development began when they were already at an older age. Even if many older people are open to digital offerings and willing to take the corresponding learning steps, there are others who, whether by choice or inability, cannot sufficiently participate in digital healthcare offerings (UNECE 2022; Federal Minister for Family Affairs, Senior Citizens, Women and Youth 2020).

However, it is to be expected that this group of people will diminish in the future because the younger generations are considered 'digital native's and might only have difficulties in this regard at an older age when limited physical or cognitive abilities make it increasingly difficult to use their existing digital skills. It can also be inspiring to consider not only the more senior stage of life but also the younger one: how can infants, children, and teenagers be appropriately integrated into digital healthcare?

It is also crucial to consider people whose physical or mental conditions, for example, due to disease, make it (increasingly) difficult for them to use digital services. There will always be individuals who, due to certain illnesses, cannot use digital services independently and, therefore, rely on support—regardless of their previous level of digital skills. Examples include individuals who experience Parkinson's disease or have limited mobility due to arthrosis and thus encounter difficulties operating smartphones or laptops manually. The accessibility of digital platforms may also be challenging for individuals with disabilities, such as visual, hearing, or motor impairments, potentially limiting their participation in digital public health initiatives.

Moreover, we have to consider those groups who might be disadvantaged or neglected in digital processes due to marginalized social categories such as gender and sexual orientation, race, or class. Structural discrimination (Young 2008) is apparent in healthcare (See, for example, Ganguli-Mitra et al. 2022; Hutler 2022) and, unfortunately, continues in digital healthcare (Baumgartner 2021; Baumgartner and Waltraud 2023). Lack of access to digital devices, internet connectivity, or affordability of technology may hinder the participation of economically disadvantaged populations in digital public health. Language and cultural barriers may impede the engagement of marginalized groups in digital public health interventions that primarily cater to mainstream populations. Trans, inter, and non-binary individuals could also face exclusion in digital health services in several ways: digital health platforms may not provide appropriate gender options or fail to consider diverse gender identities beyond the binary male/female categorization. This can result in limited or inaccurate data collection and inadequate representation of these individuals' health needs. These discriminations are already apparent in the 'analog' world, but there is a certain risk that they will be carried on and strengthened within digital contexts.

Due to some widely shared ethical values within the domain of public health ethics, we think these different groups have valid, distinctive needs and claims: for individuals who are physically unable to participate in digital processes, it is our societal responsibility to provide alternative solutions. For individuals and groups who are not adequately represented and included in the digital processes, despite wanting to, societies must make special efforts to ensure their proper integration into digital public health initiatives.

3.3 General Background: The Collective Responsibility of Societies and their Institutions

Public health ethics emphasizes, among others, the *collective responsibility of societies and their institutions to care for* the health and well-being of populations. Since the concept of collective responsibility turns groups, as opposed to their individual members, into moral agents, it has been vigorously scrutinized both methodologically and normatively in recent years (see, for example, Isaacs 2011; May and Hoffman 1991; Corlett 2001; Smiley 2017). This includes governments, health institutions, health professionals, and society at large. They all have their part to play in ensuring that no one is marginalized, excluded, or disadvantaged regarding digital healthcare and giving support, especially for those with difficulties participating in digital health services.

This societal responsibility addresses those who cannot join digital health services for being ill or lacking the necessary physical or mental abilities. Those persons and groups need to rely on a society based on solidarity and responsibility. Older, ill, and disabled persons should be given the support they need. These groups require, among other things, access to analogous infrastructures, technologies tailored to their unique needs, e.g., age-appropriate devices, and support to train digital competencies (Kurz and Richter-Kuhlmann 2023). Those marginalized or excluded for structural reasons should also have their needs recognized and be given adequate access and digital tools that fit their (health) needs and situations. This is an essential task of medical professionals, care services, and health insurance companies due to the collective responsibility of societies and their institutions (Kurz and Richter-Kuhlmann 2023).

3.4 Justice

The idea of abandoning people who are excluded from digital healthcare for various reasons does not seem just. In public health ethics, justice, here understood as equal opportunities regarding access to healthcare, is emphasized and defined in numerous ways. In general, it is assumed that efforts should be made to reduce health disparities and ensure that all people have equal access to healthcare systems and services:

> In principle, every sick person has the same right to be allocated the resources available in the given Public Health system for prevention, treatment, therapy and care according to his or her need. This corresponds to an obligation on the part of the community to ensure a sufficiently efficient Public Health system, or at least one that guarantees basic health care (Kersting 2002).

Access to digital health technologies is not equally available to all population groups today. This might be due to missing infrastructures (digital divide) (Ragnedda and Muschert 2013; Cornejo Müller et al. 2020) or due to missing competencies (digital or e-health literacy) (Griebel et al. 2018; Kramer 2017; Lee et al. 2015; Norman and Skinner 2006). Individuals and groups with limited access to infrastructures and technologies or limited digital skills might be excluded from the benefits of digitalization in healthcare, which can lead to inequalities in health (care). Here the groups of older people are addressed, as well as those who are ill and disabled. Inequalities concerning digital participation have to be eliminated, particularly for people in these groups. Individuals losing their e-health literacy and the problems that arise for those persons should be given greater attention by policymakers and healthcare institutions.

Accordingly, justice requires structural reforms and high-quality healthcare beyond digital offerings. Examples of structural reforms might include establishing sufficient consultation time in doctors' practices, support for questions and help with the use of digital offers, easily accessible telephone services in doctors' practices, health insurance companies, and health institutions, as well as help in overcoming (digital) bureaucratic hurdles.

For those who are marginalized structurally (e.g., due to gender, sexual orientation, race, or class), adequate services have to be provided by societies. Justice requires thinking about a broad range of digital and non-digital services and finding creative offers for diverse people.

Structural shortcomings, grievances, and problems within healthcare, such as overburdened physicians and other healthcare professionals, should be addressed directly. Not all of them can be solved or eliminated solely by an increased number of digital services. Thus, digitalization should not be seen as a convenient (technical) way out of structural and institutional crises and problems such as the overwork of healthcare professionals and, for example, the trend towards less time for personal communication.

3.5 Support beyond Transitions—For Health Is an Existential Good

So far, we have a collective social responsibility to support groups who cannot participate and to appropriately integrate groups who, in principle, could participate but are excluded for other reasons.

While alternatives mentioned above should be available for some time of transition, this need not always and fundamentally be the case. It's within the realm of possibility to consider that after a certain transition period, *all* members of our society—regardless of age, disease, or disabilities—should take responsibility for their own digital participation for the entire duration of their lives. Likewise, it's prudent to think in good times about who could provide care and help when limits appear in older age or, in the case of illness, organizing the transfer of digital (health) participation to trusted persons. Caring relatives, friends, or healthcare professionals might be suited to such a task. From a certain stage of digitalization processes, the responsibility for digital participation (until the end of life) might be placed entirely in the hands of the individual—just like the responsibility for their finances.

However, is this analogy convincing? Is it persuading that banks will operate solely via online banking or that railway companies will close their ticket counters, selling tickets exclusively online? Are these processes comparable? Initially, it may seem that way, but there are decisive differences. Health is not just one area of life among many others—health is a fundamental component of what is philosophically known as a *good life*:

> Health is not one good among others. Like peace, freedom, security and life itself, health is a transcendental or conditional good. It is generally true of such goods that they are not everything, but without them everything is nothing. They have an enabling character; their possession must be presupposed so that individuals can approach, pursue and expand their life projects at all with a prospect of minimal success. In times of normality they are inconspicuous, because then we are sure of their possession and do not pay much attention to them in the routine of everyday life. If, however, we run short of them and therefore find ourselves in existential borderline situations and emergencies, then they form the sole content of our concern; all other interests then fade away, the acquisition and re-acquisition of the conditional goods becomes the exclusive goal of our whole endeavor (Kersting 2002).

The field of healthcare, but especially care in cases of illness, is often associated with fears and emotions for the people affected. People are often very sensitive, uncertain, ashamed, and afraid about their bodies, health, and illness. Especially patients often want to talk to a counterpart who is aware of these feelings and notices when someone is reluctant to ask a question, express a need, or formulate a demand.

People need encouragement and the possibility to ask questions and express their feelings. It is not solely about information but also about recognition and being empathically perceived by others as a person in need.

Digital services implicate being thrown back on oneself to a certain extent, having to manage diseases and healthcare (including prevention) independently to a certain degree. Moreover, digital services require a certain degree of conformity and adaptation to predefined formats and underlying patterns of thinking and organization, which causes a certain deindividualization even if those services are supposedly tailored to meet personal needs.

Prevention and healthcare are utterly vital for all individuals. As long as people are involuntarily excluded from digital health services due to factors such as illness, disabilities, aging, lack of education, language skills, or (further) forms of structural discrimination, society should provide alternatives to digital healthcare even beyond a transitional period, because the exclusion would not be based on a decision made autonomously by the people in question. And of course, make efforts to appropriately integrate these groups into digital processes.

It is more challenging for us to decide whether this obligation to provide support, including, for example, the provision of alternative non-digital communication channels and service options, also applies to those who want to abstain from the processes of digitalization. This may be for ideological, religious, cultural, or even political reasons. In these cases, we think it is up to them to bear the consequences. This decision might be compared to those who reject the offers of conventional medicine. They should be free to make these decisions, but it might be wrong of them to expect compensation from society for these (personal) decisions. For example, those who do not use smartphones may not be reachable if necessary, and they may be unable to make phone calls while away from home. While this might not be problematic per se, there can be situations where having a smartphone would have been advantageous for them. However, it is up to them to manage these risks.

3.6 General Reasons for Retaining a Critical Stance toward Digitalization

It is also important to consider aspects that are currently being discussed in digital ethics regarding Big Data and AI-based systems (Heider et al. 2012; Yang et al. 2021; Mooney and Pejaver 2018; Vayena et al. 2015). In digital public health, justice demands that concerns about protecting sensitive health data are taken seriously. There is, for example, a risk of data breaches, misuse, or unauthorized access to personal health information (Kunz et al. 2020; Myers et al. 2008). As long as it is not guaranteed that the privacy of individuals can be adequately protected from threats of this kind—especially in the highly sensitive area of health—alternatives to digital service offerings should be an option in the healthcare system. In addition, algorithms can contain *biases* and lead to unintended discrimination, which can have dramatic consequences in healthcare (George et al. 2018; Obermeyer et al. 2019; Mason 2019). Furthermore, our lack of understanding of certain techniques, such as Machine Learning (Char et al. 2018), can be seen as another argument for providing non-digital healthcare services (see Chap. "AI Meets Digital Public Health", Steinert et al. in this handbook).

Finally, we should be aware that comprehensive digitalization in the healthcare sector would bring our technological dependence on globally operating economic corporations to an extreme. As a society, we are increasingly becoming dependent on digital infrastructures and technologies, which might implicate a growing influence of economically oriented tech companies on the field of public health.

4 Conclusion

The digitalization of public health will continue. It seems to be a success story, and many individuals seem content and happy with the new digital offerings. Digital tools and services will get better and better and will probably contribute to a high-quality healthcare system. Thus, we should be optimistic.

Presumably, people will have fewer difficulties with digital devices and offerings in the future since more and more of them will be digital natives from early on. They will grow up in a digitalized world and thus be more familiar with digital technologies.

Nevertheless, structural marginalization, discrimination and exclusion due to social categories, such as gender, race, and class, will not disappear without serious societal efforts. On the contrary, they might even be retained and—in the worst case—strengthened by digital processes. This challenge must be actively addressed by society.

From an ethical perspective, we should strive for digitalization processes in public health with a sense of proportion, namely, digitalization with an awareness of its shortcomings and necessary limits. Beyond these limits, there must be a space for alternatives and healthcare organized and operated with attention, sensitivity, and creativity.

References

Aiello AE, Renson A, Zivich PN (2020) Social media—and internet-based disease surveillance for public health. Annu Rev Public Health 41:101–118. https://doi.org/10.1146/annurev-publheal th-040119-094402

Baumgartner R (2021) Künstliche Intelligenz in der Medizin: Diskriminierung oder Fairness? In: Bauer G, Kechaja M, Engelmann S, Haug L (eds) Diskriminierung und Antidiskriminierung: Beiträge aus Wissenschaft und Praxis. transcript, Bielefeld

Baumgartner R, Waltraud E (2023) Künstliche Intelligenz in der Medizin? Intersektionale queer-feministische Kritik und Orientierung, GENDER—Zeitschrift für Geschlecht, Kultur und Gesellschaft 1-2023, 11–25. https://doi.org/10.3224/gender.v15i1.02.

Char DS, Shah NH, Magnus D (2018) Implementing machine learning in health care—addressing ethical challenges. N Engl J Med 378(11):981–983. https://doi.org/10.1056/NEJMp1714229

Chauvin J, Lomazzi M (2017) The digital technology revolution and its impact on the public's health. Eur J Public Health 27(6):947

Corlett JA (2001) Collective moral responsibility. J Soc Philos 32(4):573–584

Cornejo Müller A, Wachtler B, Lampert T (2020) Digital Divide—Soziale Unterschiede in der Nutzung digitaler Gesundheitsangebote. Bundesgesundheitsbl 63:185–191. https://doi.org/10.1007/s00103-019-03081-y

Dadaczynski K, Tolks D (2018) Digitale Public Health: Chancen und Herausforderungen internetbasierter Technologien und Anwendungen. Public Health Forum 26(3):275–278

Federal Minister for Family Affairs, Senior Citizens, Women and Youth (2020) Older people and digitisation. Findings and recommendations from the Eighth Government Report on Older People. Federal Minister for Family Affairs, Senior Citizens, Women and Youth. https://www.bmfsfj.de/resource/blob/159708/ed36ad230d6038b9f0a439fb03ddf35b/achter-altersbericht-kurzfassung-englisch-data.pdf. Accessed 22 Jun 2023.

Ganguli-Mitra A, Qureshi K, Curry GD et al (2022) Justice and the racial dimensions of health inequalities: a view from COVID-19. Bioethics 36:3. https://doi.org/10.1111/bioe.13010

George AS, Morgan R, Larson E et al (2018) Gender dynamics in digital health: overcoming blind spots and biases to seize opportunities and responsibilities for transformative health systems. J Public Health 40(2):ii6–ii11. https://doi.org/10.1093/pubmed/fdy180

Glauner P, Plugmann P, Lerzynski G (eds) (2022) Digitalization in healthcare. Implementing innovation and artificial intelligence. Springer, Cham. https://doi.org/10.1007/978-3-030-65896-0

Griebel L, Enwald H, Gilstad H et al (2018) eHealth literacy research—Quo vadis? Inform Health Soc Care 43(4):427–442. https://doi.org/10.1080/17538157.2017.1364247

Hamilton JJ, Hopkins RS (2019) Using technologies for data collection and management. In: Rasmussen SA, Goodman RA (eds) The CDC field epidemiology manual. Oxford University Press, New York

Heider D, Massanari AL et al (eds) (2012) Digital ethics—research and practice. Lang, New York

Holst A (2020) Smartphone users worldwide 2016–2021. https://www.statista.com/statistics/330695/number-of-smartphone-users-worldwide/. Accessed 30 Jun 2023.

Hutler B (2022) Causation and justice: locating the injustice of racial and ethnic health disparities. Bioethics 36:260–266. https://doi.org/10.1111/bioe.12994

Isaacs T (2011) Moral responsibility in collective contexts. Oxford University Press, Oxford

Jennings B (2007) Public health and civic republicanism: toward an alternative framework for public health ethics. In: Dawson A, Verweij M (eds) Ethics, prevention, and public health. Oxford University Press, New York, pp 30–58

Kao C-K, Liebovitz DM (2017) Consumer mobile health apps: current state, barriers, and future directions. PM&R 9. https://doi.org/10.1016/j.pmrj.2017.02.018

Kass N, Paul A, Siegel A (2015) Ethical principles and ethical issues in public health. In: Detels R et al (eds) Oxford textbook of global public health. Oxford Academic, Oxford. https://doi.org/10.1093/med/9780199661756.003.0017. Accessed 22 Jun 2023

Kenny NP, Sherwin SB, Baylis FE (2010) Re-visioning public health ethics: a relational perspective. Can J Public Health/Revue Canadienne de Santé Publique 101(1):9–11

Kersting W (2002) Egalitäre Gesundheitsversorgung und Rationierungspolitik. Überlegungen zu den Problemen und Prinzipien einer gerechten Gesundheitsversorgung. In: Kersting, W Kritik der Gleichheit. Über die Grenzen der Gerechtigkeit und der Moral. Velbrück Wissenschaft, Weilerswist.

Kramer U (2017) Selbstbestimmter Umgang mit Gesundheits-Apps? Über welche Kompetenzen müssen Verbraucher_innen verfügen? HiBiFo 2-2017, 16–30. https://doi.org/10.3224/hibifo.v6i2.02

Kunz T, Lange B, Selzer A (2020) Datenschutz und Datensicherheit in digital public health [digital public health: data protection and data security]. Bundesgesundheitsblatt, Gesundheitsforschung, Gesundheitsschutz 63(2):206–214. https://doi.org/10.1007/s00103-019-03083-w

Kurz C, Richter-Kuhlmann E (2023) Ältere und Digitalisierung. Noch viele Hürden. Deutsches Ärzteblatt 120:14
Lee K, Hoti K, Hughes JD et al (2015) Consumer use of "Dr Google": a survey on health information-seeking behaviors and navigational needs. J Med Internet Res 17(12):e288. https://doi.org/10.2196/jmir.4345
Li L, Novillo-Ortiz D, Azzopardi-Muscat N et al (2021) Digital data sources and their impact on people's health: a systematic review of systematic reviews. Front Public Health 9:645260. https://doi.org/10.3389/fpubh.2021.645260
Lupton D (2018) Digital health: critical and cross-disciplinary perspectives. Routledge, London
Marcolino MS, Oliveira JAQ, D'Agostino M et al (2018) The impact of mHealth interventions: systematic review of systematic reviews. JMIR Mhealth and Uhealth 6(1):e23. https://doi.org/10.2196/mhealth.8873
Mason M (2019) Algorithmic disability discrimination. In: Cohen IG et al (eds) (2020) Disability, health, law and bioethics. Cambridge University Press, Cambridge. Available at SSRN: https://ssrn.com/abstract=3338209
Mastroianni AC, Kahn JP, Kass NE (eds) (2019) The Oxford handbook of public health ethics, Oxford Handbooks online edn. Oxford Academic. https://doi.org/10.1093/oxfordhb/9780190245191.001.0001. Accessed 9 Jun 2023
May L, Hoffman S (1991) Collective responsibility. In: May L, Hoffman S (eds) Five decades of debate in theoretical and applied ethics. Rowman & Littlefield Publishers, Lanham
Mooney SJ, Pejaver V (2018) Big data in public health: terminology, machine learning, and privacy. Annu Rev Public Health 39(1):95–112
Myers J, Frieden TR, Bherwani KM et al (2008) Ethics in public health research. Am J Public Health 98:793–801. https://doi.org/10.2105/AJPH.2006.107706
Nievas Soriano BJ, García Duarte S, Fernández Alonso AM et al. (2019) eHealth: advantages, disadvantages and guiding principles for the future. JMIR. https://doi.org/10.2196/preprints.15366. Accessed 22 Jun 2023.
Norman CD, Skinner HA (2006) eHealth literacy: essential skills for consumer health in a networked world. J Med Internet Res 8(2):e9. https://doi.org/10.2196/jmir.8.2.e9
Obermeyer Z, Powers B, Vogeli C et al (2019) Dissecting racial bias in an algorithm used to manage the health of populations. Science 366(6464):447–453. https://doi.org/10.1126/science.aax2342
Peckham S, Hann A (eds) (2009) *Public health ethics and practice* (Bristolonline edn. Policy Press Scholarship Online), https://doi.org/10.1332/policypress/9781847421029.001.0001. Accessed 14 Jun 2023.
Pew Research Center (2021a) Mobile fact sheet. http://pewrsr.ch/2ik6Ux9. Accessed 22 Jun 2023.
Pew Research Center (2021b) Social media fact sheet. http://pewrsr.ch/2jbcwOh. Accessed 22 Jun 2023.
Public Health England (2017) Digital-first public health: public health England's digital strategy. https://www.gov.uk/government/publications/digital-first-public-health/digital-first-public-health-public-health-englands-digital-strategy. Accessed 22 Jun 2023.
Ragnedda M, Muschert GW (eds) (2013) The digital divide. The internet and social inequality in international perspective. Routledge, London. https://doi.org/10.4324/9780203069769
Roberts MJ, Reich MR (2002) Ethical analysis in public health. Lancet 359(9311):1055–1059. https://doi.org/10.1016/S0140-6736(02)08097-2
Siegel AW, Merritt MW (2019) An overview of conceptual foundations, ethical tensions, and ethical frameworks in public health. In: Mastroianni AC, Kahn JP, Kass NE (eds) The Oxford handbook of public health ethics, Oxford Handbooks, Online edn. Oxford Academic. https://doi.org/10.1093/oxfordhb/9780190245191.013.1. Accessed 14 Jun 2023
Smiley M (2017) Collective responsibility. In: Zalta EN (ed) The Stanford encyclopedia of philosophy. https://plato.stanford.edu/archives/sum2017/entries/collective-responsibility/. Accessed 30 Jun 2023
UNECE (2022) Policy brief on ageing No. 26 on ageing in the digital era. https://unece.org/sites/default/files/2022-02/ECE-WG.1-39-PB27_0.pdf. Accessed 22 Jun 2023.

Vayena E, Salathé M, Madoff LC, et al. (2015) Ethical challenges of big data in public health. PLOS. Computational Biology. https://doi.org/10.1371/journal.pcbi.1003904

Wong BLH, Maaß L, Vodden A et al (2022) European Public Health Association (EUPHA) digital health section. The dawn of digital public health in Europe: implications for public health policy and practice. Lancet Reg Health Eur 14:100316. https://doi.org/10.1016/j.lanepe.2022.100316

Yang YC, Islam SU, Noor A et al (2021) Influential usage of big data and artificial intelligence in healthcare. Comput Math Methods Med 2021:5812499. https://doi.org/10.1155/2021/5812499

Young IM (2008) Structural injustice and the politics of difference. In: Grabham E, Cooper D, Krishnadas HD (eds) Intersectionality and beyond, 1st edn. Routledge-Cavendish, Abingdon

Zeeb H, Pigeot I, Schüz B et al. (2020) Digital Public Health—ein Überblick. Bundesgesundheitsbl 63. https://doi.org/10.1007/s00103-019-03078-7.

Open Access This chapter is licensed under the terms of the Creative Commons Attribution 4.0 International License (http://creativecommons.org/licenses/by/4.0/), which permits use, sharing, adaptation, distribution and reproduction in any medium or format, as long as you give appropriate credit to the original author(s) and the source, provide a link to the Creative Commons license and indicate if changes were made.

The images or other third party material in this chapter are included in the chapter's Creative Commons license, unless indicated otherwise in a credit line to the material. If material is not included in the chapter's Creative Commons license and your intended use is not permitted by statutory regulation or exceeds the permitted use, you will need to obtain permission directly from the copyright holder.

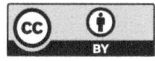

Social Media in Digital Public Health

Elida Sina, Merle Freye, Thomas Eßmeyer, Lara Reich, and Daniel Diethei

Abstract In over two decades of social media (SM) and constantly increasing user accounts, it is unquestionable that SM has taken an ever more important stand in society, combining various functions for communication and entertainment. SM represents a powerful tool to promote healthy behaviors to a larger public audience and hence, has the potential to be integrated into digital public health (DiPH). Using this potential requires a profound understanding of the potential impact of SM on health, well-being, and related behaviors. This chapter, therefore, discusses the impact of SM on DiPH, with a particular focus on the vulnerable group of children and adolescents.

This chapter considers three perspectives: First, epidemiological studies show that SM exposure has a negative impact on children's and adolescents' diets and can further contribute to addiction, psychosocial distress, and depressive symptoms. Second, from the perspective of Human-Computer Interaction (HCI), SM provides interface strategies such as dark patterns that trick users into unwanted interactions, which may lead to increased screen time, and could thus worsen the adverse health outcomes. Third, from a legislative perspective, we explore how European and mainly German laws protect vulnerable groups in the SM environment.

E. Sina (✉)
Leibniz Institute for Prevention Research and Epidemiology – BIPS, Bremen, Germany

Leibniz Science Campus Digital Public Health (LSC DiPH) Bremen, Bremen, Germany

Institute for Evidence in Medicine, Medical Faculty and Medical Center - University of Freiburg, Freiburg, Germany
e-mail: sina@leibniz-bips.de

M. Freye · L. Reich
Leibniz Science Campus Digital Public Health (LSC DiPH) Bremen, Bremen, Germany

Institute for Information, Health and Medical Law, Faculty of Law, University of Bremen, Bremen, Germany

T. Eßmeyer · D. Diethei
Leibniz Science Campus Digital Public Health (LSC DiPH) Bremen, Bremen, Germany

Faculty of Mathematics and Informatics, University of Bremen, Bremen, Germany

© The Author(s) 2025
H. Zeeb et al. (eds.), *Digital Public Health*, Springer Series on Epidemiology and Public Health, https://doi.org/10.1007/978-3-031-90154-6_15

Keywords Social media · Digital public health · Digital health interventions · Dark patterns · Regulation

Abbreviations

BGB	German Civil Code
COVID-19	Coronavirus disease 2019
DiPH	Digital public health
DSA	Digital Services Act
EDPB	European Data Protection Board
EU	European Union
FOMO	Fear of missing out
fMRI	Functional magnetic resonance imagining
GDPR	General data protection regulation
HCI	Human-computer interaction
PRISMA	Preferred reporting items for systematic reviews and meta-analyses
RCT	Randomized controlled trial
SM	Social media
UK	United Kingdom
USA	United States of America

1 Introduction

The last decades have digitally transformed various aspects of people's life. Digital transformations allow everyone with access to the internet, computers, and smart devices to maintain most of their needs from the comfort of their homes while speeding up many daily tasks. This includes things from doing the weekly grocery shopping to streaming a favorite show at any desired time, to building and keeping relationships all over the globe. As these transformations remain an ongoing process with many interpersonal interactions occurring online, it is warranted to understand the impact this contemporary digital ecosystem has on users' health and well-being. Because of their enormous scope, digital technologies yield potential benefits and risks for their users. Looking through a public health lens, benefits include the potential use of digital technologies for health promotion, disease prevention, and citizens' empowerment, which has lately led to the concept of digital public health (DiPH) (Wong et al. 2022). In contrast, risks may include dependence on the internet, smartphones, and social media (Kuss and Griffiths 2017), increased levels of upward social comparisons in the digital environment, cyberbullying (Boer et al. 2021), and poor well-being (Boers et al. 2019).

An important aggregator for DiPH is social media (SM). SM includes a wide range of social applications, such as virtual game worlds, and social networking sites like Facebook, Instagram, Snapchat, and TikTok, but also web blogs, forums, microblogs, and content communities, such as YouTube (Kuss and Griffiths 2017). SM is used for various services that include but are not limited to communication, entertainment, information access, sharing content, as well as building and maintaining social relationships. The global growth of SM is driven mainly by the increasing use of mobile devices, including smartphones and tablets. Roughly 80% of SM is used via mobile technologies (Statista 2022a). In 2020, more than 3.6 billion people were using SM worldwide, a number projected to increase to almost 4.41 billion in 2025. On average, internet users spend 147 minutes daily on SM platforms and messaging apps. This represents an increase of more than half an hour since 2015. Currently, the Philippines spend the most time on SM daily. Filipino internet users spend an average of three hours and 53 minutes daily with SM platforms (Statista 2022b). Facebook remains the most prominent social network worldwide, with 2.7 billion monthly active users, where 6.3% of its users are 13–17 years old (Statista 2022a).

In fact, the age group with the highest time spent on SM globally is adolescents and young adults (16–24 years old), with an average use of 3.34 h/day (Statista 2022c). They also have the highest number of SM accounts, an average of 9.1 accounts, to be more precise (Statista 2022c). In the United States of America (USA), 7 out of 10 adolescents reported using the internet to access Instagram, while half of adolescents reported being "almost constantly" online (Anderson and Jiang 2018). In Europe, 9- to 11-year-old children mostly use the internet to watch videos on YouTube, while older children (13–16 years) prefer to use social networking sites, such as Facebook and Instagram (Mascheroni and Ólafsson 2014). The pan-European Net Children Go Mobile study showed that 68% of 9–16-year-old children have at least one social networking profile (Smahel et al. 2020). This percentage varies by age but not by sex and very little by socio-economic status (SES). Recent data from the USA indicate that although the main SM platforms have age limitations (e.g., ≥ 13 years on Facebook and Instagram), 7 out of 10 children younger than 8 years watch SM videos on their smartphones (Rideout and Robb 2020). This indicates that age identification on SM environment does not work, and this is subsequently associated with issues such as data and consumer protection, as well as the privacy of minors, to name a few.

Given the ubiquitous presence of SM in today's world, it is unquestionable that SM represents a powerful tool to reach broader public audiences and promote healthy behaviors. Hence it represents a fundamental component of the DiPH. Also, SM can easily reach and be accepted by vulnerable groups, thus leveraging the ultimate goals of DiPH. The ubiquitous availability of SM by almost every age group calls for an urgent and profound understanding of the underlying design strategies of SM platforms and the potential impact on health, well-being, and related behaviors. Evidence from the last decade shows that the use of SM platforms is associated with a range of adverse health-related outcomes among youth, such as poor mental health (Bozzola et al. 2022) and unfavorable eating habits (Qutteina et al. 2022). Other issues have quickly emerged in the SM environment, including concerns related to privacy and cyber-security, in addition to facilitating the spreading of fake news and misinformation. In this chapter, we will focus on children and adolescents, who are considered a vulnerable group because their brain maturation is not completed until the age of 25 years (Arain et al. 2013). We will discuss the role of SM in the scope of DiPH, considering three main perspectives: (1) the impact of SM on health and well-being, (2) the problematic and unethical design patterns of SM platforms as well as fake news and misinformation sharing on SM, and (3) the related answers of European and German law. The data mentioned earlier indicate that SM has penetrated children's and adolescents' lives. Hence, it is crucial to address the role of SM exposure in health outcomes.

2 SM Environment and Health Outcomes in Children and Adolescents

Today's children and adolescents spend increasing amounts of time with SM, thanks to the broad access to mobile devices and the internet. This increasing time online offers vast opportunities for learning and self-development. First and foremost, SM is an excellent environment to help children and adolescents fulfill their need to belong, especially during times of social isolation. They use SM to connect with friends and family, get involved in community activities, but also to become part of groups with similar interests (Shychuk et al. 2022), all of which help children and adolescents to develop a sense of self, community, and the world around them. SM is useful in helping youth receive and offer emotional support and discuss mental health topics (Shychuk et al. 2022). Moreover, children and adolescents use SM to access information about local cultural and sportive events and work on school-related projects. Adolescents increasingly use SM to be up-to-date with the latest trends (e.g., fashion, music), to learn cooking recipes or craft projects, and many more (Ngqangashe et al. 2022), which helps them to develop new skills and self-representation. Adolescents, in particular, use SM to access health, dieting, or physical fitness information and, most importantly, to access information about health topics that are difficult to discuss with others, such as sexual health (Lenhart et al. 2010). Remarkably, SM has enormous benefits for health promotion, as it may reach larger target groups over a short period of time. SM is shown to be a useful and effective tool for promoting healthy nutrition and mental well-being in adolescents (Latha et al. 2020). A recent Systematic reviews have show that interventions via SM could improve fruit or vegetable intake and reduce consumption of sugar-sweetened beverages through behavioral change techniques such as social support, self-monitoring, goal setting, and feedback (Hsu et al. 2018).

2.1 Social Media and Mental Health in Children and Adolescents

Despite various benefits, SM also poses many risks for young populations. The literature examining the effects of SM on health outcomes in children and adolescents mainly focuses on SM dependence (Müller et al. 2016). A vast amount of research shows that exposure to social networking sites can contribute to addiction and psychosocial distress in adolescents and young adults (Cha and Seo 2018; Lopez-Fernandez et al. 2017). Moreover, excessive and compulsive SM use is associated with high levels of depressive symptoms (Banyai et al. 2017), mediated through poor sleeping quality (Carter et al. 2016). A recent Canadian study showed that for every hour spent using SM, adolescents showed a significant increase in depressive symptoms (Boers et al. 2019). In a representative Hungarian adolescent sample, problematic SM use—measured with the Bergen Social Media Addiction Scale— was more frequent among adolescent girls with low self-esteem and with high levels of depression symptoms (Banyai et al. 2017). Additionally, adolescent girls who regularly shared images of themselves on SM reported significantly higher overvaluation of body shape and weight, body dissatisfaction, and dietary restraint relative to those who did not (McLean et al. 2015). They also reported greater internalization of the thin ideal (McLean et al. 2019), which refers to girls' drive for thinness due to accepting the societal values of thinness and applying them to themselves (Juarascio et al. 2011). Literature suggests that the main drivers that lead to excessive use of SM are the *fear of missing out* (FOMO) and the *no mobile phone phobia* (Kuss and Griffiths 2017). FOMO is a phenomenon observed in SM, and it refers to the fear that others could be having rewarding experiences which one is missing. This fear is followed by compulsive behaviors to maintain social connections online, like checking and refreshing the SM feed to see what others are doing (Gupta and Sharma 2021). FOMO has also been related to a lack of emotional control, anxiety, poor well-being, and lack of sleep (Gupta and Sharma 2021).

Prolonged use of SM use may also lead to emotional overeating through increasing levels of anxiety (Gao et al. 2022). In fact, SM platforms are bombarded with content on health and nutrition, which promote weight loss, weight management, and even more dangerous attitudes toward eating disorders, like pro-anorexia (e.g., using hashtags #proana) and pro bulimia nervosa (e.g., #promia) related posts. Nowadays, everyone can give nutritional advice on SM, whether they have a nutritional educational background or not, including SM influencers, celebrities, user communities or culinary chefs, to name a few. Evidence shows that SM's nutrition and health content is often based on flawed assumptions due to the lack of evidence-based features (Sabbagh et al. 2020). This may lead to undermining users' efforts in managing weight and other unintended consequences, such as recurrent cycles of weight loss and regain, stress, exercise avoidance, and even depression (Marks et al. 2020). Furthermore, a study based on content analysis of *fitspiration* images on Instagram (Tiggemann and Zaccardo 2018) showed that most images contained only the thin and toned body type, which was related to adverse effects on body image for young men and women. Another study conducted on adolescents investigated the role of SM use patterns, including problematic SM use—measured as a loss of control over SM usage such that the person neglects hobbies or other daily activities due to SM—and frequency of daily SM use in relation to mental health. It was observed that problematic SM use, but not SM use frequency, was associated with decreased mental health after 1 year (Boer et al. 2021). Problematic SM use predicted increased levels of cyber-victimization, which refers to higher levels of negative experiences online, such as being insulted or receiving aggressive messages from peers. Problematic SM use also predicted higher engagement in upward social comparisons such that the person perceives their peers' appearances as superior to their own. However, the association between problematic SM use and poor mental health was not mediated by cyber-victimization nor upward social comparisons (Boer et al. 2021).

Other modifiable factors have been suggested to mediate the association between SM exposure and poor mental health. The role of offline family life and family lifestyle could moderate or mediate the association between SM exposure and youth's mental health. Preadolescents whose parents self-reported greater control over their child's time on SM described better mental health outcomes, including lower depressive symptoms and higher appearance and life satisfaction when compared to those with lower parental control (Fardouly et al. 2018). This association was mediated by preadolescents spending less time browsing and making fewer comparisons of their appearances on SM (Fardouly et al. 2018). Another study reported that a lack of family meals moderates the association between SM use and poor well-being in youth aged 16–21 (Jagtiani et al. 2019). Among those reporting no family meals, well-being scores were lower for participants using SM for longer than 4 h/day compared to those not using SM at all. In contrast, well-being scores were similar among those having more family meals but with different SM use duration. These data highlight the importance of supporting families to implement healthy media use plans and strategies to increase resilience against the negative effects of SM use.

Sex differences in the impact of SM on mental health have also been investigated. A longitudinal study among UK adolescents showed that exposure to cyberbullying, displacement of sleep, and physical activity altogether mediated 80% of the association between SM use and poor mental health in girls (Viner et al. 2019). In comparison, the mediation was only 12% in boys (Viner et al. 2019). The frequency of physical activity and difficulties getting to sleep mediated the association between SM use and poor mental health among Italian adolescent girls as well, but not among boys (Zhang et al. 2022). Findings from these studies indicate that different mechanisms appear to be operative between girls and boys. In particular, more research is warranted to understand the underlying mechanisms of the association between SM exposure and mental health in boys.

2.2 Social Media and Dietary Intake in Children and Adolescents

The ubiquitous presence of SM in children's and adolescents' lives represents a powerful tool for marketing activities. While the marketing of unhealthy commodities of alcohol and tobacco products to children is well regulated in most SM platforms, this does not hold true for unhealthy food and beverage products. As such, food companies increasingly use SM to advertise their unhealthy products to children and adolescents. These companies use various SM marketing strategies, including paid partnerships with bloggers (i.e., SM influencers), competitions based on user-generated content, marketing campaigns with celebrities, or advergames, to name a few. Some companies even allow their followers to order products directly via their SM feed. SM influencer marketing is an increasingly used strategy by food companies to promote products high in fat, sugar, and salt content, targeting children, adolescents, and young adults. In their carefully edited videos and images, SM influencers, also often referred to as internet celebrities, can influence their followers' opinions by endorsing brand products online (De Veirman et al. 2019). They are also seen as idols and role models by children and adolescents. As such, children tend to imitate influencers' behavior in their everyday life (Freeman et al. 2014).

Studies conducted in Canada (Potvin Kent et al. 2019), Australia and Belgium (Qutteina et al. 2019; Baldwin et al. 2018) examined children's and adolescents' exposure to food and beverage advertisements on SM platforms, and found that the majority of advertisements were promoting unhealthy food and beverage products. Children and adolescents are vulnerable to advertising messages, as their brain development and the cognitive ability to recognize advertisements' selling intent is not fully developed compared to adults (Rozendaal et al. 2010). Image and video-based SM platforms such as Instagram, TikTok, or YouTube, which are the platforms with the highest use among children and adolescents (Rideout and Robb 2019), have facilitated the abundance of highly appetizing, digitally-enhanced unhealthy food images and videos (Spence et al. 2016). Studies in humans have shown that mere exposure to appetizing digital food images increases neural activation in brain areas related to attention, visual processing, and reward (van Meer et al. 2015; Spence et al. 2016).

A recent comprehensive systematic review synthesized the most emerging literature examining the role of SM exposure on healthy children's and adolescents' diets (Sina et al. 2022). The review confirmed a positive relationship between SM exposure and increased intake of unhealthy foods and beverages, lowered fruit/vegetable intake, and frequent breakfast skipping. It further showed that SM exposure was associated in a dose-response manner with the daily intake of caffeine (mainly through the consumption of energy drinks) and sugar-sweetened beverages, as well as with the frequency of fast food consumption. The review identified a number of mechanisms underlying the abovementioned associations, which will be discussed in the following.

First, the association between SM exposure and dietary outcomes in children and adolescents were explained by an increased neural response in brain areas related to reward and decision-making after viewing digital food images. Randomized controlled trials (RCTs) using functional magnetic resonance imaging (fMRI) scans showed that children who were exposed to food images, compared to non-food images, had heightened brain activation in areas related to memory, reward (Allen et al. 2016), attention, and visual processing (van Meer et al. 2016; Samara et al. 2018). Two factors impacted the neural processing of food images: first, the appetitive state of children (hungry vs. satiated) when exposed to these images, and second, the portion size and energy density (high vs. low calorie) of the food depicted. Children and adolescents who were exposed to food images in a fasting state showed increased response in brain areas specialized in reward response (Charbonnier et al. 2018), and the perception and processing of sensations (Fearnbach et al. 2016). These data are particularly problematic considering that adolescents use SM as soon as they wake up and are in a fasting state (Toh et al. 2019). Exposure to unhealthy food images when hungry might lead to poor food choices for the rest of the day. Moreover, after exposure to digital food images of large rather than small portion sizes, children showed increased neural activation in brain areas related to salience and associative learning, which was associated with increased food intake (Keller et al. 2018). These results are particularly important given the abundance of food pictures shared by SM influencers and food companies, often of large portion size and high in fat, salt, and sugar content—often also called "food-porn" (Sabbagh et al. 2020).

The role of SM influencers could also explain some of the associations between SM exposure and poor dietary outcomes in children and adolescents. Remarkably, marketing of unhealthy foods by SM influencers led to a higher intake of unhealthy foods in the exposed children compared to those who were not exposed (Coates et al. 2019a, b). Food marketing with an advertising disclosure (e.g., *paid partnership* or using hashtags such as *#ad* or *#advertisement*) did not have an interaction effect with children's awareness of advertising on the actual energy intake. This suggests that SM marketing negatively impacts children's and adolescents' food intake, independent of using such advertising disclosures (Coates et al. 2019a). The emotional link and familiarity children and adolescents create with the SM influencer may lead to the perception of the advertising disclosure as a transparent act, leading to positive attitudes towards influencers (De Jans et al. 2021). Often the advertising content is also mixed with socio-cultural content, enabling misleading marketing messages (European Commission 2016). The latest evidence has illuminated that the number of followers an SM influencer has may also lead to different responses among their followers. This was investigated in a 2 × 2 experiment design, where Kay et al. compared the followers' intentions to buy a beauty product advertised by a mega-influencer (more than 100.000 followers) and micro-influencer (1.000–100.000 followers), either with or without an advertisement disclosure (i.e., *#sponsored*) (Kay et al. 2020). They observed that young consumers had higher intentions to purchase the product when exposed to the micro-influencer who disclosed the sponsorship than when exposed to the macro-influencer who did not.

This has already been recognized as a new form of marketing by companies. Further research should examine if these effects are transferable to healthy or unhealthy food products advertised to children by micro- vs. macro-influencers.

The presence of peers in the SM environment also seems to play a role in the impact of SM exposure on adolescents' diets. Adolescents exposed to peers' videos addressing barriers to healthy eating and acting as role models reported eating vegetables at least three times per day compared to adolescents not exposed to those videos (Cullen et al. 2013). Conversely, SM influencers' marketing of healthy foods on Instagram, such as bananas (Coates et al. 2019b) or red peppers (Folkvord and de Bruijne 2020), did not influence the immediate food and energy intake of children and adolescents. This indicates that marketing healthy foods via SM influencers does not improve children's food choices. Further, these data suggest that the influence of peers on SM, compared to that of SM influencers, might have a higher potential to help adolescents improve their eating habits. However, exposure to SM content did not affect nutrition literacy (Lwin et al. 2017). Further research is warranted to elucidate how SM influencers or peers can harness the effects of SM exposure to enhance nutritional outcomes in children and adolescents.

We recommend that future studies explore and evaluate emerging DiPH strategies aimed at enhancing nutrition and diet literacy among children and adolescents, thereby supporting healthier and sustainable food choices and eating habits. Moreover, strategies to make healthy foods appealing to children and adolescents are needed. The mechanisms identified, namely the role of peers and SM influencers and the portion size and energy density of foods depicted in the digital environment, may be beneficial for future DiPH interventions aiming to improve children's and adolescents' food intake and eating behaviors. Also, further research is needed to explore the potential mechanisms via which SM exposure leads to poor mental health in the long term. Understanding these mechanisms could inform future mental health interventions and policies within digital environments, especially in tackling the current adolescent mental health crisis.

3 The Problematic and Unethical Design Patterns of the SM Environment

Alone, the public health issues related to SM (namely mental and metabolic health) prompt worrisome side effects of the SM environment and its usage. Although providers of SM have started implementing mechanisms to counter adverse effects, specific problems are nested deeper in their interface designs and often rooted in the core features of SM platforms. To protect users from the health-related effects of SM usage, it is essential to understand how implemented design strategies influence users' decision-making while potentially inflicting harm. In recent years, researchers from various fields, particularly the Human-Computer Interaction (HCI) field, have increasingly investigated the effects of design strategies on SM users.

Various studies indicate a mismatch between users' ability to anticipate their time spent on an SM platform. In the case of Twitter, Schoenebek highlights a concern among users regarding the frequency with which they use SM (Schoenebeck 2014). As a last resort, many try giving up SM, with data showing that 36% of users are unable to follow through. This suggests that technological interventions may help to create better solutions for users to use the platform to their preferences. In the context of HCI, researchers have been looking at users' agency, meaning that systems should facilitate and enable users to achieve their intentions. Design interventions, for example, can be utilized to increase users' self-awareness and self-control while using SM. Interested in a similar issue as Schoenebek, Junco looks at log data of user's usage patterns for pairing actual data with users' individual perceptions (Junco 2013). Results again indicate that users are losing control as they cannot accurately state the number of times they used Facebook in a certain period. Junco shows that users tend to overestimate their time spent on Facebook. This is further confirmed by Ernala et al., who used Facebook's actual logging information to compare it to users' perceptions (Ernala et al. 2020). They found that while users overestimated the overall amount of time spent on Facebook, they significantly underestimated the number of times they opened the SM. Furthermore, they noticed that children and adolescents, in particular, showed increased difficulties in estimating their usage compared to older people. Mildner and Savino further illustrated the incongruence in users' self-reported usage behavior using a different approach but with similar outcomes (Mildner and Savino 2021). In this study, most participants acknowledged spending more time on Facebook than desired. Interestingly, a majority of participants also confirmed that they did not want to spend less time and reported satisfaction with their usage of Facebook. Together, these works highlight a serious issue related to a decrease in users' agency and self-determination on SM. Studies clearly show a problem of self-awareness when using SM platforms that needs to be addressed.

A great example of improving users' well-being in the SM environment by generating better agency for users is presented by Lukoff et al., who worked on YouTube's mobile application (Lukoff et al. 2021). Using a co-design study approach, they developed alternative interfaces to enhance available options to control the app, focusing on enabling participants to use it to their needs. A growing body of research has looked into design options to give users more agency when using SM. One established option is design nudging. Generally, the concept of nudges originates in Thaler and Sunstein's book (Thaler and Sunstein 2008). In their work, the authors describe marketing strategies that guide people's decision-making to enable more beneficial outcomes. This book further describes the underlying concept in Chap. "Ethical Implications of User Autonomy in Digital Public Health", Dassow et al. in this handbook). Utilizing the idea of nudges, Wang et al. investigated user interaction with Facebook and developed a set of interventions that offered additional information in certain situations (Wang et al. 2014, 2013). One of these interventions, for example, would remind users who will be able to see a new post. For this, they displayed a list of profile pictures of all contacts that could see the new post, nudging the user to evaluate the content before publishing it. Another intervention analyzed unpublished posts for offensive language. In doing so, they nudged the user to rethink their comment by forcing them to wait a certain amount of time before enabling them to publish their post. In a similar attempt, Lyngs and colleagues developed two design interventions that enhance the self-control of Facebook users (Lyngs et al. 2020). The first includes prompts and reminders for pre-set goals of users' intentions, and the other basically removes the *News Feed* feature of Facebook. The results of their study showed that users welcomed both strategies, positively aligning their intentions with actual usage behavior.

While nudges can help users align their expectations with their SM usage, an alarming number of negative examples have been identified in multiple instances. These so-called dark patterns describe malicious design strategies that covert or obscure interactions, potentially harming the user. Infamous in the context of cookie-consent banners (Gray et al. 2021), web developers and designers create online interfaces that mislead users into undesired actions—for example, giving consent to web hosts to access personal data that users would not have given if they were fully informed (Fig. 1) (Graßl et al. 2021). While Chap. "Ethical Implications

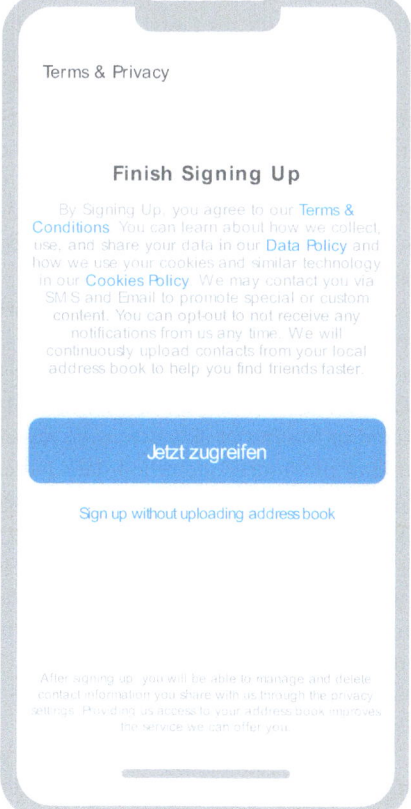

Fig. 1 When setting up a new account for SM, users are often tricked into uploading their device's local contacts using the dark patterns "interface interference" and "visual interference." Additionally, the "legalese stipulations" dark pattern can be active here, concealing how data is stored and processed

of User Autonomy in Digital Public Health", Dassow et al. in this handbook) discusses dark patterns on a more sophisticated level, the present chapter will consider their occurrence in the SM environment.

Given that dark patterns are mainly researched in the context of e-commerce, current research lacks a precise understanding of how dark patterns work in SM. Nonetheless, individual works consider SM to a certain degree allowing us to see how they adapt in this domain. Dark patterns in e-commerce are different compared to those found in SM. Where e-commerce usually wants to speed up processes such as purchasing items, the incentive of SM is to keep users engaged for long durations. This means that strategies working for online shopping systems do not necessarily apply to social networking services. As revenue is generated through users' data and advertisement, SM aims to keep users satisfied and active on their platforms for long durations. This is further shown in Mildner et al.'s work, where the researchers describe five SM-specific dark patterns within two higher strategies—engaging and governing strategies (Mildner et al. 2023). Falling under the umbrella of engaging strategies, interfaces that aim to keep users satisfied and engaged with a platform make use of these three patterns: *interactive hooks*, *social brokering*, and *decision uncertainty*. On the other hand, governing strategies are patterns that navigate users' decision-making by limiting available choices. This strategy contains the patterns of *labyrinthine navigation* and *conditional redirect*. In the context of governing strategies, Schaffner et al. studied the difficulty of account-deletion processes on SM (Brennan Schaffner and Chetty 2022). Comparing the 20 most popular SM platforms, the authors demonstrate that the option to fully delete an account often depends on whether the platform is accessed via phone or browser. At the same time, a user study shows that many users cannot complete the deletion of their accounts. The above-mentioned studies highlight the misalignment between user intentions and actual SM usage and elucidate the impact of design strategies on SM use.

A well-understood problem with dark patterns lies in their inevitability. Multiple studies have shown difficulties in users who previously proved their ability to successfully recognize dark patterns, to avoid them when encountering them on the site (Di Geronimo et al. 2020; Bongard-Blanchy et al. 2021). An explanation may be found in Mathur et al.'s extensive review (Mathur et al. 2019; Mathur et al. 2021), linking previously identified dark pattern strategies to dark pattern characteristics based on cognitive biases, which they exploit: The *default effect cognitive bias*, for instance, impacts people by convincing them to stick with preselected choices. This is because we often deem it easier to go with a pre-made suggestion than decide ourselves. The *bad default* dark pattern utilizes this bias in many applications' settings, nudging users to give more information than possibly desired (Fig. 2). Biases are often too strong to be avoided, which is emphasized in prior recognition studies with informed participants. This means that we cannot place the burden of avoiding dark patterns on the user.

However, as we cannot expect SM providers to self-regulate for the well-being of their users and avoid employing dark patterns, we have to discuss regulatory

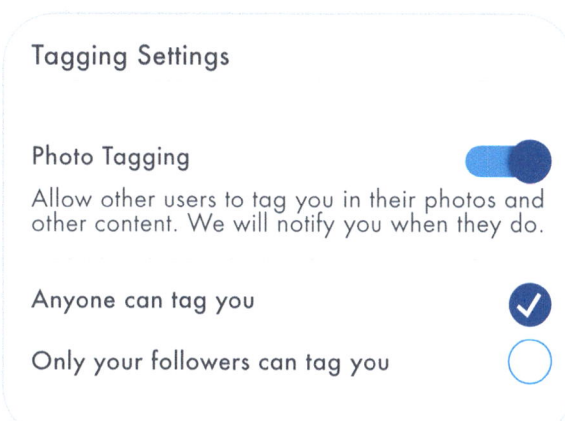

Fig. 2 Example of the "bad default" dark pattern as it appears in many SM, which allows anyone to tag the user's account by default

options that protect users' well-being and online persona. Remarkably, dark patterns make it more complicated for users to delete their SM accounts (Fig. 3). Dark patterns can support or worsen the dependence on SM by using designs that make it more difficult to stay away from social media.

While dark patterns have been shown to raise a series of severe threats to users' autonomy, misleading or fabricated content on SM has similarly become a significant challenge for public institutions and citizens. During the COVID-19 pandemic, an "epidemic of misinformation" (Zarocostas 2020) hindered pandemic control, in particular by spreading and multiplying misinformation on non-pharmaceutical interventions such as masking or social distancing, and by undermining vaccination efforts with fear and uncertainty (Imhoff and Lamberty 2020). The fact-checking collective poynter.org reports more than 15,000 unique COVID-related misinformation items as of January 2023 (Poynter 2021), which were shared repeatedly or in slight variations to create a multitude of misleading SM posts. This is particularly concerning since misinformation spreads faster and more expansively than content without false claims (Shahi et al. 2021; Vosoughi et al. 2018). Ironically, most SM platforms' architecture and algorithmic design facilitate sharing misinformation content (Charquero-Ballester et al. 2021). Moreover, these platforms' countermeasures, such as warning labels and professional fact-checking, have proven unsuitable for use at this scale (Pennycook and Rand 2021). Developing effective measures to reduce the sharing of misleading content on SM is thus a paramount issue.

In line with the overall approach by platform providers such as Twitter, previous research has shown that sharing misinformation on SM can be due to knowledge or attention deficits (Pennycook and Rand 2021), and addressing these deficits can reduce the sharing of misinformation. However, sharing misinformation (and, in

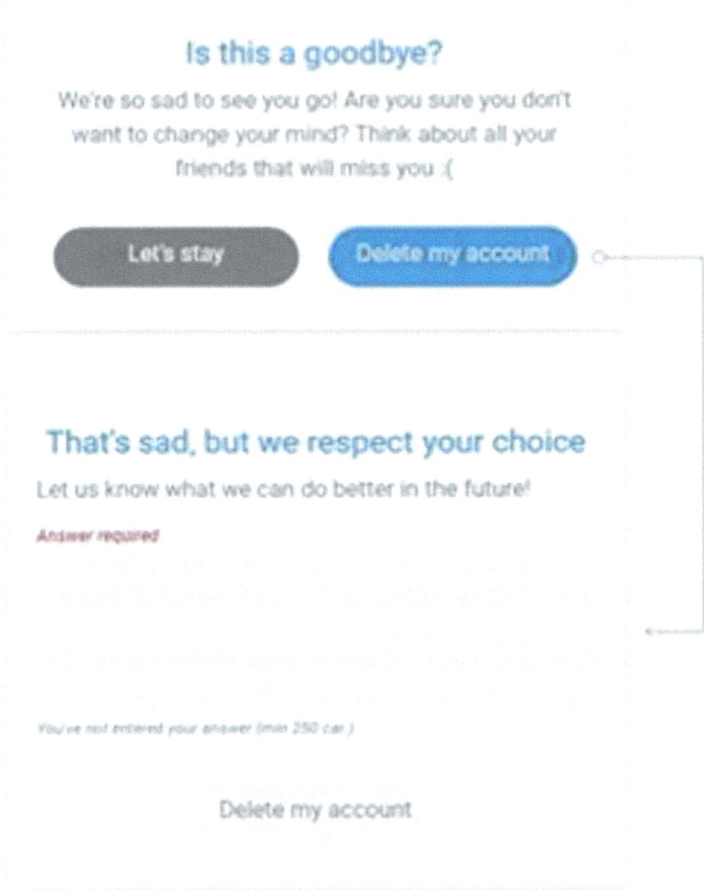

Fig. 3 An example of a dark pattern in EDPB, Guideline 3/2023 on deceptive design patterns in social media platform interfaces (Source: European Data Protection Board 2023)

fact, any information) on SM is also the result of social processes, in particular, social reinforcements accruing through, for example, "likes" (Meshi et al. 2015). Research is currently underway to address these social components of misinformation sharing by providing social reference cues for users, e.g., "in your personal Twitter network, 18 out of 20 people did not like, reply or retweet this tweet" (Jones et al. 2021). We suggest that facilitating such social references and making them a core mechanism of SM platforms has the potential to reduce the sharing of misinformation with all its associated negative consequences.

4 Legal Aspects of the SM Environment

Considering the harmful effects of SM use on children's health already presented in this chapter, one may ask whether national and international laws provide appropriate protection for this vulnerable population group. SM is an international environment; the legal reaction to SM, on the contrary, differs from country to country and even between the member states of the European Union (EU). Whether and how national and international laws protect children from adverse health effects of SM environment depends on the national perspective. Consequently, this section starts from the German perspective and, where possible, expands to the European viewpoint. Two main scenarios are addressed by law when protecting children's health in the digital environment. First, existing rules deal with whether and under which conditions children may access SM. The second scenario arises when access to SM is given. In this scenario, the law sporadically concentrates on the factors causing adverse health effects when using SM (like advertisements and manipulative design).

4.1 Regulating Access to SM

From a user's perspective, children can easily use SM in everyday life. From the standpoint of the law, access to SM is complex since the law sets several requirements. In short, two legal aspects affect children's access to SM. The first aspect is related to the user contract, which is concluded when registering in the network and is a prerequisite for its use. The German contractual law sets several rules to protect children from concluding contracts with adverse effects. The second aspect concerns user consent to data processing, which requires special conditions, especially when dealing with children's consent to data processing.

4.1.1 The German Contractual Law

By using the term "minors," the German contractual law regulates children under 18. From a legal point of view, it is decisive that minors have no or only limited legal capacity, according to §§ 104 and 106 of the German Civil Code (BGB). Nevertheless, most terms of use of SM platforms regulate that minors can also be users. For instance, Facebook's term of use states that the minimum age is 13 years (Facebook 2022). This also applies to Instagram (Instagram 2022) and TikTok (TikTok 2022b), while the minimum age on YouTube is 16 years. Nevertheless, younger children can use YouTube Kids, where content is accordingly filtered (YouTube 2022). The underlying problem is that these age limits are easy for children to circumvent due to a lack of age verification systems (Knoop 2016).

By registering, the user enters into a contract with the respective provider. This requires an effective declaration of intent by the user. Any declaration of intent from minors under 7 is void, according to § 104 BGB. The situation with children older than 7 is more complicated because those children have at least limited legal capacity. That means they need consent or ratification from their legal representatives (usually their parents). Although the terms of use allow the use by minors, the contracts are not valid without the consent or ratification of their legal representatives, § 107 BGB.

However, there are exceptions to these legal principles. According to § 107 BGB, a declaration of intention of the minor is effective if the minor merely obtains a legal advantage through it. The legal transaction must, therefore, exclusively improve the legal position of the minor (Spickhoff 2021, marginal no. 37). However, access to SM does not improve the legal position of the minor. Although the minor does not pay money, the disadvantage lies in the data processing and the acceptance of the terms of use. These terms often deviate negatively from the legal provisions and therefore constitute a disadvantage for minors (Jandt and Roßnagel 2011). Thus, the exception of § 107 BGB is not applicable, and the contract is still invalid without the approval or consent of a legal representative. A second exception to an invalid contract is regulated in § 110 BGB. Accordingly, a contract concluded by a minor shall be valid even if the minor performs the service with means provided to him for this purpose or at his free disposal by his legal representatives. In practice, this means that a contract concluded by the minor without their parent's consent becomes valid if the minor pays with their pocket money. Regarding SM, the minor does not pay with money but with their personal data. According to § 327 (3) BGB, this is, in principle, not a legal problem. However, these data were not given to the minors by their parents. Thus, the paragraph is not applicable either (Bräutigam 2012).

In summary, the agreements of minors are only effective with the approval or consent of their legal representatives. However, this is only in theory. In practice, there is no effective control by the SM networks. When using TikTok, for example, the user can enter any date of birth. The proof is not required (TikTok 2022a). Hence, every user can make themselves older than they are. In the end, contracts are often invalid from the perspective of contractual law. However, this does not stop children from using SM.

4.1.2 Data Protection Law

Even if a contract is effective, the question arises whether the data of minors is accurately protected from the perspective of data protection law. Article 8 of the General Data Protection Regulation (GDPR) states that processing a child's personal data should be lawful when the child is at least 16 years old. Younger children need the consent of their legal representatives. The article aims to protect children who are not sufficiently aware of the risks and consequences of processing their personal data (Kampert 2022). According to Recital 38 of the GDPR, specific protection should apply, in particular, to the use of children's personal data for marketing purposes, for creating personality or user profiles, and for the collection of children's personal data when using services offered directly to a child. That means that for children under 16, the legal representatives must consent not only to the declaration of the minor's will (see above) but also to the data processing.

According to Art. 8 (2) GDPR, the controller, in this case, the provider, shall make reasonable efforts to verify that the consent is given or authorized by the holder of parental responsibility over the child, taking into consideration available technology. That means the provider must check the age and, if necessary, parental consent. Nevertheless, the question is what technical means can be considered adequate. Simply clicking on a check box to confirm age is not sufficient (Taeger 2021). Instead, what would be necessary is for the provider to contact the holder of parental responsibility (Frenzel 2021, marginal no. 13). Suppose this is done most easily using a simple email with a confirmation link. In that case, the subsequent problem arises because it cannot be ensured that it is really the parents responding and not the minor themselves (Möhrke-Sobolewski and Klas 2016). This procedure must also be judged as unsuitable because of the high risk of abuse from third parties (Taeger 2021). For the operators of SM platforms, creativity is, therefore, required regarding verifiable parental consent to ensure the protection of minors in practice (Möhrke-Sobolewski and Klas 2016). Thus, the legal framework is clear, but the biggest problem is the lack of adequate age verification regarding both the contract's effectiveness as well as the privacy of minors.

4.2 Regulating Dark Patterns in SM

Another aspect that needs attention by law is dark patterns. The current regulation of dark patterns in Europe is in constant flux and multi-dimensional. Dark patterns have recently drawn the attention of European regulators (European Data Protection Board 2023; European Commission 2022), who tend to explicitly address design patterns and refer to the buzzword "dark patterns" in new regulatory frameworks. Besides these recent attempts, older laws already regulate several dark patterns without using the terms "dark patterns" or "design" but referring to a prohibited misleading action/omission or an aggressive commercial practice. Identifying the applicable law for dark patterns becomes even more difficult as design patterns can be subject to different areas of law (like data protection law, consumer law, and competition law), depending on their impact on consumers, traders, and personal data. Especially in Europe, extensive reports and articles deal with the demanding question under which conditions dark patterns fall and under the scope of which laws (Leiser and Caruana 2021; Martini et al. 2021). These debates are also fueled by the different legal acts of the EU. Some European laws are directly applicable in each European country with little space to create national deviation (so-called *regulations* like the GDPR) (European Union 2022). Besides, European *directives* contain specific results that must be achieved, but each member state can decide how to transpose directives into national laws. It's important to note that there is a complex structure of laws that come from different areas and apply to the phenomenon of dark patterns. However, protecting vulnerable groups like children and adolescents in the SM environment is often only briefly mentioned. Fortunately, two European documents have recently addressed the interface between SM, minors, and dark patterns: the guidelines of the European Data Protection Board (EDPB) and the Digital Services Act (DSA).

With regard to the processing of personal data, the GDPR establishes rules for processing personal data by processors who offer services or goods to individuals in the EU or monitor their behavior in the EU. In 2023 the EDPB adopted guidelines on dark patterns in SM platform interfaces (European Data Protection Board 2023). These provide best practices and recommendations and refer to the articles of the GDPR that specific dark patterns could violate. The guidelines emphasize the vulnerable position of children when using SM since children may be less aware of the risks and consequences of data processing (European Data Protection Board 2023). Dark patterns may influence children to share more information because imperative expressions can make them feel obliged to do so to appear popular among peers. Besides this general statement, the guidelines highlight that dark patterns and especially emotional steering when registering with an SM platform may have a high impact, especially on children. Therefore, SM platforms should ensure that the language used, including its tone and style, is appropriate so that children easily understand the information provided (European Data Protection Board 2023).

Although the GDPR has binding legal force throughout every member state and enters into force on a set date in all the member states, the guidelines are only guidelines and, thus, non-binding (European Union 2022). Additionally, the guidelines do not show examples of dark patterns that specifically affect and manipulate children. Whether a particular design pattern unlawfully affects a child's choices is not clear but depends on the circumstances of the individual case and the person who applies the law. Consequently, the guidelines provide an essential starting point on the one hand but need clarification and binding force on the other.

Another European attempt that directly addresses dark patterns in SM concerning children is the DSA, which is directly applicable in all EU member states. This European regulation focuses on a legal framework for the digital market and contains uniform rules, duties, and responsibilities for online marketplaces and SM platforms. During the ordinary legislative procedure, the European Parliament proposed Article 13a No 3, which states: "Where applicable, providers of intermediary services shall adapt their *design features* to ensure a high level of safety, security and privacy by design for minors" (European Parliament 2022). Nevertheless, the final version of DSA does not contain Art. 13a anymore. Instead, Art. 28 DSA addresses the online protection of minors in general. Accordingly, providers of online platforms accessible to minors shall put appropriate and proportionate measures in place to ensure a high level of safety, security, and privacy for minors on their service (European Commission 2022). Nevertheless, this regulation does not answer the question of which specific dark patterns are forbidden when dealing with minors. Understandably, not all forms of currently identified dark patterns can be listed in the DSA since the digital environment knows many multifarious design patterns and rapidly spawns new ones. Figuratively speaking, the law lags behind the rapid development of dark patterns. Consequently, the solution lies between banning dark patterns in general and constantly updating a blocklist with concrete and current examples. This general procedure is described in Art. 25 DSA, which focuses on all users but not explicitly on minors. The Commission's guidelines pursuant to Art. 28 DSA are expected to specify dark patterns that specifically target minors. Due to the interplay of Art. 25 and 28 DSA, the DSA is a first step towards protecting children from dark patterns in SM. The regulation of dark patterns in SM, as well as the regulation of access to SM, emphasize that regulation is time-consuming and that not all problems are solved yet.

5 Conclusion

SM has many benefits for the self- and social development of children and adolescents. However, increasing evidence shows that SM use is linked to adverse health outcomes and unfavorable health behaviors in children and adolescents, namely poor mental health, deteriorated food intake, and harmful eating habits. Several mechanisms may explain this negative impact. First, the social mechanisms, such as upward social comparisons with peers or internet celebrities and the marketing of unhealthy foods via SM influencers. Second, the physiological mechanisms, including the displacement of sleep, physical activity, and impact on circadian rhythms as well as the heightened neural response after exposure to digital food images. Third, the technological mechanisms, where the architecture and design issues of SM platforms, like dark patterns, may also play a crucial role. Dark patterns affect the duration of using SM and could worsen the adverse impact of SM use on the health outcomes of its users, especially in children and adolescents. Therefore, this age group needs special attention. Although further research is required to understand the full influence of dark patterns on users' well-being, the EU recently launched specific legislation on dark patterns, where the impact on children is already recognized. While the law lags behind the technological advancements regarding dark patterns, in the case of minors' access to SM, it is the other way around: the legal framework is clear, but there is a lack of practical technical feasibility, which needs to be tackled urgently.

Finally, we acknowledge that SM environment raises questions for several disciplines. Whereas specific questions could only be solved within expert knowledge in each domain, we see space for a potential interaction of the epidemiology, HCI, and law disciplines. The evidence from epidemiology acts as a starting point and alert for stakeholders to prevent users' poor well-being in the online environment. HCI becomes the first instance to avoid these adverse outcomes by employing design. As a second instance (i.e., ultima ratio), the law can set binding rules for protection from negative consequences by incorporating research findings in HCI and epidemiology.

References

Allen HA, Chambers A, Blissett J, Chechlacz M, Barrett T, Higgs S, Nouwen A (2016) Relationship between parental feeding practices and neural responses to food cues in adolescents. PLoS One 11(8):e0157037. https://doi.org/10.1371/journal.pone.0157037

Anderson M, Jiang J (2018) Teens, social media & technology 2018. Pew Research Center 31(2018):1673–1689

Arain M, Haque M, Johal L, Mathur P, Nel W, Rais A, Sandhu R, Sharma S (2013) Maturation of the adolescent brain. Neuropsychiatr Dis Treat 9:449–461. https://doi.org/10.2147/ndt.S39776

Baldwin HJ, Freeman B, Kelly B (2018) Like and share: associations between social media engagement and dietary choices in children. Public Health Nutr 21(17):3210–3215. https://doi.org/10.1017/s1368980018001866

Banyai F, Zsila A, Kiraly O, Maraz A, Elekes Z, Griffiths MD, Andreassen CS, Demetrovics Z (2017) Problematic social media use: results from a large-scale nationally representative adolescent sample. PLoS One 12(1):e0169839. https://doi.org/10.1371/journal.pone.0169839

Boer M, Stevens GWJM, Finkenauer C, de Looze ME, van den Eijnden RJJM (2021) Social media use intensity, social media use problems, and mental health among adolescents: investigating directionality and mediating processes. Comput Hum Behav 116:106645. https://doi.org/10.1016/j.chb.2020.106645

Boers E, Afzali MH, Newton N, Conrod P (2019) Association of screen time and depression in adolescence. JAMA Pediatr 173(9):853–859. https://doi.org/10.1001/jamapediatrics.2019.1759

Bongard-Blanchy K, Rossi A, Rivas S, Doublet S, Koenig V, Lenzini G (2021) I am definitely manipulated, even when I am aware of it. It's ridiculous!—dark patterns from the end-user perspective. Paper presented at the DIS '21: designing interactive systems conference 2021, 28 June–2 July 2021

Bozzola E, Spina G, Agostiniani R, Barni S, Russo R, Scarpato E, Di Mauro A et al (2022) The use of social media in children and adolescents: scoping review on the potential risks. Int J Environ Res Public Health 19:16. https://doi.org/10.3390/ijerph19169960

Bräutigam P (2012) Das Nutzungsverhältnis bei sozialen Netzwerken - Zivilrechtlicher Austausch von IT-Leistung gegen personenbezogene Daten. MMR 15(10):635–641

Brennan Schaffner NAL, Marshini Chetty (2022) Understanding account deletion and relevant dark patterns on social media. In the 25th CSCW2 Proceedings of the ACM on Human-Computer Interaction, 8–22 November 2022

Carter B, Rees P, Hale L, Bhattacharjee D, Paradkar MS (2016) Association between portable screen-based media device access or use and sleep outcomes: a systematic review and meta-analysis. JAMA Pediatr 170(12):1202–1208. https://doi.org/10.1001/jamapediatrics.2016.2341

Cha S-S, Seo B-K (2018) Smartphone use and smartphone addiction in middle school students in Korea: prevalence, social networking service, and game use. Health Psychol Open 5(1):2055102918755046. https://doi.org/10.1177/2055102918755046

Charbonnier L, van Meer F, Johnstone AM, Crabtree D, Buosi W, Manios Y, Androutsos O et al (2018) Effects of hunger state on the brain responses to food cues across the life span. NeuroImage 171:246–255

Charquero-Ballester M, Walter JG, Nissen IA, Bechmann A (2021) Different types of COVID-19 misinformation have different emotional valence on twitter. Big Data Soc 8(2):1–11. https://doi.org/10.1177/20539517211041279

Coates AE, Hardman CA, Halford JCG, Christiansen P, Boyl EJ (2019a) The effect of influencer marketing of food and a "protective" advertising disclosure on children's food intake. Pediatr Obes 14(10):e12540

Coates AE, Hardman CA, Halford JCG, Christiansen P, Boyland EJ (2019b) Social media influencer marketing and children's food intake: a randomized trial. Pediatrics 143(4):e20182554. https://doi.org/10.1542/peds.2018-2554

Cullen KW, Thompson D, Boushey C, Konzelmann K, Chen T-A (2013) Evaluation of a web-based program promoting healthy eating and physical activity for adolescents: teen choice: food and fitness. Health Educ Res 28(4):704–714

De Jans S, Spielvogel I, Naderer B, Hudders L (2021) Digital food marketing to children: how an influencer's lifestyle can stimulate healthy food choices among children. Appetite 162:105182. https://doi.org/10.1016/j.appet.2021.105182

De Veirman M, Hudders L, Nelson MR (2019) What is influencer marketing and how does it target children? A review and direction for future research. Front Psychol 10:2685. https://doi.org/10.3389/fpsyg.2019.02685

Di Geronimo L, Braz L, Fregnan E, Palomba F, Bacchelli A (2020) UI dark patterns and where to find them. Paper presented at the CHI '20: proceedings of the 2020 CHI conference on human factors in computing systems, Honolulu, HI, USA, 25–30 April 2020

Ernala SK, Burke M, Leavitt A, Ellison NB (2020) How well do people report time spent on Facebook? An evaluation of established survey questions with recommendations. Paper presented at the CHI '20: proceedings of the 2020 CHI conference on human factors in computing systems, Honolulu, HI, USA, 25–30 April 2020

European Commission (2016) Directive 2005/29/EC of the European Parliament and of the Council concerning unfair business-to-consumer commercial practices in the internal market and amending Council Directive 84/450/EEC, Directives 97/7/EC, 98/27/EC and 2002/65/EC of the European Parliament and of the Council and Regulation (EC) No 2006/2004 of the European Parliament and of the Council ('Unfair Commercial Practices Directive'). https://eur-lex.europa.eu/legal-content/EN/TXT/PDF/?uri=CELEX:02005L0029-20220528. Accessed 05 Jul 2023

European Commission (2022) Regulation (EU) 2022/2065 of the European Parliament and of the Council on a Single Market For Digital Services (Digital Services Act) and amending Directive 2000/31/EC. https://eur-lex.europa.eu/legal-content/EN/TXT/PDF/?uri=CELEX:32022R2065. Accessed 5 Jul 2023

European Data Protection Board (2023) Guidelines 3/2022 on deceptive design patterns in social media platform interfaces: how to recognise and avoid them. https://edpb.europa.eu/system/files/2022-03/edpb_03-2022_guidelines_on_dark_patterns_in_social_media_platform_interfaces_en.pdf. Accessed 5 Jul 2023

European Parliament (2022) Amendments adopted by the European Parliament on 20 January 2022 on the proposal for a regulation of the European Parliament and of the Council on a Single Market For Digital Services (Digital Services Act) and amending Directive 2000/31/EC. https://www.europarl.europa.eu/doceo/document/TA-9-2022-0014_EN.html. Accessed 5 Jul 2023

European Union (2022) Types of regulation. https://european-union.europa.eu/institutions-law-budget/law/types-legislation_en. Accessed 19 Oct 2022

Facebook (2022) Terms of service. https://www.facebook.com/legal/terms/update. Accessed 7 Jul 2022

Fardouly J, Magson NR, Johnco CJ, Oar EL, Rapee RM (2018) Parental control of the time preadolescents spend on social media: links with preadolescents' social media appearance comparisons and mental health. J Youth Adolesc 47(7):1456–1468. https://doi.org/10.1007/s10964-018-0870-1

Fearnbach SN, English LK, Lasschuijt M, Wilson SJ, Savage JS, Fisher JO, Rolls BJ, Keller KL (2016) Brain response to images of food varying in energy density is associated with body composition in 7- to 10-year-old children: results of an exploratory study. Physiol Behav 162:3–9

Folkvord F, de Bruijne M (2020) The effect of the promotion of vegetables by a social influencer on adolescents' subsequent vegetable intake: a pilot study. Int J Environ Res Public Health 17:7

Freeman B, Kelly B, Baur L, Chapman K, Chapman S, Gill T, King L (2014) Digital junk: food and beverage marketing on Facebook. Am J Public Health 104(12):e56–e64. https://doi.org/10.2105/AJPH.2014.302167

Frenzel M (2021) Art. 8. In: Paal B, Pauly D (eds) DSGVO BDSG, 3rd edn. C.H. Beck, München

Gao Y, Ao H, Hu X, Wang X, Huang D, Huang W, Han Y et al (2022) Social media exposure during COVID-19 lockdowns could lead to emotional overeating via anxiety: the moderating role of neuroticism. Appl Psychol Health Well Being 14(1):64–80. https://doi.org/10.1111/aphw.12291

Graßl P, Schraffenberger H, Borgesius FZ, Buijzen M (2021) Dark and bright patterns in cookie consent requests. J Digit Soc Res 3(1):1–38. https://doi.org/10.33621/jdsr.v3i1.54

Gray CM, Santos C, Bielova N, Toth M, Clifford D (2021) Dark patterns and the legal requirements of consent banners: an interaction criticism perspective. Paper presented at the CHI '21: Proceedings of the 2021 CHI Conference on Human Factors in Computing Systems, Yokohama, Japan, 8–13 may 2021

Gupta M, Sharma A (2021) Fear of missing out: a brief overview of origin, theoretical underpinnings and relationship with mental health. World J Clin Cases 9(19):4881–4889. https://doi.org/10.12998/wjcc.v9.i19.4881

Hsu MSH, Rouf A, Allman-Farinelli M (2018) Effectiveness and behavioral mechanisms of social media interventions for positive nutrition behaviors in adolescents: a systematic review. J Adolesc Health 63(5):531–545. https://doi.org/10.1016/j.jadohealth.2018.06.009

Imhoff R, Lamberty P (2020) A bioweapon or a hoax? The link between distinct conspiracy beliefs about the coronavirus disease (COVID-19) outbreak and pandemic behavior. Soc Psychol Personal Sci 11:1110–1118. https://doi.org/10.1177/1948550620934692

Instagram (2022) Terms of service. https://help.instagram.com/581066165581870?cms_id=581066165581870&maybe_redirect_pol=true&published_only=true&force_new_ighc=false. Accessed 19 Oct 2022

Jagtiani MR, Kelly Y, Fancourt D, Shelton N, Scholes S (2019) #StateOfMind: family meal frequency moderates the association between time on social networking sites and Well-being among U.K. young adults. Cyberpsychol Behav Soc Netw 22(12):753–760. https://doi.org/10.1089/cyber.2019.0338

Jandt S, Roßnagel A (2011) Social Networks für Kinder und Jugendliche: Besteht ein ausreichender Datenschutz? MMR 14(10):637–642

Jones CM, Diethei D, Schöning J, Shrestha R, Jahnel T, Schüz B (2021) Social reference cues can reduce misinformation sharing behaviour on social media. PsyArXiv 2021. https://doi.org/10.31234/osf.io/v6fc9

Juarascio AS, Forman EM, Timko CA, Herbert JD, Butryn M, Lowe M (2011) Implicit internalization of the thin ideal as a predictor of increases in weight, body dissatisfaction, and disordered eating. Eat Behav 12(3):207–213. https://doi.org/10.1016/j.eatbeh.2011.04.004

Junco R (2013) Comparing actual and self-reported measures of Facebook use. Comput Hum Behav 29(3):626–631. https://doi.org/10.1016/j.chb.2012.11.007

Kampert D (2022) Artikel 8: Einwilligung eines Kindes in Bezug auf Dienste der Informationsgesellschaft. In: Sydow G, Marsch N (eds) Datenschutz-Grundverordnung (DSGVO). Nomos

Kay S, Mulcahy R, Parkinson J (2020) When less is more: the impact of macro and micro social media influencers' disclosure. J Mark Manag 36(3–4):248–278. https://doi.org/10.1080/0267257X.2020.1718740

Keller KL, English LK, Fearnbach SN, Lasschuijt M, Anderson K, Bermudez M, Fisher JO et al (2018) Brain response to food cues varying in portion size is associated with individual differences in the portion size effect in children. Appetite 125:139–151

Knoop M (2016) Digitaler Nachlass—Vererbbarkeit von Konten (minderjähriger) Nutzer in sozialen Netzwerken. NZFam 3(21):966–970

Kuss DJ, Griffiths MD (2017) Social networking sites and addiction: ten lessons learned. Int J Environ Res Public Health 14(3):311

Latha K, Meena KS, Pravitha MR, Dasgupta M, Chaturvedi SK (2020) Effective use of social media platforms for promotion of mental health awareness. J Educ Health Promot 9:124. https://doi.org/10.4103/jehp.jehp_90_20

Leiser MR, Caruana M (2021) Dark patterns: light to be found in Europe's consumer protection regime. J Eur Consum Market Law:237–251

Lenhart A, Purcell K, Smith A, Zickuhr K (2010) Social media & mobile internet use among teens and young adults. Millennials Pew internet & American life project https://eric.ed.gov/?id=ED525056 Accessed 7 Jul 2022

Lopez-Fernandez O, Kuss DJ, Romo L, Morvan Y, Kern L, Graziani P, Rousseau A et al (2017) Self-reported dependence on mobile phones in young adults: a European cross-cultural empirical survey. J Behav Addict 6(2):168–177. https://doi.org/10.1556/2006.6.2017.020

Lukoff K, Liao JV, Choi J, Fan K, Munson SA, Hiniker A (2021) How the design of YouTube influences user sense of agency. Paper presented at the CHI '21: Proceedings of the 2021 CHI conference on human factors in computing systems, Yokohama, Japan, 8–13 May 2021

Lwin MO, Malik S, Ridwan H, Sum Au CS (2017) Media exposure and parental mediation on fast-food consumption among children in metropolitan and suburban Indonesian. Asia Pac J Clin Nutr 26(5):899–905

Lyngs U, Lukoff K, Slovak P, Seymour W, Webb H, Jirotka M, Zhao J et al (2020) 'I just want to hack myself to not get distracted': evaluating design interventions for self-control on Facebook. Paper presented at the CHI '20: Proceedings of the 2020 CHI conference on human factors in computing systems, Honolulu, 25–30 April 2020

Marks RJ, De Foe A, Collett J (2020) The pursuit of wellness: social media, body image and eating disorders. Child Youth Serv Rev 119:105659. https://doi.org/10.1016/j.childyouth.2020.105659

Martini M, Drews C, Seeliger P, Weinzierl Q (2021) Dark patterns. ZfDR 2021(1):47–41

Mascheroni G, Ólafsson K (2014) Net children go mobile: risks and opportunities. https://eprints.lse.ac.uk/55798/. Accessed 7 Jul 2023

Mathur A, Acar G, Friedman MJ, Lucherini E, Mayer J, Chetty M, Narayanan A (2019) Dark patterns at scale. Findings from a crawl of 11K shopping websites. Proc. ACM Hum.-Comput. Interact. 3, CSCW, article 81 (November 2019), 32 pages. https://doi.org/10.1145/3359183

Mathur A, Mayer J, Kshirsagar M (2021) What makes a dark pattern ... dark? Design attributes, normative considerations, and measurement methods. Paper presented at the CHI '21: Proceedings of the 2021 CHI conference on human factors in computing systems, Yokohama, Japan, 8–13 May 2021

McLean SA, Paxton SJ, Wertheim EH, Masters J (2015) Photoshopping the selfie: self photo editing and photo investment are associated with body dissatisfaction in adolescent girls. Int J Eat Disord 48(8):1132–1140. https://doi.org/10.1002/eat.22449

McLean SA, Jarman HK, Rodgers RF (2019) How do "selfies" impact adolescents' Well-being and body confidence? A narrative review. Psychol Res Behav Manag 12:513–521. https://doi.org/10.2147/PRBM.S177834

Meshi D, Tamir DI, Heekeren HR (2015) The emerging neuroscience of social media. Trends Cogn Sci 19(12):771–782

Mildner T, Savino G-L (2021) Ethical user interfaces: exploring the effects of dark patterns on Facebook. Paper presented at the extended abstracts of the 2021 CHI conference on human factors in computing systems, Yokohama, Japan, 8–13 may 2021

Mildner T, Savino GL, Doyle P R, Cowan BR, Malaka R. (2023) About engaging and governing strategies: a thematic analysis of dark patterns in social networking services. Paper presented at the proceedings of the 2023 CHI conference on human factors in computing systems, Hamburg, Germany, 23–28 April 2023

Möhrke-Sobolewski C, Klas B (2016) Zur Gestaltung des Minderjährigendatenschutzes in digitalen Informationsdiensten. K&R 6:373–378

Müller KW, Dreier M, Beutel ME, Duven E, Giralt S, Wölfling K (2016) A hidden type of internet addiction? Intense and addictive use of social networking sites in adolescents. Comput Hum Behav 55:172–177. https://doi.org/10.1016/j.chb.2015.09.007

Ngqangashe Y, Maldoy K, Backer CJSD, Vandebosch H (2022) Exploring adolescents' motives for food media consumption using the theory of uses and gratifications. Communications 47(1):73–92. https://doi.org/10.1515/commun-2019-0164

Pennycook G, Rand DG (2021) The psychology of fake news. Trends Cogn Sci 25(5):388–402. https://doi.org/10.1016/j.tics.2021.02.007

Potvin Kent M, Pauzé E, Roy EA, de Billy N, Czoli C (2019) Children and adolescents' exposure to food and beverage marketing in social media apps. Pediatr Obes 14(6):e12508

Poynter (2021) Covid-19 misinformation. https://www.poynter.org/ifcn-covid-19-misinformation/

Qutteina Y, Hallez L, Mennes N, De Backer C, Smits T (2019) What do adolescents see on social media? A diary study of food marketing images on social media. Front Psychol 10:2637. https://doi.org/10.3389/fpsyg.2019.02637

Qutteina Y, Hallez L, Raedschelders M, De Backer C, Smits T (2022) Food for teens: how social media is associated with adolescent eating outcomes. Public Health Nutr 25(2):290–302. https://doi.org/10.1017/s1368980021003116

Rideout VJ, Robb MB (2019) The common sense census: media use by tweens and teens. Common Sense Media, San Fransisco, CA

Rideout V, Robb MB (2020) The common sense census: media use by kids age zero to eight, 2020. Commen Sense Media, San Fransisco, CA

Rozendaal E, Buijzen M, Valkenburg P (2010) Comparing children's and adults' cognitive advertising competences in The Netherlands. J Child Media 4(1):77–89. https://doi.org/10.1080/17482790903407333

Sabbagh C, Boyland E, Hankey C, Parrett A (2020) Analysing credibility of UK social media influencers' weight-management blogs: a pilot study. Int J Environ Res Public Health 17(23). https://doi.org/10.3390/ijerph17239022

Samara A, Li X, Pivik RT, Badger TM, Ou X (2018) Brain activation to high-calorie food images in healthy normal weight and obese children: a fMRI study. BMC Obes 5(1):31

Schoenebeck SY (2014) Giving up twitter for lent: how and why we take breaks from social media. Paper presented at the CHI '14: Proceedings of the SIGCHI conference on human factors in computing systems, Toronto, Ontario, Canada, 26 April–1 may 2014

Shahi GK, Dirkson A, Majchrzak TA (2021) An exploratory study of COVID-19 misinformation on twitter. Online Soc Netw Media 22:100104. https://doi.org/10.1016/j.osnem.2020.100104

Shychuk M, Joseph N, Thompson LA (2022) Social media use in children and adolescents. JAMA Pediatr 176(7):730–730. https://doi.org/10.1001/jamapediatrics.2022.1134

Sina E, Boakye D, Christianson L, Ahrens W, Hebestreit A (2022) Social media and children's and adolescents' diets: a systematic review of the underlying social and physiological mechanisms. Adv Nutr 13:913–937. https://doi.org/10.1093/advances/nmac018

Smahel D, Machackova H, Mascheroni G, Dedkova L, Staksrud E, Ólafsson K, Livingstone S, Hasebrink U (2020) EU Kids Online 2020: survey results from 19 countries. EU Kids Online. https://doi.org/10.21953/lse.47fdeqj01ofo. Accessed 07 Jul 2022

Spence C, Okajima K, Cheok AD, Petit O, Michel C (2016) Eating with our eyes: from visual hunger to digital satiation. Brain Cogn 110:53–63. https://doi.org/10.1016/j.bandc.2015.08.006

Spickhoff A (2021) § 107. In: Schubert C (ed) Münchener Kommentar zum Bürgerlichen Gesetzbuch Band 1: §§ 1–240, 9th edn. C.H. Beck, München

Statista (2022a) Social media—statistics & facts. Statista. https://www.statista.com/topics/1164/social-networks/#topicHeader__wrapper. Accessed 7 Jul 2022

Statista (2022b) Social media: global daily usage by territory Q4 2020. Statista. https://www.statista.com/statistics/270229/usage-duration-of-social-networks-by-country/. Accessed 7 Jul 2022

Statista (2022c) Social media- statistics and facts. https://www.statista.com/topics/1164/social-networks/. Accessed 15 Dec 2022

Taeger J (2021) Einwilligung von Kindern gegenüber Diensten der Informationsgesellschaft. ZD 11(9):505–508

Thaler RH, Sunstein CR (2008) Nudge: improving decisions about health, wealth, and happiness. Yale University Press, New Haven

Tiggemann M, Zaccardo M (2018) 'Strong is the new skinny': a content analysis of #fitspiration images on Instagram. J Health Psychol 23(8):1003–1011. https://doi.org/10.1177/1359105316639436

TikTok (2022a) Sign-in. https://www.tiktok.com/signup/phone-or-email/phone. Accessed 19 Oct 2022

TikTok (2022b) Terms of service. https://www.tiktok.com/legal/terms-of-service-eea?lang=de. Accessed 19 Oct 2022

Toh SH, Howie EK, Coenen P, Straker LM (2019) "From the moment I wake up I will use it...Every day, very hour": a qualitative study on the patterns of adolescents' mobile touch screen device use from adolescent and parent perspectives. BMC Pediatr 19(1):30. https://doi.org/10.1186/s12887-019-1399-5

van Meer F, van der Laan LN, Charbonnier L, Viergever MA, Adan RA, Smeets PA, Consortium obotIF (2016) Developmental differences in the brain response to unhealthy food cues: an fMRI study of children and adults. Am J Clin Nutr 104(6):1515–1522. https://doi.org/10.3945/ajcn.116.137240

van Meer F, van der Laan LN, Adan RA, Viergever MA, Smeets PA (2015) What you see is what you eat: an ALE meta-analysis of the neural correlates of food viewing in children and adolescents. Neuroimage 2015, 104:35–43

Viner RM, Gireesh A, Stiglic N, Hudson LD, Goddings A-L, Ward JL, Nicholls DE (2019) Roles of cyberbullying, sleep, and physical activity in mediating the effects of social media use on mental health and wellbeing among young people in England: a secondary analysis of longitudinal data. Lancet Child Adolesc Health 3(10):685–696. https://doi.org/10.1016/S2352-4642(19)30186-5

Vosoughi S, Roy D, Aral S (2018) The spread of true and false news online. Science 359(6380):1146–1151. https://doi.org/10.1126/science.aap9559

Wang Y, Leon PG, Scott K, Chen X, Acquisti A, Cranor LF (2013) Privacy nudges for social media: an exploratory Facebook study. In: proceedings of the 22nd international conference on world wide web, Rio de Janeiro, 13–17 May 2013. P 763-770

Wang Y, Leon PG, Acquisti A, Cranor LF, Forget A, Sadeh N (2014) A field trial of privacy nudges for facebook. Paper presented at the proceedings of the SIGCHI conference on human factors in computing systems, Toronto, Ontario, Canada, 26 April–1 may 2014

Wong BLH, Maaß L, Vodden A, van Kessel R, Sorbello S, Buttigieg S, Odone A (2022) The dawn of digital public health in Europe: implications for public health policy and practice. Lancet Reg Health—Europe 14. https://doi.org/10.1016/j.lanepe.2022.100316

YouTube (2022) Terms of service. https://www.youtube.com/static?gl=DE&hl=de&template=terms. Accessed 7 Jul 2022

Zarocostas J (2020) How to fight an infodemic. Lancet 395(10225):676. https://doi.org/10.1016/S0140-6736(20)30461-X

Zhang J, Marino C, Canale N, Charrier L, Lazzeri G, Nardone P, Vieno A (2022) The effect of problematic social media use on happiness among adolescents: the mediating role of lifestyle habits. Int J Environ Res Public Health 19:5. https://doi.org/10.3390/ijerph19052576

Open Access This chapter is licensed under the terms of the Creative Commons Attribution 4.0 International License (http://creativecommons.org/licenses/by/4.0/), which permits use, sharing, adaptation, distribution and reproduction in any medium or format, as long as you give appropriate credit to the original author(s) and the source, provide a link to the Creative Commons license and indicate if changes were made.

The images or other third party material in this chapter are included in the chapter's Creative Commons license, unless indicated otherwise in a credit line to the material. If material is not included in the chapter's Creative Commons license and your intended use is not permitted by statutory regulation or exceeds the permitted use, you will need to obtain permission directly from the copyright holder.

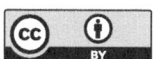

Digital Technology to Serve Key Public Health Functions

Surveillance of Population Health and Well-being (EPHO 1)

Wolfgang Ahrens and Iris Pigeot

Abstract According to the World Health Organization, public health surveillance is a continuous process of collecting, analyzing, and interpreting health data such that the results can be directly disseminated to responsible actors to take immediate action if necessary. Although disease surveillance has its roots in managing infectious diseases, it has also become essential for tracking non-communicable diseases (NCDs) as well as health-related behaviors and contextual factors. Due to the increasing digitalization of the health space, traditional methods of data collection are being complemented by digital information such as Electronic Health Records or self-generated internet data, e.g., on social media. In this chapter, we will first define the term surveillance before introducing different approaches that are used depending on whether the focus is on infectious diseases or NCDs. Here, we will distinguish two major threads that underline the huge impact of digitalization on surveillance systems, i.e., the usage of digital technologies for primary data collection and the usage of routinely collected available digital data. We will then provide some prominent examples of surveillance systems before we conclude by highlighting the importance of the FAIR guiding principles for data sharing and of record linkage for disease surveillance.

Keywords Disease surveillance · Electronic health records · Social media · FAIRification of research data · Record linkage

Abbreviations

CHS	Community Health Survey
COSI	Childhood Obesity Surveillance Initiative
DiPH	Digital public health

W. Ahrens (✉) · I. Pigeot
Leibniz Institute for Prevention Research and Epidemiology – BIPS, Bremen, Germany

University of Bremen, Faculty of Mathematics and Computer Science, Bremen, Germany
e-mail: ahrens@leibniz-bips.de

DPHS	Digital public health surveillance
EC	European Commission
EHDS	European Health Data Space
EHRs	Electronic Health Records
EPHOs	Essential Public Health Operations
FAIR	Findable, accessible, interoperable, reusable
GPS	Global Positioning System
HPV	Human Papilloma Virus
NCDs	Non-communicable diseases
NYC	New York City
NYC HANES	NYC Health and Nutrition Examination Survey
PCIP	NYC Health Department's Primary Care Information Project
PIA	Prospective Monitoring and Management App
PPH	Precision public health
STEPS	STEPwise approach to noncommunicable disease risk factor surveillance
WHO	World Health Organization

1 Introduction

According to Wong et al. (2022), the central aim of digital public health (DiPH) is improving the health of populations from the individual to the population level by using information and communications technologies. Applying this broad definition to digital public health surveillance (DPHS) would include the use of digital tools in data collection and any digital data source that provides health-related data on exposures and outcomes that are relevant for the planning, implementation, and evaluation of public health practice.

In 2012, the World Health Organization published an action plan for Europe to strengthen public health services and capacity (World Health Organization Regional Office for Europe 2012). This action plan consists of ten Essential Public Health Operations (EPHOs). They are closely linked with the increasing digitalization of the health sector and will be discussed in ten chapters of this handbook, each devoted to one EPHO. The present chapter will concentrate on "Surveillance of population health and well-being" (EPHO 1).

Instead of a roll-out of these EPHOs through vertical programs, the WHO aims at an integrated approach, as visualized in Fig. 1 (World Health Organization Regional Office for Europe 2012), where related EPHOs are clustered to facilitate delivery. All EPHOs are subdivided into two groups of five, the so-called core EPHOs and the enabler EPHOs. The core EPHOs are further subdivided into two sub-clusters where EPHO 1 and EPHO 2, "Monitoring and response to health hazards and emergencies," are the main components of the public health intelligence cluster together with EPHO 10 "Research."

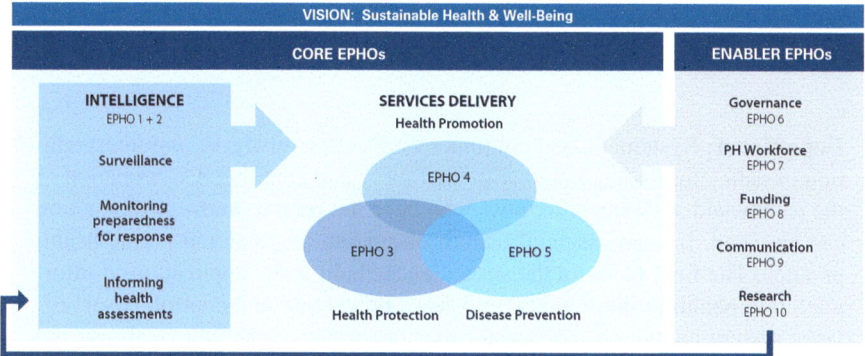

Fig. 1 Clustering and interdependencies of EPHOs (Source: World Health Organization Regional Office for Europe 2012)

To disentangle EPHO 1 and 2, we will first define the term surveillance and differentiate it from monitoring in order to provide a common understanding in Sect. 2. Here, we will also address the different necessary approaches depending on whether the focus is on infectious or non-communicable diseases (NCDs). In addition, we will introduce the two major threads that underline the huge impact of digitalization on approaches for surveillance, i.e., the usage of digital technologies for primary data collection and the usage of available (secondary) digital data. Section 3 will illustrate surveillance systems by giving some prominent examples before Sect. 4 concludes with the importance of sharing data according to the FAIR guiding principles. This will include an outlook that will critically appraise the set-up of the European Health Data Space and the potential information gained by using record linkage of different data sources while balancing data protection and health protection.

2 General Concepts of Digital Public Health Surveillance

2.1 Scope and Definition of Health Surveillance and Monitoring

The terms surveillance and monitoring are often used with different meanings and connotations. Sometimes they are even considered synonyms, depending on the context and professional background in which they are used. Here, we argue that monitoring and surveillance should not be considered synonymous since surveillance refers to a continuous activity, whereas monitoring to an episodic activity. The fact that both terms are often used interchangeably may be due to different definitions found in the literature. The Dictionary of Epidemiology (Porta 2008) offers two definitions of surveillance and monitoring, each depending on the data source and the context of interest, respectively. The definitions of surveillance are as follows:

> **Definition 1:** Systematic and continuous collection, analysis, and interpretation of data, closely integrated with the timely and coherent dissemination of the results and assessment to those who have the right to know so that action can be taken. It is an essential feature of epidemiological and public health practice. The final phase in the surveillance chain is the application of information to health promotion and to disease prevention and control. A surveillance system includes a functional capacity for data collection, analysis, and dissemination linked to public health programs. It is often distinguished from monitoring by the notion that surveillance is continuous and ongoing, whereas monitoring tends to be more intermittent or episodic.
>
> **Definition 2:** Continuous analysis, interpretation, and feedback of systematically collected data, generally using methods distinguished by their practicality, uniformity, and rapidity rather than by accuracy or completeness. By observing trends in time, place, and persons, changes can be observed or anticipated and appropriate action, including investigative or control measures, can be taken. Sources of data may relate directly to disease or to factors influencing disease. Thus they may include mortality and morbidity reports based on death certificates, hospital records, general practice sentinels, or notifications; laboratory diagnoses; outbreak reports; vaccine uptake and side effects; sickness absence records; changes in disease agents, vectors, or reservoirs; serological surveillance through serum banks. The latter can also be seen as an example of biological monitoring.

Both definitions have four essential elements in common: (1) Surveillance requires continuity; it is an ongoing activity with (regularly) repeated cycles; (2) Data are continuously obtained, analyzed, interpreted, and communicated; (3) Temporal trends, regional variations, and population distributions of diseases and factors related to them can be assessed; (4) The information gained is used to take action on disease prevention or control. The main difference between both definitions lies in the data sources used. While Definition 1 focuses on primary data that are repeatedly collected for the purpose of a given surveillance system, Definition 2 relates to the exploitation of existing secondary data that may have been recorded for other purposes. In this chapter, we will consider both data sources.

Both definitions are in agreement with the WHO definition of public health surveillance: "Public health surveillance is the continuous and systematic collection, orderly consolidation and evaluation of pertinent data with prompt dissemination of results to those who need to know, particularly those who are in a position to take action." (WHO 2023a).

The Dictionary of Epidemiology also offers two definitions for the term monitoring (Porta 2008):

> **Definition 1:** The intermittent performance and analysis of measurements aimed at detecting changes in the health status of populations or in the physical or social environment. In principle, it is different from surveillance, which is often a continuous process, although surveillance techniques are used in monitoring. It may also imply intervention in the light of observed measurements and analysis of the effect of the intervention (e.g., on the health status of a population or on an environmental compartment). The process of collecting and analyzing information about the implementation and effects of a public health program.
>
> **Definition 2:** In management, the episodic oversight of the implementation of an activity, seeking to ensure that input deliveries, work schedules, targeted outputs, and other required actions are proceeding according to plan.

According to both definitions, the main difference between surveillance and monitoring is the sporadic character of monitoring as opposed to the ongoing and continuous data acquisition and reporting that characterizes surveillance systems. Accordingly, disease monitoring may be accomplished by sporadic cross-sectional studies while a surveillance system that relies on primary data collection requires repeated surveys, i.e., a series of cross-sectional data collections, in random samples of a defined target population which are drawn sequentially and independently of each other. While such a series of surveys provide data on temporal trends of the health-related states or events of interest on a population level, it must not be confused with a longitudinal epidemiological study. A study that provides information on longitudinal changes in a group of individuals, i.e., the members of a cohort, is a study where the same individuals are followed and repeatedly assessed concerning health outcomes over a defined time period. Observational cohort studies are designed to investigate the etiology of health outcomes and the determinants or predictors of diseases, which allows for the estimation of disease risks. The cross-sectional design of surveillance systems is best suited for descriptive purposes. Surveillance can provide prevalence data on temporal trends, geographic variations, and the population distribution of health outcomes, health behaviors, risk factors, or utilization of health care. This information is needed for the planning of health systems as well as for the evaluation of programs aimed at health promotion, disease prevention, or disease control. In this chapter, we will use the term surveillance according to the above definitions and discuss its potential with regard to digitalization to meet the aforementioned purposes. Since a comprehensive overview would go beyond the scope of this chapter, we will focus on recent reviews and highlight selected current developments in this field.

2.2 Disease Surveillance Based on Electronic Health Records

In the past, public health surveillance heavily relied on reported cases, i.e., on patients with a given disease, and less on risk factors such as health-related behaviors. The reported cases needed to be confirmed using standard tools such as telephone or fax to learn about the diagnosis and disease severity and understand transmission risk factors and potential comorbidities. As Birkhead et al. (2015) underline, public health surveillance may be significantly advanced by using Electronic Health Records (EHRs). The use of which "should increase further the timeliness and completeness of surveillance."

According to Birkhead et al. (2015), infectious diseases such as smallpox, cholera, typhoid, and tuberculosis were a major driver of public health surveillance in the nineteenth century. In the 1930s, surveillance of sexually transmitted diseases further developed the field. Later, with the development of vaccines, the surveillance of vaccine-preventable diseases and immunization played a major role. Surveillance systems for chronic diseases were only put in place after the implementation of surveillance systems for infectious diseases. Finally, "syndromic" surveillance systems have been developed that are close to real-time reporting systems and that should enable rapid reporting to detect, e.g., a terrorist attack or an influenza outbreak.

However, traditional surveillance systems face several limitations, including incompleteness of information and lack of timeliness, non-accurate coding of data, missing information on risk factors, and high data collection costs. Here, EHRs or data from regional health information organizations could improve the quality of existing surveillance systems and increase their efficiency. We will see later that utilizing these data is not without limitations and challenges. Birkhead et al. (2015) report that EHRs are mainly used for communicable disease surveillance, whereas chronic disease surveillance based on EHRs has been reported less frequently. Examples are, among others, estimating the prevalence of asthma in Wisconsin, and assessing the validity of estimated smoking prevalence in England.

At the same time, disease surveillance using EHRs faces characteristic challenges. In a systematic literature review by Aliabadi et al. (2020), 50 studies were screened for challenges and solutions when using EHRs for disease surveillance. Most of the studies were conducted in the United States (78%), Canada (8%), and Europe (8%); one study each was reported from Australia, Thailand, and China. The challenges these studies faced (Table 2 in Aliabadi et al. 2020) can be summarized in six main groups: (1) policy and regulations including data security, privacy, confidentiality, and informed consent, lack of legal authority to create a unique health identifier facilitating record linkage on the level of individuals, lack of legal authority to collect and use EHR data for research, and policies restricting the dissemination of collected data and anonymous data sharing; (2) technical factors such as the fact that EHR data are unstructured and different EHR systems are in use; (3) managerial factors such as the inadequate population coverage of EHR providers, along with a lack of user training and of mutual understanding between medical and technical communities; (4) standardization, i.e., lack of interoperable standards and of data on social variables and risk factors in the EHR system; (5) financial factors related, for example, to the high costs of using unstructured data, the time-consuming and thus expensive process of customizing disease surveillance systems, and the development and maintenance costs; (6) poor data quality, differences in quality across different EHRs, and problems with reliability and validity of unstructured EHR data.

Aliabadi et al. (Table 3) also list solutions to overcome these problems: (1) using natural language processing and machine learning for unstructured data; (2) using appropriate technical solutions for data retrieval, extraction, identification, and visualization; (3) the collaboration of health and clinical departments to access data; (4) standardizing EHR data for public health purposes; and (5) using a unique individual health identifier. In conclusion, Aliabadi et al. (2020) state that disease surveillance based on EHRs may be a powerful tool that can lead to improved disease surveillance. However, its implementation is a time-consuming process requiring a long-term strategic plan and the enacting of appropriate laws, regulations, and standards.

2.3 *Disease Surveillance Based on User-Generated Data*

Here, we refer to data that users of smartphones and internet platforms generate for primary purposes other than health surveillance. The COVID-19 pandemic, if nothing else, has made clear in an impressive and alarming way that traditional approaches to detect and follow-up the outbreak of an infectious disease are no longer sufficient to cope with the speed of such an outbreak due to the high mobility of individuals. Traditional approaches, such as conducting interviews with infected persons and their contacts to trace their movements, have been shown to be much too time-consuming, inefficient, and slow. Traditional approaches are also, as Schlosser and Brockmann (2021) point out, error-prone and might lead to infections being overlooked or falsely identified. Thus, the authors suggest the use of Global Positioning System (GPS) data automatically generated by mobile phones together with an algorithm that is able to scan movement trajectories for locations shared by infected individuals. Thus, this approach requires access to historical movement data of individuals who are known to be infected. Such data are highly sensitive, and careful procedures have to be applied to gather these data under consideration of data protection regulations. The authors claim that data from only four individuals are sufficient to identify the time and place where the outbreak originated with high accuracy.

While the above algorithm is based on a parsimonious set of data that are automatically generated by smartphones connected to mobile phone networks, other tools rely on more diverse and rich data that internet users voluntarily generate on a huge variety of platforms such as Twitter, Facebook, and Google Trends. Data provided on these platforms were, for instance, used to profile vaccine criticisms, track disease outbreaks geospatially, and assess the clustering of behavioral risk factors like substance use, physical inactivity, and poor diet (Shakeri Hossein Abad et al. 2021). Such data may complement traditional data collection for digital public health surveillance (DPHS). Accordingly, in their recent review, Shakeri Hossein Adab et al. propose an alternative definition of DPHS that is restricted to the use of "digital data voluntarily generated by the public, regardless of the main objectives of the task at hand." This definition of DPHS explicitly excludes the traditional approach of surveillance systems with specified goals that generate data through online surveys or include digital content that is not publicly available such as Electronic Health Records. An alternative definition, which we will use in this section, has a restricted scope as it does not fully embrace the widely established definition of surveillance given above.

The number of publications exploring health-related user-generated content available via various internet and social media platforms has increased substantially in recent years. These data allow the investigation of public health aspects not previously covered by health surveillance systems, such as the assessment of the sources and content of misinformation distributed via the internet that may require targeted counter-action. In their scoping review, Shakeri Hossein Abad et al. (2021) have identified 755 articles published between 2005 and 2020 covering 16 prominent public health themes. Even though the studies did not yet include the COVID-19 pandemic, communicable disease was the theme with the highest number of publications (25%). The majority of these studies (69%) were related to identifying disease outbreaks caused, for example, by (Avian) Influenza, Ebola, Zika, or Norovirus. Twitter, Google (Flu) Trends, and Facebook were the three most common digital platforms used. The second most common theme was related to behavioral risk factors, with smoking-related topics like E-cigarettes, vaping, and little cigars and cigarillos in first place (89%). Seventy-five percent of these publications showed the prevalence of advertising smoking behavior (note: prevalence, in this case, refers to the web-based frequency, not the population prevalence), and 19% explored the marketing strategies of smoking vendors on internet platforms. The publication by Smith et al. (2023) may serve as an example of such studies. They undertook a content analysis of narrative post content as well as audio and video content on Instagram and YouTube and found that 87% of Instagram posts and 66% of YouTube videos portrayed vaping as positive, while only 43% of YouTube videos and only 20% of Instagram posts contained an age warning.

Returning to the Shakeri Hossein Abad review—with regards to vaccine surveillance, a majority of studies (48%) explored public opinion and sentiment towards immunization, which show, for example, that men are far more likely to express negative opinions about HPV immunization than women and that being more often exposed to negative opinions increases the likelihood of posting negative messages.

These examples illustrate the different scope of this relatively new means of analyzing publicly available user-generated data on digital platforms to answer questions relevant to public health. While these data seem to provide new opportunities to investigate health-seeking behavior, novel marketing strategies, and misinformation, their usefulness for the primary purpose of surveillance is limited. Time, place, demographic characteristics, and representativeness of the population under study are key factors to be considered here. However, thirty-two percent of the studies included in the review did not capture any variable related to age, sex, or place, and only 25% of them explored the extent to which the assessed characteristics are representative of the target population (Shakeri Hossein Abad et al. 2021). Moreover, since it is difficult to distinguish subjective self-reported information from generic content (i.e., content originating from sources other than the users themselves), only 20% of the studies considered whether or not their results were related to the users' personal experience. Thus the validity and generalizability of social media and internet data remain questionable. None of the studies assessed digital media usage among vulnerable (e.g., low-income) population sub-groups. Therefore, these studies cannot provide insights on the (potentially detrimental) effects of digital media exposure on health behaviors or outcomes, e.g., concerning the massive exposure of children to unhealthy food and sugar-sweetened beverages through influencers on social media platforms, product placements, and advertisements on digital platforms.

Exploiting social media to gather health information for disease surveillance is facing further challenges as relevant information has to be extracted from unstructured data that come along with large amounts of irrelevant content and noise. Also, as described by Khedo et al. (2020), "the short length of the tweets, the large number of spelling and grammatical errors as well as the frequent use of informal, irregular and abbreviated words, and the use of improper sentence structure and mixed language" make it extremely difficult to detect the relevant information for disease surveillance and the identification of outbreaks. In this context, natural language processing seems to be a promising approach to extract and process data from social media (Farzindar and Inkpen 2020). Khedo et al. (2020) suggest a crowdsourcing approach by collecting data via a dedicated smartphone application (see below).

2.4 *Implementation of Digital Tools for Disease Surveillance*

Smartphone applications are a novel tool for data collection that may allow a close to real-time identification of disease outbreaks by collecting disease-related information from patients on a regular basis. Khedo et al. (2020) describe the methodology, design, implementation, and results of such a mobile crowdsourcing application to monitor infectious disease outbreaks in Mauritius, a setting without a routine health information system. Specific algorithms were developed to analyze and visualize the collected data in real time and to identify temporal and regional spikes of disease occurrence. The authors conclude that the novel system can aid outbreak detection as the data corresponded well to existing data from previous years (Khedo et al. 2020).

A similar tool was developed in Germany to assess infectious diseases on a population level (Ortmann et al. 2023). According to the authors, their Prospective Monitoring and Management App (PIA) "allows researchers to implement questionnaires on any topic and to manage biosamples." If short and designed in a user-friendly manner, the implementation of such smartphone applications may help to overcome the problem of (nowadays) often low participation in population-based studies by reducing the threshold for participation and offering the option for immediate feedback to provide personal benefits to participants. Correspondingly, the authors report high acceptability of their app and exceptionally high participation in women over 60 and men under 40 years of age. They conclude that their app is a useful tool for deploying regular short questionnaires in epidemiological studies (Ortmann et al. 2023).

3 Examples

In the following, we will give three examples of surveillance systems based on different types of data sources, use different types of data, and serve different purposes.

3.1 The WHO European Childhood Obesity Surveillance Initiative (COSI)

The WHO European Childhood Obesity Surveillance Initiative (COSI) (WHO 2023b) is an example of a more traditional surveillance system based on primary data collection (questionnaires and anthropometric measurements), which is increasingly extended by digital tools to collect the information of interest (see below).

It was set up in response to the WHO European Ministerial Conference on Counteracting Obesity, held in Istanbul, Turkey, in 2006. This harmonized surveillance system among primary school children aged 6–9 years has been established to observe the alarming trend in the prevalence of childhood obesity and to inform policy-makers about necessary actions to counterbalance this trend. The political commitment to COSI was reinforced in the Vienna Declaration on Nutrition and Noncommunicable Diseases in the Context of Health 2020, adopted in 2013, and the European Food and Nutrition Action Plan 2015–2020, adopted in 2014. COSI is based on the collection of primary data via national surveys under the responsibility of one institution that is nominated by the respective country, and that signs a collaborative agreement with WHO/Europe. Even though COSI does not afford too many resources, European countries are encouraged to integrate COSI into their existing national systems, if possible. Data entry is now facilitated via a tool for online data collection. WHO/Europe also offers technical support as well as training and assistance in the conduct of the survey.

The first COSI round took place during the 2007–2008 school year; 45 member states and almost 411,000 primary school children participated in the fifth round, and the sixth round is currently ongoing. In each country, parents are fully informed about the study protocol; informed consent is also requested from children and schools.

Based on a common protocol, countries must provide children's measured weight and height, date of birth (or age), and sex. While these variables are mandatory, further information may be provided on a voluntary basis. Of central importance is the optional family record form, which is completed by parents. Here, data on children's dietary, physical activity, and sedentary behavior are collected, as well as on families' socioeconomic characteristics and comorbid conditions related to obesity. This recording form is available as an online survey tool, using LimeSurvey (LimeSurvey GmbH, Hamburg, Germany), to allow families to complete it online and to choose a preferred language for multilingual countries. Last but not least, the schools are asked to provide information on the frequency of physical education classes, the availability of school playgrounds, the availability of specific food items and beverages at the school premises, and any school-based initiatives that promote a healthy lifestyle. For more details on the study instruments and the implementation of COSI, we refer to Breda et al. (2021).

3.2 STEPwise Approach to Noncommunicable Disease Risk Factor Surveillance (STEPS)

The WHO STEPwise approach to noncommunicable disease risk factor surveillance (STEPS) (WHO 2023c) is another survey-based approach where primary data on key NCD risk factors are collected using standardized instruments in participating households. Similar to COSI, this more traditional surveillance system is taking advantage of the increasing availability and decreasing costs of digital tools (see below). For instance, tools such as a **sample size calculator** and a **sampling workbook** are provided by the WHO to assist **each country in** determining an adequate sample size and scientifically selecting an appropriate sample. Typically, country-specific samples consist of around 5000 households.

The STEPS approach is based on three steps where information on the core aspects of each risk factor should be collected in each step. Complementary, expanded instruments are also offered in a standardized format if a country needs more detailed information. The key element is, of course, that comparability of the data collected is guaranteed to allow monitoring of temporal trends and comparisons across countries.

In Step 1, trained interviewers collect information on demographics and behavioral risk factors via face-to-face interviews. Since 2009, eSTEPS has been used to collect data via a handheld PC, which provided major benefits compared to the previously used paper-pencil method: (1) It allows immediate error-checking during data collection; (2) It provides real-time tracking of fieldwork; (3) It allows data to be sent to a centralized server as soon as it is collected; (4) Interviewers need to carry fewer materials; (5) No data-entry is required (World Health Organization

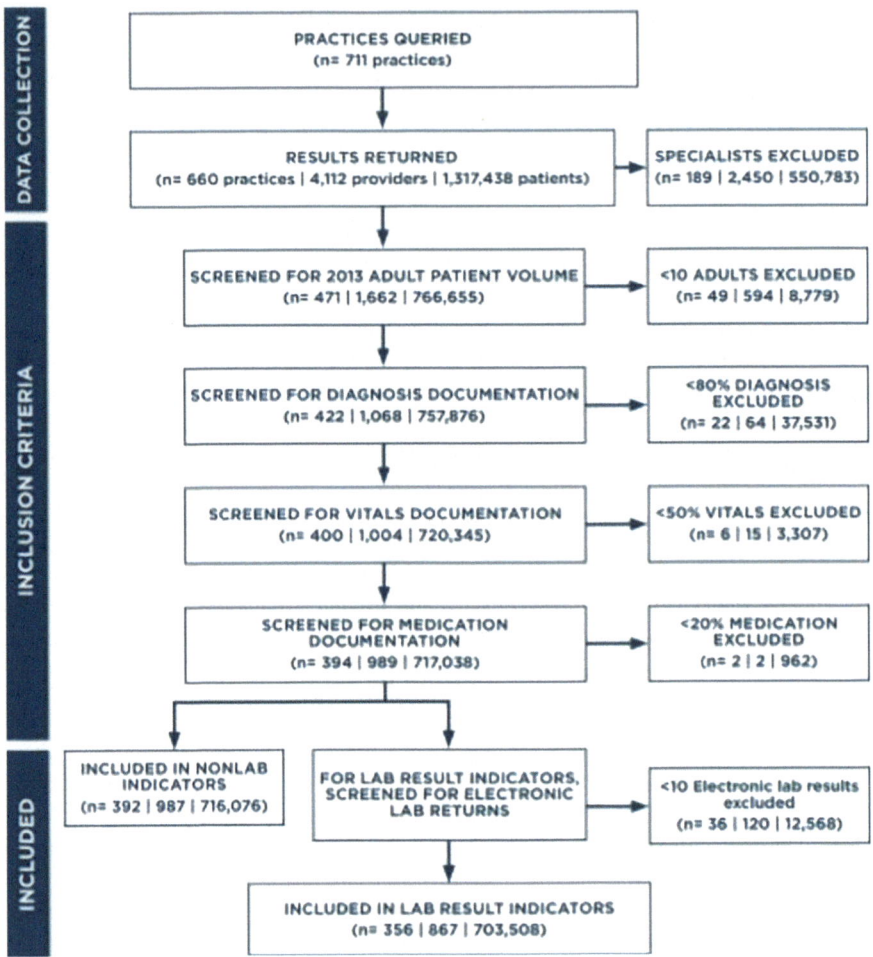

Fig. 2 Inclusion criteria and sample selection for the 2014 NYC Macroscope (Source: Newton-Dame et al. 2016; CC-BY NC ND License 3.0)

2023c). In late 2015, eSTEPS also started enabling data collection via Android devices (Riley et al. 2016).

As reported by Riley et al. (2016), the information collected in Step 1 covers tobacco use, alcohol consumption, dietary behaviors, physical inactivity, as well as the history of NCDs and related conditions such as elevated blood pressure, diabetes, elevated cholesterol, and cardiovascular diseases. In Step 2, height, weight, waist circumference, and blood pressure are measured. Hip circumference and heart rate may be additionally measured. In Step 3, biochemical measurements of fasting blood glucose, total cholesterol levels, and urinary sodium are typically taken at a local clinic or health center. Additionally, triglycerides and high-density lipoprotein cholesterol levels may be measured. Further standardized optional modules are provided by WHO to capture cervical cancer, drug use, household energy use, violence and injury, mental health and suicide, oral health, sexual health, and tobacco control policy (WHO 2023c).

According to Riley et al. (2016), STEPS was piloted in 2002 and 2003. In 2015, 112 of 122 countries (42 countries of the WHO African Region, 21 countries of the WHO Region of the Americas, 16 countries of the WHO Eastern Mediterranean Region, 6 countries of the WHO European Region, 11 countries of the WHO South-East Asia Region, 26 countries of the WHO Western Pacific Region) completed all three steps of the STEPS survey and ten countries completed only Step 1 and 2. For more details we refer to Fig. 1 of Riley et al. (2016).

3.3 The New York City (NYC) Macroscope

The NYC Macroscope is an example of the potential use of secondary data for surveillance. In particular, it was set up to explore the usefulness of Electronic Health Records (EHRs) provided by a network of ambulatory care practices for health surveillance of adults visiting a healthcare provider in the preceding year. For this purpose, aggregate EHR data were requested from outpatient practices in New York City that had agreed to share data with the NYC Health Department's Primary Care Information Project (PCIP). Participating practices, concentrated in low-income neighborhoods, provide their data through the Hub Population Health System (Buck

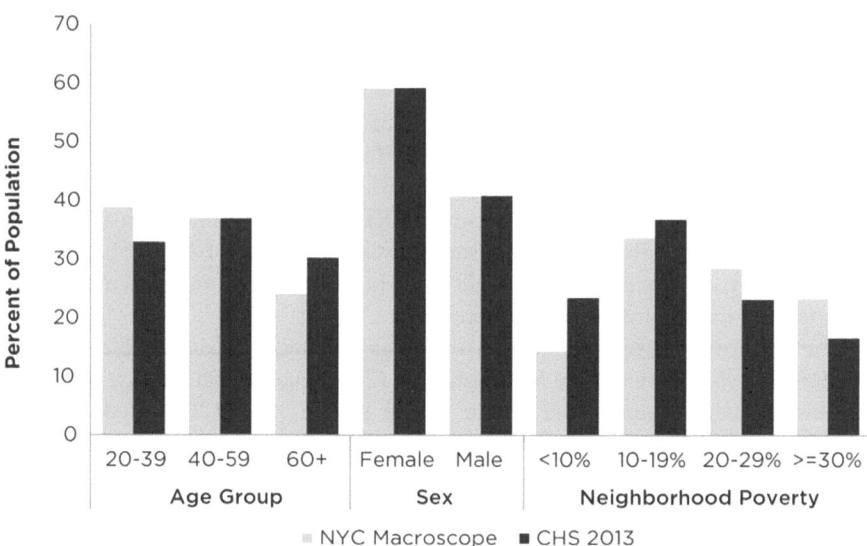

Fig. 3 Distribution of unweighted data from the 2014 NYC Macroscope compared with the 2013 Community Health Survey (CHS) estimations of the population in care (Source: Newton-Dame et al. 2016; CC-BY NC ND License 3.0)

et al. 2012) using a uniform EHR platform. The Health Department collects data via SQL queries to participating practices, which then automatically return aggregate counts to a secure database. No patient-identifying data are transferred. These data are primarily used by requesting providers to increase the delivery of preventive care, track chronic disease, and improve disease management. For the NYC Macroscope, all 711 practices connected to the Hub were approached. The returned data were transformed and filtered according to predefined quality and inclusion criteria, as illustrated in Fig. 2.

Information on seven health domains (i.e., prevalence, treatment, and control of (1) diabetes, (2) hypertension and (3) hyperlipidemia, prevalence of (4) smoking, (5) obesity and (6) depression, and (7) uptake of influenza vaccination) was collected from the adult population 20 years and older visiting a doctor in the preceding year. The estimates obtained from the NYC Macroscope were then validated against the 2013–2014 NYC Health and Nutrition Examination Survey (NYC HANES) and the 2013 Community Health Survey (CHS). A working group of epidemiologists and clinical experts selected the above-listed seven domains as primary drivers of morbidity and mortality. They then drafted indicators to assess the performance of the NYC Macroscope, which was finally approved by content experts and an external scientific advisory group. All indicators were stratified by age, sex, and neighborhood poverty. More details on the indicators and the design of the NYC Macroscope can be found in Newton-Dame et al. (2016) (see also Fig. 2).

When assessing the representativeness and completeness of their data, the authors concluded that they could finally obtain estimates based on data from 9.7% of primary care providers covering 15% of the adult NYC patient population in 2013, penetrating most neighborhoods by more than 10%. Major deviations were observed with respect to age, where the 20–23-year-olds were over- and the 60+-year-olds underrepresented, and income with an overrepresentation of neighborhoods with higher poverty (see Fig. 3), indicating the necessity of an appropriate weighting scheme. Weights had to be obtained for each indicator based on age, sex, and neighborhood poverty from NYC Health and Nutrition Examination Survey (HANES) and Community Health Survey (CHS), respectively, to maximize comparability with each of these reference surveys. Completeness of NYC Macroscope data varied greatly by domain, from 98% for blood pressure among patients with hypertension to 33% for depression screening.

The validity of the results obtained according to domain is described in detail in two further publications where McVeigh et al. (2016) focused on obesity, smoking, depression, and influenza vaccination, while Thorpe et al. (2016) reported the respective results for metabolic outcomes. McVeigh et al. (2016) fixed five statistical criteria to assess the performance of the NYC Macroscope estimates compared to NYC HANES survey estimates: statistical equivalence, statistical difference, absolute prevalence difference, prevalence ratio, and internal consistency. In summary, the prevalence estimates for both smoking and obesity of the weighted NYC Macroscope data fell between the corresponding estimates of NYC HANES and CHS. Regarding the five criteria, smoking fulfilled all five and obesity three. Based on a subsample of 48 NYC HANES participants who were also included in the NYC Macroscope, the sensitivity and specificity of being a smoker ($n = 43$) or being obese ($n = 44$) were both above 90%. However, the results were less convincing for depression and influenza vaccination, where the NYC Macroscope resulted in prevalence estimates that were more than 10 percentage points lower than those of the two other surveys. In addition, sensitivity for depression was 31% and for influenza 64%, while specificity was, again, higher than 90%. With respect to metabolic outcomes, Thorpe et al. (2016) reported that the NYC Macroscope prevalence estimates for hypertension were highly concordant with NYC HANES estimates. Concordance was also high for diagnosed diabetes but less so when accounting for the laboratory results. Prevalence estimates for hypercholesterolemia were less concordant. The authors found a poor agreement for treatment and control of all of these metabolic outcomes.

Main limitations discussed by Newton-Dame et al. (2016) related, among others, to the fact that access was only provided to aggregated data, information on the practice documentation and workflows in the primary care practices was missing, and access to socio-economic variables was limited. Nevertheless, McVeigh et al. (2017) concluded "that many of the EHR-based surveillance indicators developed and validated for the NYC Macroscope are generalizable for use in other EHR surveillance systems," which might help to pave the way for making better use of such data for surveillance purposes.

4 Outlook: Precision Public Health

When focusing on non-communicable diseases (NCDs), which are still the largest public health threat globally, the term precision public health plays an increasingly important role. Precision public health "(PPH) seeks to create an agile, responsive and data-driven public health system that strengthens current evidence-based approaches. PPH aims to improve population health by integrating data and digital technology to guide precision decisions, interventions and policy." (Canfell et al. 2022a). According to Muin J Khoury, Director of the Office of Public Health Genomics at the Centers for Disease Control and Prevention "precision public health is about populations. It is essentially about delivering `the right intervention at the right time, every time to the right population." in contrast to precision medicine which is about the individual, i.e., "in lay terms, precision medicine can be thought of as giving "the right treatments at the right time, every time to the right person." (Khoury 2018).

In creating a precision public health system, real-world data from different sources such as electronic medical records, personal health records, genomics, claims data, mobile health, digital wearables, and social media need to be exploited, i.e., data that are collected "automatically," routinely and in real time (Canfell et al. 2022a). For this purpose, the authors suggest a strategic road map towards precision public health with three components: (1) digital public health workflows; (2) population health data and analytics; (3) precision public health.

In a scoping review, Canfell et al. (2022b) aim to understand how real-world and traditional data are aggregated to support precision public health for NCDs. They identified six studies that fulfilled their inclusion criteria: three were conducted in the United States, two in Canada, and one in China. This review is referenced here because the included studies aim to describe the development of a population health surveillance platform, for instance, PopHR, a Big Data platform in Canada (Shaban-Nejad et al. 2017). Among these six studies, one study aligned with component 1, five with component 2, and none with component 3. The authors conclude that the overall focus was "building digital public health foundations through integrating real-world data and traditional data into surveillance platforms (component 1)" and "creating basic population health analytics as a foundation for improving policy and practice decisions (component 2)" and that the major challenge in the future will be to achieve a shared vision of component 3.

5 Conclusion

The digitalization of the health sector has had an enormous impact on the amount of health data that are potentially useful to guide political decisions that foster population health. However, not only data generated in the health sector can be used for DPHS. As we have shown above, multiple data sources provide automatically or voluntarily generated data on health and health-related behaviors that may be exploited for DPHS. For instance, public health researchers are currently exploring the usefulness of satellite data for public health surveillance, and it seems as if data collected by earth observation satellites may become a powerful tool for this purpose when it comes to the identification and tracking of, for example, outbreaks of infectious diseases. This has particular potential for waterborne diseases such as cholera and typhoid, which are closely related to climate change, or vector-borne diseases such as malaria and dengue fever, whose vectors are influenced by factors such as temperature, vegetation, and land cover (for more details, see Skyrora 2023). Taubenböck et al. (2020) describe in detail the potential of satellite data to assess, for example, environmental exposure to air pollution or characteristics of the physical environment that may shape physical activity and other health behaviors. Such data have a huge potential for health surveillance and health research if they can be linked to geocodes of places of residence or work of study participants in order to provide objective exposure data while reducing the need to collect subjective self-reported data, thereby reducing the effort and burden for participants.

Unfortunately, data such as Electronic Health Records are typically not generated, managed, and stored according to the FAIR guiding principles (Wilkinson et al. 2016), where FAIR stands for data being findable, accessible, interoperable, and reusable. The *findability* of digital health data is usually limited since metadata

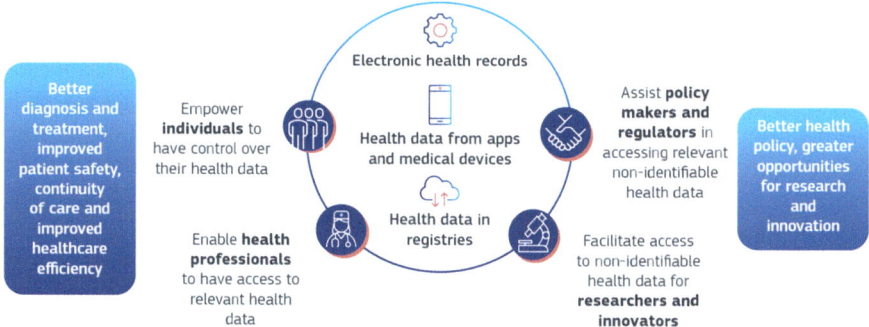

Fig. 4 Objectives of the European Health Data Space (Source: European Commission 2022, © European Union 2022; CC-BY License 4.0)

that describe the datasets appropriately are mostly missing. Even if metadata are provided, they do not follow a common metadata schema. Missing or non-harmonized metadata hamper a structured search for adequate health-related datasets. In addition, their *access* may be strongly restricted if the respective health data are person-related and, therefore, highly sensitive. In such cases, their use must observe strict data protection regulations and comply with ethical requirements. Moreover, access may be denied by data holders due to legal restrictions, property rights, or lack of willingness to share data. The *interoperability* of data from different data sources may be impaired because data holders use different classification systems and variable formats. *Reuse* of existing data may be further impeded by insufficient documentation of data and their provenance. In Sect. 2 of this chapter, the importance of the FAIR guiding principles for setting up surveillance systems became apparent, particularly in the review of Aliabadi et al. (2020).

Aliabadi et al. (2020) also stress that an accurate record linkage of different health records of one individual over time and from different EHR systems is a major challenge in public health surveillance that can be appropriately addressed by creating a unique health identifier that is recorded by all EHRs. Such an identifier would significantly decrease the costs and effort and, at the same time, facilitate accurate patient identification for record linkage, which is currently not often feasible.

The authors also mention the major ethical concerns when using Electronic Health Records for surveillance purposes. These are closely related to data protection issues. Here, clear regulations and laws are missing that allow access to EHR data for surveillance purposes and health research without the informed consent of insurants. Otherwise, the representativeness of an EHR-based surveillance system is compromised if insurants deny the use of their EHR data for surveillance purposes.

The necessity to improve the sharing of health data has also been acknowledged by the European Commission (EC), which proposes a regulation to set up a European Health Data Space (EHDS). The latter should (1) "facilitate access to non-identifiable health data for researchers and innovators," (2) "assist policymakers and regulators in accessing relevant non-identifiable health data," (3) "enable health professionals to have access to relevant health data," and (4) "empower individuals to have control over their health data" where the ultimate goals are "better diagnosis and treatment, improved patient safety, continuity of care and improved healthcare efficiency" as well as "better health policy" and "greater opportunities for research and innovation" (see Fig. 4, European Commission 2022). For this purpose, access to health care records, health data from apps and medical devices, and health data in registries should be enabled for the benefit of public health. However, this EC proposal focuses on patient data and thus seems to miss the opportunity to take advantage of surveillance as an integral part of the EHDS. Therefore, the above listing should be extended beyond clinical data to include population-based surveillance data that are needed for policy evaluation and public health planning.

The value of existing data would be further enhanced if the various sources could be linked to create a full picture of all factors causing a certain disease such that adequate prevention measures can be developed and implemented in the general public. This would, however, require not only a change in the legal framework of possibilities for record linkage in Germany compared to other European countries (see Sect. 3 of this chapter) but also improved interoperability of different databases by employing, for example, a unified classification system (see also Aliabadi et al. 2020). Interoperability of the various databases would also facilitate easy reuse of these data and improve population health surveillance.

This work was conducted as part of the NFDI4Health Consortium (www.nfdi4health.de). We gratefully acknowledge the financial support of the German Research Foundation (DFG)—project number 442326535.

References

Aliabadi A, Sheikhtaheri A, Ansari H (2020) Electronic health record-based disease surveillance systems: a systematic literature review on challenges and solutions. J Am Med Inform Assoc 27(12):1977–1986

Birkhead GS, Klompas M, Shah NR (2015) Uses of electronic health records for public health surveillance to advance public health. Annu Rev Public Health 36:345–359

Breda J, McColl K, Buoncristiano M, Williams J, Abdrakhmanova S, Abdurrahmonova Z, Ahrens W, Akhmedova D, Bakacs M, Boer JMA, Boymatova K, Brinduse LA, Cucu A, Duleva V, Endevelt R, Sant'Angelo VF, Fijałkowska A, Hadžiomeragić AF, García-Solano M, Grøholt EK, Gualtieri A, Hassapidou M, Hejgaard T, Hyska J, Kelleher CC, Kujundžić E, Mäki P, Markidou Ioannidou E, Melkumova M, Moyersoen I, Milanović SM, Nurk E, Ostojic SM, Peterkova V, Petrauskienė A, Pudule I, Rito AI, Russell Jonsson K, Rutter H, Salanave B, Seyidov N, Shengelia L, Silitrari N, Spinelli A, Spiroski I, Starc G, Stojisavljević D, Tanrygulyyeva M, Tichá Ľ, Usupova Z, Weghuber D, Yardim N, Zamrazilová H, Zbanatskyi V, Branca F, Weber M, Rakovac I (2021) Methodology and implementation of the WHO European Childhood Obesity Surveillance Initiative (COSI). Obes Rev 22(Suppl 6):e13215

Buck MD, Anane S, Taverna J, Amirfar S, Stubbs-Dame R, Singer J (2012) The hub population health system: distributed ad hoc queries and alerts. J Am Med Inform Assoc 19(e1):e46–e50

Canfell OJ, Davidson K, Woods L, Sullivan C, Cocoros NM, Klompas M, Zambarano B, Eakin E, Littlewood R, Burton-Jones A (2022a) Precision public health for non-communicable diseases: an emerging strategic roadmap and multinational use cases. Front Public Health 10:854525

Canfell OJ, Kodiyattu Z, Eakin E, Burton-Jones A, Wong I, Macaulay C, Sullivan C (2022b) Real-world data for precision public health of noncommunicable diseases: a scoping review. BMC Public Health 22(1):2166

European Commission (2022) Factsheet—European Health Data Space. https://ec.europa.eu/commission/presscorner/detail/en/fs_22_2713. Accessed 2 Feb 2023.

Farzindar AA, Inkpen D (2020) Natural language processing for social media, 3rd edn. Morgan & Claypool Publishers, San Rafael, California

Khedo K, Baichoo S, Nagowah SD, Mungloo-Dilmohamud Z, Cadersaib Z, Cheerkoot-Jalim S, Nagowah L, Sookha L (2020) DOT: a crowdsourcing mobile application for disease outbreak detection and surveillance in Mauritius. Health Technol (Berl) 10(5):1115–1127

Khoury MJ (2018) Precision public health: what is it? Centers for Disease Control and Prevention, Genomics and Precision Health, May 15, 2018. https://blogs.cdc.gov/genomics/2018/05/15/precision-public-health-2/. Accessed 1 May 2023.

McVeigh KH, Newton-Dame R, Chan PY, Thorpe LE, Schreibstein L, Tatem KS, Chernov C, Lurie-Moroni E, Perlman SE (2016) Can electronic health records be used for population health surveillance? Validating population health metrics against established survey data. EGEMS (Wash DC) 4(1):1267

McVeigh KH, Lurie-Moroni E, Chan PY, Newton-Dame R, Schreibstein L, Tatem KS, Romo ML, Thorpe LE, Perlman SE (2017) Generalizability of indicators from the New York City Macroscope Electronic Health Record Surveillance System to systems based on other EHR platforms. EGEMS (Wash DC) 5(1):25

Newton-Dame R, McVeigh KH, Schreibstein L, Perlman S, Lurie-Moroni E, Jacobson L, Greene C, Snell E, Thorpe LE (2016) Design of the New York City Macroscope: innovations in population health surveillance using electronic health records. EGEMS (Wash DC) 4(1):1265

Ortmann J, Heise JK, Janzen I, Jenniches F, Kemmling Y, Frömke C, Castell S (2023) Suitability and user acceptance of the eResearch system "Prospective Monitoring and Management App (PIA)"—the example of an epidemiological study on infectious diseases. PLoS One 18(1):e0279969

Porta M (2008) A dictionary of epidemiology, 5th edn. Oxford University Press, New York

Riley L, Guthold R, Cowan M, Savin S, Bhatti L, Armstrong T, Bonita R (2016) The World Health Organization STEPwise approach to noncommunicable disease risk-factor surveillance: methods, challenges, and opportunities. Am J Public Health 106:74–78

Schlosser F, Brockmann D (2021) Finding disease outbreak locations from human mobility data. EPJ Data Science 10:52

Shaban-Nejad A, Lavigne M, Okhmatovskaia A, Buckeridge DL (2017) PopHR: a knowledge-based platform to support integration, analysis, and visualization of population health data. Ann N Y Acad Sci 1387(1):44–53

Shakeri Hossein Abad Z, Kline A, Sultana M, Noaeen M, Nurmambetova E, Lucini F, Al-Jefri M, Lee J (2021) Digital public health surveillance: a systematic scoping review. NPJ Digit Med 4(1):41

Skyrora (2023) Applying satellite technology in detecting and managing disease outbreak. https://www.skyrora.com/applying-satellite-technology-in-detecting-and-managing-disease-outbreak/. Accessed 7 May 2023.

Smith MJ, Buckton C, Patterson C, Hilton S (2023) User-generated content and influencer marketing involving e-cigarettes on social media: a scoping review and content analysis of YouTube and Instagram. BMC Public Health 23(1):530

Taubenböck H, Schmich P, Erbertseder T, Müller I, Tenikl J, Weigand M, Staab J, Wurm M (2020) Satellitendaten zur Erfassung gesundheitsrelevanter Umweltbedingungen: Beispiele und interdisziplinäre Potenziale [satellite data for recording health-relevant environmental conditions: examples and interdisciplinary potential]. Bundesgesundheitsblatt, Gesundheitsforschung, Gesundheitsschutz 63(8):936–944. https://doi.org/10.1007/s00103-020-03177-w

Thorpe LE, McVeigh KH, Perlman S, Chan PY, Bartley K, Schreibstein L, Rodriguez-Lopez J, Newton-Dame R (2016) Monitoring prevalence, treatment, and control of metabolic conditions in New York City adults using 2013 primary care electronic health records: a surveillance validation study. EGEMS (Wash DC) 4(1):1266

Wilkinson MD, Dumontier M, Aalbersberg IJ, Appleton G, Axton M, Baak A et al (2016) The FAIR guiding principles for scientific data management and stewardship. Sci Data 3(1):1–9

Wong BLH, Maaß L, Vodden A, van Kessel R, Sorbello S, Buttigieg S, Odone A, on behalf of the European Public Health Association (EUPHA) Digital Health Section (2022) The dawn of digital public health in Europe: implications for public health policy and practice. Lancet Reg Health Eur 14:100316

World Health Organization (2023a) Public health surveillance. https://www.emro.who.int/health-topics/public-health-surveillance/index.html. Accessed 1 May 2023.

World Health Organization (2023b) WHO European Childhood Obesity Surveillance Initiative (COSI). https://www.who.int/europe/initiatives/who-european-childhood-obesity-surveillance-initiative-(cosi). Accessed 3 Feb 2023.

World Health Organization (2023c) Noncommunicable Disease Surveillance, Monitoring and Reporting. https://www.who.int/teams/noncommunicable-diseases/surveillance. Accessed 3 Feb 2023.

World Health Organization Regional Office for Europe (2012) Strengthening public health services and capacity: an action plan for Europe: promoting health and well-being now and for future generations. https://apps.who.int/iris/handle/10665/340447. Accessed 4 July 2023.

Open Access This chapter is licensed under the terms of the Creative Commons Attribution 4.0 International License (http://creativecommons.org/licenses/by/4.0/), which permits use, sharing, adaptation, distribution and reproduction in any medium or format, as long as you give appropriate credit to the original author(s) and the source, provide a link to the Creative Commons license and indicate if changes were made.

The images or other third party material in this chapter are included in the chapter's Creative Commons license, unless indicated otherwise in a credit line to the material. If material is not included in the chapter's Creative Commons license and your intended use is not permitted by statutory regulation or exceeds the permitted use, you will need to obtain permission directly from the copyright holder.

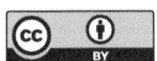

Monitoring and Response to Health Hazards and Emergencies (EPHO2)

Corona-Warn-App: A Digital Tool in the SARS-CoV-2 Pandemic

Göran Kirchner, Robin Houben, Justus Benzler, Tobias R. K. Heller, Tim Einbeck, Katrin Werth, and Patrick Schmich

Abstract In this chapter, the Corona-Warn-App (CWA), a digital contact tracing tool developed during the SARS-CoV-2 pandemic, will be outlined as an example of a digital tool supporting Essential Public Health Operation (EPHO) 2. The CWA was the official contact tracing app in Germany, commissioned by the Robert Koch Institute, developed by SAP, and run on infrastructure set up by T-Systems. During the first months of the pandemic, decision-makers feared that manual contact tracing would not be sufficient to end infection chains. It turned out that with digital contact tracing, a slight paradigm shift—from tracing contact persons to tracing contact—was established. This, in turn, changes the vantage point for future measures in monitoring and response to health hazards and emergencies.

Germany's contact tracing app had a very high uptake in the German population. The decision to follow a data-protection-friendly path was warmly welcomed by the German civil society and might have had an impact on the positive opinion towards the app, thus helping to improve its efficacy.

The Corona-Warn-App followed three main aims: (1) Provide test results (quickly), (2) warn other users (by sharing), and (3) determine potential risks (correctly).

Despite the limitations of its underlying technology, the Corona-Warn-App has shown to be an effective digital tool which has probably helped to reduce the number of infected persons and deaths during the SARS-CoV-2 pandemic.

Keywords Digital public health · Corona-Warn-App · CWA · Digital contact tracing · COVID-19

G. Kirchner · R. Houben · J. Benzler · T. R. K. Heller · T. Einbeck · K. Werth · P. Schmich (✉)
Robert Koch Institute, Berlin, Germany
e-mail: schmichp@rki.de

Abbreviations

BLE	Bluetooth Low Energy/Bluetooth LE
CCC	Chaos Computer Club
COVID-19	Coronavirus Disease 19
DCT	Digital contact tracing
EDUS	Event-driven user survey
ENF	Exposure Notification (GAEN) framework
EU DCC	EU Digital COVID-19 Certificates (DCC)
MCT	Manual contact tracing
PPA	Privacy-Preserving Analytics
RKI	Robert Koch Institute
RPI	Rolling Proximity Identifier
SARS-CoV-2	Severe acute respiratory syndrome coronavirus type 2

1 Introduction

1.1 Purpose of the Chapter

This chapter investigates the significance of digital epidemiology (Salathé 2023) when responding to a health hazard through the example of a digital contact tracing app, the German Corona-Warn-App (CWA). It comprehensively summarizes the app's creation, features, and utilization, along with its possible advantages and drawbacks. Additionally, the broader implications of the app, including the challenges and prospects it poses, will be discussed. By analyzing Germany's experience with the CWA, the chapter seeks to enhance comprehension of digital technologies' role in combating infectious disease outbreaks and the potential of digital tools and processes in epidemiology and public health. The chapter provides both a retrospective and a prospective view.

1.2 History of the Corona-Warn-App

During SARS-CoV-2 pandemic, the CWA was the official digital contact tracing (DCT) app in Germany (Fig. 1), commissioned by the country's public health institute, the Robert Koch Institute (RKI), developed by SAP and run on infrastructure set up by T-Systems. It was available for download in Germany from June 16, 2020, and in many other countries in seven languages (German, English, Turkish, Bulgarian, Polish, Romanian, and Ukrainian) since early July 2020. The CWA existed alongside manual contact tracing (MCT) conducted by local health authorities.

Fig. 1 Examples of a Corona-Warn-App campaign: "Doesn't know you. But still helps you," "Tells you if things get serious" (Source: Corona-Warn-App, RKI 2020)

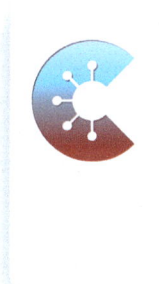

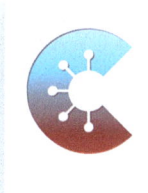

In the early phase of the COVID-19 pandemic, there were concerns that manual contact tracing would be insufficient to contain the spread of SARS-CoV-2. Initially, leaders of the federal government and federal states preferred a centralized approach for a DCT tool conceptualized by the Heinrich Hertz Institute (Fraunhofer). However, following controversial discussions within civil society and due to the progress of other endeavors in the scientific community (DP-3T 2020), the government decided on April 14, 2020, to adopt a decentralized approach.

Google and Apple provided the Exposure Notification (GAEN) framework, which allowed for a decentralized contact tracing app that could work between iPhones and smartphones from other manufacturers operating on Android systems. These companies provided the necessary interface for Bluetooth-based distance and duration measurements, making it possible to gather information about encounters between devices. A more in-depth explanation of how the CWA works is provided later in this chapter.

By the end of April 2020, it was decided that the Robert Koch Institute, as a public health institute, would be the publisher of the CWA. Two weeks later, the source code was published online on GitHub (Corona-Warn-App documentation 2020–2023) to involve civil society and allow tech-oriented citizens to review the code and provide valuable feedback to the developers.

Germany's contact tracing app became one of the most frequently downloaded apps worldwide, reaching nearly 20 million downloads in the first 100 days[1] and totaling over 48 million downloads.[2] At its peak, it was actively used by more than 35 million people[3] and offered not only contact tracing by proximity measurement but also an event check-in feature, the transmission of test results, statistics on the pandemic situation in Germany, and storage of EU digital COVID certificates. Within its ecosystem, 59 million PCR test results and 183 million rapid antigen test results were provided to potential CWA users.

In the event of a positive test result, users could immediately warn their contacts through the CWA, which was done nearly nine million times. Due to the decentralized and privacy-preserving design of the CWA, the exact number of warnings received by users is unknown. However, thanks to approximately 13 million (at its peak 17 million) voluntary data donors,[4] it is estimated that users were warned more than 253 million times. Research conducted by the CWA team at the RKI (Kirchner G, Benzler J et al. 2021–2022) showed that one in five people who received an increased risk warning via their CWA subsequently tested positive.[5]

The Corona-Warn-App has been adapted and improved in numerous releases, with information on selected releases detailed in Table 1.

2 Digital Epidemiology and the Corona-Warn-App

2.1 *Aims and Purposes of the Corona-Warn-App*

The aims of the Corona-Warn-App are defined in the Data Protection Impact Assessment (*Datenschutzfolgenabschätzung, DSFA*) in which the adequacy of the use of personal data (albeit pseudonymized) is to be questioned and answered with the help of a continuous evaluation process.

In this regard, the Corona-Warn-App has three main aims:

1. Provide test results (quickly): people tested for SARS-CoV-2 should receive their test results as soon as possible.
2. Warn other users (by sharing): people who have received a positive test result should be able to inform or warn other people who have been in their immediate vicinity of the increased risk of infection.

---

[1] https://www.coronawarn.app/en/blog/2020-09-23-100-tage-positive-bilanz. Accessed 28 Jun 2023
[2] https://www.coronawarn.app/en/analysis. Accessed 28 Jun 2023
[3] https://www.coronawarn.app/en/science/2022-03-03-science-blog-5. Accessed 28 Jun 2023
[4] https://www.coronawarn.app/en/science/2021-10-15-science-blog-4. Accessed 28 Jun 2023
[5] https://www.coronawarn.app/en/science/2021-10-15-science-blog-4/#65-association-between-risk-assessment-and-infection. Accessed 28 Jun 2023

Table 1 Selected releases of the CWA and their main functional enhancements. (Source: own table)

Release	Functions implemented in the CWA
1.0	Core functionalities: Proximity tracing via Bluetooth LE, sharing of positive Corona test results, warning other users
1.5	Support for the European Federation Gateway
1.7	Risk status updates several times a day
1.9	Update to GAEN framework v2
1.10	Contact diary
1.11	Key figures re. the pandemic (newly reported infections etc.)
1.13	Voluntary data donation (Privacy-Preserving Analytics (PPA))
1.15	Interoperability with Swiss app
2.0	Event registration (check-in)
2.1	Integration of rapid antigen tests
2.3	Support for EU digital COVID (vaccination) certificates (EU DCC)
2.4	Support for EU digital test certificates
2.5	Support for EU digital certificates of recovery
2.6	Check travel validity for certificates
2.9	Event hosts can warn for others representatively
2.16	Current status evidence of DCCs (2G, 3G, etc.)
2.27	Adjusted immunity status according to new regulations
3.0	Warn without a QR code or a TAN, warn with a positive self-test
3.2	Prepared the app for its shutdown

3. Determine risks (correctly): People who have been in the immediate vicinity of a person with SARS-CoV-2 should be informed or warned of the increased risk of infection.

These three aims are interconnected and depend on each other for their effect. Persons who have been in the immediate vicinity of someone with SARS-CoV-2 can only be informed or warned that they were at an *increased risk of infection* (Aim 3) if the person who received the positive test result can inform or warn them and actually does so, *sharing the positive test result* (Aim 2). Moreover, if this is to happen quickly enough to break the infection chain: persons who tested positive for SARS-CoV-2 must *receive their test results as soon as possible* (Aim 1).

As its evaluation shows, the CWA can be assumed to be contributing towards its purpose of combating the pandemic if it fulfills these three aims (see Sect. 2.3).

2.2 Challenges in the Development of the Corona-Warn-App

The initial version of the Corona-Warn-App was developed in the spring of 2020 when it became evident that COVID-19 posed a significant threat to public health and that contact tracing was crucial. Initially, policymakers leaned towards a centralized approach for a DCT app, which would store all users' contact tracing data on a central server. However, concerns from civil society and data privacy experts made the acceptance of a centralized app uncertain. Following the GAEN framework's publication in May 2020, policymakers decided to build the German app using this technology, which employs a decentralized approach, only storing users' contact tracing data locally on their devices (see also Chap. "Open Data for DiPH Research Versus Data Protection", Freye and Buchner, in this handbook).

It took approximately 6 weeks from the announcement to the app's first release, including development and coordination between governmental organizations and industrial partners, specifically SAP and Telekom. The initial version included essential features such as receiving warnings and, if tested positive, warning contacts who were close, as measured via the Bluetooth signal, for an extended period. Moreover, the app allowed users to receive their PCR test results by scanning a QR code.

The app's development continued after the initial release, and numerous new features were incorporated into the CWA. A list of selected features can be found in Table 1.

By the end of 2022, in line with the German government's general decision on how to address the ongoing pandemic, it was decided to discontinue the CWA's development. The app's full functionality was available until April 30, 2023, while the development officially ended on May 31, 2023. The app remained usable but with reduced functionality and without further maintenance.

The development of the Corona-Warn-App was quite a challenge in multiple ways. Its first version was required to be released as soon as possible. After the decision to develop a decentralized contact tracing app, the industrial partners SAP and Telekom developed an initial version of the app in about 7 weeks.

But just developing an app that traces contacts was not enough. For the system to work and fulfill its purpose, it needed the following further ingredients:

- Adoption: to detect contacts, people have to use the app. Therefore, civil society must *trust* the app. Thus, an extensive public relations campaign was initiated at the app's release to reach as many people as possible and explain its privacy-preserving features. This campaign included analog and digital advertising. To further strengthen its credibility and empower everyone to participate in its development, the source code was released on GitHub as an *open-source project*. A cherished *user community* and an efficient *hotline and FAQ* have helped to find and mitigate problems as early as possible.
- Interoperable integration: laboratories and test sites should be enabled to quickly integrate their systems and provide the test results.
- Calibration: to correctly estimate the risk during exposure, the Bluetooth Low Energy (BLE) measurements provided by the GAEN framework should be well understood. Here Fraunhofer IIS, SAP, and RKI have made many test runs, which helped to calibrate the system (Kirchner et al. 2020; Meyer et al. 2021).
- Continuous evaluation and improvements: during the pandemic, many new political decisions (e.g., the introduction of behavioral rules) and measurements (e.g.,

vaccination) were made, and lots of changes in the situation have occurred (e.g., new strains and variants of the virus). Thus, a flexible design and the possibility to adapt fast and preview possible changes assisted in these situations.
- International collaboration: finally, an exchange with partners abroad has helped a lot in identifying improvements, preventing pitfalls, and being prepared for upcoming changes (see Lueks et al. 2021; Rivest et al. 2021; World Health Organization, and European Centre for Disease Prevention and Control, Geneva 2021).

2.3 How the App Worked

To reduce the spread of COVID-19, it was necessary to inform people about their proximity to individuals who tested positive. Without the use of digital solutions, health departments and affected individuals could only identify possibly infected individuals in personal conversations based on each individual's memory. This led to a high number of unknown connections, e.g., when using public transport or visiting public places.

The Corona-Warn-App pursued two main objectives:

1. It supported individuals in finding out whether they had been exposed to a person who later tested positive.
2. It received the result of a SARS-CoV-2 test on a user's mobile phone through an online system. This helped reduce the time until necessary precautions, e.g., contact reduction and testing, could be taken.

The basic workflow in using the app is shown in Fig. 2a, b below.

2.3.1 Basic Functionalities and User Interface

The Corona-Warn-App measures the distance between people who have installed and activated the app using Bluetooth technology and allows the smartphone to remember these encounters. The devices exchange temporary encrypted random codes (Bluetooth IDs) with each other. These temporary random codes are derived multiple times per hour cryptographically from the random device key of the smartphone. The random device keys are generated anew every day.

The Corona-Warn-App thus uses two types of random codes, a random device key and a short-lived random Bluetooth ID derived from the random device key and exchanged between adjacent mobile devices. Both random codes cannot be assigned to a specific person without additional knowledge and are automatically deleted when they are 14 days old.

If a user of the app tests positive for the coronavirus, they can choose to share their device keys for comparison. The device keys of the person who tested positive for SARS-CoV-2 are uploaded to the Corona-Warn-App server. All active

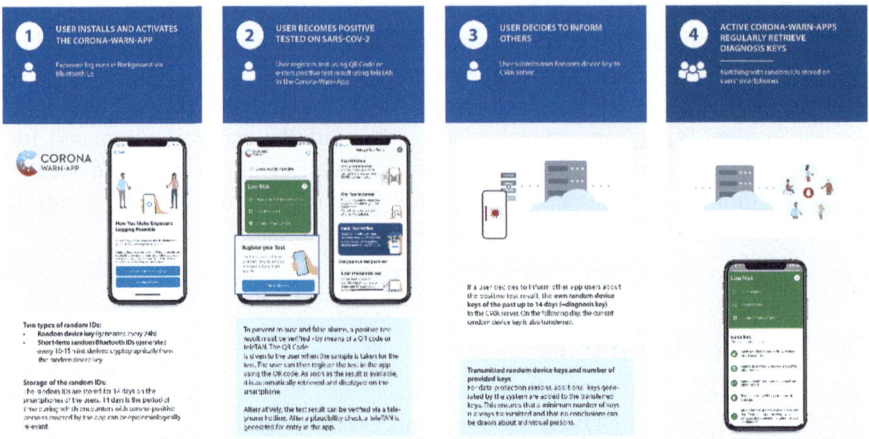

Fig. 2 (**a**) Overview of steps and processes in the use of the CWA, part I (Source: RKI, own figure). (**b**) Overview of steps and processes in the use of the CWA, part II (Source: RKI, own figure)

Corona-Warn-Apps regularly download those published on the CWA server and pass them on to the operating system via an interface. The system checks whether recorded random codes match a random code of the person who tested positive for SARS-CoV-2.

If there is a match, a multi-stage process is used to determine the transmission risk, and, if defined threshold values have been exceeded, the user is informed about the possible risk assessment. At no time does this process allow any conclusions to be drawn about the user or their location.

2.3.2 Contact Tracing Architecture and Data Protection

The Corona-Warn-App, shown centrally in Fig. 3, enables individuals to trace their personal exposure risk via their mobile phones. The Corona-Warn-App uses a framework provided by Apple and Google (GAEN: Exposure Notification Framework). The framework employs Bluetooth Low Energy mechanics. BLE lets the individual mobile phones act as beacons meaning that they constantly broadcast a temporary identifier called Rolling Proximity Identifier (RPI) that is remembered and, at the same time, lets the mobile phone scan for identifiers of other mobile phones. This is shown on the right side of Fig. 3.

The Corona-Warn-App meets the highest standards of data protection and security.

In order to prevent misuse, individuals need to provide proof that they have tested positive before they can upload their keys. Through this integrated approach, the verification needed to upload the diagnosis keys does not require any further action

Monitoring and Response to Health Hazards and Emergencies (EPHO2) 337

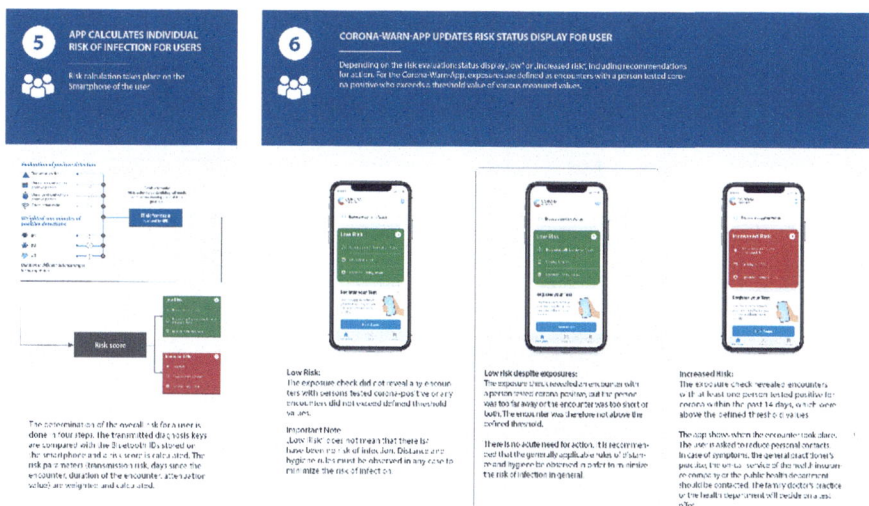

Fig. 17.2 (continued)

from the users. They only have to confirm in the app and for the Exposure Notification Framework that they agree to share their diagnosis keys.

Manual verification is also possible if the lab that performed the testing does not support the direct electronic transmission of test results to the users' mobile phones or if users have decided against the electronic transmission of their test results.

During the development of the app, experts from the Federal Office for Information Security (Bundesamt für Sicherheit in der Informationstechnik; BSI) and the Federal Commissioner for Data Protection and Freedom of Information (Bundesbeauftragter für den Datenschutz und die Informationsfreiheit; BfDI) were involved from the beginning; the individual development steps were published and closely monitored by representatives of the data protection community.

All data, such as information about encounters with other users, is encrypted and stored exclusively on the user's own smartphone. If a user tests positive, they can decide whether to release the random codes stored on their smartphone from the past 14 days to warn potential contacts. If they choose to be notified, they will not find out who was informed, and the contacted individuals will not know who tested positive.

After a positive test result, various verification steps prevent false notifications from being triggered. Misuse or unauthorized access to the app will be prosecuted to the extent possible under criminal law. It is important to note that the persons exposed to a positive-tested individual are not informed by a central instance, but the risk of exposure is calculated locally on their phones. The information about the exposure remains on the user's mobile phone and is not shared.

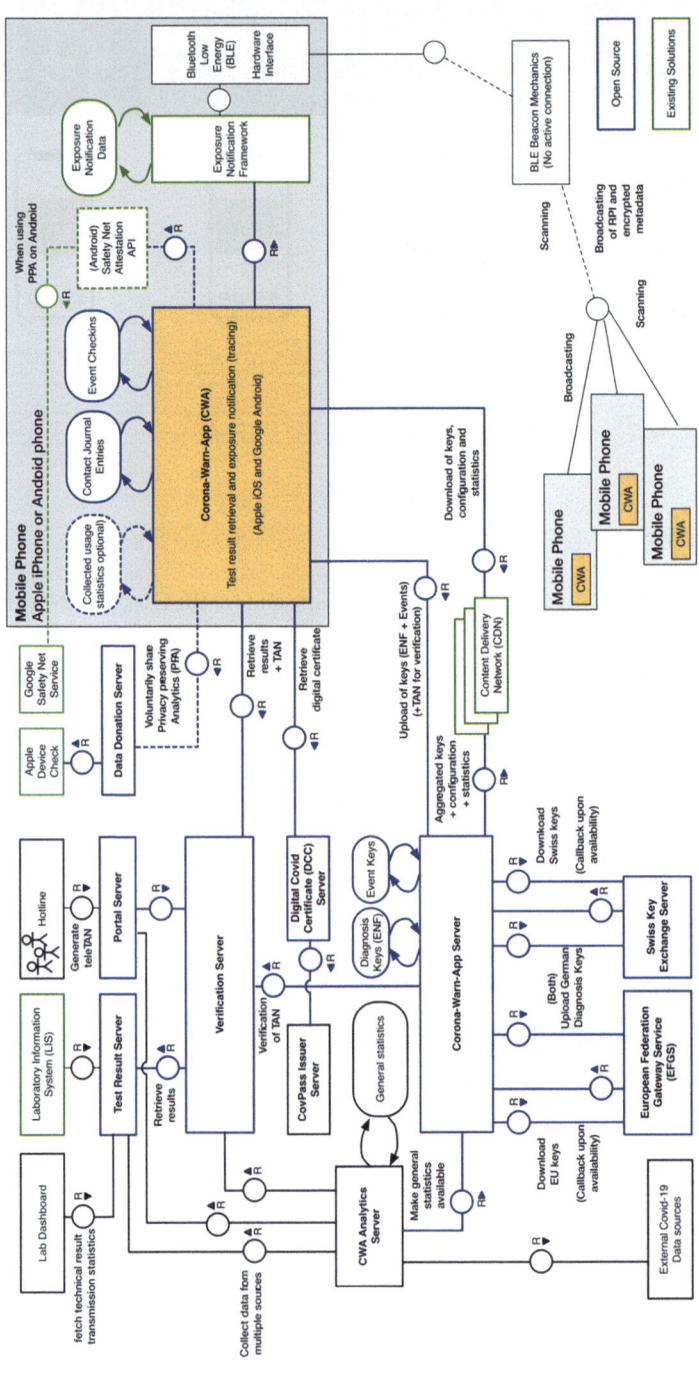

Fig. 3 Architecture of the Corona-Warn-App (Source: RKI, own figure)

2.3.3 Estimation of the Infection Risk

Figure 4 displays how the total risk score is calculated from the exposure windows. The application is provided with a set of parameters. Those parameters are regularly downloaded from the CWA Server, which means they can be modified without requiring a new version of the application.

In the first step, each exposure window is processed individually. The duration of each scan instance is weighted according to its attenuation, i.e., its proximity. When those weighted durations are summed up, they are multiplied by the "transmission risk value." The result is a normalized exposure time on a specific day (e.g., "10 normalized exposure minutes on May 3 in a 30-minute window"). The app uses this

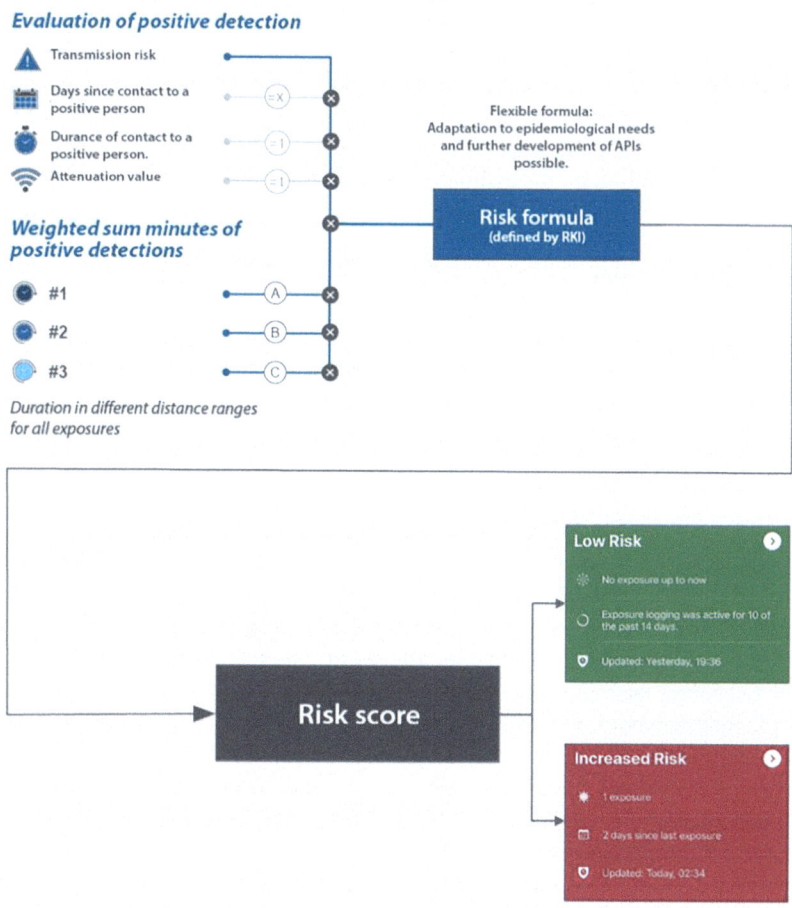

Fig. 4 Exposure risk estimation algorithm (Source: RKI, own figure)

information to determine if an individual encounter (i.e., exposure window) by itself is a low- or high-risk exposure.

In the second step, the normalized exposure times are summed up by day (e.g., "20 normalized exposure minutes on May 3"). The app uses this information to determine if the sum of all encounters on a given day is a low- or high-risk exposure.

The transmission risk is part of the shared key of a positive tested person. It takes into account when the first symptoms have occurred and estimates the infectiousness of that person on the given day.

2.4 Usage and Evaluation of the Corona-Warn-App

The Corona-Warn-App was downloaded approx. 48.8 million times and was one of the most successful and widely used DCT apps worldwide. It was the most downloaded contact tracing app in Europe. This shows that, in general, German society was very open to a new, digital approach to tackling the pandemic and the everyday problems that arise during a pandemic (certification of vaccination, test result management, etc.). During the peak of its usage, there were about 32.8–35.4 million active users, depending on the estimation method.

2.4.1 Data Collection

To answer questions about the functionality, effectiveness, and use of the CWA, besides operational data from the CWA backend and Google and Apple's app stores, app users were invited to provide additional data on a voluntary basis. User data have been collected in this manner in two ways:

- an event-driven user survey (*EDUS*), and
- a privacy-preserving data donation.

An online survey was undertaken among users who received a notification indicating they were at "increased risk" between the beginning of March and the beginning of May 2021. The users were asked about their behavior before receiving the risk notification and their planned behavior afterward. The second part of the survey was conducted 5 days later and aimed to determine whether these users had implemented their planned behavior. One of the goals of the survey, therefore, was to find out whether the risk notification provided by the CWA actually led users to change their behavior. The evaluation also involves an event-independent analysis of technical usage data on the function and usage of the CWA. These data are collected from app users via voluntary data donation. Privacy-Preserving Analytics (PPA)—the analysis of usage data while preserving privacy—has helped provide a better understanding of how the CWA was used and has enabled its functions and user-friendliness to be continuously improved. Relevant data have been collected since the beginning of March 2021.

2.4.2 Facts and Figures on the Corona-Warn-App

Some key facts and figures on the CWA (additional information can be retrieved from the website https://coronawarn.app):

- Downloads: 48.8 million
- Active users: 32.8 to 35.4 million (40% of total, 50% of target population)
- Connected labs and test facilities: 270 labs and 20.000 test sites results provided: 242.4 million, 29.2 million positive
  - PCR tests: 59.1 million, 21.2 million positive
  - rapid antigen tests: 183.3 million, eight million positive
- Registered positive test results: 12.3 million
- Shared positive test results: nine million (74% sharing rate)
- Daily PPA data donations: 17.2 Mio. (mean: 13.2 million, median: 14.6 million)
  - PCR test result: received within 16.2 h after test registration (median: 10 h)
  - Warning: received about 3.9 d after exposition (median 4 d). Warned persons get tested about 5.5 d after the warning (median 1.8 d)
  - Risk assessment: the positivity rate was always higher after a high-risk warning (red) than after a low-risk warning with exposure (green)
- Costs for development and operation: 210 million EUR (i.e., about 2 EUR per user and year)

2.4.3 Evaluation

As the key figures show, the Corona-Warn-App detects possible risks of infections precisely and quickly and has supplemented conventional MCT. It has achieved its aims.

A simple heuristic might illustrate this further: in 14 days, contact with a contact person occurs at about 5% in a household, 35% to known people, and 60% in public places, transport, etc. About 30% of contacts can be detected via MCT since only known contact persons can be identified, and remembrance is confined. Furthermore, due to an overload of local health authorities in times of high incidences, delays in processing might occur. During these times, conventional MCT was often replaced by informal contact tracing (ICT), i.e., when friends and acquaintances were non-officially informed. With the adoption of the CWA by about half the target population and a sharing rate of 75%, the effective proportion of detected contact persons is approximately 20% ($0.5^2 \cdot 0.75 = 0.19$). Even if an overlap of 50% might be assumed, an additional 10% of all contacts can still be identified. The contribution is higher since the processes of the CWA are as fast as in ICT. This establishes an important overall contribution in preventing the further spread of COVID-19.

In addition, DCT scales easily and without further significant efforts and costs: more users—fewer infections. With an adoption rate of 80% of the population, the effective proportion of detected contacts would have been 50% ($0.8^2 \cdot 0.75 = 0.48$), with the overlap of 24% (80% of 30% from MCT) the CWA (together with ICT) could have replaced MCT almost completely. This heuristic is well supported by various modeling studies (see, for example, Boldrini et al. 2022; Burdinski et al. 2022; Ferretti et al. 2020).

2.5 Communication and Open Source

The Corona-Warn-App received significant media attention in Germany upon its launch. Media outlets extensively covered its release, with headlines highlighting its potential to assist in contact tracing and breaking the chains of infection. On the release date, several German ministers and the president of the RKI gathered for a press conference, which received a wide media echo. The app's main functionality, using Bluetooth technology to anonymously notify users if they had been in close proximity to someone infected with the virus, sparked debates and discussions across various platforms. The media played a pivotal role in disseminating information about the app's features and privacy measures, thus encouraging widespread adoption. While initial enthusiasm was met with concerns about data protection and low utilization rates, the media continued to monitor its progress, reporting on updates, user feedback, and improvements. Overall, the media attention surrounding the Corona-Warn-App in Germany demonstrated the nation's keen interest in leveraging technology to combat the pandemic and keep citizens informed.

From the beginning on, the Corona-Warn-App was developed as open source. For a long time, civil society in Germany has requested open-source coding of governmental projects, which was well appreciated, for example, by the Chaos Computer Club (CCC, a renowned German hacker collective and computer security organization that champions digital civil liberties). Here, trust could be built as interested people could have a close look into the code of the Corona-Warn-App and give valuable feedback to the programmers.

3 Conclusions

Despite the limitations of its underlying technology, the Corona-Warn-App has shown to be an effective digital contact tracing tool and has probably helped to reduce the number of infected persons and deaths during the SARS-CoV-2 pandemic.

We can conclude that digital tools can effectively help improve conventional processes in support of EPHO 2 by supplementing and partially replacing them. To achieve this, the design should reflect people's privacy concerns and might shift or change the objectives of consideration (e.g., with DCT, *contacts* are traced, whereas, with MCT, *contact persons* are traced). The focus of efforts should not reside on the tooling, the technology, or established processes but rather on the user's capabilities and common public health goals. Trust and transparency are prerequisites and result in success with digital solutions. We are convinced that digital tools such as the CWA, even though it slightly changes traditional approaches, will be indispensable to monitor and respond to health hazards and emergencies in the future. We have proven that a privacy-compliant and governmental app could help millions of users to assess their risk and adjust their behavior accordingly.

Digitalization has yet to unleash its full potential: due to heterogeneous contributions, many key features are not readily (if at all) available in conventional processes. Especially the means of evaluation, like operational or anonymous data donations and user surveys, should be used to continuously measure and improve performance and experience. They should be planned and taken seriously right from the beginning. In plans for pandemic preparedness, these lessons should be integrated and reflected accordingly (Rivest et al. 2021).

All in all, the Corona-Warn-App was an ambitious project around a tool that has proven effective in tackling the SARS-CoV-2 pandemic and breaking infection chains. This tool was an easy, scalable, and flexible instrument, especially in high-incidence times when MCT reached its limits. German society has shown to be open to adopting new digital tools. Furthermore, the project has demonstrated that open and transparent communication between decision-makers, developers, and the public community is necessary and fruitful.

References

Boldrini C, Passarella A, Conti M (2022) Models for digitally contact-traced epidemics. IEEE Access 10:106180–106190. https://doi.org/10.1109/ACCESS.2022.3211425

Burdinski A, Brockmann D, Maier BF (2022) Understanding the impact of digital contact tracing during the COVID-19 pandemic. PLOS Digit Health 1(12):e0000149. https://doi.org/10.1371/journal.pdig.0000149

Corona-Warn-App, RKI (2020) is misleading. The promotional images are from a public campaign by the federal government. Its elements can still be found here: https://web.archive.org/web/20220810173537/https://styleguide.bundesregierung.de/sgde/basiselemente/programmmarken/corona-warn-app.

Corona-Warn-App documentation (2020–2023) https://github.com/corona-warn-app/cwa-documentation. Accessed 28 Jun 2023.

DP-3T (2020). https://github.com/DP-3T/documents. Accessed 28 Jun 2023.

Ferretti L et al (2020) Quantifying SARS-CoV-2 transmission suggests epidemic control with digital contact tracing. Science 368. https://doi.org/10.1126/science.abb6936

Kirchner G, Benzler J et al (2021–2022) Corona-Warn-App Science Blog. https://www.coronawarn.app/de/science/. Accessed 21 Jun 2023.

Kirchner G, Weidemann F, Höhle M, Benzler J, Schumacher D (2020) Epidemiological motivation of the transmission risk level, https://github.com/corona-warn-app/cwa-documentation/blob/main/transmission_risk.pdf. Accessed 28 Jun 2023.

Lueks W, Benzler J, Bogdanov D, Kirchner G, Lucas R, Oliveira R, Preneel B, Salathé M, Troncoso M, von Wyl V (2021) Toward a common performance and effectiveness terminology for digital proximity tracing applications, front. Digit. Health, Aug. 2021, Sec. Health Technology Implementation, Volume 3–2021. https://doi.org/10.3389/fdgth.2021.677929.

Meyer S, Windisch T, Perl A, Dzibela D, Marzilger R, Witt N, Benzler J, Kirchner G, Feigl T, Mutschler C. (2021) Contact tracing with the exposure notification framework in the German Corona Warn-App, 2021 International Conference on Indoor Positioning and Indoor Navigation (IPIN), Lloret de Mar, Spain, 29 November–2 December 2020, p 1–8. https://doi.org/10.1109/IPIN51156.2021.9662591.

Rivest R et al. (2021) Automated exposure notification for COVID-19, ImPACT 2021 workshop, Lincoln Laboratory TR-1288, a joint technical report of MIT Lincoln Laboratory and MIT CSAIL. https://hdl.handle.net/1721.1/148149

Salathé M (2023) Digital epidemiology. https://www.digitalepibook.com/. Accessed 27 May 2023.

World Health Organization and European Centre for Disease Prevention and Control, Geneva (2021) Indicator framework for the evaluation of the public health effectiveness of digital proximity tracing solutions. Licence: CC BY-NC-SA 3.0 IGO. https://www.ecdc.europa.eu/en/publications-data/indicator-framework-evaluate-public-health-effectiveness-digital-proximity. Accessed 27 May 2023.

Open Access This chapter is licensed under the terms of the Creative Commons Attribution 4.0 International License (http://creativecommons.org/licenses/by/4.0/), which permits use, sharing, adaptation, distribution and reproduction in any medium or format, as long as you give appropriate credit to the original author(s) and the source, provide a link to the Creative Commons license and indicate if changes were made.

The images or other third party material in this chapter are included in the chapter's Creative Commons license, unless indicated otherwise in a credit line to the material. If material is not included in the chapter's Creative Commons license and your intended use is not permitted by statutory regulation or exceeds the permitted use, you will need to obtain permission directly from the copyright holder.

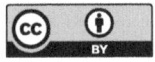

Health Protection, Including Environmental and Food Safety (EPHO 3)

Anna Förster, Gibson Kimutai, Myat Su Yin, Peter Haddawy and Urte Klink

Abstract Health protection encompasses measures and practices that protect individuals, groups, or populations in order to prevent and mitigate the effects of infectious disease, environmental, chemical, or other threats. Digital tools and approaches increasingly shape the field covered by this essential public health operation, namely infectious disease control, as experienced during the COVID-19 pandemic. Here, we provide various perspectives and two specific examples of digitalization: infectious disease vector monitoring as an environmental health topic and food safety. These examples exemplify the broad range of topics the EPHO covers. We highlight the potential as well as limitations of digital tools to support these areas.

Keywords Environmental monitoring · Internet of things · Machine learning · Workplace preotection · Mosquito counting · Mosquito identification

---

A. Förster (✉)
Sustainable Comminucatiom Networks, University of Bremen, Bremen, Germany
e-mail: anna.foerster@uni-bremen.de

G. Kimutai
Department of Mathematics, Physics and Computing, Moi University, Eldoret, Kenya

M. S. Yin
Mahidol University, Bangkok, Thailand

P. Haddawy
Sustainable Comminucatiom Networks, University of Bremen, Bremen, Germany

Mahidol University, Bangkok, Thailand

U. Klink
Institute for Public Health and Nursing Research, University of Bremen, Bremen, Germany

1 Introduction

Health protection is a rather generic term encompassing measures and practices that protect individuals, groups, or populations to prevent and mitigate the effects of infectious disease, environmental, chemical, or other threats (Ghebrehewet et al. 2016). Health protection is one of the key fields of public health and an essential public health operation (EPHO3), with environmental and occupational health protection and food safety being key drivers of implementing health-related regulatory policies historically and in current times. Digital technologies have increasingly shaped the field of health protection, and there are numerous examples of new applications and technological solutions to support health protection functions in all domains. This chapter highlights the potential of digital technologies for this public health function using examples of infectious disease prevention through environmental mosquito monitoring, and digital tools for food safety.

1.1 ICT-Supported Mosquito Identification and Counting

One prominent example of using modern ICT technologies for health protection is the automatic detection and classification of mosquitoes. The goal is to be able to produce counts of mosquitoes of different species since different species serve as vectors of different diseases. This is a very important health protection issue, associated mainly with Sustainable Development Goal 3 (Good Health and Well Being), and could significantly contribute to better control of some widely spread diseases, such as malaria, dengue, zika, and West Nile virus. These diseases are currently mainly encountered in tropical countries, but with climate change, they are expected to propagate to other areas too, and have already been discovered in parts of Europe (Madeira and south of Italy). Currently, state-of-the-art research focuses on the automatic detection and classification of specific species of mosquitoes. Practical, large-scale use in the field is very rare and very challenging. In the next few paragraphs, we will first discuss the algorithms to detect and classify mosquitoes before discussing the challenges associated with deployments and some examples of their potential usage.

Obtaining accurate counts of mosquitoes by species is important for estimating risk, focusing disease control efforts (e.g., dissemination of bed nets, installation of screens, elimination of mosquito breeding sites), and monitoring results of mosquito vector control efforts. Different ways exist to classify mosquitoes automatically (Spitzen and Takken 2018; Joshi and Miller 2021). The first and most coarse approach is to detect actual or potential breeding sites. The next level is to detect mosquitoes without identifying their precise species. The highest precision level is achieved when the exact species can be identified.

The second problem is counting the mosquitoes. Again, several levels of detail are possible: from fuzzy and approximate, like "high number" or "low number," to exact counts. Different algorithms enable different levels of detail for each of the two problems (identification and counting). In the next paragraphs, we will step through the available techniques of how to identify mosquitoes and will discuss the levels of detail of each of the techniques and other properties of digital technologies, such as the cost and their real-world applicability.

1.2 Identification of Breeding Sites

Apart from manual surveys, breeding sites are usually identified via images. Two possible sources of images have been proposed: street view images (as taken from a normal human perspective) and aerial images.

Street view images are easy to take, and even some open sources can be used, like Google Street View Images (Haddawy et al. 2019). The technical approach is to train a machine learning model to identify various types of water containers, such as pots, vases, old tires, and trash bins. A drawback of using street view images is that they only cover areas along roads and thus miss containers in yards, fields, and indoors. In addition, containers may be occluded by other objects. One should also consider their timeliness when using image sources like Google Street View, as those sources are updated only very irregularly. This can be partially addressed using crowd-sourced images like those from Mapillary or Open Street Cam. This approach can be used with citizen science to acquire data from end users and their smartphones. Despite the limitations of using street view images, the generated container counts have been shown to have a good correlation with larval counts and to improve the accuracy of predictive models of dengue in studies conducted in Thailand (Yin et al. 2021) (Fig. 1).

Aerial images are typically taken by drones—autonomously or remotely (Passos et al. 2022; Bravo et al. 2021; Amarasinghe 2017; Carrasco-Escobar et al. 2022). Drones are able to survey very large areas in a very short time and "see" also

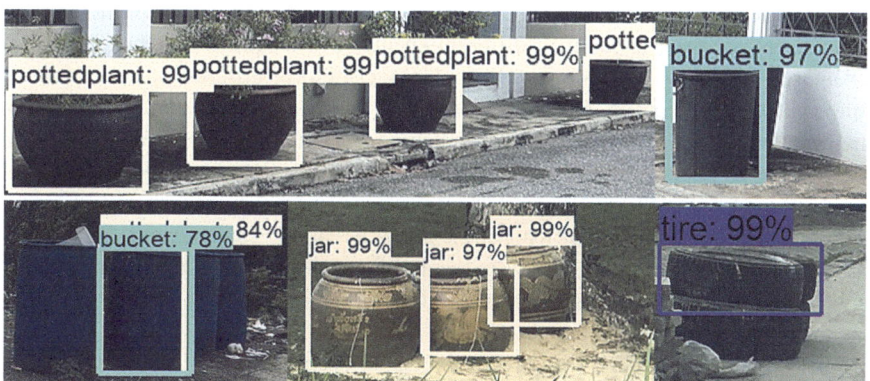

Fig. 1 Street view images of containers with an accuracy of breeding site predictions (Image reproduced with permission from Haddawy et al. (2019))

otherwise hidden areas like gardens or fields. However, this approach also has some disadvantages. First, data privacy is an issue when taking images of private properties. Second, trees and bushes can largely obstruct the view. Last but not least, one needs drones, which are expensive, especially for developing countries. Satellite images can also be used but are usually not timely (Knoblauch et al. 2023) and may not have sufficient resolution to detect many relevant containers.

Both methods also suffer from usual machine learning-related problems. First, only a priori known types of containers can be identified, and new, unexpected ones cannot be easily integrated into the machine learning model on the fly, although they can be added with additional training data. Second, the accuracy is usually high, but false negatives and positives also exist. For example, one problem with street view images is that tires attached to cars are also recognized as tires but are not, in fact, water reservoirs. This can be solved with sufficient training data or by detecting the car's presence (Haddawy et al. 2019).

One possible extension to these methods is to identify larvae in the water directly (instead of identifying only water container tanks). For example (Arista-Jalife et al. 2020), work uses deep learning methods to analyze pictures of water tanks and identify mosquito larvae. The authors achieved a very good classification accuracy of over 90%. However, the images of each tank need to be of high enough resolution to detect the larva, which is, for example, typically not the case for street-view images.

In summary, identifying breeding sites via ICT is a very promising and relatively cheap (even with drones) alternative to manual surveys. One big advantage is that citizens can be involved, which also increases the knowledge about the problem and thus also its possible counteractions.

1.3 Image Processing for Mosquito Identification

Image processing can be used to identify mosquitoes and differentiate them from other insects or even to identify different species of mosquitoes. For example, in (Okayasu et al. 2019) the authors collected images of three different species of mosquitoes (*Aedes albopictus*, *Anopheles stephensi*, and *Culex pipiens pallens*) in a lab environment and implemented various machine learning methods to classify them. They managed to achieve 95% accuracy with a deep learning model. However, one should consider that the results are based on high-quality images clearly showing the mosquito. This is different when working in a realistic environment. Moreover, the deep learning model developed by the authors is quite processing-intensive and requires the images to be processed in a rich environment, such as a powerful desktop or cloud service.

This approach has been further developed by (Semwal et al. 2022), where the authors use a mobile robot to attract, trap and classify mosquitoes. The robot attracts the mosquitoes towards an isolated chamber with good lighting conditions and a camera. The cues used include Ultra Violet (UV) Light-Emitting Diode (LED) at

368 nm, octanol, and lactic acid, and the robot's motion mimics the movement of a living creature. Additionally, a fan pulls the mosquitoes towards the isolated chamber with a yellow glue surface. There, a camera takes pictures of an area of many mosquitoes at once, and image preprocessing is applied to cut out individual mosquitoes. Then, a similar approach with deep learning is developed and applied to differentiate between Aedes Aegypti, Aedes Albopictus, and Culex. Even in an outdoor real environment, the authors achieve more than 80% accuracy, which is sufficient for coarse and large-scale surveys. However, the authors do not discuss the issue of attracting other, potentially protected insects into the trap. Another practical drawback is that mobile robots need a flat surface on which to move around. One immediate idea would be to use drones instead of mobile robot, but it is still being determined whether the air fluctuations around the drone will allow trapping the mosquitoes at all. Of course, the approach can also be used without any robots or other moving elements and attract mosquitoes, similar to any conventional mosquito trap.

1.4 Acoustic and Optoacoustic Identification of Mosquitoes

Mosquito wingbeats possess distinct and recognizable flight tones, making them an effective tool for monitoring and surveilling mosquito populations. This includes detecting the presence of mosquitoes, accurately counting their numbers, and identifying the species and sex of individual mosquitoes (Joshi and Miller 2021). Mosquito species and sex classification using wingbeat frequency data can be divided into two groups: those using microphones to collect audio recordings of sound pressure waves and those using opto-acoustics obtained through audification of mosquito wingbeats interacting with a light source (Hermann et al. 2011). Audio input data can be presented as a raw signal, a power spectral distribution, or a spectrogram image (Fanioudakis et al. 2018; Yin et al. 2021), to name a few. Chen et al. (2014) applied the Discrete Fourier Transform to an audio recording snippet/segments corresponding to a flying mosquito and fitted a Gaussian distribution for each wingbeat frequency histogram to achieve 95.23% accuracy in classifying six insect sounds (including mosquitoes) which were equally distributed. Ouyang et al. (2015) employed the EM algorithm to create Gaussian mixture models for mosquito species and gender classification, achieving 87.9% accuracy. Vasconcelos et al. (Vasconcelos et al. 2019; 2024) presented various signal features to detect mosquitoes in the field and controlled lab environments. Meanwhile, Ziemer and colleagues (2022) have suggested extracting features from the mosquito sound to mimic the sound processing in the mosquito antenna.

Low-cost automated devices and machine-learning techniques have also been used for mosquito species detection based on acoustic signals (Genoud et al. 2018 ; Kimutai and Förster 2023). Potamitis (2014) constructed a codebook of power spectral density patterns for each mosquito species using the sonification of a signal from a sensor device embedded in an insect trap. Deep learning models for image classification have been used to extract features from spectrogram representations of wingbeat recordings for species and sex identification. Luna-Gonzalez et al. (2020) extracted audio features, transformed them into a color image and applied a CNN to achieve 90.75% accuracy in classifying mosquito species from optical sensor samples. Yin and colleagues (Yin 2021–2) built a 1D-CNN model and a 1D-CNN with LSTM model for mosquito classification based on raw audio waveforms and achieved an accuracy of over 93% on a dataset of pure audio recordings of males and females of five mosquito species. Fanioudakis et al. (2018) experimented with several deep-learning network architectures, XgBoost, and lightGBM, to classify mosquito species. They found that DenseNet121, trained with spectrograms, achieved the highest accuracy of 96%. Kiskin et al. (2021) presented a Bayesian Convolutional Neural Network (BCNN) pipeline to automatically record, detect, and archive mosquito sounds from recordings made with mobile phones.

Similarly, Yin et al. (2023) developed a deep learning-based pipeline for detecting and classifying four mosquito species in Thailand based on acoustic signals. Recently, there have been quite successful attempts to compress the models to be run on low-cost microcontrollers, for example, with the help of TinyML (Altayeb et al. 2022). Smartphones can also be sensors (Mukundarajan et al. 2017; Sinka et al. 2021). This makes these solutions low-cost and thus usable in resource countries where mosquitoes breed more because of the unhygienic environments.

1.5 Potential Applications of Mosquito Identification and Counting

There are only very few real-world applications of ICT-supported mosquito identification or counting. Most of the work presented so far has been only tested in lab or testbed environments, and many challenges remain before they can be used in real applications. However, the first results are highly promising, and thus in this section, we discuss the potential applications.

The most often discussed application is to estimate mosquito vector counts and to estimate the proportions of species. Such an application can be a real game changer for pest control, with much lower costs than manual surveys and much bigger precision (time and area) of the acquired data. Once fully developed, such applications have the potential for low-cost implementation in areas at the highest risk for mosquito-vector disease, as they can be realized at low cost, low required training, and scalable dissemination. It is also possible to immediately eliminate mosquitoes when using a trap. This is, for example, very useful for private gardens, schools, sporting facilities, etc.

Another currently discussed application is the automatic distribution of mosquito repellents. Repellants are usually distributed automatically, but in a simple way, by releasing them in regular intervals. However, the repellants are also a health risk by themselves and are costly. Thus, a more intelligent release based on really present mosquitoes of the dangerous species will be very beneficial. The information about the repellent usage can also be easily provided to the end users, e.g., for re-fill or general information.

1.6 Challenges of Real-World Applications

For image-based methods, one of the challenges is the quality of the images, especially when taken by end users and their smartphones. They often need to be clearer, of low resolution, with bad lighting conditions, the area of interest in not in focus, and many more. Another problem is their availability, for example, from private grounds. Yet another problem is their timeliness (e.g. when using satellite images or sources like Google Streetview) and the obstruction from foliage. What is needed is a high-resolution, regular screening of areas of interest, including private grounds and badly accessible areas. One of the simplest and cost-efficient ways of acquiring such data is currently citizen science and empowering all citizens to contribute. This will require developing very user-friendly services adapted for children, handicapped persons, and illiterate persons. Citizen science also requires extensive information campaigns and incentives to participate, which need to be developed and run by the authorities.

When using traps with acoustic methods, the main challenge remains the noisy environment. Here, more data from real environments must be gathered to improve the algorithms and make them more robust against background noise. The cost of the systems will remain high as long as only a few traps are used. However, if the traps prove practical and accurate enough, the cost savings will still be significant compared to manual work, which will also push the costs of the individual sensors down.

However, there is another challenge with counting mosquitoes with traps. The so-called sensor range is very limited, i.e., the mosquito needs to be very close to the trap, and thus a very small area can be monitored. Installing more traps will not necessarily improve the situation, at least not much. Thus, research must focus more on attracting mosquitoes into the traps and avoiding attracting other insects. Current methods include the use of heat, odors, and CO_2. The method used must be cost-efficient and must only require a refill sometimes.

The last challenge comes from the used ICT methods themselves. The most accurate current models for mosquito detection and classification are deep learning models. But these require large amounts of training data, which is labor intensive to gather in the case of mosquito wingbeat data. Deep learning models also require large amounts of memory and processing power. Thus, it is not trivial to deploy them in a cost-efficient and power-efficient way.

2 Digital Approaches for Food Safety Measures

Food safety is a major concern worldwide as harmful substances in food can pose significant health risks and negatively impact economies. Digital applications can potentially improve food safety testing and keep food provision chains safe. The World Health Organization states that foodborne diseases account for 420,000 deaths yearly (WHO 2015). Despite strict legislation and standard methods for chemical and microbiological/pathogen food safety testing, food-related scandals still occur, posing threats to consumer health and the food economy (Tsagkaris et al. 2019). Food scandals, such as dioxins in eggs (Kupferschmidt 2011) and aflatoxins in dairy (Popovic et al. 2017), have highlighted the need for improved and innovative methods for monitoring contaminants. Typically, high-performance liquid or gas chromatography coupled with mass spectrometry is used for chemical food safety testing, while culture plate analysis is often used for microbiological/pathogen testing. Despite their high reliability, these methods are expensive, time-consuming, and require trained personnel (Jafari et al. 2021). Therefore, cheaper, portable, fast analytical tools are needed to ensure consumer safety and minimize health risks and economic losses.

New mobile sensing approaches are being developed to address the limitations of traditional food safety testing methods. These devices offer faster testing, lower costs, ease of use, and minimal equipment requirements. Sensing technologies can be integrated with smartphones to create platforms for food safety analysis that function as lab-on-smartphones (Rateni et al. 2017). Smartphones have various components such as a processor, camera, wireless connectivity, and display, making them useful for measurement and detection. However, they need to be augmented by other accessories to function as laboratory instruments. Many external sensor modules have been designed and integrated with smartphones, extending their capabilities for extracting more sophisticated diagnostic information (Zhang and Liu 2016). These comparatively inexpensive devices can run routine tests rapidly and on-site, provide personalized diagnostic options and enable rapid inspection of suspected contamination. For instance, smartphones can help allergic individuals by providing personalized health information capability or allowing quick detection of contamination from foodborne pathogens or other harmful substances (Rateni et al. 2017; Zhang and Liu 2016).

Smartphone-based methods for food analysis can be classified as either lab-on-smartphone biosensors or smartphone optical and spectroscopy methods (Zhang and Liu 2016).

Smartphone-based biosensors benefit from the optical capabilities of smartphones, such as the camera acting as a photodetector and the light source (Jafari et al. 2021). Biosensors integrate bio-receptors and a transduction method to detect target analytes. The analyte and receptor interaction produces a measurable signal, allowing for direct detection and high selectivity. However, prior sample treatment is necessary for transduction. Biosensors offer affordable and fast analysis in a portable and miniaturized format. Combining smartphone technology with adapted biochemical assays can create biosensor-based analytical systems for on-site detection of various analytes, including contaminants, drugs, pesticide residues, and foodborne pathogens (Rateni et al. 2017).

Various methodologies are used for lab-on-smartphone biosensors, including fluorescence imagining, colorimetric assay, and electroanalytical methods (Rateni et al. 2017). An example of smartphone-based colorimetric readers includes the development by Levin et al., who created a smartphone-based colorimeter to screen groundwater for excess fluoride that can be used in areas affected by fluorosis, an ongoing challenge in India. The colorimeter used a commercially available reagent and an easy-fit, compact sample chamber adapter but required each phone's calibration due to color sensing variation. A software program was developed to analyze the red-green-blue color of the image, resulting in fluoride estimation comparable to expensive laboratory methods without technical expertise (Levin et al. 2016).

Spectroscopy involves analyzing the different wavelengths of light absorbed, emitted, or scattered by a material to gather information about its properties, such as composition, structure, and physical state. As such, spectroscopy is a valuable tool for non-invasive analysis in various industries, such as food quality assessment, but most setups are expensive and cumbersome, limiting their use in laboratory settings. Recent advancements in micro-technologies have allowed the development of portable spectrometers that are cost-effective and small in size. However, miniaturized systems must provide reliable results without intervention from trained technicians. The goal is to integrate spectrometers into smartphones to provide real-time sensitive and specific spectroscopic information (Bouyé et al. 2016; Rateni et al. 2017).

An example of smartphone-based spectroscopy includes a handheld fluorescence-based imagining device developed by Oh et al. to enhance visual detection of fecal contamination on red meat, fat, and bone surfaces of beef under varying luminous intensities. This device comprises four 405-nm 10 W LEDs for fluorescence excitation, a charge-coupled device camera, an optical filter at 670 nm, and a Wi-Fi transmitter for sending real-time data to a smartphone or tablet. The system successfully identified the localization of most fecal contamination spots on beef surfaces by detecting chlorophyll metabolites discharging fluorescence near 670 nm, and results suggest that this method can effectively assist in visually inspecting and detecting fecal contamination (Oh et al. 2016).

Although these smartphone-based food diagnostic technologies show potential and new techniques and methodologies are constantly developed, several limitations must be addressed. These technologies often require peripherals for analysis, which limit their practicality in field conditions. The analytical procedures required for obtaining meaningful results may involve instruments and materials typically found only in laboratories. Time-consuming and multi-stage sample preparation procedures can discourage potential end-users, particularly those without training. The repeatability, selectivity, and limit of detection of proposed methods must be thoroughly tested and confirmed while considering the complexity of food matrices. It is important to note that smartphone cameras may have default settings optimized for photography, and color readouts may not be transferable across different smartphone models (Kalinowska et al. 2021). Despite technological advancements, some of these devices are still at the proof-of-concept stage and require more testing before being introduced (Jafari et al. 2021). Additionally, legal challenges may arise in implementing such devices, as analytical methods must meet regulatory requirements (Tsagkaris et al. 2019). Societal and ethical impacts also need to be considered (see Chap. "Ethical Implications of User Autonomy in Digital Public Health", Dassow et al. in this handbook).

Nevertheless, smartphones and other digital devices can change the current food testing concept by allowing farmers and consumers to conduct food safety analysis with a simple sample preparation protocol and smartphone application. Users can receive a fast answer directly from their phone, and the online connectivity of smartphones can be used as a quality assurance feature. If a sample is contaminated, the user could alert an expert group responsible for confirmatory analysis (Tsagkaris et al. 2019). Due to the complexity of the food matrix and recent developments in the field, particularly biosensors utilizing microfluidics and bioassays may be used for smartphone-based food analysis in the future. Such solutions of on-site analytical techniques will make food quality assessment more accessible, convenient, and readily available (Kalinowska et al. 2021). Ultimately, these innovative technologies can help reduce the risk of foodborne diseases.

3 Concluding Remarks

The examples provided in this chapter only offer a first insight into the broad range of digital applications and systems increasingly shaping the field of health protection from environmental, occupational, nutritional, and other risks. Many of these applications are still in their infancy, and so are the insights into the positive and negative consequences of novel digital and/or AI tools with relevance for health protection. As in many other fields, there is an urgent need to accomplish sound evaluations of new approaches to strengthen those that build up the toolbox of digital technologies in support of the health protection of the population.

References

Altayeb A, Zennaro M, Rovai M (2022) Classifying mosquito wingbeat sound using TinyML. ACM International Conference Proceeding Series (9 2022): 132–137. https://doi.org/10.1145/3524458.3547258.

Amarasinghe A (2017) A machine learning approach for identifying mosquito breeding sites via drone images. Proceedings of the 15th ACM Conference on Embedded Network Sensor Systems, Delft Netherlands November 6–8. ACM New York https://doi.org/10.1145/3131672.

Arista-Jalife A, Nakano M, Garcia-Nonoal Z et al (2020) Aedes mosquito detection in its larval stage using deep neural networks. Knowl-Based Syst 189:104841. https://doi.org/10.1016/j.knosys.2019.07.012

Bouyé C, Kolb H, d'Humières B (2016) Mini and micro spectrometers pave the way to on-field advanced analytics. Proc. SPIE 9754, Photonic Instrumentation Engineering III, 975408. https://doi.org/10.1117/12.2212384.

Bravo DT et al (2021) Automatic detection of potential mosquito breeding sites from aerial images acquired by unmanned aerial vehicles. Comput Environ Urban Syst 90:101692

Carrasco-Escobar G et al (2022) The use of drones for mosquito surveillance and control. Parasit Vectors 15:473

Chen Y, Why A, Batista G, Mafra-Neto A, Keogh E (2014) Flying insect classification with inexpensive sensors. J Insect Behav 27:657–677

Fanioudakis E, Geismar M, Potamitis I (2018) Mosquito wingbeat analysis and classification using deep learning. 2018 26th European Signal Processing Conference (EUSIPCO): 2410–2414.

Genoud AP, Basistyy R, Williams GM, Thomas BP (2018) Optical remote sensing for monitoring flying mosquitoes, gender identification and discussion on species identification. Appl Phys B Lasers Optics 124:46. https://dl.acm.org/doi/10.1145/3582515.3609514

Ghebrehewet S, Stewart AG, Rufus I (2016) What is health protection? In: Ghebrehewet S et al (eds) Health protection: principles and practice (Oxford, 2016; online edn). Oxford Academic. https://doi.org/10.1093/med/9780198745471.003.0001. accessed 25 Apr. 2023

Haddawy P, Wettayakorn P, Nonthaleerak B et al (2019) Large scale detailed mapping of dengue vector breeding sites using street view images. PLoS Negl Trop Dis 13:e0007555

Hermann T, Hunt A, Neuhoff JG (2011) The sonification handbook, vol 1. Logos Verlag, Berlin

Jafari S et al (2021) Assured point-of-need food safety screening: a critical assessment of portable food analyzers. Food 10(6):1399. https://doi.org/10.3390/foods10061399

Joshi A, Miller C (2021) Review of machine learning techniques for mosquito control in urban environments. Ecol Inform 61:101241

Kalinowska K, Wojnowski W, Tobiszewski M (2021) Smartphones as tools for equitable food quality assessment. Trends Food Sci Technol 111:271–279. https://doi.org/10.1016/j.tifs.2021.02.068

Kimutai G, Förster A (2023) A low-cost TinyML model for mosquito detection in resource-constrained environments. In GoodIT '23: Proceedings of the 2023 ACM conference on information technology for social good. pp 23–30. https://dl.acm.org/doi/10.1145/3582515.3609514

Kiskin I, Cobb AD, Sinka M, Willis K, Roberts SJ (2021) Automatic acoustic mosquito tagging with Bayesian neural networks. Machine learning and knowledge discovery in databases. Appl Data Sci Track 351–366. Lecture Notes in Computer Science. https://doi.org/10.1007/978-3-030-86514-6_22

Knoblauch S, Li H, Lautenbach S, Elshiaty Y et al (2023) Semi-supervised water tank detection to support vector control of emerging infectious diseases transmitted by Aedes Aegypti. Int J Appl Earth Observ Geoinform 119:103304. https://doi.org/10.1016/j.jag.2023.103304

Kupferschmidt K (2011) Dioxin scandal triggers food debate in Germany. Can Med Assoc J 183(4):E221–E222. https://doi.org/10.1503/cmaj.109-3801

Levin S, Krishnan S, Rajkumar S, Halery N, Balkunde P (2016) Monitoring of fluoride in water samples using a smartphone. Sci Total Environ 551-552:101–107. https://doi.org/10.1016/j.scitotenv.2016.01.156

Luna-Gonzalez JA, Robles-Camarillo D, Nakano-Miyatake M, Lanz-Mendoza H, Meana HMP (2020) A CNN-based mosquito classification using image transformation of wingbeat features. Front Artif Intell Appl 327:127–137. https://doi.org/10.3233/FAIA200559

Mukundarajan H, Hol FJH, Araceli Castillo E, Newby C, Prakash M (2017) Using mobile phones as acoustic sensors for high-throughput mosquito surveillance. eLife 6:e27854

Oh M, Lee H, Cho H, Moon SH, Kim EK, Kim M (2016) Detection of fecal contamination on beef meat surfaces using handheld fluorescence imaging device (HFID). Proc. SPIE 9864, Sensing for Agriculture and Food Quality and Safety VIII, 986411 https://doi.org/10.1117/12.2227184.

Okayasu K, Yoshida K, Fuchida M, Nakamura A (2019) Vision-based classification of mosquito species: comparison of conventional and deep learning methods. Appl Sci 9(18): 3935. https://www.mdpi.com/2076-3417/9/18/3935

Ouyang TH, Yang EC, Jiang JA, Lin TT (2015) Mosquito vector monitoring system based on optical wingbeat classification. Comput Electron Agric 118:47–55

Passos WL, Araujo GM, de Lima AA, Netto SL, da Silva EAB (2022) Automatic detection of Aedes aegypti breeding grounds based on deep networks with spatio-temporal consistency. Comput Environ Urban Syst 93:101754. ISSN 0198-9715

Popovic R, Radovanov B, Dunn JW (2017) Food scare crisis: the effect on Serbian dairy market. Int Food Agribus Manag Rev 20(1):113–127. https://doi.org/10.22434/ifamr2015.0051

Potamitis I (2014) Classifying insects on the fly. Ecol Inform 21:40–49

Rateni G, Dario P, Cavallo F (2017) Smartphone-based food diagnostic technologies: a review. Sensors (Switzerland) 17(6):1453. https://doi.org/10.3390/s17061453
Semwal A, Melvin LMJ, Mohan RE, Ramalingam B, Pathmakumar (2022) AI-enabled mosquito surveillance and population mapping using dragonfly robot. Sensors 22(13): 4921. https://www.mdpi.com/1424-8220/22/13/4921
Sinka ME et al (2021) HumBug–an acoustic mosquito monitoring tool for use on budget smartphones. Methods Ecol Evol 12:1848–1859
Spitzen J, Takken W (2018) Keeping track of mosquitoes: a review of tools to track, record and analyse mosquito flight. Parasit Vectors 11:1–11
Tsagkaris AS, Nelis JLD, Ross GMS, Jafari S, Guercetti J, Kopper K, Zhao Y, Rafferty K, Salvador JP, Migliorelli D, Salentijn GI, Campbell K, Marco MP, Elliot CT, Nielen MWF, Pulkrabova J, Hajslova J (2019) Critical assessment of recent trends related to screening and confirmatory analytical methods for selected food contaminants and allergens. TrAC—Trends Anal Chem 121:115688. https://doi.org/10.1016/j.trac.2019.115688
Vasconcelos D, Nunes N, Ribeiro M, Prandi C, Rogers A (2019) LOCOMOBIS: a low-cost acoustic-based sensing system to monitor and classify mosquitoes. 2019 16th IEEE Annual Consumer Communications Networking Conference (CCNC): 1–6. https://www.sciencedirect.com/science/article/pii/S0010482523012520.
Vasconcelos D, Nunes NJ, Förster A, Gomes JP (2024) Optimal 2D audio features estimation for a lightweight application in mosquitoes species: ecoacoustics detection and classification purposes. Comput Biol Med 168: 107787. https://www.sciencedirect.com/science/article/pii/S0010482523012520
WHO (2015) WHO estimates of the global burden of foodborne diseases: executive summary. World Health Organization. https://apps.who.int/iris/handle/10665/200046. Accessed July 2023
Yin MS, Haddawy P, Nirandmongkol B. (2021). A lightweight deep learning approach to mosquito classification from wingbeat sounds. Proceedings of the ACM GoodIT conference. Rom, Italy 9–11 September https://doi.org/10.1145/3462203.3475908.
Yin MS et al (2023) A deep learning-based pipeline for mosquito detection and classification from wingbeat sounds. Multimed Tools Appl 82(4):5189–5205
Zhang D, Liu Q (2016) Biosensors and bioelectronics on smartphone for portable biochemical detection. Biosens Bioelectron 75:273–284. https://doi.org/10.1016/j.bios.2015.08.037
Ziemer T, Wetjen F, Herbst A (2022) The antenna base plays a crucial role in mosquito courtship behavior. Front Trop Dis 3:803611. https://doi.org/10.3389/fitd.2022.803611. [Original source: https://studycrumb.com/alphabetizer]

Open Access This chapter is licensed under the terms of the Creative Commons Attribution 4.0 International License (http://creativecommons.org/licenses/by/4.0/), which permits use, sharing, adaptation, distribution and reproduction in any medium or format, as long as you give appropriate credit to the original author(s) and the source, provide a link to the Creative Commons license and indicate if changes were made.

The images or other third party material in this chapter are included in the chapter's Creative Commons license, unless indicated otherwise in a credit line to the material. If material is not included in the chapter's Creative Commons license and your intended use is not permitted by statutory regulation or exceeds the permitted use, you will need to obtain permission directly from the copyright holder.

Health Promotion, Including Action to Address Social Determinants and Health Inequity (EPHO 4)

Digital Interventions for Health Behavior Promotion

Laura M. König

Abstract Digital health behavior interventions have the potential to reach many people at low cost and in remote locations, contributing to promoting health for all. However, the reach of digital health behavior interventions is currently limited, and many interventions are quickly abandoned, which limits their effectiveness. A number of factors contribute to the limited uptake of and engagement with digital health behavior interventions, including limited availability and access, psychological factors (e.g., knowledge, motivation), the technology itself (e.g., usability, privacy), and social influences (e.g., recommendations, stigmatization). Stakeholders, including intervention developers and policymakers, can use this knowledge to identify strategies to overcome these barriers and design improved digital health behavior interventions that attract more users and engage them for prolonged periods. In this vein, they will help to promote health behaviors at scale.

Keywords Digital public health · Ehealth · Health behavior change · Health psychology · Mhealth

1 Introduction

A website to record caloric intake, a bracelet to record steps, or a smartphone application (app) to track the menstrual cycle—digital media and tools are increasingly used to promote health at the individual level. According to the World Health Organization (WHO), health promotion is defined as "the process of enabling people to increase control over, and to improve their health" (World Health

---

L. M. König (✉)
Faculty of Life Sciences: Food, Nutrition and Health, University of Bayreuth, Bayreuth, Germany

Faculty of Psychology, University of Vienna, Vienna, Austria
e-mail: laura.koenig@univie.ac.at

© The Author(s) 2025
H. Zeeb et al. (eds.), *Digital Public Health*, Springer Series on Epidemiology and Public Health, https://doi.org/10.1007/978-3-031-90154-6_19

Organization 1986). Interventions for health promotion traditionally have been and continue to be delivered face-to-face; however, technological advances increasingly allow for interventions to be delivered digitally. This has led to the emergence of the field of eHealth, i.e., the development and use of "health services and information delivered or enhanced through the internet and related technologies" (Eysenbach 2001). The first instances of eHealth interventions were used as early as the 1970s: due to their use of telecommunication services such as telephone and videoconferencing services, including remote consultations (Moore 1999); the field is also referred to as telemedicine. Since then, digital technologies continuously developed, which was also reflected in health promotion and healthcare services.

Digital health interventions have the potential to reach large numbers of people at relatively low cost and also in remote locations. They allow to track behaviors continuously and in daily life and to provide continued care independent of time and location (Fischer et al. 2016). Some technologies even allow tailoring of the intervention content and timing to suit the individual's needs, allowing for highly individualized support, so-called Just-in-Time Adaptive Interventions (JITAIs; Nahum-Shani et al. 2018) that may be associated with increased intervention effectiveness (Wang and Miller 2020). Accordingly, the WHO stated that digital health interventions may accelerate the progress toward reaching health-related Sustainable Development Goals (World Health Organization 2021).

Indeed, internet access and computer and mobile phone ownership are increasing worldwide (The World Bank 2023), potentially allowing more and more people to use digital health behavior interventions to benefit their health. However, research is accumulating that casts doubt on the WHO's statement. For example, digital interventions for physical activity promotion are much less effective in populations with a low socio-economic status (SES) than in high SES populations (Western et al. 2021). Similarly, eHealth interventions for weight loss may be less effective in low-income groups (Clark et al. 2023). Finally, a range of social determinants, including age, gender, place of residency, and occupation, may impact engagement with and effectiveness of mobile interventions for weight-related behaviors (König et al., 2025a; Szinay et al. 2023). To date, digital interventions for health promotion thus risk widening, instead of reducing, health disparities; this phenomenon is also called the digital health divide (Müller et al. 2020) (see Chap. "Digital Health Inequalities", Brand et al. in this handbook). Furthermore, digital health behavior interventions are not widely used. For instance, in Germany, only 8% to 25% of the population uses digital tools for health promotion, depending on the targeted behavior (Ernsting et al. 2017; König et al. 2018). In sum, the impact of digital tools on public health and health promotion is currently limited. Improvements are necessary to facilitate the uptake of and engagement with digital interventions for health behavior promotion to boost their effectiveness and unleash their full potential.

This chapter will provide an overview of the current landscape of digital health behavior interventions and their effectiveness before reviewing the literature regarding uptake of and engagement with digital interventions, which are important prerequisites for intervention effectiveness. Based on the presented evidence, the chapter will then provide recommendations for improving digital tools in public health and health promotion to increase uptake and engagement and boost effectiveness. It will focus on diet and physical activity since these behaviors are not only among the behaviors most frequently targeted by digital interventions (Sama et al. 2014) but also cause a large share of the global burden of disease and so require urgent attention to promote public health (Afshin et al. 2019; Strain et al. 2020).

2 Digital Tools Used for Health Behavior Promotion

A variety of digital tools are used for health behavior promotion. Computer-based programs and websites are frequently used (Stark et al. 2022), which is partly due to the fact that these technologies are already relatively old. However, newer technologies such as mobile phones, smartphones, social media, and games are quickly catching up. Each technology has a specific set of advantages and disadvantages (e.g., regarding populations that may be reached and use of resources), and some technologies may be more suited for targeting some behaviors than for others due to the fit between functionalities of the tools and characteristics of the behavior (see, e.g., König et al. 2018, for a discussion). In the following, some of the most frequently used digital tools for health behavior promotion are briefly reviewed regarding their potential reach and effectiveness as digital behavior change interventions.

2.1 Computer-based Programs and Websites

Before the widespread availability of the internet, computer-based health behavior promotion programs were often distributed via CD-ROM, which made interactive lessons available to the users. Other interventions used touchscreens to allow users to interact with the content. Later, websites became increasingly popular; static websites can be used to deliver information via text and media (e.g., videos), while dynamic websites allow for tailoring and interaction (see, e.g., Jacobs et al. 2016 for an overview). Today, website-based interventions can also be used on smartphones or tablets, increasing potential users. The majority of published interventions showed beneficial effects for a wide range of behaviors, including healthy eating (Jacobs et al. 2016; Rodriguez Rocha and Kim 2019) or physical activity (Hamel et al. 2011), especially when interventions were tailored. Overall effects, however, remain small.

2.2 Text Messaging

Due to the increased popularity of mobile phones, many text messaging interventions have been developed for a wide range of behaviors. Text messages allow the delivery of a range of behavior change techniques (BCTs), including self-monitoring, feedback, and goal setting. However, other BCTs may be more difficult to deliver via text messaging (e.g., the cluster "scheduled consequences") or cannot be delivered via text messaging at all (Doğru et al. 2022). Overall, text messaging interventions are an effective tool for promoting a variety of health behaviors, including physical activity and smoking cessation, and significantly contribute to weight loss (Hall et al. 2015). Interestingly, interventions focusing solely on text messaging are equally effective as interventions including other components delivered through other means; accordingly, text messaging interventions may be relatively cost-effective (Head et al. 2013). In recent years, text messaging has become less popular, amongst others, because of short messaging services such as WhatsApp, which allow users to send free messages that do not require a carrier (as long as wireless internet is available), including the sending of voice messages, photos, and videos.

2.3 Social Media

Since the early 2000s, an increasing number of social networks have been launched, and more and more people are using social media. To date, Facebook is still the largest social media globally, followed by the video platform YouTube, the messaging service WhatsApp, and the photo-sharing platform Instagram (Statista 2023). Each social media emphasizes different media formats—WhatsApp, for instance, is largely text-based, while YouTube focuses on videos and Instagram on photos and short video clips—providing opportunities for different intervention content. In the health domain, social media is often criticized for promoting unrealistic ideals and body disturbance (Mingoia et al. 2017); during the COVID-19 pandemic, social media has also been criticized because of the unhindered spread of misinformation regarding public health issues, which may negatively impact health (Rocha et al. 2021; Suarez-Lledo and Alvarez-Galvez 2021). At the same time, multiple studies underline the potential of social media to distribute health-related information (Weiß and König 2022), debunk health-related misinformation (König 2023; Kotz et al. 2023), and promote health behavior change (Laranjo 2016; Maher et al. 2014). Their potential lies in the fact that they allow interventions to reach a large number of people and thus allow them to provide social support at a low cost. Research is still lacking, however, on how social media can best be harnessed to provide this support (Jane et al. 2018), which is complicated by the fact that social media is a rapidly evolving field of study.

2.4 Smartphone and Tablet Apps

Apps for smartphones and tablets are especially popular in the domain of health promotion and, thus, are increasingly commercialized. Across countries and platforms, more than 350,000 health apps are available for users to download (IQVIA

2021). However, many available apps are of low quality, and their effectiveness is often not evaluated (BinDhim et al. 2015), which makes it difficult for health professionals to recommend appropriate apps to their patients (Boudreaux et al. 2014). Also, more and more health apps are developed and tested in research settings. Although they potentially allow the inclusion of a wide range of BCTs, most app-based interventions (e.g., for promoting weight-related behaviors) focus on goal-setting and planning, feedback and self-monitoring, social support, and shaping knowledge (Middelweerd et al. 2014; Villinger et al. 2019), which is mainly in line with what potential users expect from this type of intervention (DeSmet et al. 2019). App-based interventions are generally effective in promoting health behaviors such as diet and physical activity (Schoeppe et al. 2016; Villinger et al. 2019). Some studies conclude that app-based interventions are as effective as face-to-face interventions (Villinger et al. 2019), which are more costly to deliver; other studies, however, indicate that multi-component interventions that use apps as one of multiple modalities to deliver intervention content may be more effective than exclusively app-based interventions (Schoeppe et al. 2016).

2.5 Wearables

Portable trackers are very popular for tracking components of physical activity, such as steps or exercise. They are available either as standalone devices or, more recently, included in smartwatches. Consumers can purchase wearable activity trackers at a relatively low cost (Degroote et al. 2020). At the same time, meta-analyses have repeatedly shown that they are effective in promoting physical activity and inducing weight loss across age groups; in a systematic review of meta-analyses, Ferguson et al. (2022) concluded that wearables may induce approx. 40 min/day more walking and reductions of approx. 1 kg in body weight during the intervention (which typically lasted 3 months or less), which may have a small but tangible impact on public health.

2.6 Health Games

By including gamified elements in digital health behavior interventions, intervention developers aim to sustain engagement, e.g., by including challenges, points, or other rewards (Lister et al. 2014; Johnson et al. 2016; Sardi et al. 2017) or by allowing users to interact with (or compete against) other players (Cromjongh et al. 2023; König et al., 2025b). Other interventions, however, are much more game-like or even marketed as a game rather than a health intervention. One of the most famous examples is Pokémon Go, which requires users to go for a walk in their neighborhood to find and catch Pokémon, which leads to statistically and clinically relevant increases in step counts (Khamzina et al. 2020). Another example is the Nintendo

Switch game Ring Fit Adventure, where users must walk or jog to advance through the virtual world and fight monsters using exercises. Ring Fit Adventure improves physical fitness as well as psychological well-being (Wu et al. 2022). Some health games, like Pokémon Go, are free to play and only require low-cost technology (e.g., smartphone), while others, like Ring Fit Adventure, require a more expensive gaming console and to buy the game itself. Thus, despite their potential positive effects on healthy lifestyles (DeSmet et al. 2014), the public health impact may be limited due to relatively high costs.

2.7 Virtual Reality

Although Virtual Reality (VR) as a concept has been discussed since the 1980s, it has only been popularized in the 2010s, with multiple companies selling VR headsets to consumers. Since VR is immersive and may require users to stand relatively still to reduce the risk of falling, VR is currently more frequently applied for educational purposes (Dhar et al. 2021) or for the treatment of mental health issues, e.g., to substitute or prepare real-life exposures in exposure therapy (Valmaggia et al. 2016). A small but increasing number of studies, however, applied VR to the promotion of healthy dietary behaviors (Fuentes et al. 2020) or physical activity (Faric et al. 2019) and provided important starting points for improvement. Amongst others, they highlight the high costs of VR systems, which may limit the usefulness of VR interventions for health behavior promotion at the population level.

3 Uptake of and Engagement with Digital Interventions

For any behavior change intervention to be effective, it must be taken up and engaged with until the new behavior becomes habitual. Often, uptake of digital health behavior interventions is already low (Siopis et al. 2023; König et al. 2018; Baretta et al. 2019), which for digital health behavior interventions typically refers to purchasing or installing the intervention (Szinay et al. 2020). In the context of many health behaviors, including diet and physical activity, forming a new habit may require months of continued engagement with the intervention (Gardner et al. 2022). Accordingly, sustained engagement with digital health interventions—as for any other intervention—is crucial for their success. In the literature, engagement with digital health interventions has been defined objectively (i.e., via the extent of use, including frequency and duration of using intervention components) as well as subjectively (i.e., as attention, interest, and affect (i.e., positive or negative emotional states when using an intervention, see also König et al. 2021) towards the intervention (Perski et al. 2017; see also Short et al. 2018, for a detailed review of measures)). Somewhat independent of how engagement with digital health interventions is measured, several factors have been identified that may be beneficial for uptake and engagement, while others might be hindering. Barriers and facilitators operate on different levels; however, it is important to note that these factors relate to both the psychological processes and the digital health tools at hand (Perski et al. 2017; Yardley et al. 2016). In the following, these factors are reviewed with the aim of identifying guidelines for promoting the uptake of and engagement with digital health behavior interventions for different stakeholders in the sphere of digital health promotion (see Table 1 for a summary).

Table 1 Factors influencing digital health behavior intervention uptake and engagement and resulting recommendations for stakeholders (intervention developers, educators, health professionals, policymakers)

Factor	Recommendation	For
Availability of and access to required technology	Ensure that intervention uses technology that is widely available at no or low cost. Provide devices if needed	Intervention developers, health professionals, policymakers
Availability of and access to culturally appropriate intervention content in users' native languages	Ensure that intervention is developed to reflect cultural values and requirements (incl. language) of the target population, e.g., through co-creation. Point out relevant interventions to individuals	Intervention developers, health professionals
Awareness of digital health behavior interventions and knowledge about their benefits and functionalities	Promote eHealth literacy across the population. Provide guidance on how to use the digital health behavior intervention	Educators, health professionals, policymakers
Risk perception and motivation to change behavior	Promote awareness of the need to change behavior and how this may be achieved with digital health behavior interventions	Educators, health professionals
The fit of goals to intervention	Design distinct interventions for different goals or allow for tailoring to goal	Intervention developers
Sustained motivation to achieve goal	Include intervention features that sustain engagement, e.g., through introducing novel components	Intervention developers
Forming a tracking habit	Include features that support habit formation, e.g., reminders to track	Intervention developers
Usability of intervention as a whole and of tracking features	Implement features that reduce user burden. Pilot test the intervention to ensure ease of use	Intervention developers
Accuracy of collected data	Ensure that tracked data is accurate	Intervention developers
Design and comfort considerations	Offer different designs. Ensure the device is comfortable to wear	Intervention developers
Expectations regarding intervention content	Include self-monitoring, feedback, and knowledge provision. Carefully consider the use of reminders, gamification, and social comparison	Intervention developers

(continued)

Table 1 (continued)

Factor	Recommendation	For
Customization	Allow users to customize the intervention. Implement algorithms that continuously adjust the intervention	Intervention developers
Data security and privacy	Be transparent about data use and storage. Allow users to choose with whom data will be shared	Intervention developers
Negative anticipated and experienced outcomes of intervention	Minimize potential harms of the intervention. Communicate measures implemented to reduce harm	Intervention developers, health professionals
Positive anticipated and experienced outcomes of intervention	Maximize positive outcomes including cognitive and emotional outcomes. Communicate benefits beyond health promotion	Intervention developers, health professionals
Recommendations via health professionals	Provide training for health professionals on how to identify effective interventions. Identify quality criteria and labels	Educators, policymakers

3.1 Opportunity and Resources

Essential prerequisites for the uptake of digital health behavior interventions are the availability of and access to the intervention and, particularly regarding digital interventions, the required digital technology. Most digital health behavior interventions cannot be used without the required device and mobile data or Wi-Fi connection (Szinay et al. 2020; Whitelaw et al. 2021). Furthermore, it is important to consider that digital technology is quickly developing, but not everyone has the means to keep up to date with these developments—both in terms of skill (c.f. eHealth literacy; Norman and Skinner 2006) and ownership. Populations who tend to report higher levels of eHealth literacy are younger, better educated, and have a higher income compared to populations who report lower levels of eHealth literacy (Guo et al. 2021), mirroring established findings regarding health literacy and health outcomes (Bittlingmayer et al. 2021). Regarding ownership of digital devices, new versions of smartphone operating systems are released regularly, but older devices may not receive updates anymore. Ultimately, this may lead to apps not working as intended, or not at all, on older smartphones, which constitutes a barrier to intervention access. Similarly, when system requirements for an intervention are not fulfilled, malfunctions may occur, which may hinder intervention uptake and engagement (König et al. 2021; Simblett et al. 2018). Finally, intervention accessibility may also be limited due to language and culture. If an intervention is unavailable in the user's native language and does not reflect their cultural values (Aljuraiban 2019), uptake will be less likely.

Moreover, costs might be an issue, especially for low-income populations (König et al. 2021; Simblett et al. 2018; Szinay et al. 2020). Direct costs include the costs of buying the intervention, e.g., when having to pay for an app, but also required equipment such as wearables. In some cases, health insurances might offer programs that cover at least parts of the costs. Furthermore, in Germany, digital interventions may be prescribed for certain diagnoses, which will also lead to the costs being covered by insurance. It is important to note, however, that existing regulations in Germany only cover secondary and tertiary prevention (Sauermann et al. 2022; Schliess et al. 2022), which excludes interventions aiming at improving health behaviors as a measure to prevent disease.

3.2 Psychological Processes

As with any behavior change process, the uptake and continued use of digital health behavior interventions is also influenced by a range of psychological factors. As described by König et al. (2018), using a digital health behavior intervention can itself be described by psychological stage models such as the Precaution Adoption Process Model (Weinstein 1988). This model divides the behavior change process into distinct stages (see Fig. 1) through which people pass during the behavior change process. In the different stages, different psychological processes play an important role in progressing to the next stage; the most important, as identified by several literature reviews, are summarized below.First, it is imperative that potential users are aware of the existence of digital health behavior interventions and know about the opportunities, but also potential harms for achieving health-related goals (Szinay et al. 2020; König et al. 2021; Pywell et al. 2020). This also extends to knowledge about how to use these interventions, which may impact uptake and use directly (Szinay et al. 2020) and indirectly by boosting people's self-efficacy in the long term (Boswell 2013). Providing guidance within the digital intervention or, for example, supplied via training sessions or companion materials may thus promote both uptake and later engagement.

Second, potential users have to feel the need to change their behavior and perceive the intervention as helpful for this endeavor. As with any intervention, this requires them to be generally motivated to change their behavior; if they are not interested in changing their behavior, it is unlikely that they will start using the intervention (König et al. 2021). The use of digital vs. traditional in-person interventions adds another layer of complexity to this issue: without seeing the need for

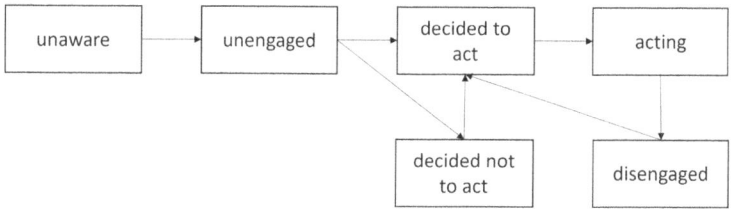

Fig. 1 Adaptation of the Precaution Adoption Process Model for the uptake and continued use of digital health behavior intervention (Source: based on König et al. 2018)

a digital health behavior intervention, it is unlikely that an individual will form the intention to use the intervention if it is only available in a digital format.

Once they decide to use a digital health behavior intervention, potential users must identify an intervention best suited to their goals. Goals that potential users may want to achieve are diverse; in the context of diet and nutrition apps, for instance, goals may range from tracking dietary behaviors to better understanding patterns through automated feedback, including identifying foods that may cause allergic reactions to restricting food intake to lose weight and increasing the intake of specific macronutrients to gain muscle mass and receiving related tailored advice at their convenience (König et al. 2021).

If individuals identify an intervention that fits their goals and needs, engagement with the intervention is likely, at least as long as the goal is maintained. However, if the goal is abandoned in favor of other goals or because it does not seem important anymore, the likelihood of abandoning the intervention increases (Attig and Franke 2020; König et al. 2021). Users may be retained, among other things, by keeping the intervention interesting and novel (Lyzwinski et al. 2018; Perski et al. 2017), e.g., by automatically providing access to additional features as time progresses. Furthermore, forming a habit of using the intervention is crucial. Most digital interventions rely on self-monitoring of behavior (see, e.g., Rhodes et al. (2020); Sediva et al. (2022); Villinger et al. (2019) for analyses of behavior change techniques in digital health behavior interventions), not only because it is an effective behavior change technique (Michie et al. 2009), but also because the tracked data is used in other intervention components such as providing feedback (Krukowski et al., 2024), judging whether goals were achieved, or automatically tailoring intervention components to behaviors or context variables. This often requires users to actively track their behavior. In the context of dietary behaviors, users typically need to complete food diaries, which may be more effortful than remembering to put on an activity tracker in the morning to record physical activity (König et al. 2018). In any case, however, a tracking routine needs to be established to allow for continued engagement and the intervention to provide meaningful insights (König et al. 2021). Moreover, tracking routines need to be compatible with existing daily routines. If the tracking routine is disrupted or incompatible with other daily routines, abandonment of the intervention becomes more likely (Attig and Franke 2020; Simblett et al. 2018).

3.3 Technological Factors

The impact of characteristics of the technology underlying the intervention is frequently discussed in the digital health literature. Most often, usability concerns play a role. Of course, the intervention needs to be easy to set up and to use, ideally also for potential users who report relatively low levels of digital literacy (Attig and Franke 2020; König et al. 2021; Sharpe et al. 2017; Simblett et al. 2018). Instructions on how to use the intervention may help promote both uptake and engagement

(Szinay et al. 2020). Since self-monitoring is an integral part of many digital health behavior interventions, it may be especially crucial for sustained engagement that tracking features are easy to use. This may be an important consideration when detailed manual tracking is required, as in many dietary interventions. Research suggests that instead of using databases that often provide too much or too little choice and asking users to estimate portion sizes, which may lead to considerable estimation errors (König et al. 2019; König et al., 2024), photo-based recording may be preferred (Boushey et al. 2017; König et al. 2021) due to its low user burden (Turner-McGrievy et al. 2021; Allmeta et al. 2025). The use of photo-based recording, however, is still in its early stages since identifying foods via Artificial Intelligence is still relatively difficult (Allegra et al. 2020).

Design and comfort considerations are also important depending on the type of digital interventions. This refers not only to the design of smartphone or web applications but also to the physical design of digital tools such as wearables or VR equipment. If wearing the equipment is uncomfortable, it is likely to be abandoned (Attig and Franke 2020). Since digital tools such as smartwatches and wearables demonstrate a certain lifestyle, visual design considerations may also be necessary for some users (Attig and Franke 2020). For example, offering different colors or patterns for wristbands may be an important lever to boost uptake.

Users of digital health behavior interventions also likely have expectations regarding the intervention content, including behavior change techniques employed in the intervention. Most users expect self-monitoring and feedback features and to receive information they otherwise would not have. This includes both general information about the behavior and its consequences as well as statistics about their own behavior (Baer et al. 2022; König et al. 2021; Lyzwinski et al. 2018; Perski et al. 2017; Sharpe et al. 2017; Szinay et al. 2020; Cao et al. 2022). The information provided should be understandable and prove useful to the user. In addition, the collected data should be accurate and reflect the users' subjective experiences; if this is not the case, disengagement is likely (Attig and Franke 2020; Sharpe et al. 2017). However, disagreements have been reported in the literature regarding the use of other behavior change techniques and intervention features such as reminders and gamification. While some people seem to be easily annoyed by reminders, others feel they are necessary to maintain their interest in the intervention (Szinay et al. 2020; König et al. 2021). Similarly, some people appreciate the use of gamified elements such as points and leaderboards because it maintains their interest, while others feel that these elements are unnecessary (König et al. 2021). Across intervention components, an interactive and supportive tone may be necessary to maintain engagement (Lyzwinski et al. 2018; Szinay et al. 2020).

Essentially independent of which behavior change techniques and features are implemented in the interventions, most people wish for digital health behavior interventions to be customizable (Cao et al. 2022; Lyzwinski et al. 2018; Sharpe et al. 2017). The flexibility of digital interventions is often seen as a significant advantage by health professionals and users alike (Marcu et al. 2022). Users can indicate their preferences to adjust the intervention to their needs, for instance, during setup or via changing settings, including aspects such as the frequency of reminders or message tone. Customization can also be implemented in the use of different intervention features, such as providing a list of goals to choose from when asked to set goals, to which the intervention then automatically adapts (König et al. 2021; Perski et al. 2017). Customization preserves freedom of choice and feelings of autonomy and may thus be considered an important tool for promoting long-term engagement (Flaherty et al. 2019). In addition, interventions should ideally tailor the content automatically based on user input and collected data to improve the user experience. Due to advances in technology, automated tailoring of interventions has become increasingly popular and easier to achieve; this is, for instance, indicated by the rising interest in JITAIs, which allow the tailoring of the intervention content to input data and context variables and constant tuning of the intervention according to the individual's progress (Chevance et al. 2021) (see also Simons et al. 2023), for a summary of the usefulness of JITAIs for health behavior change). This, however, may require technical expertise that data scientists, Artificial Intelligence experts, and app developers need to bring to an interdisciplinary project team.

For digital health behavior interventions to work, they often require users to disclose personal health-related information. Contrary to in-person interventions, where information may be shared verbally with a trusted individual and confidentiality is implied in an implicit social contract, digital health behavior interventions are usually a black box regarding where data is stored and with whom it is shared. Although data protection statements are typically required, these are very difficult to understand for laypersons (Powell et al. 2018). Reluctance to share health-related data with a larger group of people or even publicly may contribute to hesitation to start using a digital intervention, especially if it is unclear how the data is going to be stored and used; concerns include the data to be shared without permission with third parties for advertising purposes or on social media (Attig and Franke 2020; Baer et al. 2022; König et al. 2021). Users tend to trust digital applications more if they were (co-)created by health professionals compared to commercial companies (Dennison et al. 2013; Peng et al. 2016). Understandable data usage and privacy statements, as well as allowing users to choose with whom data will be shared, may be important levers to promote trust in the intervention and, consequently, uptake and engagement (König et al. 2021).

3.4 Anticipated or Experienced Outcomes of Intervention Use

Before taking up any intervention, potential users are likely to have expectations of outcomes of intervention use. If these expectations are largely positive, uptake is more likely than when outcome expectations are negative (Molloy et al. 2021; Zhang et al. 2019). Similarly, after using a digital health behavior intervention, the valence of experiences made will likely impact whether the intervention will be used continuously or quickly abandoned (König et al. 2021). Accordingly, it is vital to shape positive outcome expectancies regarding the intervention, including but not limited to the intervention's effectiveness in changing the behavior. Additionally, cognitive and emotional outcomes are important. In the context of digital weight-related interventions, potential users may be afraid of developing an obsession with calorie counting or being overly engaged with their behaviors, which may turn into eating disorders or other mental disorders. They may also fear receiving negative feedback if they repeatedly fall short of reaching their goals, which is generally seen as demotivating (Attig and Franke 2020; König et al. 2021). When developing a digital health behavior intervention, it is thus essential to anticipate potential negative outcomes or stereotypes about digital health behavior interventions and prevent them, and highlight these measures in communication materials to take away potential users' worries.

At the same time, positive cognitive and emotional expectations and experiences may be powerful in promoting intervention uptake and engagement. For example, a digital health behavior intervention may increase motivation to engage in healthy behaviors and induce feelings of pride and accountability when goals are achieved, which may boost self-efficacy. In addition, digital health behavior interventions have the potential to induce positive emotions about the targeted behavior, including demonstrating that health behaviors are associated with feeling energized and happy (König et al. 2021; Wahl et al. 2017). These positive outcomes can be harnessed in conversation and advertising to promote the uptake of digital health behavior interventions.

3.5 Social Influence

Finally, the social environment contributes substantially to the uptake, engagement, and effectiveness of digital health behavior interventions. Many people turn to cues in their social environment to decide whether to use such an intervention and identify a suitable one. In addition to using ratings, comments, and reviews in app stores and on websites, conversations with friends and family members may be important sources of information (König et al. 2021; Szinay et al. 2020). Adverse reactions from the social environment may discourage the use of digital health behavior interventions, for example, if they stigmatize tracking and subsequently induce feelings of embarrassment (König et al. 2021). Moreover, health professionals and healthcare providers are important gatekeepers since they may be considered expert sources and may also recommend the use of a digital health behavior intervention as part of a treatment plan (König et al. 2021). However, this task may be difficult for health professionals and healthcare providers since little information regarding effectiveness is available for many apps (Marcu et al. 2022), and to date, there are no quality scores or labels for digital health behavior interventions which would be important in guiding choice (Wood et al. 2022). A labeling scheme for the European market is currently being developed (Hoogendoorn et al. 2023), which will be a welcome guide for health professionals, healthcare providers, and potential users alike. Furthermore, many health professionals are still hesitant to recommend digital interventions at all because they believe that digital approaches are inferior to traditional forms of treatment and are unsure of how to integrate digital components into routine care (Hennemann et al. 2017). The social environment, thus, is an important contributor to digital health behavior intervention use and nonuse, depending on existing knowledge and attitudes.

Intervention components harnessing social influence to promote engagement and behavior change are frequently used in digital health behavior interventions. Social interactions and competition may promote behavior change and encourage continued tracking (Attig and Franke 2020; König et al. 2021; Szinay et al. 2020). Social interactions may be promoted directly in the intervention or by allowing users to connect the intervention with their social media profiles (Szinay et al. 2020), thereby promoting interaction and an exchange of knowledge (Baer et al. 2022). However, it is important to note that there are interindividual differences in the acceptance and effectiveness of social comparison in health behavior change, so this might not be a "one size fits all" approach (Arigo et al. 2020, 2021; König et al., 2025b). Instead of promoting competition, some digital health behavior interventions focus on providing social support, which may also contribute to intervention engagement (Cao et al. 2022; König et al. 2021; Perski et al. 2017; Sharpe et al. 2017). While potentially beneficial, intervention components relying on the social environment need to be carefully crafted and potentially closely monitored and tested to maximize benefits.

4 Recommendations for Digital Health Promotion

Based on the extensive literature available on barriers and facilitators of using digital behavior change interventions for health promotion, several recommendations for advancing the practice of digital health promotion can be derived, which are listed in Table 1. These recommendations do not only target intervention developers, but also educators, health professionals, and policymakers. Most importantly, the recommendations highlight the need for interdisciplinary and intersectoral collaboration in the development and implementation of digital health behavior interventions. Naturally, many recommendations target intervention developers; ideally, teams developing digital health behavior interventions should be composed of different areas of expertise. This includes psychologists and behavioral scientists to ensure that theoretical determinants and mechanisms of action are appropriately targeted; computer and data scientists to ensure that technological components are appropriately designed and that data is collected, analyzed, and displayed accurately; finally, healthcare professionals to ensure the compatibility of the intervention with care and patient requirements.

Moreover, partnerships between researchers in academia and the private sector may be helpful to ensure that interventions can be scaled up and maintained in the long term. These collaborations, however, are often difficult to instigate and maintain for a number of reasons. Different academic disciplines may have different expectations regarding outcomes and timelines in which these outcomes are achieved (Sucala et al. 2021). Especially when a collaboration is newly established, a common vocabulary and trust in each other may be lacking (Blandford et al. 2018). Finally, public funding for interdisciplinary research projects that use co-creation and iterative design processes is lacking. A culture shift towards interdisciplinary and intersectoral research is needed to boost the public health impact of digital health behavior interventions (Nordgreen et al. 2021).

In addition, involving potential users at every step of the intervention development process has been beneficial when developing in-person interventions (Leask et al. 2019), and the same holds true for developing digital interventions. Patient and public involvement may be highly beneficial to ensure that the needs of the target group are adequately reflected and addressed (Chen et al. 2023; Hochmuth et al. 2020) (see also Chap. "Participatory Approaches for Digital Public Health", Shresta et al. in this handbook). The utility of this approach is, amongst others, reflected in the Path to Health study (Solar et al. 2022), which aims to support weight management among urban public housing developments in the US who are primarily low-income and from racial/ethnic minority groups. The design of the intervention was supported by a community advisory board, which ensured that the intervention components developed fit the needs of the target group. This included the development of text messages in English and Spanish since many public housing residents' native language is Spanish. In addition, the intervention includes counseling sessions delivered by community health workers, who were recruited from the study population and trained to support the intervention users in their attempts to change their behavior. In this vein, cultural appropriateness is achieved, which allows study participants to relate better to the intervention content and is expected to promote engagement and effectiveness (Quintiliani et al. 2021).

Finally, adequate conditions must be created to roll out digital interventions at scale. Most importantly, this requires addressing policymakers who may facilitate access to digital technology by providing relevant infrastructure (e.g., Kalichman et al. (2002)) and digital intervention uptake through legislation. An example is the Digital Healthcare Act in Germany, which allows medical professionals to prescribe digital interventions as part of treating an increasing number of medical conditions, including but not limited to obesity. Health insurances reimburse the costs, thus promoting the use of digital interventions independent of income and simultaneously stimulating investment in digital interventions (Gehde et al. 2022). To date, however, prescriptions are only covered if they are used for treating specific physical or mental illnesses; the costs for digital interventions for primary prevention and health promotion currently need to be covered by the users themselves, which risks widening existing health inequalities (Jensen et al. 2010). Similar models for covering the costs of digital interventions may also be needed for primary prevention to promote health at scale.

In addition, educators will need to promote eHealth literacy in the population to ensure that people are equipped with the required knowledge to be able to engage with digital interventions meaningfully; this also requires the promotion of digital literacy starting from an early age, among other measures (Azzahra and Amanta 2021), since this is a core component of eHealth literacy (Norman and Skinner

2006). This also includes educating the public about the potential benefits that digital technology may offer to changing health behaviors and promoting physical (and mental) health, as well as providing guidance on how to identify the most helpful intervention for their needs. Lastly, healthcare professionals, including general practitioners, nutritionists, and physiotherapists, need to be trained to identify the most effective digital interventions and communicate the benefits and risks of these interventions to their patients (Virtanen et al. 2021). Only through an interdisciplinary and intersectoral effort can digital health promotion move forward to reach its full potential.

5 Conclusion

Digital interventions for health promotion have the potential to improve a range of health behaviors, including diet and physical activity at scale due to their potential reach. However, they currently do not fulfill their potential. Despite the availability of many different digital tools that can potentially be used in interventions, many populations still have limited access to digital health behavior interventions. In addition, a variety of factors may contribute to digital health behavior interventions not yet being used at all or long enough to achieve meaningful behavior change. These factors operate on different levels and include barriers at the level of the technology (e.g., usability, malfunctions, privacy concerns), the individual (e.g., motivation to change behaviors, lack of knowledge about digital health behavior interventions), their interaction that may result in positive or negative consequences, and the social environment. To properly harness digital interventions in health promotion, these barriers need to be addressed by different stakeholders. Naturally, many obstacles need to be addressed by intervention developers, who ideally work in multidisciplinary and intersectoral teams and involve potential end users in the development process; however, policymakers need to create conditions under which effective interventions can be developed, distributed, and used, and health professionals and educators need to increase awareness and needed skills in the population to engage with digital health behavior interventions effectively. In this vein, digital health behavior interventions can be a driver of behavior change at the population level, contributing to achieving health for all.

Acknowledgement I thank Dr. Lisa Quintiliani for her comments on an earlier version of the manuscript.

References

Afshin A, Sur PJ, Fay KA, Cornaby L, Ferrara G, Salama JS, Mullany EC et al (2019) Health effects of dietary risks in 195 countries, 1990–2017: a systematic analysis for the Global Burden of Disease Study 2017. Lancet 393(10184):1958–1972

Aljuraiban GS (2019) Use of weight-management mobile phone apps in Saudi Arabia: a web-based survey. JMIR Mhealth Uhealth 7(2):e12692

Allegra D, Battiato S, Ortis A, Urso S, Polosa R (2020) A review on food recognition technology for health applications. Health Psychol Res 8:3

Allmeta A, Sutton S, König LM (2025) The same, only different: Smartphone-based dietary Ecological Momentary Assessment tools vary in complexity, usability, and active information processing. https://doi.org/10.31234/osf.io/j3xbg_v1

Arigo D, Brown MM, Pasko K, Suls J (2020) Social comparison features in physical activity promotion apps: scoping meta-review. J Med Internet Res 22(3):e15642

Arigo D, Mogle JA, Smyth JM (2021) Relations between social comparisons and physical activity among women in midlife with elevated risk for cardiovascular disease: an ecological momentary assessment study. J Behav Med 44(5):579–590

Attig C, Franke T (2020) Abandonment of personal quantification: a review and empirical study investigating reasons for wearable activity tracking attrition. Comput Hum Behav 102:223–237

Azzahra NF, Amanta F (2021) Promoting digital literacy skill for students through improved school curriculum. Policy Brief. https://www.cips-indonesia.org/publications/promoting-digital-literacy-skill-for-students-through-improved-school-curriculum. Accessed July 2023

Baer N-R, Vietzke J, Schenk L (2022) Middle-aged and older adults' acceptance of mobile nutrition and fitness apps: a systematic mixed studies review. PLoS One 17(12):e0278879

Baretta D, Perski O, Steca P (2019) Exploring users' experiences of the uptake and adoption of physical activity apps: longitudinal qualitative study. JMIR Mhealth Uhealth 7(2):e11636

BinDhim NF, Hawkey A, Trevena L (2015) A systematic review of quality assessment methods for smartphone health apps. Telemed e-Health 21(2):97–104

Bittlingmayer UH, Harsch S, Islertas Z (2021) Health literacy in the context of health inequality–a framing and a research overview. In: Saboga-Nunes LA, Bittlingmayer UH, Orkan O, Sahrai D (eds) New approaches to health literacy: linking different perspectives. Springer VS Wiesbaden, pp 11–43

Blandford A, Gibbs J, Newhouse N, Perski O, Singh A, Murray E (2018) Seven lessons for interdisciplinary research on interactive digital health interventions. Digital Health 4:2055207618770325

Boswell SS (2013) Undergraduates' perceived knowledge, self-efficacy, and interest in social science research. J Eff Teach 13(2):48–57

Boudreaux ED, Waring ME, Hayes RB, Sadasivam RS, Mullen S, Pagoto S (2014) Evaluating and selecting mobile health apps: strategies for healthcare providers and healthcare organizations. Transl Behav Med 4(4):363–371

Boushey CJ, Spoden M, Zhu F, Delp E, Kerr D (2017) New mobile methods for dietary assessment: review of image-assisted and image-based dietary assessment methods. Proc Nutr Soc 76:283–294. https://doi.org/10.1017/S0029665116002913

Cao W, Milks MW, Liu X, Gregory ME, Addison D, Zhang P, Li L (2022) mHealth interventions for self-management of hypertension: framework and systematic review on engagement, interactivity, and tailoring. JMIR Mhealth Uhealth 10(3):e29415

Chen Y, Hosin AA, George MJ, Asselbergs FW, Shah AD (2023) Digital technology and patient and public involvement (PPI) in routine care and clinical research—a pilot study. PLoS One 18(2):e0278260

Chevance G, Perski O, Hekler EB (2021) Innovative methods for observing and changing complex health behaviors: four propositions. Transl Behav Med 11(2):676–685

Clark TL, Savin KL, Perez-Ramirez P, Valdez T, Toba G, Gallo LC (2023) eHealth weight loss interventions for adults with low income: a systematic review. Health Psychol 42(6):353–367. https://doi.org/10.1037/hea0001278

Cromjongh R, Van Reenen Q, König L, Kanning M, Reips U-D, Feuchtner T, Hauptmann H (2023) Group adapted avatar recommendations for exergames. In: Adjunct proceedings of the 31st ACM conference on user modeling, adaptation and personalization. ACM, New York, pp 283–290

Degroote L, Hamerlinck G, Poels K, Maher C, Crombez G, De Bourdeaudhuij I, Vandendriessche A et al (2020) Low-cost consumer-based trackers to measure physical activity and sleep duration among adults in free-living conditions: validation study. JMIR Mhealth Uhealth 8(5):e16674

Dennison L, Morrison L, Conway G, Yardley L (2013) Opportunities and challenges for smartphone applications in supporting health behavior change: qualitative study. J Med Internet Res 15(4):e86. https://doi.org/10.2196/jmir.2583

DeSmet A, Van Ryckeghem D, Compernolle S, Baranowski T, Thompson D, Crombez G, Poels K et al (2014) A meta-analysis of serious digital games for healthy lifestyle promotion. Prev Med 69:95–107. https://doi.org/10.1016/j.ypmed.2014.08.026

DeSmet A, De Bourdeaudhuij I, Chastin S, Crombez G, Maddison R, Cardon G (2019) Adults' preferences for behavior change techniques and engagement features in a mobile app to promote 24-hour movement behaviors: cross-sectional survey study. JMIR Mhealth Uhealth 7(12):e15707

Dhar P, Rocks T, Samarasinghe RM, Stephenson G, Smith C (2021) Augmented reality in medical education: students' experiences and learning outcomes. Med Educ Online 26(1):1953953

Doğru OC, Webb TL, Norman P (2022) Can behavior change techniques be delivered via short text messages? Transl Behav Med 12(10):979–986

Ernsting C, Dombrowski SU, Oedekoven M, Lo J, Kanzler M, Kuhlmey A, Gellert P (2017) Using smartphones and health apps to change and manage health behaviors: a population-based survey. J Med Internet Res 19(4):e101. https://doi.org/10.2196/jmir.6838

Eysenbach G (2001) What is e-health? J Med Internet Res 3(2):e833

Faric N, Potts HW, Hon A, Smith L, Newby K, Steptoe A, Fisher A (2019) What players of virtual reality exercise games want: thematic analysis of web-based reviews. J Med Internet Res 21(9):e13833

Ferguson T, Olds T, Curtis R, Blake H, Crozier AJ, Dankiw K, Dumuid D et al (2022) Effectiveness of wearable activity trackers to increase physical activity and improve health: a systematic review of systematic reviews and meta-analyses. Lancet Digit Health 4(8):e615–e626

Fischer F, Aust V, Krämer A (2016) eHealth: Hintergrund und Begriffsbestimmung. eHealth in Deutschland: Anforderungen und Potenziale innovativer Versorgungsstrukturen:3–23

Flaherty SJ, McCarthy MB, Collins AM, McAuliffe FM (2019) A different perspective on consumer engagement: exploring the experience of using health apps to support healthier food purchasing. J Mark Manag 35(3–4):310–337

Fuentes EM, Varela-Aldás J, Palacios-Navarro G, García-Magariño I (2020) Immersive virtual reality app to promote healthy eating in children. In: HCI international 2020-posters: 22nd international conference, HCII 2020, Copenhagen, Denmark, July 19–24, 2020, proceedings, part II 22, 2020. Springer, pp 9–15

Gardner B, Rebar AL, Lally P (2022) How does habit form? Guidelines for tracking real-world habit formation. Cogent Psychol 9(1):2041277

Gehde KM, Rausch F, Leker J (2022) Business model configurations in digital healthcare—a German case study about digital transformation. Int J Innov Manag 26(03):2240018

Guo Z, Zhao SZ, Guo N, Wu Y, Weng X, Wong JY-H, Lam TH, Wang MP (2021) Socioeconomic disparities in eHealth literacy and preventive behaviors during the COVID-19 pandemic in Hong Kong: cross-sectional study. J Med Internet Res 23(4):e24577

Hall AK, Cole-Lewis H, Bernhardt JM (2015) Mobile text messaging for health: a systematic review of reviews. Annu Rev Public Health 36:393–415

Hamel LM, Robbins LB, Wilbur J (2011) Computer- and web-based interventions to increase preadolescent and adolescent physical activity: a systematic review. J Adv Nurs 67(2):251–268

Head KJ, Noar SM, Iannarino NT, Harrington NG (2013) Efficacy of text messaging-based interventions for health promotion: a meta-analysis. Soc Sci Med 97:41–48

Hennemann S, Beutel ME, Zwerenz R (2017) Ready for eHealth? Health professionals' acceptance and adoption of eHealth interventions in inpatient routine care. J Health Commun 22(3):274–284

Hochmuth A, Exner AK, Dockweiler C (2020) Implementierung und partizipative Gestaltung digitaler Gesundheitsinterventionen. Bundesgesundheitsblatt Gesundheitsforschung Gesundheitsschutz 63:2

Hoogendoorn P, Versluis A, van Kampen S, McCay C, Leahy M, Bijlsma M, Bonacina S et al (2023) What makes a quality health app—developing a global research-based health app quality assessment framework for CEN-ISO/TS 82304-2: Delphi study. JMIR Form Res 7:e43905

IQVIA (2021) Digital health trends 2021. https://www.iqvia.com/insights/the-iqvia-institute/reports/digital-health-trends-2021. Accessed July 2023

Jacobs RJ, Lou JQ, Ownby RL, Caballero J (2016) A systematic review of eHealth interventions to improve health literacy. Health Inform J 22(2):81–98

Jane M, Hagger M, Foster J, Ho S, Pal S (2018) Social media for health promotion and weight management: a critical debate. BMC Public Health 18:1–7

Jensen JD, King AJ, Davis LA, Guntzviller LM (2010) Utilization of internet technology by low-income adults: the role of health literacy, health numeracy, and computer assistance. J Aging Health 22(6):804–826

Johnson D, Deterding S, Kuhn K-A, Staneva A, Stoyanov S, Hides L (2016) Gamification for health and wellbeing: a systematic review of the literature. Internet Interv 6:89–106

Kalichman S, Weinhardt L, Benotsch E, Cherry C (2002) Closing the digital divide in HIV/AIDS care: development of a theory-based intervention to increase internet access. AIDS Care 14(4):523–537

Khamzina M, Parab KV, An R, Bullard T, Grigsby-Toussaint DS (2020) Impact of Pokémon go on physical activity: a systematic review and meta-analysis. Am J Prev Med 58(2):270–282

König LM (2023) Debunking nutrition myths: An experimental test of the 'truth sandwich' text format. Brit J Health Psych 28(4):1000–1010. https://doi.org/10.1111/bjhp.12665

König LM, Sproesser G, Schupp HT, Renner B (2018) Describing the process of adopting nutrition and fitness apps: behavior stage model approach. JMIR Mhealth Uhealth 6(3):e55

König LM, Ziesemer K, Renner B (2019) Quantifying actual and perceived inaccuracy when estimating the sugar, energy content and portion size of foods. Nutrients 11(10):2425. https://doi.org/10.3390/nu11102425

König LM, Attig C, Franke T, Renner B (2021) Barriers to and facilitators for using nutrition apps: systematic review and conceptual framework. JMIR Mhealth Uhealth 9(6):e20037. https://doi.org/10.2196/20037

König LM, Schupp HT, Renner B (2024) A matter of the metric? Sugar content overestimation is less pronounced in sugar cubes versus grams. Nutrition Research 131:111–120.

König LM, Western MJ, Denton AH, Krukowski RA (2025a) Umbrella review of social inequality in digital interventions targeting dietary and physical activity behaviors. npj Digital Medicine 8(1):11.

König LM, Kanning M, Hauptmann H, Feuchtner T, Arigo D (2025b) Who is willing to play skill-adapted exergames? Influences of sociodemographic factors and social comparison processes. Computers in Human Behavior 165:108562.

Kotz J, Giese H, König LM (2023) How to debunk misinformation? An experimental online study investigating text structures and headline formats. Brit J Health Psych 28(4):1097–1112 https://doi.org/10.1111/bjhp.12670

Krukowski RA, Denton AH, & König LM (2024). Impact of feedback generation and presentation on self-monitoring behaviors, dietary intake, physical activity, and weight: a systematic review and meta-analysis. International Journal of Behavioral Nutrition and Physical Activity 21(1):3.

Laranjo L (2016) Social media and health behavior change. In: Syed-Abdul S, Gabarron E, Lau AYS (eds) Participatory health through social media. Elsevier, Amsterdam, pp 83–111

Leask CF, Sandlund M, Skelton DA, Altenburg TM, Cardon G, Chinapaw MJ, De Bourdeaudhuij I et al (2019) Framework, principles and recommendations for utilising participatory methodologies in the co-creation and evaluation of public health interventions. Res Involv Engage 5(1):1–16

Lister C, West JH, Cannon B, Sax T, Brodegard D (2014) Just a fad? Gamification in health and fitness apps. JMIR Serious Games 2(2):e3413

Lyzwinski LN, Caffery LJ, Bambling M, Edirippulige S (2018) Consumer perspectives on mHealth for weight loss: a review of qualitative studies. J Telemed Telecare 24(4):290–302

Maher CA, Lewis LK, Ferrar K, Marshall S, De Bourdeaudhuij I, Vandelanotte C (2014) Are health behavior change interventions that use online social networks effective? A systematic review. J Med Internet Res 16(2):e40

Marcu G, Ondersma SJ, Spiller AN, Broderick BM, Kadri R, Buis LR (2022) The perceived benefits of digital interventions for behavioral health: qualitative interview study. J Med Internet Res 24(3):e34300

Michie S, Abraham C, Whittington C, McAteer J, Gupta S (2009) Effective techniques in healthy eating and physical activity interventions: a meta-regression. Health Psychol 28(6):690–701. https://doi.org/10.1037/a0016136

Middelweerd A, Mollee JS, van der Wal CN, Brug J, te Velde SJ (2014) Apps to promote physical activity among adults: a review and content analysis. Int J Behav Nutr Phys 11(1):97. https://doi.org/10.1186/s12966-014-0097-9

Mingoia J, Hutchinson AD, Wilson C, Gleaves DH (2017) The relationship between social networking site use and the internalization of a thin ideal in females: a meta-analytic review. Front Psychol 8:1351

Molloy A, Ellis DM, Su L, Anderson PL (2021) Improving acceptability and uptake behavior for internet-based cognitive-behavioral therapy. Front Digit Health 3:653686

Moore M (1999) The evolution of telemedicine. Futur Gener Comput Syst 15(2):245–254

Müller AC, Wachtler B, Lampert T (2020) Digital Divide–Soziale Unterschiede in der Nutzung digitaler Gesundheitsangebote. Bundesgesundheitsblatt Gesundheitsforschung Gesundheitsschutz 63(2):185

Nahum-Shani I, Smith SN, Spring BJ, Collins LM, Witkiewitz K, Tewari A, Murphy SA (2018) Just-in-time adaptive interventions (JITAIs) in mobile health: key components and design principles for ongoing health behavior support. Ann Behav Med 52(6):446–462

Nordgreen T, Rabbi F, Torresen J, Skar YS, Guribye F, Inal Y, Flobakk E et al (2021) Challenges and possible solutions in cross-disciplinary and cross-sectorial research teams within the domain of e-mental health. J Enabl Technol 15(4):241–251

Norman CD, Skinner HA (2006) eHealth literacy: essential skills for consumer health in a networked world. J Med Internet Res 8(2):e506

Peng W, Kanthawala S, Yuan S, Hussain SA (2016) A qualitative study of user perceptions of mobile health apps. BMC Public Health 16(1):1–11

Perski O, Blandford A, West R, Michie S (2017) Conceptualising engagement with digital behaviour change interventions: a systematic review using principles from critical interpretive synthesis. Transl Behav Med 7(2):254–267

Powell A, Singh P, Torous J (2018) The complexity of mental health app privacy policies: a potential barrier to privacy. JMIR Mhealth Uhealth 6(7):e9871

Pywell J, Vijaykumar S, Dodd A, Coventry L (2020) Barriers to older adults' uptake of mobile-based mental health interventions. Digit Health 6:2055207620905422

Quintiliani LM, Whiteley JA, Murillo J, Lara R, Jean C, Quinn EK, Kane J et al (2021) Community health worker-delivered weight management intervention among public housing residents: a feasibility study. Prev Med Rep 22:101360

Rhodes A, Smith AD, Chadwick P, Croker H, Llewellyn CH (2020) Exclusively digital health interventions targeting diet, physical activity, and weight gain in pregnant women: systematic review and meta-analysis. JMIR Mhealth Uhealth 8(7):e18255

Rocha YM, de Moura GA, Desidério GA, de Oliveira CH, Lourenço FD, de Figueiredo Nicolete LD (2021) The impact of fake news on social media and its influence on health during the COVID-19 pandemic: a systematic review. J Public Health:1–10

Rodriguez Rocha NP, Kim H (2019) eHealth interventions for fruit and vegetable intake: a meta-analysis of effectiveness. Health Educ Behav 46(6):947–959

Sama PR, Eapen ZJ, Weinfurt KP, Shah BR, Schulman KA (2014) An evaluation of mobile health application tools. JMIR Mhealth Uhealth 2(2):e19. https://doi.org/10.2196/mhealth.3088

Sardi L, Idri A, Fernández-Alemán JL (2017) A systematic review of gamification in e-Health. J Biomed Inform 71:31–48

Sauermann S, Herzberg J, Burkert S, Habetha S (2022) DiGA–a chance for the German healthcare system. J Eur CME 11(1):2014047

Schliess F, Affini Dicenzo T, Gaus N, Bourez J-M, Stegbauer C, Szecsenyi J, Jacobsen M et al (2022) The German fast track toward reimbursement of digital health applications (DiGA): opportunities and challenges for manufacturers, healthcare providers, and people with diabetes. J Diabet Sci. Techn:19322968221121660

Schoeppe S, Alley S, Van Lippevelde W, Bray NA, Williams SL, Duncan MJ, Vandelanotte C (2016) Efficacy of interventions that use apps to improve diet, physical activity and sedentary behaviour: a systematic review. Int J Behav Nutr Phys 13(1):127. https://doi.org/10.1186/s12966-016-0454-y

Sediva H, Cartwright T, Robertson C, Deb SK (2022) Behavior change techniques in digital health interventions for midlife women: systematic review. JMIR Mhealth Uhealth 10(11):e37234

Sharpe EE, Karasouli E, Meyer C (2017) Examining factors of engagement with digital interventions for weight management: rapid review. JMIR Res Protoc 6(10):e6059

Short CE, DeSmet A, Woods C, Williams SL, Maher C, Middelweerd A, Müller AM et al (2018) Measuring engagement in eHealth and mHealth behavior change interventions: viewpoint of methodologies. J Med Internet Res 20(11):e292

Simblett S, Greer B, Matcham F, Curtis H, Polhemus A, Ferrão J, Gamble P, Wykes T (2018) Barriers to and facilitators of engagement with remote measurement technology for managing health: systematic review and content analysis of findings. J Med Internet Res 20(7):e10480

Simons M, Ligtenberg A, Naughton F, Murphy SA, König LM, Winkens L (2023) Personalised context-aware digital health interventions: crossing boundaries between data science, geoscience and health psychology. European Health Psychologist, 23(1):1035–1041

Siopis G, Moschonis G, Eweka E, Jung J, Kwasnicka D, Asare BY-A, Kodithuwakku V et al (2023) Effectiveness, reach, uptake, and feasibility of digital health interventions for adults with hypertension: a systematic review and meta-analysis of randomised controlled trials. Lancet Digit Health 5(3):e144–e159

Solar C, Nansubuga A, Murillo J, Ranker L, Borrelli B, Bowen DJ, Xuan Z et al (2022) Mobile health plus community health worker support for weight management among public housing residents (path to health): a randomized controlled trial protocol. Contemp Clin Trials 119:106836

Stark AL, Geukes C, Dockweiler C (2022) Digital health promotion and prevention in settings: scoping review. J Med Internet Res 24(1):e21063

Statista (2023) Most popular social networks worldwide as of January 2023, ranked by number of monthly active users https://www.statista.com/statistics/272014/global-social-networks-ranked-by-number-of-users/. Accessed 27 Feb 2023

Strain T, Brage S, Sharp SJ, Richards J, Tainio M, Ding D, Benichou J, Kelly P (2020) Use of the prevented fraction for the population to determine deaths averted by existing prevalence of physical activity: a descriptive study. Lancet Glob Health 8(7):e920–e930

Suarez-Lledo V, Alvarez-Galvez J (2021) Prevalence of health misinformation on social media: systematic review. J Med Internet Res 23(1):e17187

Sucala M, Cole-Lewis H, Arigo D, Oser M, Goldstein S, Hekler EB, Diefenbach MA (2021) Behavior science in the evolving world of digital health: considerations on anticipated opportunities and challenges. Transl Behav Med 11(2):495–503

Szinay D, Jones A, Chadborn T, Brown J, Naughton F (2020) Influences on the uptake of and engagement with health and well-being smartphone apps: systematic review. J Med Internet Res 22(5):e17572

Szinay D, Forbes CC, Busse H, DeSmet A, Smit ES, König LM (2023) Is the uptake, engagement, and effectiveness of exclusively mobile interventions for the promotion of weight-related behaviors equal for all? A systematic review. Obes Rev:e13542

The World Bank (2023) World development indicators [version: 17 February 2023]. https://datacatalog.worldbank.org/search/dataset/0037712/World-Development-Indicators. Accessed 27 Feb 2023

Turner-McGrievy GM, Yang C-H, Monroe C, Pellegrini C, West DS (2021) Is burden always bad? Emerging low-burden approaches to mobile dietary self-monitoring and the role burden plays with engagement. J Technol Behav Sci:1–9

Valmaggia LR, Latif L, Kempton MJ, Rus-Calafell M (2016) Virtual reality in the psychological treatment for mental health problems: An systematic review of recent evidence. Psychiatry Res 236:189–195

Villinger K, Wahl DR, Boeing H, Schupp HT, Renner B (2019) The effectiveness of app-based mobile interventions on nutrition behaviours and nutrition-related health outcomes: a systematic review and meta-analysis. Obes Rev 20(10):1465–1484

Virtanen L, Kaihlanen A-M, Laukka E, Gluschkoff K, Heponiemi T (2021) Behavior change techniques to promote healthcare professionals' eHealth competency: a systematic review of interventions. Int J Med Inform 149:104432

Wahl DR, Villinger K, König LM, Ziesemer K, Schupp HT, Renner B (2017) Healthy food choices are happy food choices: evidence from a real life sample using smartphone based assessments. Sci Rep 7:17069. https://doi.org/10.1038/s41598-017-17262-9

Wang L, Miller LC (2020) Just-in-the-moment adaptive interventions (JITAI): a meta-analytical review. Health Commun 35(12):1531–1544

Weinstein ND (1988) The precaution adoption process. Health Psychol 7(4):355–386. https://doi.org/10.1037/0278-6133.7.4.355

Weiß K, König LM (2022) Does the medium matter? Comparing the effectiveness of videos, podcasts and online articles in nutrition communication. Appl Psychol Health Well Being 15(2):669–685. https://doi.org/10.1111/aphw.12404

Western MJ, Armstrong ME, Islam I, Morgan K, Jones UF, Kelson MJ (2021) The effectiveness of digital interventions for increasing physical activity in individuals of low socioeconomic status: a systematic review and meta-analysis. Int J Behav Nutr Phys 18(1):1–21

Whitelaw S, Pellegrini DM, Mamas MA, Cowie M, Van Spall HG (2021) Barriers and facilitators of the uptake of digital health technology in cardiovascular care: a systematic scoping review. Eur Heart J Digit Health 2(1):62–74

Wood GM, van Boom S, Recourt K, Houwink EJ (2022) FHH quick app review: how can a quality review process assist primary care providers in choosing a family health history app for patient care? Genes 13(8):1407

World Health Organization (1986) Ottawa charter for health promotion. World Health Organization, Copenhagen

World Health Organization (2021) Global strategy on digital health 2020–2025. World Health Organization, Geneva

Wu Y-S, Wang W-Y, Chan T-C, Chiu Y-L, Lin H-C, Chang Y-T, Wu H-Y et al (2022) Effect of the Nintendo Ring Fit Adventure exergame on running completion time and psychological factors among university students engaging in distance learning during the COVID-19 pandemic: randomized controlled trial. JMIR Serious Games 10(1):e35040

Yardley L, Spring BJ, Riper H, Morrison LG, Crane DH, Curtis K, Merchant GC et al (2016) Understanding and promoting effective engagement with digital behavior change interventions. Am J Prev Med 51(5):833–842

Zhang C-Q, Zhang R, Schwarzer R, Hagger MS (2019) A meta-analysis of the health action process approach. Health Psychol 38(7):623

Open Access This chapter is licensed under the terms of the Creative Commons Attribution 4.0 International License (http://creativecommons.org/licenses/by/4.0/), which permits use, sharing, adaptation, distribution and reproduction in any medium or format, as long as you give appropriate credit to the original author(s) and the source, provide a link to the Creative Commons license and indicate if changes were made.

The images or other third party material in this chapter are included in the chapter's Creative Commons license, unless indicated otherwise in a credit line to the material. If material is not included in the chapter's Creative Commons license and your intended use is not permitted by statutory regulation or exceeds the permitted use, you will need to obtain permission directly from the copyright holder.

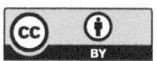

Disease Prevention, Including Early Detection of Illnesses (EPHO5)

Applying Health Equity Principles Across the Life Cycle of Digital Disease Prevention Interventions: The *GetCheckedOnline* Experience

Ihoghosa Iyamu, Devon Haag, Heather Pedersen, and Mark Gilbert

Abstract Digital public health (DiPH) interventions have been used to achieve public health disease prevention goals. As a practical example, we describe GetCheckedOnline, a publicly funded web-based testing service for sexually transmitted and blood-borne infections (STBBI) in British Columbia, Canada. This service has gained increasing relevance, especially among people experiencing marginalization who bear a disproportionate burden of STBBIs. It continues to contribute to the secondary and tertiary disease prevention of STBBIs by facilitating early diagnoses and treatment of infections, thereby disrupting their community transmission. In this chapter, we highlight the importance of applying the fundamental public health principle of health equity across the life cycle of DiPH interventions and suggest that a focus on health equity inevitably ensures the achievement of overarching disease prevention goals. We reflect on practical considerations for health equity across various phases of the planning and development, implementation, scale-up, adaptation, sustainment, and maintenance of these DiPH interventions. Further, we demonstrate the central and complementary roles that human-centered design and embedded research and evaluation play in prioritizing health equity across the phases of DiPH interventions. We also highlight key challenges encountered when implementing DiPH interventions that focus on health equity.

Keywords Digital health equity · Disease prevention · Online sexual health · Sexually transmitted and blood-borne infections · Web-based STI testing

---

I. Iyamu · M. Gilbert (✉)
School of Population and Public Health, University of British Columbia, Vancouver, BC, Canada

BC Centre for Disease Control (BCCDC), Vancouver, BC, Canada
e-mail: mark.gilbert@bccdc.ca

D. Haag · H. Pedersen
BC Centre for Disease Control (BCCDC), Vancouver, BC, Canada

Abbreviations

BC	British Columbia
BCCDC	British Columbia Centre for Disease Control
DiPH	Digital Public Health
GBMSM	Gay, Bisexual, and other Men who have Sex with Men
HCV	Hepatitis C Virus
HEIA	Health Equity Impact Assessment
NAT	Nucleic Acid Testing
PHN	Public Health Numbers
RE-AIM	Reach, Effectiveness, Adoption, Implementation and Maintenance
STBBI	Sexually Transmitted and Blood-Borne Infections
STI	Sexually Transmitted Infections

1 Introduction

Digital technologies have the potential to significantly improve public health outcomes by ensuring access to quality care services, especially among people who face challenges in timely access to "bricks and mortar" health services (World Health Organization 2021). Digital technologies can help achieve disease prevention goals by expanding access and utilization of health services that ensure early diagnosis and treatment of diseases (Budd et al. 2020; World Health Organization 2021). This is especially true for the prevention and control of sexually transmitted and blood-borne infections (STBBI) because evidence suggests that late diagnosis and delayed treatment increase the spread of infections and result in greater health systems costs (Gilbert et al. 2016; Wilson et al. 2017; Moore et al. 2021). Therefore, public health organizations have prioritized health education as a primary prevention strategy with multiple sexual health education interventions being implemented (Wadham et al. 2019). Public health organizations have also promoted routine STBBI screening based on testing recommendations, especially among populations with a higher prevalence of infections for earlier diagnosis and treatment (Gilbert et al. 2016; Moore et al. 2021). The combination of early diagnoses and treatment can be considered as secondary and tertiary prevention strategies that prevent clinical complications and further transmission of STBBIs (Moore et al. 2021). Digital technologies can facilitate efforts to limit the transmission of infections and reduce the burden of disease within communities while empowering individuals to take control of their health (Gilbert et al. 2017b).

Empowering individuals and communities is essential because STBBIs disproportionately affect communities and individuals who experience social and health inequities based on their age, race, ethnicity, gender, sexual orientation, socio-economic factors, and other social factors (Canadian Public Health Association 2014; Gilbert et al. 2019b). These equity deserving populations experience multiple barriers in accessing STBBI testing and treatment, including individual-level barriers like suboptimal knowledge of testing locations, experiences of stigma, fear of discrimination, and discomfort with healthcare professionals (Wilson et al. 2017; Gilbert et al. 2019b). Similarly, provider-level barriers like inaccurate healthcare provider perceptions of risk and discomfort with questions about sexual behaviors have been noted in addition to health system-level factors present in clinics and healthcare like unavailability of appropriate sexual health services, prolonged wait times, limited clinic hours and travel requirements to access testing (Gilbert et al. 2016, 2019b). Given that current recommendations for STBBI screening and linkage to treatment rely mainly on opportunistic screening in clinical settings like primary health care, these barriers continue to be perpetuated for those most in need, who may not readily access these clinical settings (Moore et al. 2021).

Digital public health (DiPH) interventions have been implemented assuming that they circumvent barriers in accessing clinic-based STBBI testing, thereby promoting *health equity* (Spielberg et al. 2014; Gilbert et al. 2017b; Kersaudy-Rahib et al. 2017; Wilson et al. 2017). For example, web-based testing services that do not require a clinician's consultation and laboratory requisition (Gilbert et al. 2017b), online self-sample collection and postal (Wilson et al. 2017), and online supervised self-testing services have gained popularity in recent years (Anand et al. 2017). We define health equity as the absence of systematic, avoidable, and unjust differences in the health of groups and communities occupying unequal positions in society that are determined by the conditions in which people are born, grow, live, work, and age (Solar and Irwin 2010). Despite health equity being an underpinning focus of many DiPH interventions, practitioners are realizing that digital technologies may in themselves reinforce existing health inequities and even create new inequities if attention is not paid to health equity during the planning, implementation, and evaluation of these interventions (Crawford and Serhal 2020; Rodriguez et al. 2020; World Health Organization 2021; Gómez-Ramírez et al. 2021b; Lyles et al. 2021). For example, multiple DiPH interventions have only benefited those with access to digital technologies, including smartphones and stable internet services (Rodriguez et al. 2020; Iyamu et al. 2023b).

1.1 Digital Health Equity as an Emerging Field of Public Health Interest

Interest in ensuring health equity in digital health interventions only started around 2009 (Iyamu et al. 2021). This interest in digital health equity heightened during the COVID-19 pandemic as digital technologies were implemented at scale across the healthcare sector in attempts to address disruptions in access to health services resulting from public health restrictions (Crawford and Serhal 2020; Rodriguez et al. 2020; Gómez-Ramírez et al. 2021b). The discourse on digital health equity has primarily focused on two main areas, including differential *digital access* (i.e., access to digital technologies—more commonly referred to as the "digital divide") and differential *digital health literacy*, which is used to refer to systematic differences in people's ability to seek, appraise and understand digital information, and act on the information to improve their health status (Rodriguez et al. 2020; Lawrence 2022). More recently, the term *"digital determinants of health"* has been used to refer to people's capacities and experiences with digital technologies that affect their health and health risks and their ability to use and benefit from digital health ecosystems (Crawford and Serhal 2020; Lawrence 2022; Richardson et al. 2022).

Few theoretical models have been developed to explain digital health equity (Antonio and Petrovskaya 2019; Crawford and Serhal 2020). The digital health equity framework draws on Dover and Belon's health equity framework (DHEF) to describe multi-level factors that explain the intended and unintended health equity impacts of digital interventions (Crawford and Serhal 2020). The DHEF describes systemic and social contexts that influence equity in digital health interventions. The intersection of race, gender, sexual orientation, and other health equity factors effectively determine the social location of potential digital health users, influencing the impact that health, social policies, and health care resourcing (i.e., health system factors) can have on them. Intermediate user-level factors, including health beliefs and behaviors and risk appraisal, are often determined by a user's social location. This location also determines their material circumstances, which in turn influence *digital determinants of health*, including access to digital technologies, use patterns and habits with digital technologies, and digital skills, including digital literacy, confidence, and self-efficacy. Additional digital determinants of health include users' beliefs and attitudes towards digital technologies (for example, their perception of its usability and usefulness), trust, and experiences with technological bias. These digital determinants of health differentially influence users' uptake of digital interventions. The complexity of this process emphasizes the need to apply equity-focused perspectives during the design, implementation, and evaluation of DiPH interventions (Lyles et al. 2021; Lee et al. 2022).

Many have called for a socio-ecological approach to designing and implementing DiPH interventions. This approach considers the contexts in which populations experiencing marginalization engage with digital technologies and how previously described multi-level factors may interact to address, propagate, or create new health inequities through the interventions (Lyles et al. 2021; Lee et al. 2022). Considerations for DiPH interventions must extend beyond usability testing at the individual level to include design and implementation dimensions for multiple contexts (Gómez-Ramírez et al. 2021b; Lyles et al. 2022). Such considerations must blend digital and in-person supports, leveraging human-centered design and codesign principles within communities of interest, that demonstrate the effectiveness of the interventions at a population and systems level (Gómez-Ramírez et al. 2021b; Iyamu et al. 2022; Lee et al. 2022). Advocacy efforts must also facilitate expanded access to broadband internet technologies, digital devices, accessibility standards, and reimbursement strategies to foster equitable access to digital public health interventions (Crawford and Serhal 2020; Lyles et al. 2021; Iyamu et al. 2022).

Summarily, these recommendations call for a holistic view of how we design, implement, and evaluate digital public health interventions with a clear focus on fostering equitable public health outcomes.

In this chapter, we use an equity lens to reflect on our experiences of planning, designing, implementing, adapting, scaling up, and maintaining a DiPH disease prevention service called GetCheckedOnline in British Columbia (BC), Canada (Farrell 2012; Gilbert et al. 2016). We draw on our experiences and perspectives operating in dual roles as public health implementers and applied public health researchers with a focus on digital health equity. We highlight practical strategies that can promote equitable outcomes for digital public health interventions. Here, we refer to DiPH interventions as interventions that address at least one of the essential public health functions using digital technologies (Wienert et al. 2021). Our description of GetCheckedOnline aligns with this definition, given that it addresses the vertical public health function of disease prevention through early STBBI diagnosis and treatment. However, we acknowledge the interrelationship between public health and primary health care services and the potential confusion between these fields of practice, especially in relation to digital health. We situate our work at the intersection of public health and primary care functions, including disease screening, early preventive interventions, and advocacy for healthy communities, equity, and access (Levesque et al. 2013). Our position is that adopting a central focus on health equity in digital disease prevention programs to promote early diagnoses and prevention of STBBIs, inevitably addresses public health prevention goals (Gómez-Ramírez et al. 2021c).

2 An Introduction to GetCheckedOnline as a Digital Disease Prevention Service and its Foundational Strategies

2.1 GetCheckedOnline—A Digital Disease Prevention Service

GetCheckedOnline was launched as Canada's first publicly funded comprehensive internet-based testing service by the British Columbia Centre for Disease Control (BCCDC) in 2014 and offers testing for chlamydia, gonorrhea, syphilis, HIV, and hepatitis C virus (HCV). Its three main objectives are to: (1) increase the uptake and frequency of STBBI testing and early diagnosis; (2) reach populations with greater prevalence of STBBIs and those facing barriers to testing; (3) increase the capacity of the STI clinic services and improve the use of clinician resources (by diverting asymptomatic screening to online testing) (Gilbert et al. 2016, 2017a). Additionally, GetCheckedOnline's implementers embedded research and evaluation throughout all phases of program implementation. This decision aimed to facilitate evidence-informed action in developing a novel program and knowledge generation in a field without many comparable programs at the time of its development. Currently, GetCheckedOnline provides access to free online STBBI testing in nine cities in BC (large urban, urban, and rural). The program model has been described in detail elsewhere (Gilbert et al. 2016). Summarily, to access online STBBI testing through GetCheckedOnline, users create an account, complete a risk assessment and consent to testing, download the laboratory requisition form, visit a partner laboratory to submit specimens (including blood, urine, and swab), and receive results online (if negative) or by phone (if any of STBBI tests are positive) with linkage to appropriate treatment services being facilitated virtually by public health nurses at BCCDC (Fig. 1) (Gilbert et al. 2016). This current program model has evolved from the original model designed during the planning and development of GetCheckedOnline (Hottes et al. 2012). For example, the current model includes options for collecting throat and rectal swab specimens, supports the use of mobile devices through responsive design, and uses 2D barcodes on electronic lab requisitions that can be scanned to auto-populate the laboratory information system at the point of specimen collection, among other user-experience and design improvements to the model.

Since its launch, there has been growth in the number of users accessing STBBI tests through GetCheckedOnline. Between September 2014 and December 2023, over 75,000 online accounts had been created, over 72,000 tests had been completed, and over 6600 positive infections (including 3500 chlamydia, 235 syphilis and 23 HIV) were diagnosed through GetCheckedOnline. After a short initial decline in March 2020 resulting from the COVID-19 pandemic restrictions, GetCheckedOnline's userbase has increased significantly, and its share of all STBBI tests in communities where it is available increased up to 15% higher than prepandemic trends (Iyamu et al. 2023a).

2.2 A Health Equity-Focused Approach across the Life Cycle of the GetCheckedOnline.com Project

Although the idea of health equity was implied in GetCheckedOnline's objective to reach populations with a greater prevalence of STBBIs and those facing barriers to testing, the focus on digital health equity as a defining principle of the program evolved over time. During the planning and development phase, we identified the need for a health equity framing of the program to ensure both the program's intended and unintended consequences improved outcomes, especially for people experiencing marginalization (Farrell 2012). This made sense considering the burden of STBBIs was more in this population. Over the years, our embedded research and evaluation findings have highlighted the need to apply a health-equity lens in planning, implementing, and evaluating DiPH interventions.

The overwhelming majority of DiPH interventions have been implemented as pilot projects or as vertical interventions in research contexts, with little to no integration with existing health systems (Huang et al. 2017; Iyamu et al. 2022). There have been calls to develop digital public health interventions at a scale that ensures

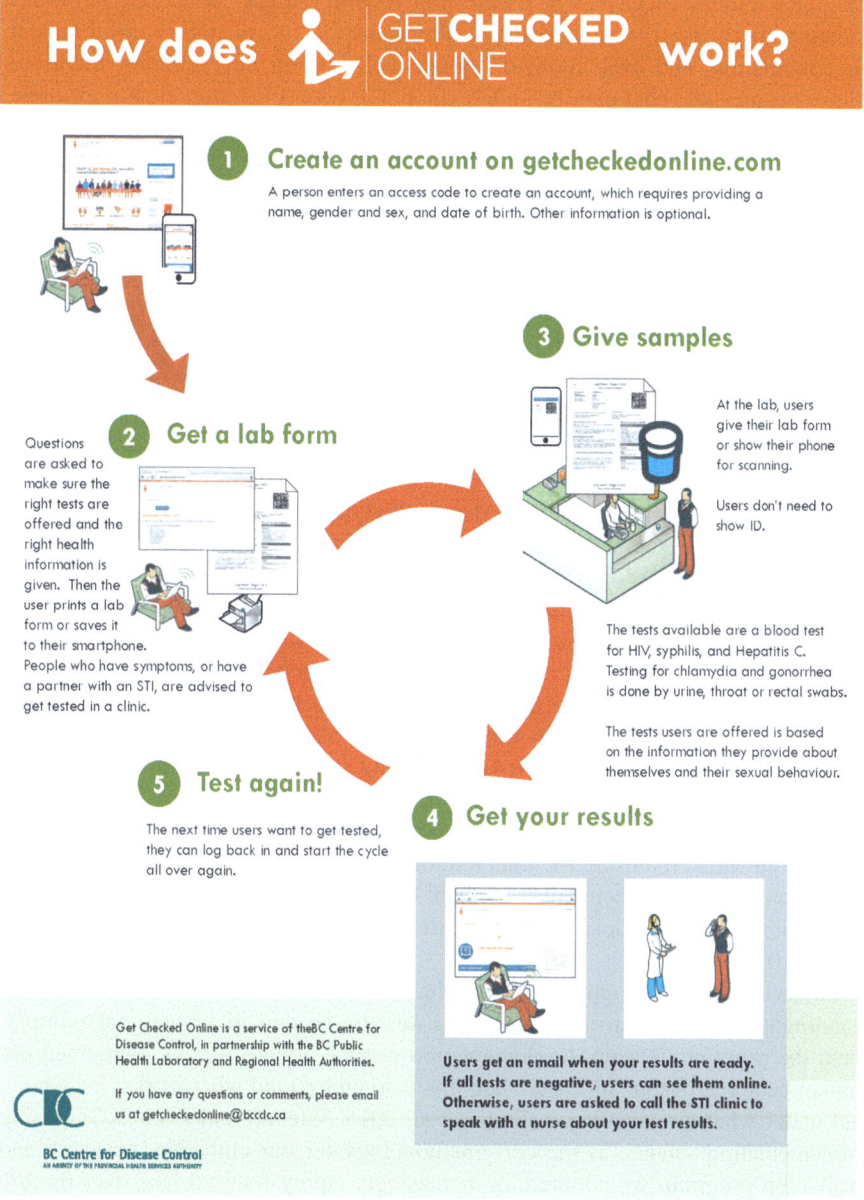

Fig. 1 How does GetCheckedOnline work? (Source: BC Centre for Disease Control)

public health benefits (Iyamu et al. 2022). GetCheckedOnline is a digital public health intervention that was designed and planned for implementation at scale. It has successfully spanned the initial implementation and scale-up phases and is now integrated into the BCCDC's STBBI testing system. Using GetCheckedOnline as a demonstrative case for considering health equity in the planning, development, implementation, and evaluation of digital public health interventions, therefore, allows perspectives that may be underexplored in other pilot studies. For example, considering the implementation of digital public health interventions at scale implies that practitioners must consider challenges to scale up and sustain DiPH interventions.

2.2.1 Promoting Health Equity Through a Foundation of Human-Centered Design and Implementation Science

It is important to highlight foundational factors that have reinforced the central focus on health equity for GetCheckedOnline. Throughout this program, human-centered design and implementation science have played fundamental, consistent, and complementary roles in ensuring that GetCheckedOnline remains attuned to the needs of those requiring the service the most. Human-centered design is a systematic approach to systems design and development that emphasizes a deep understanding of users, user needs, challenges, and contexts with the aim of creating interactive systems that are more usable and effective (Giacomin 2014; Roberts et al. 2016). The key features of human-centered design include the adoption of interdisciplinary skills and perspectives, explicit understanding of users, tasks and environments, user-centered evaluation-driven design, holistic consideration of user experience, involvement of users throughout design and development, and iterative design approaches (Giacomin 2014). Designing DiPH interventions based on the needs of those requiring these interventions may ensure its uptake and facilitate health equity goals. Therefore, human-centered design and co-design approaches are recommended to ensure the interventions draw on and appeal to the lived realities of potential users (Vechakul et al. 2015; UNICEF Health Section Implementation Research and Delivery Science Unit and the Office of Innovation Global Innovation Centre 2018).

An evidence-based approach to implementing GetCheckedOnline and understanding its impact on various populations was also needed, given our goal to implement the program at scale. Implementation science effectively complemented our human-centered design approach, helping us to understand what works, for whom, and under what circumstances (Bauer et al. 2015; Wienert and Zeeb 2021) Using implementation science as the core methodology for our embedded research and evaluation program, we adopted an increasingly equity-focused lens over the life cycle of GetCheckedOnline. We applied an interdisciplinary approach involving various research and provider disciplines while engaging stakeholders and potential users throughout the process. This process involved continuous and systematic evaluations using robust mixed methods research that integrated quantitative and qualitative data (Gilbert et al. 2016). We also established a public health-research partnership between BCCDC program implementers and researchers at the Youth Sexual Health Team at the University of British Columbia, which was influential in leading to our integrated research and evaluation approach from the outset of the planning and development process (Shoveller and Gilbert 2013). This also contributed to our use of an integrated knowledge translation model (i.e., where knowledge translation principles are applied to the entire research process, with the involvement of knowledge users as equal partners) (Gilbert et al. 2016; Boland et al. 2020).

Finally, GetCheckedOnline was positioned as a complementary service to clinic-based STBBI testing (i.e., a virtual extension of low-barrier sexual health clinics). This positioning was key to the design of GetCheckedOnline. For instance, GetCheckedOnline was designed to closely mimic in-person testing, including the use of similar screening questions and test requisition processes across systems. It also follows guidelines for practice in STBBI testing and management, facilitating follow-up through the central STI clinic for people with positive test results. Our approach to implementation and scale-up emphasized the importance of in-person and digital options in facilitating access to STBBI testing among underserved people.

2.3 Health Equity-Focused Work Across each Implementation Phase of a Digital Disease Prevention Program

Figure 2 describes the life cycle of GetCheckedOnline to date. We describe three sequential phases, including the planning and development phase, initial implementation (synonymous with pilot phases in other contexts), and the scale-up of the service. In addition, we describe three concurrent phases implemented after the planning and development phases, which span the project's life cycle. These include the project's adaptation, maintenance, and sustainability phases, which are also central to its health equity goals.

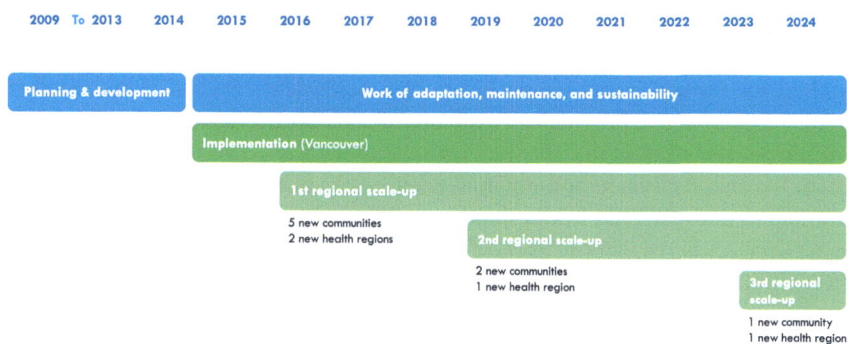

Fig. 2 Implementation phases of GetCheckedOnline (Source: GetCheckedOnline)

2.3.1 Planning and Development—2009 to 2013

Other authors have described principles of digital health design for underserved populations and the human-centered design approach that espouses equitable design of interventions, all of which were evident in our work (UNICEF Health Section Implementation Research and Delivery Science Unit and the Office of Innovation Global Innovation Centre 2018; Lee et al. 2022). Our descriptions of the steps taken during the planning and implementation phase to promote health equity largely align with these principles.

Step 1: Identifying and Consulting with Stakeholder Groups and Potential Users

We established a community consultation working group that served in an external advisory capacity and consisted of community organizations working in sexual health and STBBI prevention. It was important that the community advisory group consisted of people with lived experiences of marginalization and disparate barriers in accessing STBBI testing. This group would support GetCheckedOnline's governance by highlighting community perspectives to inform pragmatic adaptations to promote health equity.

Step 2: Understanding and Responding to User Needs

In keeping with the human-centered design approach, we consulted with potential users of the service through three research studies with youth, gay, bisexual, and other men who have sex with men (GBMSM) and STI clinic clients (identified as groups who may experience challenges accessing testing). We found high acceptability of the service but concerns about privacy and security, as well as anxiety about receiving positive results (Shoveller et al. 2012; Hottes et al. 2012; Gilbert et al. 2013). We elicited suggestions for mitigating these concerns, which were then implemented in the development phase. For example, we described the security measures of the website upfront, restricted data collection only to information required for testing while making other data fields like city and phone numbers optional for users, and provided an explicit rationale for the data being collected and how it would be used in the service's privacy policy and terms of use (Hottes et al. 2012). We also facilitated non-nominal testing (i.e., testing without using real user information and personal health numbers). This ensured the perception of a low-barrier service. In response to user concerns about receiving adequate support when receiving positive STBBI test results, we designed the system to send discrete email notifications to clients with links to access results on the service portal if the results were negative. Positive test results would only be provided over phone calls made to the user by public health nurses. Finally, we highlighted the privacy and convenience of GetCheckedOnline and its delivery by the BCCDC in promotional efforts to boost user confidence.

Step 3: Conducting a Health Equity Impact Assessment

Critiques of digital health have highlighted the role of technological optimism and determinism in perpetuating health inequities (i.e., overly enthusiastic implementation of technologies as the singular way to improve health outcomes) (McIntyre 2003; Gómez-Ramírez et al. 2021b). To mitigate this challenge, we conducted a preliminary health equity impact assessment (HEIA), a process and tool that helps policymakers, programs, and organizations understand how their programs or initiatives will impact different population groups (Canadian Public Health Association 2014). Through our HEIA, we identified ways that GetCheckedOnline could reinforce or create health inequities, especially for historically underserved populations disparately affected by STBBIs. For example, the HEIA explored concerns about GetCheckedOnline only reaching cisgender and downtown Vancouver populations that already had access to STBBI testing (Farrell 2012). Therefore, we collected additional information on ethnicity and gender identity to track uptake among various populations while avoiding normative and stigmatizing language and images.

Step 4: Redesigning the Informed Consent Process

Another equity consideration was to ensure that consent to use the service was truly informed. For most digital health services, the consent process is viewed as another short step toward accessing services in what is sometimes referred to as "click and go" models (Gilbert et al. 2017a). Users also expressed concerns about the comprehensiveness of pretest counseling, emphasizing their need to be fully aware of the services they are consenting to (Hottes et al. 2012). Through our human-centered design approach, we created alternative informed consent processes. First, we reviewed the existing policies and guidelines to determine the core requirements for informed consent. Then, we created reframed versions of informed consent forms with short summary statements that users had to attest to (using checkboxes). Additional information was provided as drop-down content if needed. We conducted usability tests to understand how users appraised the revised process. We found that using checkboxes to disrupt the routinization of informed consent helped users focus on the essential information needed to provide consent. Our simple framing of consent statements and additional explanations ensured that users with lower literacy levels and internet access were not excluded (Gilbert et al. 2017a).

2.3.2 Initial Implementation 2014 and Onwards

Step 5: Focusing Initial Efforts on Populations with a Higher Prevalence of STBBIs

Starting in 2014, we implemented GetCheckedOnline in Vancouver (our "pilot") with a focus on reaching GBMSM. This step was informed by evidence that this population disparately experienced barriers to clinic-based STBBI testing compared to the general population. We used the initial uptake of the service as a proof of concept of its acceptability and feasibility (Gilbert et al. 2016). One of the ways we promoted the service was through social marketing campaigns focusing on GBMSM in Vancouver. Early during the program, our evaluation found that GetCheckedOnline users were more likely to be GBMSM who had previously delayed testing due to more frequent experiences of STBBI testing access barriers (Gilbert et al. 2019b). This demonstrated the early health equity impacts of the program in addition to its feasibility.

Step 6: Using an Evidence-Informed Approach to Guide the Initial Implementation

Our integrated research approach also helped us compare the impacts of different social marketing strategies, including promotions through local advertisements in print or video displayed at gay venues or events, ads on queer news websites, and ads on social media websites and apps (Gilbert et al. 2019a). We found that online ads were not the most cost-effective way of gaining new and diverse users to the service, despite general perceptions of their usefulness in promoting digital disease prevention interventions, and these were stopped.

2.3.3 Scale-Up

Until the COVID-19 pandemic in 2020, only a few DiPH interventions were implemented at scale. GetCheckedOnline's scale-up began in 2016. Scale-up refers to our process of expanding the geographic reach of GetCheckedOnline by introducing the service to new geographic regions in partnership with BC health authorities.

Step 7: Using Available Evidence to Guide and Evaluate Equity-Focused Scale-Up

During the scale-up, we used integrated implementation science approaches to understand how communities were taking up these digital services, what sociodemographic groups benefited most, and what additional communities would be best served by our expansion strategy. Communities for scale-up were chosen by partnering health authorities based on local surveillance and testing data and the availability of in-person testing services. We conducted community surveys among GBMSM to understand the awareness of and intention to use GetCheckedOnline in communities where the service was available to tailor promotional efforts (Dulai et al. 2021).

The second scale-up phase was also informed by analyses of regional differences in the barriers that STBBI testers faced within each of the first phase communities. The analyses revealed generalized barriers in testing with no significant differences in the barriers experienced in each community (Ablona et al. 2019b). However, positivity rates for STBBIs were high, with testers reporting STBBI risk factors including condomless sex with multiple partners and younger age, suggesting that the scale-up of the service was reaching those most in need of STBBI testing (Ablona et al. 2019c).

2.3.4 Adaptation, Maintenance, and Sustainability Phases

We consider the adaptation, maintenance, and sustainability phases of GetCheckedOnline to be conceptually distinct but overlapping, occurring concurrently across the implementation period after the initial planning and development phase. We describe equity-focused steps taken across these three phases, referring to the most relevant steps in each phase.

Adaptation

The adaptation phase describes our commitment to continuously modifying GetCheckedOnline's features in response to ongoing needs and feedback from users, health providers, and implementers using our evaluation and research findings. This phase also reflects our commitment to human-centered design's key characteristic of iteration, following cycles of empathizing with users (generating evidence to understand user needs within the context), defining the core problems, ideating to find potential solutions, prototyping and testing solutions (Giacomin 2014). Our integrated implementation science approach complemented the human-centered design approach, ensuring that ongoing adaptation remained evidence-informed, responsive to the context, and equity-focused. Some adaptations to promote health equity are described below.

Step 8: Introducing Self-Collected Rectal and Throat Swab Sampling

Rectal and throat swabs were initially planned to be introduced to the service over time in keeping with best practices. However, this process was accelerated based on feedback from healthcare providers who expressed concerns about the clinical safety of GetCheckedOnline with missed infections. Therefore, we introduced self-collected rectal and throat swabs in addition to urine nucleic acid testing (NAT) for gonorrhea and chlamydia. GetCheckedOnline was adapted to recommend rectal swabs for GBMSM who reported receptive anal sex in the past 3 months, while GBMSM reporting giving oral sex in the past 3 months had throat swabs recommended as part of their package of tests. Our analyses of the data in 2018 revealed that approximately 75% of chlamydia and gonorrhea infections among GBMSM would have been missed if rectal and throat swabs were not included during the adaptation (Ablona et al. 2019a).

Step 9: Fostering an Inclusive and Equitable Digital Public Health Intervention

Additional changes were made to promote inclusion and equity on GetCheckedOnline. For instance, in designing instructional materials for self-collected rectal swabs, we explored existing examples of clinical instructions and how they may be perceived as biased and exclusionary to people who historically experience marginalization (Farrell et al. 2015). We consulted with users and developed new clinical instruction materials that used more inclusive language and imagery. The resulting materials were assessed as more inclusive in user testing (Farrell et al. 2015). The work of adapting GetCheckedOnline to foster inclusion is constant, and needs may change over time. For example, account creation questions related to gender and sex have evolved in relation to user feedback and a robust engagement and consultation process with trans and gender-diverse people, communities, and organizations. GetCheckedOnline was also included in the Making Space Project, an initiative undertaken by BCCDC's Clinical Prevention Services division to improve the Indigenous cultural safety of our clinical and online services. Other planned adaptations to foster inclusion include considerations for minority language populations (Cantonese, Mandarin, and Punjabi speaking) and the incorporation of self-collected specimen kits to reach people who face testing barriers and do not live in a city with a referral laboratory. The ongoing nature of this work reemphasizes the importance of iteration in promoting health equity through DiPH interventions.

Step 10: Eliminating Paper-Based Laboratory Requisitions

While the laboratories and health systems routinely rely on paper-based and faxed requisitions, users reported that the requirement for printed requisitions introduced an additional access barrier. Therefore, we adapted to allow lab requisitions to be presented on users' mobile phones. This was the first time that referral laboratories allowed testing without paper-based requisitions. Further, we included 2D codes that allowed laboratory staff to auto-populate their laboratory information systems with user-provided information on the requisition forms from GetCheckedOnline.

Maintenance

In terms of maintenance, which we use to describe ongoing operations required to run GetCheckedOnline, key steps were taken to foster health equity, some of which required adaptations of the service itself.

Step 11: Ensuring Human Resource Capacity to Run GetCheckedOnline

While GetCheckedOnline seems to ease STBBI testing from users' perspectives, some of the burden was transferred to the health workers running the service. Additional time was required from public health nurses and clinic staff to facilitate administrative tasks exceeding the time that would have been required for clinic-based STBBI testing. Tasks like manual data entry became relevant due to interoperability conflicts between GetCheckedOnline and the laboratory information systems. This remains an ongoing challenge that is further complicated by GetCheckOnline's decision not to collect Public Health Numbers (PHN)—the unique identifier relevant to the province's single-payer health system. PHN collection was excluded to allay user concerns about privacy and ensure low-barrier testing (Hottes et al. 2012). An alphanumeric code (i.e., a QQ sign-up code linked to user email addresses) generated by GetCheckedOnline was used instead to identify users and ensure non-nominal testing, while healthcare providers were assigned the responsibility of transferring records (i.e., test results) from the laboratory information system to the GetCheckedOnline platform. Excluding PHN collection and the resulting interoperability challenges is an example of how design choices promoting health equity may constitute a barrier to integrated services.

Step 12: Adapting to Organizational Information Technology Standards while Maintaining Equitable Access to STBBI Testing

One feature that users needed was the ability to review their STBBI testing history through GetCheckedOnline, requiring retention of user health records. To meet enterprise security requirements while providing users access to testing history, two-step security verification measures were added as an optional feature for users to further secure their accounts. Implementers had to find a low-barrier solution to ensure that all users, especially those with low levels of digital literacy and those with unstable internet or mobile-only access, continued to have good experiences with the service. This represented one of many adaptations of organizational requirements and processes to allow for an iterative approach to GetCheckedOnline's implementation that ensured that the health equity focus of the program remained intact.

Sustainability

The sustainability phase refers to our efforts to ensure the sustainment of the service over the medium and long term and is a phase that is not well evaluated in the DiPH literature. During this phase, our primary concerns were managing challenges and maintaining a balance between continued equitable scale-up of the service and ensuring sustainable funding of the service.

Step 13: Collecting Personal Health Numbers

As described, GetCheckedOnline was designed not to collect PHNs to maintain a low-barrier and equity-serving approach to testing. However, our post-implementation research demonstrated that a majority of GetCheckedOnline clients are comfortable using their PHN to test. Including the option to provide a PHN has been identified as a key strategy to improve sustainability by permitting testing to be conducted at a broader range of laboratories and enhancing integration with primary care and with clinical and laboratory information systems. Our team is currently engaging with private and public laboratory stakeholders to understand how the inclusion of PHNs might work. We have also planned to engage users and other stakeholders to communicate changes and to generate strategies to foster users' trust in the platform despite PHN collection.

Step 14: Adding Options to Self-Collect STBBI Test Specimens

GetCheckedOnline's current model requires in-person visits to local laboratories for urine and serology specimen collection, which is a barrier for people in rural and remote communities, given their longer travel times and higher costs of accessing laboratories (Shoveller et al. 2009; Iyamu et al. 2024). Online postal sexually transmitted infection services have been implemented in other jurisdictions to bridge gaps in access in similar contexts (Wilson et al. 2017, 2019). Our preliminary stakeholder and user engagements have suggested that self-collection of samples is highly acceptable to sexual health clinics and GetCheckedOnline clients. We are doing more work to identify appropriate and sustainable strategies to facilitate the integration of the self-collection of STBBI test specimens with GetCheckedOnline, especially for rural and remote communities.

Across the adaptation, maintenance, and sustainability phases, additional research and evaluation work is being undertaken to understand how users are experiencing the service. For example, we are exploring user behaviors on the website using clickstream data (i.e., data tracking time spent on the website and elements of the website that users interact with) (Moe and Fader 2004). Of particular interest is understanding the experiences of people who experience missed opportunities on the GetCheckedOnline website (i.e., those who have the intention to test when using the website but do not complete the testing process). Evidence from this work may inform further adaptation of the web experience to optimize outcomes for those most in need of the service.

Digital health equity in disease prevention is an evolving field. Some health equity goals and adaptations for GetCheckedOnline have yet to be implemented. We still encounter challenges securing funding to expand GetCheckedOnline to more underserved communities. This highlights the need for concurrent financial planning while planning and implementing digital disease prevention interventions. We have also experienced challenges increasing awareness about the service among underserved sub-populations, especially those without access to healthcare providers and our usual promotion channels. We have found that awareness of GetCheckedOnline is associated with having connections to the gay community and access to a provider (not priority groups for raising awareness as most are expected to have access to testing already) (Dulai et al. 2021). Moreover, GetCheckedOnline is only available in English, in select communities, and to people with some level of digital literacy despite multiple adaptations. These challenges hint at the need to critically explore the impacts of the service beyond traditional program metrics like the number of service users and other similar metrics.

3 Advancing Digital Health Equity Across the Life Cycle of Digital Disease Prevention Interventions: Lessons Learned

Most DiPH prevention interventions have been implemented as pilot programs, often in specific circumstances that may not be representative of real-world contexts (Huang et al. 2017). Further, many have not considered health equity as a core component of the design, implementation, and evaluation process for these digital public health interventions. In this chapter, we have drawn on our experience of implementing GetCheckedOnline, including and beyond the initial design and implementation phases, to include the scale-up, adaptation, maintenance, and sustainability of this digital public health intervention on a provincial level. We have also highlighted the importance of adapting human-centered design and integrated research and evaluation approaches that leverage implementation science in promoting health equity as a foundational principle of public health through digital tools (Canadian Public Health Association et al. 2017). We posit that this central focus on health equity is one key distinguishing factor between digital health and DiPH interventions. For digital disease prevention interventions like GetCheckedOnline, significant resources, including manpower, financing, and effort, must be dedicated to upholding this principle, particularly when integrated within health systems that are potentially siloed. Below we summarize key lessons we have learned regarding equity considerations over the life cycle of an intervention.

1. Integrate health equity considerations early in the planning and development of DiPH interventions: To achieve equitable outcomes, health equity considerations must not be an afterthought. For example, the global health sector strategy on HIV, hepatitis, and sexually transmitted infections recommends defining the

populations most affected by STBBIs and reaching them with more precise strategies that prioritize equity (World Health Organization 2022). This focus on health equity is reflected in most disease prevention programs, and our experience suggests that it applies to digital disease prevention interventions, which must reach populations at the lower end of the social gradient. Early and ongoing health equity considerations can inform strategies to engage the right stakeholders and identify opportunities for equitable scale-up and program sustainment, program financing, and evaluation. These considerations can also dissuade technologically deterministic and optimistic implementation of digital disease prevention programs (Gómez-Ramírez et al. 2021b). Rather, these considerations guide implementers to understand the short- and long-term impacts of their interventions across social gradients and inform proactive steps to address inequities. The use of HEIAs is one effective way to stimulate these conversations, as it helped our team highlight health equity issues to address during the initial planning and development.
2. Ensuring DiPH interventions achieve equitable outcomes requires significant and ongoing resourcing and planning: Adequate resourcing must be allocated towards efforts and strategies to promote health equity through DiPH interventions. As we have described, human resources, materials, and equipment are required to conduct repeated exploratory research cycles to understand users and their contexts and support service adaptation to meet users' needs, especially those most affected by STBBIs. Resources are also required to make organizational changes that facilitate the iterative approach to improving the service, particularly within health organizations that are perhaps slower and less amenable to change than is necessary to foster health equity. In our case, additional funding for some of this work was obtained through research grants and other partnerships. Early health equity considerations will allow implementers to identify resources to support this process.
3. Human-centered design principles can engender digital health equity: Digital health equity can be achieved by grounding the design of interventions in users' realities, ensuring usability and pleasant experiences of the intervention among populations most affected by the disease (Lawrence 2022). The WHO's people-centered approach supports this view and seeks to organize health systems around the needs of people and communities to increase efficiency and patient engagement. The human-centered design of DiPH interventions involves considering digital access through low-barrier technological interventions that sometimes require adaptation of organizational systems. For example, creating simplified low-barrier login systems required the revision of our organizational data protocols. Human-centered design also involves considering digital literacy, other digital determinants of health, and perceptions of the service among people who historically have experienced marginalization and fear discrimination even through digital intervention (Lawrence 2022). Human-centered design addresses this concern through iteration and refinement based on learnings about users, their tasks, and contexts.

4. Equity-focused research and evaluation complement human-centered design to promote digital health equity: We found that integrating equity-focused research and evaluation complements human-centered design by fostering a rigorous exploration of user contexts. Embedding equity-focused research and evaluation allows DiPH interventions to understand how diverse users are experiencing the intervention and potentially mitigate inequities that the intervention may create or reinforce. New solutions may be designed and tested to assuage equity concerns while improving the efficiency of DiPH interventions, especially in the context of disease prevention. For instance, our decision to accelerate the integration of throat and rectal swabs with clear and friendly instructions, based on stakeholder and user feedback, reduced the likelihood of excluding specific populations. Further, it is important to consider health equity outcomes in addition to demonstrating overall efficacy or effectiveness during evaluation. Our experience of using implementation science frameworks in engendering health equity-focused approaches corroborates recommendations for frameworks, like the Reach, Effectiveness, Adoption, Implementation, and Maintenance (RE-AIM) framework, which can demonstrate health equity impacts of digital health interventions in real-world contexts (Lawrence 2022).
5. Interdisciplinary perspectives are crucial in developing, implementing, and evaluating DiPH interventions to promote health equity: We have previously noted the importance of interdisciplinary perspectives and partnerships in developing effective DiPH interventions (Iyamu et al. 2022). Similarly, these interdisciplinary perspectives and skills (including health psychology, community-based research, institutional ethnography, sociology, etc.) are needed to design evaluations that appropriately identify and highlight issues affecting important subpopulations. Facilitating these perspectives will require the implementers to create partnerships that ensure the complementarity of skillsets and experiences (Iyamu et al. 2022). Our partnerships with research groups helped establish the integrated research and evaluation program to inform the development of GetCheckedOnline using human-centered design principles. Such partnerships should also consider technical (information technology) skills, as integrating these skills within the implementing team may represent a significant learning curve (Gómez-Ramírez et al. 2021a). Other experts have recommended that considerations for team building must consider the diverse experiences of the team to promote equity (Lawrence 2022).

Overall, our lessons align with Lee et al.'s proposed five key principles to ensure optimized usability through human-centered design considerations for digital health interventions while paying attention to the wider socio-ecological contexts in which these digital public health interventions are being experienced by target populations (Lee et al. 2022). These principles include developing a strategic road map to address communication inequalities; engaging multiple stakeholders throughout the program; designing with usability (i.e., readability and navigability) in mind; building privacy safeguards into digital health interventions and communicating privacy-utility trade-offs in simplicity; and striving for an optimal balance between open science aspirations and protection of underserved groups. We found that close consideration of users' social context implies more thoughtful planning, implementation, and evaluation of digital public health interventions to promote equitable outcomes (Baumann and Ylinen 2017).

4 Conclusion

DiPH interventions have only recently gained traction, especially with their increased prominence during the COVID-19 pandemic, and this explains the suboptimal attention to health equity within these interventions. To effectively address public health goals of disease prevention, DiPH interventions must prioritize health equity as this position can help them more effectively reach populations most in need of services. Through our experiences, we have identified specific strategies that can engender health equity and suggest that health equity must not be an afterthought for DiPH interventions. Early considerations for health equity, ensuring complementary integration of human-centered design and research and evaluation, and promoting interdisciplinary perspectives through health equity-focused partnerships can help DiPH interventions live up to their potential, especially in the context of disease prevention. The work to produce GetcheckedOnline has been a long and hard labor of love from a large team of people, too numerous to mention, who are deeply passionate about improving sexual health equity using digital technology. Specifically, we would like to acknowledge the contributions of the GetCheckedOnline operations team, which has demonstrated a constant desire to learn and adapt the program to foster health equity. We would also like to appreciate the input of the GetCheckedOnline research team, whose various contributions have provided the insight necessary to write this book chapter.

References

Ablona A, Grennan T, Hart T et al (2019a) The impact of including throat and rectal swabs for chlamydia and gonorrhea testing online in British Columbia, Canada. Sex Transm Infect 95:A277. https://doi.org/10.1136/sextrans-2019-sti.696

Ablona A, Grennan T, Salway T et al (2019b) Regional differences in STI testing barriers among online testers in British Columbia, Ccanada. Sex Transm Infect 95:A97. https://doi.org/10.1136/sextrans-2019-sti.248

Ablona A, Korol E, Gauthier B et al (2019c) Regional differences in use of getcheckedonline and client characteristics across British Columbia, Canada. Sex Transm Infect 95:A98. https://doi.org/10.1136/sextrans-2019-sti.249

Anand T, Nitpolprasert C, Kerr SJ et al (2017) Implementation of an online HIV prevention and treatment cascade in Thai men who have sex with men and transgender women using Adam's Love Electronic Health Record system. J Virus Erad 3:15–23

Antonio MG, Petrovskaya O (2019) Towards developing an eHealth equity conceptual framework. Stud Health Technol Inform 257:24–30. https://doi.org/10.3233/978-1-61499-951-5-24

Bauer MS, Damschroder L, Hagedorn H et al (2015) An introduction to implementation science for the non-specialist. BMC Psychol 3:1–12. https://doi.org/10.1186/S40359-015-0089-9

Baumann LC, Ylinen A (2017) Prevention: primary, secondary, tertiary. In: Gellman M, Turner JR (eds) Encyclopedia of behavioral medicine. Springer, New York, NY, pp 1–3

Boland L, Kothari A, McCutcheon C, Graham ID, Gray M (2020) Building an integrated knowledge translation (IKT) evidence base: colloquium proceedings and research direction. Health Res Policy Syst. 18(1):8. https://doi.org/10.1186/s12961-019-0521-3

Budd J, Miller BS, Manning EM et al (2020) Digital technologies in the public-health response to COVID-19. Nat Med 26:1183–1192. https://doi.org/10.1038/s41591-020-1011-4

Canadian Public Health Association (2014) Sexually transmitted infections and other blood-borne infections, including HIV, (STBBI) Health Equity Impact Assessment (HEIA) Tool https://www.cpha.ca/sites/default/files/uploads/resources/stbbi/HEIA_tool_EN.pdf. Accessed July 3 2023

Canadian Public Health Association, The Canadian Public Health Association, Canadian Public Health Association (2017) Public health: a conceptual framework. https://www.cpha.ca/public-health-conceptual-framework. Accessed July 3 2023

Crawford A, Serhal E (2020) Digital health equity and COVID-19: the innovation curve cannot reinforce the social gradient of health. J Med Internet Res 22:e19361. https://doi.org/10.2196/19361

Dulai J, Salway T, Thomson K et al (2021) Awareness of and intention to use an online sexually transmitted and blood-borne infection testing service among gay and bisexual men in British Columbia, two years after implementation. Can J Public Health 112:78–88. https://doi.org/10.17269/s41997-020-00323-4

Farrell J, Haag D, Bondyra M, et al (2015) Should your visuals be wearing blue, pink or yellow pants (or no pants at all)? Developing specimen self-collection instructions that are more sensitive to the needs of traditionally marginalized and underserved client populations. Paper presented at: Gay & Lesbian Medical Association 33rd Annual Conference; September 24–26, 2015; Portland, Oregon

Farrell JE (2012) Health equity and GetChecked: how can we make an online testing service that works for everyone? https://dishiresearch.ca/resource/health-equity-and-getchecked-how-can-we-make-an-online-testing-service-that-works-for-everyone/ Accessed July 3 2023

Giacomin J (2014) What is human centred design? Des J 17:606–623. https://doi.org/10.2752/175630614X14056185480186

Gilbert M, Bonnell A, Farrell J et al (2017a) Click yes to consent: acceptability of incorporating informed consent into an internet-based testing program for sexually transmitted and blood-borne infections. Int J Med Inform 105:38–48. https://doi.org/10.1016/j.ijmedinf.2017.05.020

Gilbert M, Haag D, Hottes TS et al (2016) Get checked… where? The development of a comprehensive, integrated internet-based testing program for sexually transmitted and blood-borne infections in British Columbia, Canada. JMIR Res Protoc 5:e186. https://doi.org/10.2196/resprot.6293

Gilbert M, Hottes TS, Kerr T et al (2013) Factors associated with intention to use internet-based testing for sexually yransmitted infections among men who have sex with men. J Med Internet Res 15:e254. https://doi.org/10.2196/jmir.2888

Gilbert M, Salway T, Haag D et al (2017b) Use of GetCheckedOnline, a comprehensive web-based testing service for sexually transmitted and blood-borne infections. J Med Internet Res 19:e81. https://doi.org/10.2196/jmir.7097

Gilbert M, Salway T, Haag D et al (2019a) Assessing the impact of a social marketing campaign on program outcomes for users of an internet-based testing service for sexually transmitted and blood-borne infections: observational study. J Med Internet Res 21:e11291. https://doi.org/10.2196/11291

Gilbert M, Thomson K, Salway T et al (2019b) Differences in experiences of barriers to STI testing between clients of the internet-based diagnostic testing service GetCheckedOnline.com and an STI clinic in Vancouver, Canada. Sexually Transmitted Infections 95:151–156. https://doi.org/10.1136/sextrans-2017-053325

Gómez-Ramírez O, Gilbert M, Grace D (2021a) Beyond initial implementation: barriers and facilitators to the scale-up, adaptation, maintenance and sustainability of GetCheckedOnline. Digital Sexual Health Initiative. https://dishiresearchca/resource/beyond-initial-implementation-barriers-and-facilitators-to-the-scale-up-adaptation-maintenance-sustainability-of-getcheckedonline/ Accessed July 3 2023

Gómez-Ramírez O, Iyamu I, Ablona A et al (2021b) On the imperative of thinking through the ethical, health equity, and social justice possibilities and limits of digital technologies in public health. Can J Public Health 112:412–416. https://doi.org/10.17269/s41997-021-00487-7

Gómez-Ramírez O, MacKinnon KR, Bannar-Martin S et al (2021c) Caught between HIV exceptionalism and health service integration: making visible the role of public health policy in the scale-up of novel sexual health services. Health Place 72:102696. https://doi.org/10.1016/j.healthplace.2021.102696

Hottes TS, Farrell J, Bondyra M et al (2012) Internet-based HIV and sexually transmitted infection testing in British Columbia, Canada: opinions and expectations of prospective clients. J Med Internet Res 14:e41. https://doi.org/10.2196/jmir.1948

Huang F, Blaschke S, Lucas H (2017) Beyond pilotitis: taking digital health interventions to the national level in China and Uganda. Glob Health 13:49. https://doi.org/10.1186/s12992-017-0275-z

Iyamu I, Gómez-Ramírez O, Xu AXT et al (2021) Defining the scope of digital public health and its implications for policy, practice, and research: protocol for a scoping review. JMIR Res Protoc 10:e27686. https://doi.org/10.2196/27686

Iyamu I, Gómez-Ramírez O, Xu AX et al (2022) Challenges in the development of digital public health interventions and mapped solutions: findings from a scoping review. Digit Health 8:20552076221102256. https://doi.org/10.1177/20552076221102255

Iyamu I, Pedersen H, Ablona A, Chang HJ, Worthington C, Grace D, Grennan T, Wong J, Salmon A, Koehoorn M, Gilbert M. (2023a) Evaluating the impact of the COVID-19-related public health restrictions on access to digital sexually transmitted and blood-borne infection testing in British Columbia, Canada: an interrupted time series analysis. Sex Transm Dis. Sep 1; 50(9):595–602. https://doi.org/10.1097/OLQ.0000000000001833. PMID: 37195276; PMCID: PMC10430673

Iyamu I, Sierra-Rosales R, Estcourt CS, et al (2023b) Differential uptake and effects of digital sexually transmitted and bloodborne infection testing interventions among equity seeking groups: a scoping review Sexually Transmitted Infections 99:554–560

Iyamu I, Kassam R, Worthington C, et al. (2024) Missed opportunities to provide sexually transmitted and blood-borne infections testing in British Columbia: An interpretive description of users’ experiences of Get Checked Online's design and implementation. DIGITAL HEALTH, 10. https://doi.org/10.1177/20552076241277653

Kersaudy-Rahib D, Lydie N, Leroy C et al (2017) Chlamyweb study II: a randomised controlled trial (RCT) of an online offer of home-based chlamydia trachomatis sampling in France. Sex Transm Infect 93:188–195. https://doi.org/10.1136/sextrans-2015-052510

Lawrence K (2022) Digital health equity. In: Linwood SL (ed) UCR Health and UCR School of Medicine, Riverside, CA, USA. Digital Health. Exon Publications, Brisbane, pp 121–130

Lee EW, McCloud RF, Viswanath K (2022) Designing effective eHealth interventions for underserved groups: five lessons from a decade of eHealth intervention design and deployment. J Med Internet Res 24:e25419. https://doi.org/10.2196/25419

Levesque J-F, Breton M, Senn N et al (2013) The interaction of public health and primary care: functional roles and organizational models that bridge individual and population perspectives. Public Health Rev 35:14. https://doi.org/10.1007/BF03391699

Lyles CR, Aguilera A, Nguyen O, Sarkar U (2022) Bridging the digital health divide: how designers can create more inclusive digital health tools. CHCF Issue Brief 9 https://www.chcf.org/wp-content/uploads/2022/02/BridgingDigitalDivideDesigners.pdf. Accessed July 3 2023

Lyles CR, Wachter RM, Sarkar U (2021) Focusing on digital health equity. JAMA 326:1795. https://doi.org/10.1001/jama.2021.18459

McIntyre D (2003) Technological determinism: a social process with some implications for ambulance paramedics. Australas J Paramed 7:1. https://doi.org/10.33151/ajp.1.3.197

Moe WW, Fader PS (2004) Capturing evolving visit behavior in clickstream data. J Interact Mark 18:5–19. https://doi.org/10.1002/dir.10074

Moore A, Traversy G, Reynolds DL et al (2021) Recommendation on screening for chlamydia and gonorrhea in primary care for individuals not known to be at high risk. Can Med Assoc J 193:E549–E559. https://doi.org/10.1503/cmaj.201967

Richardson S, Lawrence K, Schoenthaler AM, Mann D (2022) A framework for digital health equity. npj Digit Med 5:119. https://doi.org/10.1038/s41746-022-00663-0

Roberts JP, Fisher TR, Trowbridge MJ, Bent C (2016) A design thinking framework for healthcare management and innovation. Healthcare 4:11–14. https://doi.org/10.1016/j.hjdsi.2015.12.002

Rodriguez JA, Clark CR, Bates DW (2020) Digital health equity as a necessity in the 21st Century Cures Act era. JAMA 323:2381–2382. https://doi.org/10.1001/jama.2020.7858

Shoveller J, Gilbert M (2013) Applied public health chair feature science and partnership: informing BC'S online sexual health services. In: Canadian Institutes of Health Research—POP News—Spring 2013, Volume 2, Issue 5. https://cihr-irsc.gc.ca/e/46868.html#a2. Accessed 24 Aug 2022

Shoveller J, Johnson J, Rosenberg M et al (2009) Youth's experiences with STI testing in four communities in British Columbia, Canada. Sex Transm Infect 85:397–401. https://doi.org/10.1136/sti.2008.035568

Shoveller J, Knight R, Davis W et al (2012) Online sexual health services: examining youth's perspectives. Can J Public Health 103:14–18. https://doi.org/10.1007/BF03404062

Solar O, Irwin A (2010) A conceptual framework for action on the social determinants of health: social determinants of health discussion paper 2 (policy and practice). Report. Geneva, World Health Organization

Spielberg F, Levy V, Lensing S et al (2014) Fully integrated e-services for prevention, diagnosis, and treatment of sexually transmitted infections: results of a 4-county study in California. Am J Public Health 104:2313–2320. https://doi.org/10.2105/AJPH.2014.302302

UNICEF Health Section Implementation Research and Delivery Science Unit and the Office of Innovation Global Innovation Centre (2018) Designing digital interventions for lasting impact: a human-centred guide to digital health deployment. UNICEF, Geneva, Switzerland

Vechakul J, Patel B, Jaspal S (2015) Human-centered design as an approach for place-based innovation in public health : a case study from Oakland , California. Matern Child Health J 19:2552–2559. https://doi.org/10.1007/s10995-015-1787-x

Wadham E, Green C, Debattista J et al (2019) New digital media interventions for sexual health promotion among young people: a systematic review. Sex Health 16:101–123

Wienert J, Jahnel T, Maaß L (2021) What are digital public health interventions? First steps towards a definition and an intervention classification framework (preprint). J Med Internet Res 24:e31921. https://doi.org/10.2196/31921

Wienert J, Zeeb H (2021) Implementing health apps for digital public health—an implementation science approach adopting the consolidated framework for implementation research. Front Public Health 9:610237. https://doi.org/10.3389/fpubh.2021.610237

Wilson E, Free C, Morris TP et al (2017) Internet-accessed sexually transmitted infection (e-STI) testing and results service: a randomised, single-blind, controlled trial. PLoS Med 14:e1002479. https://doi.org/10.1371/journal.pmed.1002479

Wilson E, Leyrat C, Baraitser P, Free C (2019) Does internet-accessed STI (e-STI) testing increase testing uptake for chlamydia and other STIs among a young population who have never tested? Secondary analyses of data from a randomised controlled trial. Sex Transm Infect 95:569–574. https://doi.org/10.1136/sextrans-2019-053992

World Health Organization (2021) Global strategy on digital health 2020–2025. World Health Organization, Geneva, Switzerland

World Health Organization (2022) Global health sector strategies on, respectively, HIV, viral hepatitis and sexually transmitted infections for the period 2022–2030. World Health Organization, Geneva, Switzerland

Open Access This chapter is licensed under the terms of the Creative Commons Attribution 4.0 International License (http://creativecommons.org/licenses/by/4.0/), which permits use, sharing, adaptation, distribution and reproduction in any medium or format, as long as you give appropriate credit to the original author(s) and the source, provide a link to the Creative Commons license and indicate if changes were made.

The images or other third party material in this chapter are included in the chapter's Creative Commons license, unless indicated otherwise in a credit line to the material. If material is not included in the chapter's Creative Commons license and your intended use is not permitted by statutory regulation or exceeds the permitted use, you will need to obtain permission directly from the copyright holder.

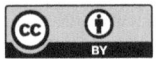

Assuring Governance for Health and Well-Being (EPHO 6)

Digital Public Health Governance: Navigating Complex Structures

Sarah Forberger

Abstract Health and health systems have been undergoing rapid changes in recent years. Digital health, using information and communication technologies in the health system, is a crucial building block for universal health coverage and achieving health-related Sustainable Development Goals. However, to develop its full potential, the individual aspects of the digital health governance structure must be known, and the appropriate governance structures should be accompanied by mechanisms for equitable, sustainable, and high-quality health systems. The World Health Organization has identified six building blocks of a health system (service delivery, health workforce, health information systems, access to essential medicines, financing, and leadership/governance) for strengthening health systems, forming the basis for digital health governance. They must naturally be combined with the core elements of good governance (transparency, accountability, participation, integrity, and capacity). Using both analytical frameworks to analyze the state of digital health governance in Germany, for example, we get a first impression of where Germany stands in digitizing its health system. That information is essential, as health systems worldwide are increasingly faced with digitalization and digital transformation. Thus developing and providing strong governance, as exemplified in this chapter, will be necessary to harvest benefits and reduce unnecessary errors and negative trends worldwide health systems may take.

Keywords Health governance · Health systems · Digital health · Health information systems · Digital public health

S. Forberger (✉)
Department of Prevention and Evaluation, Leibniz Institute for Prevention Research and Epidemiology—BIPS, Bremen, Germany

Leibniz Science Campus Digital Public Health Bremen (LSC), Bremen, Germany
e-mail: forberger@leibniz-bips.de

Abbreviations

AI	Artificial Intelligence
DiGA	Digital health application
DVPMG	Law on Digital Modernization of Healthcare and Nursing
eGK	electronic health card
EHR	Electronic Health Records
eMP	electronic medication plan
EPHS	Essential Public Health Services
ePKA	Patient summary record
GDPR	General Data Protection Regulation
GSAV	Act for Greater Security in the Supply of Medicines
ICT	Information and communications technology
ML	Machine learning
PDSG	Patient Data Protection Act
TAPIC	Transparency, Accountability, Participation, Integrity, and Capacity framework
TSVG	Appointment Service and Supply Act

1 Introduction

Health and health systems have been undergoing rapid changes in recent years. These changes have been driven by several factors, including technological advances, consumerism, and the need to address rising healthcare costs. Technology has enabled healthcare providers to deliver more efficient and effective care while giving patients more access to information and resources. Consumerism has increased the focus on patient experience, quality of care, value, and the need for transparency and cost-effectiveness. Additionally, rising healthcare costs have necessitated cost-containment measures, such as value-based care and alternative payment models. These changes have had a significant impact on the way health systems are structured, and the way care is delivered. As a result, health systems are increasingly focusing on patient-centered care and population health. Health systems have been adopted by using Electronic Health Records (EHRs), telemedicine, and mobile health applications. Health systems have placed greater emphasis on patient experience, leading to an increased focus on patient satisfaction, communication, and engagement. Further, health systems have shifted their focus from individual patient care to population health, including prevention, chronic disease management, and public health initiatives.

Furthermore, external pressures like a health and environmental crisis, climate, and demographic change continue to pressure the health sector, which is responding with reforms and transformations. These events underscore the necessity for an interdisciplinary approach in health governance, combining innovations from various fields to create resilient and adaptive systems. For instance, climate change is having a significant impact on the health system. As temperatures rise, air pollution increases, and extreme weather events become more frequent; the health system faces an increased disease burden. Additionally, the aging population is more vulnerable to the effects of climate change, such as heat waves and extreme weather events. This can lead to an increased demand for healthcare services and an increased risk of chronic diseases. Health systems must be prepared to address these challenges to ensure their populations' health and well-being. Furthermore, the COVID-19 pandemic has significantly impacted the health system. It has placed an unprecedented strain on healthcare resources and increased service demand. Further, the pandemic has disrupted care delivery and increased the risk of infection for healthcare workers. Health systems have had to rapidly adapt to the changing landscape, including the implementation of telemedicine, virtual visits, and other innovative solutions. Consequently, health systems must remain agile and adaptive to respond to the pandemic effectively. Therefore, it is unsurprising that interdisciplinary public health questions have recently been at the forefront of addressing crises (Greer et al. 2015). This goes along with dynamic, flexible, and adaptive health governance structures as the role of the Ministry of Health shifted from direct provision of health to overall stewardship of the health sector (Bigdeli et al. 2020).

Digital health, using information and communication technologies in the health system, is a crucial building block to universal health coverage and the health-related Sustainable Development Goals by the United Nations (World Health Organization 2016, 2021a, b). The WHO defines digital health as "The field of knowledge and practice associated with developing and using digital technologies to improve health. Digital health expands the concept of eHealth to include digital consumers, with a wider range of smart devices and connected equipment" (World Health Organization Regional Committee for Europe 2022). Digital health is the use of digital technologies to improve health and healthcare. This includes using digital tools such as mobile apps, wearables, telemedicine, and Electronic Health Records (EHRs) to monitor, diagnose, treat, and manage health and healthcare. Digital health also includes using Artificial Intelligence (AI) and machine learning (ML) to improve health outcomes. It covers all health sectors, like prevention and health care, and emphasizes a close interlinkage. The central goal of digital public health is to advance the improvement of population health through the application of new technologies at the individual, community, and global levels (Darmann-Finck et al. 2020), with a focus on the development, application, and insight interest in the field of public health and thus also on prevention and health promotion (Zeeb et al. 2020). Digital public health also involves using data to inform public health decisions, such as population health trends and behaviors. Data can inform public health policy, identify health disparities, and develop targeted interventions to improve health outcomes. Digital health and digital public health are components of a digital health system.

Digital health systems encompass, e.g., digital disease surveillance systems, digital prevention approaches, electronic medical records, and social health insurance payment processes. They also contains user satisfaction, need assessments, interoperability of the digital systems, dual data use, workforce education, the role of literacy, and the digital divide. Digital health initiatives outside the healthcare system is also known as consumer health or self-care. This includes using digital tools like fitness trackers, nutrition apps, and telemedicine to monitor and manage health and wellness. Following this line, digital public health is part of a more comprehensive health system. In the broadest sense, the health system covers primary, secondary, and tertiary healthcare, public health and preventive services, and self-care. In addition, as an intersectoral action, it addresses the broader determinants of health (World Health Organization 2021b).

Therefore, good digital governance is needed to govern all processes involved. Applying these principles specifically to digital health ensures that new technologies are used responsibly and ethically, maximizing benefits while minimizing risks. Following the 10 Essential Public Health Services (EPHS), EPHS 6 covers legal and regulatory actions designed to improve and protect the public's health. With the increasing use of digital approaches in public health, these principles also apply to digital solutions. Digital policies exploit and promote digitalization opportunities, including regulating digital and electronic communications, network and information security, spectrum policy and broadband access, and digital infrastructure issues, but also dual data use, data protection, data linkage, and profiling. This means that digital policy provides the structure for using digital public health. This requires the coordination of stakeholders and policies to develop, implement, and maintain a well-functioning and comprehensive health system and to combine analogy and digital structures (Carnicero and Serra 2020). In general, health governance is the capacity of the health system to cope with everyday challenges and those arising from new problems (Greer et al. 2016a). It works every day, every time, with and without a leader, and is the combination of rules and institutions that determine what is possible within the health sector (Greer et al. 2016a). These governance models must be adapted to address digital health's specific challenges, including data privacy, interoperability, and reaching underserved populations. This also means that we know what is considered possible in a society and a health system as a component of a digital public health system.

It is essential to analyze health governance, keeping sight of the health system's power and not leaving it to its own devices, hoping it will develop as it evolves. Without analysis and attention to the governance of health and health systems, function and integrity are at risk in many ways.

For example, a European Union study of corruption showed that the healthcare sector could be prone to corruption problems, and improved pharmaceutical policy governance was crucial to improved health system performance (European Commission 2013, 2014). Generally speaking, the quality of the health sector's governance affects the health system's ability to be sustainable, universal, and of high quality. That, in turn, affects the ability of the whole society to pursue social goods. Further, bad governance, in particular high corruption, increases inequality. Unfortunately, there is a link between the quality of governance and inequality. Bad governance is best addressed by making affected people more independent. However, policies that address dependency and reduce inequality are more prone to bad governance (Rothstein 2011; Svallfors 2012). Therefore, appropriate governance goes along with mechanisms for transparency, accountability, participation, integrity, and capacity (Greer et al. 2019). Further, it should be designed and tailored to capture all relevant changes within the (digital) health transformation pathway (Ricciardi et al. 2019).

Analyzing digital public health governance is paramount for leveraging and scaling up digital transformation for better health and aligning digital technology investment decisions with their health system needs while fully respecting the values of equity, solidarity, and human rights (World Health Organization Regional Committee for Europe 2022). These analytical frameworks facilitate a comprehensive assessment of digital health governance models, allowing stakeholders to identify areas for improvement and adapt strategies to evolving healthcare landscapes. Digital health governance manages, protects, and regulates digital health technologies and data. It involves the implementation of policies, procedures, and systems that ensure that digital health technologies and data are used securely and responsibly while still meeting the needs of the healthcare system, not only in a technical-administrative sense but also against the background of the needs of the individual members of society.

To understand what digital health governance entails, the chapter starts with the definition of governance (Sect. 2: What is governance). Then, it explains the five fundamental determinants considered to be critical components of good governance which resonates with the WHO guiding principles for appropriate and sustainable adoption of digital health solutions within the context of national health sectors and health and digital transformation strategies (World Health Organization Regional Committee for Europe 2022). Section 2 introduces the TAPIC framework (transparency, accountability, participation, integrity, and capacity) as an example of good governance's core elements (Greer et al. 2019). After explaining what governance means, the concept is applied to digital governance in Sect. 3 (Digital public health governance). The digitalization of health systems should ensure the quality, efficiency, effectiveness, and safety of modern health systems that deal with numerous challenges like disease burden, demographic change, scarce resources, and pandemic challenges. Sound digital health governance includes all the demands that are made on health governance (TAPIC) applied to the six building blocks of a health system (service delivery, health workforce, health information systems, access to essential medicines, financing, and leadership/governance) (World Health Organization and International Telecommunication Union 2012). Both aspects allow the mapping of all areas touched by a national eHealth strategy, which is essential to consider when looking at digital public health governance. The map helps get an overview but allows zooming in and out for more detailed or overview-driven analyses. The grit is the basis for an exemplary analysis of the state of digital public health governance in Germany, as exemplified in Sect. 4 (Case study: Germany). Finally, Sect. 5 concludes with a brief outlook.

2 What Is Governance?

Governance is a broad and complex topic with overlapping definitions, frameworks, and recommendations. It serves as the oundation for health systems. For example, the World Health Organization defines governance as "the careful and responsible management of the population's well-being" (World Health Organization 2000).

Governance is foundational to the entire health system, including digital public health. Governance structures determine how decisions are made; whether the decisions are evidence-informed and alternatives analyzed beforehand; whether they are elaborated legally, financially, and practically; how implementation, monitoring, evaluation, and enforcement are organized; and how all parts of society are integrated (Greer et al. 2019). Governance determines how conflicts are managed and authority and power are exerted (Fox 2010). It is the systematic, patterned way decisions are made and implemented daily, mostly automatically (Greer et al. 2016b).

While health systems may be diverse, the agenda for health policy-making often looks the same (Greer et al. 2019; Quaglio et al. 2018). Ministries, managers, and other stakeholders seek efficient population health and health care without cutting beneficial treatments. However, the desired outcome, sound and sustainable health for all, depends on good decisions and effective and efficient implementation, or, in other words, good governance (Greer et al. 2019).

Good governance means that processes and institutions produce results that meet the needs of society while making the best use of resources at their disposal (European Commission for Democracy through Law (Venice Commission) 2011; United Nations Economic and Social Commission for Asia and the Pacific). This covers (a) the organization of the political system (selection of the government, monitoring, and accountability by the general public), (b) the capacity of the government (resource management, formulation, implementation, and enforcement of policies, and (c) respect of the citizens and trust in the governance of social and economic interactions (Kaufmann et al. 2009).

Governance for digital health can be defined as the exercise of political, administrative, and technical authority to manage everything associated with the health information system in all areas of a national health system. This governance structure consists of the mechanisms, processes, and institutions through which all stakeholders articulate their interests, exercise their rights, meet their obligations, resolve their differences, and oversee the operation of the health information system (Smith et al. 2013). Applying the broader concept of governance to digital health includes managing specific rights, regulations, responsibilities, and risks associated with health data and information systems.

Applying this concept to digital health governance includes rights, regulations, responsibilities, and risks in areas such as the internet and health, the use of health data, and information systems. In addition, sound digital health governance involves participation, transparency, accountability to society, fairness, integrity, and effectiveness in the context of population health.

While the definition of governance is highly diverse, transparency (Table 1), accountability (Table 2), participation (Table 3), integrity and capacity (Table 4) form five overarching key determinants found repeatedly in the various concepts (Greer et al. 2016b, 2019; Mikkelsen-Lopez et al. 2011).

Each attribute has a series of different associated policy and administrative tools. These tools should be properties of the system and the individual organizations (Table 1).

Table 1 Transparency

Mechanism	Examples
Transparency	
Transparency means that institutions inform the public and other actors of upcoming decisions and decisions that have been made and of the process and grounds on which decisions are being made (Greer et al. 2016b)	Watchdog committees, inspectorates, regular reporting, Freedom of Information legislation, performance managing/reporting/assessment, and clear and valuable public information (e.g., open meetings, clarity about key personnel, and information presented in clear and usable formats)

Source: Based on Greer et al. (2016b)

Table 2 Accountability

Mechanism	Examples
Accountability	
Accountability ensures that everyone who acts is accountable for their actions to the appropriate other actors who may reward or punish them. Accountability is promoted through clear mandates and reporting Accountability involves explanation and sanction (Weale 2011). Therefore, actions must be explained, and, in particular, consequences must be applied when the mandate has been violated	Contracts; other financial instruments, such as performance-based pay; laws that set goals, reporting, and tools; competitive bidding; organizational separation; conflict of interest policies; regulation; delegated regulation; standards; codes of conduct; electoral mechanisms (Meijer and Schillemans 2009; Schillemans 2008)

Source: Based on Weale (2011), Meijer and Schillemans (2009), and Schillemans (2008)

Table 3 Participation

Mechanism	Examples
Participation	
Participation ensures that people affected by a decision can express their views about it in a way that ensures they are at least heard. Ideally, however, they are part of the whole decision-making process	Stakeholder forums, consultations, elections, appointed representatives, appeals, electoral mechanisms, advisory committees (ad hoc or otherwise), partnerships, surveys, pooled budgets, joint workforces, participatory budgets (Seekings 2013), and citizen juries (Bevir 2013)

Source: Based on Seekings (2013) and Bevir (2013)

Public perceptions of transparency do not always correlate with actual transparency (de Fine Licht 2014). While transparency involves the availability and accessibility of information, accountability ensures that individuals and organizations are held responsible for their actions. Both are crucial for effective governance but address different aspects of trust and compliance. Therefore, transparency for health (services, products, prevention strategies) often should mean that data and decisions are available to experts who can challenge a decision and the decision-making process, as well as simple explanations of decisions and their justification for the public.

Table 4 Integrity and capacity

Mechanism	Examples
Integrity	
Integrity means that representation, decision-making, and enforcement processes should be clearly defined. All members should be able to understand and predict how an institution's decisions are made and implemented; individual members should have a transparent allocation	Solid and well-rewarded internal career paths that allow high-ranking civil servants to be rewarded for their service rather than for profit or positions outside government, internal audit (to ensure that funds are flowing correctly), personnel policies (recruitment, job descriptions, procedures for weeding out erring individuals), legislative mandate, budget, procedures (e.g., document management, the conduct of the board, minutes of meetings), audit, clear organizational roles, and purposes
Capacity	
Capacity employs the necessary expertise to assist policy-making in avoiding, diagnosing, and remedying policy failures and unintended consequences, and the capacity to develop a policy aligned with resources in pursuit of goals (Greer et al. 2016b, 2019) Policy capacity refers to developing policies aligned with resources to pursue objectives. It is part of the government and its bodies that transforms ideas into workable, well-designed policies. If it succeeds, it can allow governments to formulate innovative and effective policies for health in the face of resistance (Forest et al. 2015)	Intelligence on performance and process (e.g., understanding of legal and budgetary issues and the system that is being changed), research/analysis capacity (e.g., trained staff with skills such as research and the ability to identify and work with valuable outsiders), staff training to improve their technical policy capacity, hiring procedures to enhance the quality of the policy bureaucracy, methods to incorporate specialist advice into policy formulation and recommendations, sufficient in-house capability to manage contractors such as consultancy firms as required (Greer et al. 2016b)

Source: Based on Greer et al. (2019, 2016b) and Forest et al. (2015)

At its best, transparency produces available, helpful, and accurate information so that it can be used by those who would rely on, plan with, or seek to influence the organization. The result is trust. Suppose patients, citizens, investors, and other organizations know how, when, and why decisions are made. In that case, they can plan accordingly and work out how to contribute their views and knowledge or challenge the policy-makers (Greer and Lillvis 2014). As health systems increasingly integrate digital technologies, it is essential to apply traditional governance principles, such as those outlined in TAPIC, to ensure digital health solutions are both effective and equitable. However, in the digital age, relevant information travels very fast, and transparency in health governance may be questioned at any time in the decision-making process. Therefore, managing this rapid information flow is crucial for maintaining trust and effectiveness in health governance.

While transparency focuses on openness and accessibility, accountability shifts the emphasis to responsibility and consequences for actions within the health system. However, transparency should be distinct from accountability (Table 2).

Table 2 provides a comprehensive overview of mechanisms that promote accountability, highlighting practical examples of how this principle is applied within healthcare governance.

The mechanisms work differently and not all equally well. An essential question in this context is to whom one is accountable. This question is necessary to understand the functions and power structure. Many of the actors working in the health care system are involved in a network of accountability, as opposed to mere delegation or fiduciary relationships (Tuohy 2003). Understanding this mechanisms is crucial for tailoring effective governance strategies that address the complex interdependencies among stakeholders (Table 3).

Effective participation processes improve implementation through various aspects. Participation, as detailed in Table 3, ensures that stakeholder voices are integrated into decision-making processes, which enhances legitimacy and effectiveness across governance activities. First, the link between participation, legitimacy, and key actors' involvement increases the implementation quality. Second, participation increases the uptake of information in the policy-making process. Third, participatory approaches have the advantage of including other points of view and thus making the policy more equitable and supporting of horizontal integration (Peters 2016; Tosun and Treib 2018; Wu et al. 2018). Fourth, by bringing in more diverse information, participation also impacts effectiveness. Finally, the information improves implementation processes and knowledge about effects (Fung 2006) and supports health equity (Francés and Daniel 2019). These participatory processes ensure that policies do not only reflect expert opinions but also incorporate insights from those directly affected by them, leading to more robust and accepted health policies.

However, it is also important to note that participation may reveal conflicts. Despite its benefits, participation can reveal conflicts and is sometimes difficult to facilitate, particularly when patient groups are fragmented or individuals lack interest in engagement. Sometimes no consensus can be reached, and, therefore, there are both winners and losers. It is also sometimes difficult to find representatives. For example, patient groups are highly fragmented, and their possibility to participate needs to be improved, or opportunities for participation need to be given. Sometimes, only some people also want to participate (Greer et al. 2014a, b). Moreover, participation mechanisms are lengthy, time-consuming, and sometimes cost-intensive (Greer et al. 2016b) (Table 4). Addressing these challenges requires carefully designed mechanisms that ensure representation and inclusivity without imposing excessive burdens on participants.

All five aspects of the framework can improve a health system's effectiveness, creativity, efficiency, and flexibility. However, it's also important to stress that the framework is not prescriptive. The five categories are not 'ingredients of good governance' as the authors put it, but boxes that tell us what needs to be addressed. While simply seeking more of one of the categories may not necessarily be better, there may also be trade-offs and conflicts between the different categories. Therefore, strong governance of health systems is characterized by appropriate investment in adequate institutional arrangements and capacities, suitable regulatory measures, and effective community engagement in health decision-making, aiming to enhance transparency, accountability, and responsiveness to public expectations. That also entails inclusive and participatory mechanisms, emphasizing the importance of engaging a broad range of stakeholders to ensure the health system is reflective of public needs.

All those concepts are central to and apply to digital health governance and resonate with the WHO principles for appropriate and sustainable adoption of digital health solutions within the context of national health sectors and health and digital transformation strategies (World Health Organization Regional Committee for Europe 2022).

The guiding principles are:

- Place the individual at the center of trustworthy care delivered digitally
- Understand health system challenges, including health needs and trends, and acknowledge the edge, the needs, and expectations of citizens and health workers
- Recognize the need for policy decision-making based on data, evidence, and lessons learned while allowing for continuous learning, adaptation, and innovation
- Leverage digital transformation to reimagine the future of health systems
- Recognize that the institutionalization of digital health requires a long-term commitment and an integrated care approach (World Health Organization Regional Committee for Europe 2022)

3 Digital Public Health Governance

Information and communication technologies have been incorporated with the digital transformation of the health system in the last few years. However, the change also requires the uptake of new issues in the governance of health systems that address rights, regulations, responsibilities and risks, health data usage, and information systems (Carnicero and Serra 2020).

Digital governance adds the "digital" to governance. It should ensure the quality, efficiency, effectiveness, and safety of modern health systems that deal with numerous challenges like disease burden, demographic change, scarce resources, and pandemic challenges. Sound digital health governance covers participatory processes, transparency, societal accountability, fairness, and effectiveness (Carnicero and Serra 2020). It includes all the demands that are also made on health governance (TAPIC), plus the challenges that arise from the use of information and communication technologies. By navigating these challenges, digital governance can effectively support the transition towards a more integrated health ecosystem. If developed and implemented correctly, digitalization can unfold its benefits and help put people at the center of prevention, care delivery, and empowerment. It can help to shift the focus from cure to prevention, thus strengthening public health (Odone et al. 2019).

Digital health governance needs a clear digital strategy and architectural support based on a country's overarching vision for the organization of its (public) health sector. Strong governance explicitly identifies and names each actor's specific roles and responsibilities and ensures legislation and policies. Furthermore, standards are applied across all digital health enterprises, suitable coordinating mechanisms and decision-making are promoted, and digital health solutions are encouraged and incentivized (Marcelo et al. 2018). As for good health governance, good digital governance has to ensure at all levels throughout the whole health information system to support equitable access, delivery of quality and affordable health, and the principles of TAPIC are applied. For that, digital health governance needs stable structures, strategy funding, guarantees of the rights of all involved, and connectivity (Carnicero and Serra 2020). However, what can such an architecture look like? Developing a robust framework will require collaboration among policymakers, technologists, and healthcare professionals to establish adaptable and resilient systems. Such an architecture should be designed to accommodate emerging technologies and evolving health needs, while ensuring equitable access and quality care for all.

3.1 Health System Building Blocks

The building blocks for digital health governance follow the structure of the WHO framework that describes health systems in terms of six core components or "building blocks": (i) service delivery, (ii) health workforce, (iii) health information systems, (iv) access to essential medicines, (v) financing, and (vi) leadership/governance (World Health Organization 2007; World Health Organization and International Telecommunication Union 2012). These blocks are the core areas of the health system and are, therefore, strongly affected by the transformation of the health system into the digital age (Fig. 1). By integrating digital capabilities into these building blocks, health systems can enhance their capacity to deliver efficient and effective care, manage resources, and respond to public health challenges.

The building blocks can be grouped into three tiers:

1. The first tier is leadership, governance, and multi-sector engagement. Without this in place, no system-wide decisions can be made. This layer represents the

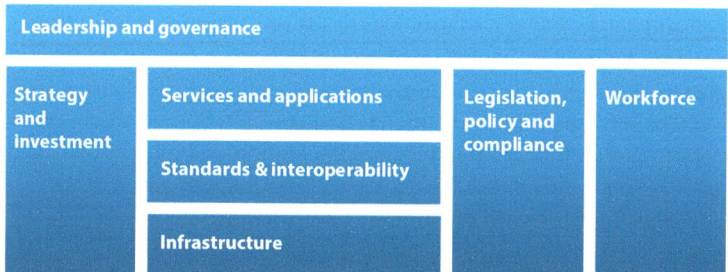

Fig. 1 National eHealth strategy: six health system building blocks. (Source: World Health Organization and International Telecommunication Union 2012)

framework's steering and stakeholder coordination function (direct, coordinate digital health, align with health goals, engage stakeholders, implement, and monitor).
2. The second tier covers the governance process (legislation, policy, and compliance), which creates the enabling environment to ensure IT policies are aligned across sectors and the country and that laws are enforced. This is crucial to establishing trust and protection for the public and the health sector workforce. It includes, for example, regulations and policies on data standards, privacy, and security.
3. The third tier is strategy and investment, ensuring financing priorities are aligned across governments, donor agencies, and the private sector. As part of the governance framework, a national digital health strategy should be defined by the national health strategy, policies, and plans. This strategy defines the digital health enterprise goal. Once this strategic vision is established, a strong and functional governance structure can be implemented.

Those three tiers primarily define how to govern a digital health system. Workforce, standards and interoperability, infrastructure and service, and applications can be subsumed under what to govern, which is determined by the "how." Workforce use of ICT and the information generated, stored, and retrieved must be included as components of digital health, which require governance (Marcelo et al. 2018; World Health Organization and International Telecommunication Union 2012) (Table 5).

Only a combination of all building blocks would span all sectors affected by digital health governance and allow a whole-of-society approach to digital health governance. This holistic approach ensures that no sector is left unaddressed and that synergies between different components are maximized. The building blocks can be used as a starting point to map all policy fields influenced by a national digital strategy in the health sector and thus show the bigger picture. Figure 2 (World Health Organization and International Telecommunication Union 2012) shows what that entails and which policy fields are affected by digital public health governance. The map is an example of a national eHealth strategy, illustrating what this can include, and what should be covered in a digital health governance strategy. The components must be coordinated individually in their fields and with each other, aligning with the requirements of the TAPIC framework. This alignment ensures consistency and coherence across different levels of governance. The detailed component map can be used to identify and assess eHealth components. The map can also be used to check existing structures, map them, and see which aspects are missing or should be thought of in an interconnected way. This process helps reveal gaps and overlaps that may hinder effective implementation. Rippling effects and skewing can also be reproduced, which occur when individual subfields are adjusted without considering the overall picture.

Table 5 Role of eHealth components

	Component	Role	Description
How	Leadership, governance, and multi-sector engagement	Enabling environment	• Direct and coordinate eHealth at the national level; ensure alignment with health goals and political support; promote awareness and engage stakeholders • Use mechanisms, expertise, coordination, and partnerships to develop or adopt eHealth components (e.g., standards) • Support and empower required change, implementation of recommendations, and monitor results for delivery of expected benefits
	Strategy and investment	Enabling environment	• Ensure a responsive strategy and plan for the national eHealth environment. Lead planning, with the involvement of major stakeholders and sectors • Align financing with priorities; donor, government, and private sector funding identified for a medium-term
	Legislation, policy, and compliance	Enabling environment	• Adopt national policies and legislation in priority areas; review sectoral policies for alignment and comprehensiveness; establish regular policy reviews • Create a legal and enforcement environment to establish trust and protection for consumers and industry in eHealth practice and systems
What	Workforce	Enabling environment	• Make eHealth knowledge and skills available through internal expertise, technical cooperation, or the private sector • Build national, regional, and specialized networks for eHealth implementation • Establish eHealth education and training programs for health workforce capacity building
	Standards and interoperability	Enabling environment	• Introduce standards that enable consistent and accurate collection and exchange of health information across health systems and services
	Infrastructure	ICT environment	• Form the foundations for electronic information exchange across geographical and health-sector boundaries. This includes the physical infrastructure (e.g., networks), core services, and applications that underpin a national eHealth environment
	Services and applications	ICT environment	• Provide tangible means for enabling services and systems; access to, exchange, and management of information and content. Users include the general public, patients, providers, and insurance. The means may be supplied by the government or commercially

Adapted from WHO and ITU (2012) (World Health Organization and International Telecommunication Union 2012)

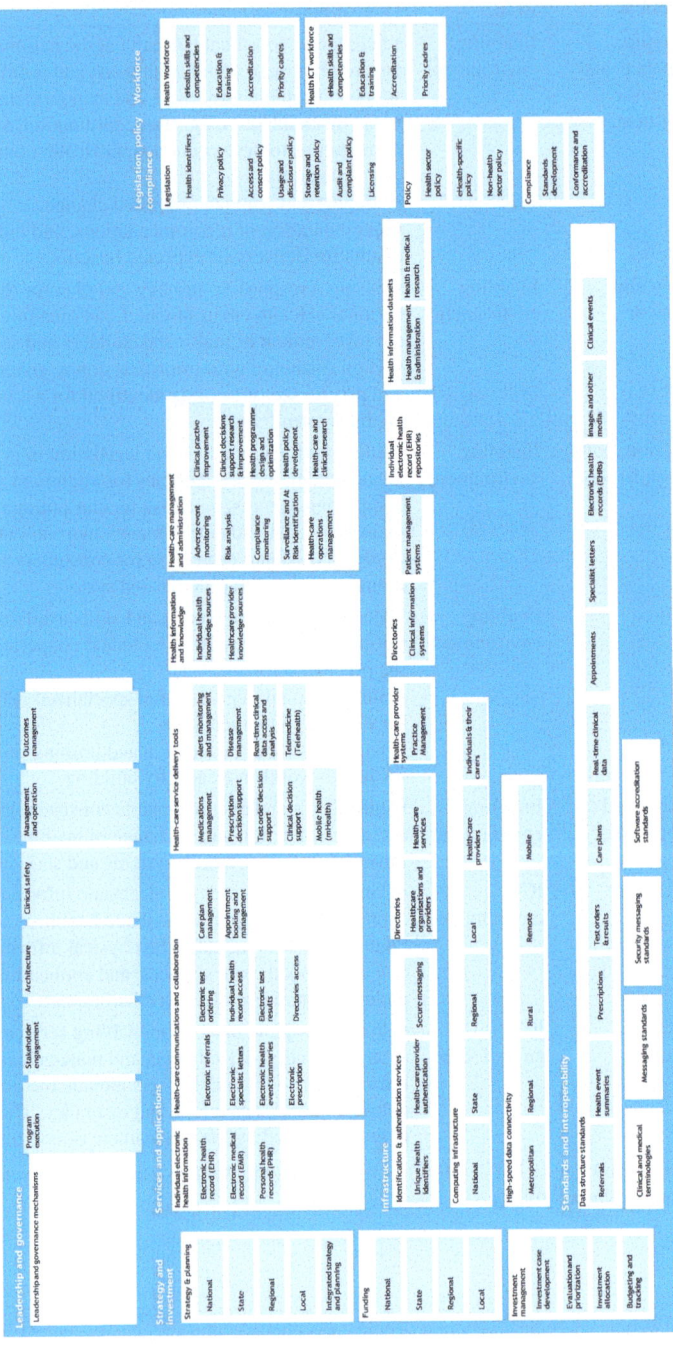

Fig. 2 Example of a National eHealth component map. (Source: World Health Organization and International Telecommunication Union 2012)

4 Case Study: Germany

Based on the example of a national eHealth component map from Fig. 2, Germany's digital health structure will be described, thus providing a concrete overview of current digital health governance in an industrialized country. Note that some countries may have progressed much faster, while others must catch up in developing and implementing their digitalization strategy.

4.1 Leadership and Governance

In November 2019, the consultation processes for developing a "Digital Health 2025" strategy for Germany began (Bundesministerium für Gesundheit 2020). The "Digital Health 2025" process aims to create a shared understanding of a digitalized healthcare system and to implement measures in a pragmatic and coordinated manner by 2025. Service providers, patient representatives, research and industry representatives, and governmental actors have participated. With its identified needs for action, the current result can and should be understood as a starting point. Furthermore, the identified needs for action can be harmonized with other processes, such as the roadmap for developing and implementing innovative e-health solutions (Bundesministerium für Gesundheit 2020).

The Digital Health Strategy is part of the Federal Government's digitalization strategy, forming Germany's digital progress until 2030. Digitization is a cross-sectional task on which all federal ministries work together. Therefore, the Federal Government's digital strategy forms a common umbrella for the ministries' digital policy priorities and goals. It is divided into three fields of action: "Connected and digitally sovereign society," "Innovative economy, working world, science and research," and "Learning, digital state" (Bundesregierung 2023).

The concrete results up to 2025 also include concrete goals of the Ministry of Health's digitization strategy for health and care, which was presented in March 2023 and contained the results of the consultation process permitted in 2019 (Bundesministerium für Gesundheit 2022, 2023).

Both strategies (target end of 2025) stipulate that the electronic patient file is used by at least 80% of the statutory health insurers and that e-prescriptions are established as a standard (Bundesministerium für Gesundheit 2023; Bundesregierung 2023).

Furthermore, the following goals were formulated in the digitization strategy in the health sector: (a) consistent focus on people, patient sovereignty, and enthusiasm; (b) improvement of the quality of care; and (c) increasing cost-effectiveness and efficiency. That should be achieved through the three central fields of action for the digital transformation in the health and care sector: digitally supported care processes (contains the goals on the patient file and e-prescription), use of health data, and benefit-oriented technologies and applications.

4.2 Legislation, Policy, Compliance

The Secure Digital Communications and Applications in Health Care Act (E-Health Act) set the initial course for developing the secure telematics infrastructure (TI) and introducing medical applications. Towards the end of 2015, the Statute for Secure Digital Communication and Applications in the Health Sector (eHealth Act) came into force. It can be seen as formal guidelines for establishing a data culture roadmap in establishing digital health (Bundesministerium für Gesundheit 2022). It focuses on the following:

- Creating incentives for the rapid introduction and use of medical applications (modern insurance master data management, emergency data, electronic doctor's letter, and uniform medication plan),
- Opening up the TI and perspective development towards an authoritative and secure infrastructure for the German health care system
- Creation of an interoperability directory to improve communication between different IT systems in the health system,
- Promotion of telemedical services (online video consultation, teleconsiliary assessment of X-ray images)

Since then, the digitization of the health care system has been driven forward by various legal measures, for example, the Appointment Service and Supply Act (TSVG), the Act for Greater Security in the Supply of Medicines (GSAV), the Digital Supply Act (DVG), the Patient Data Protection Act (PDSG) as well as Law on Digital Modernization of Healthcare and Nursing (DVPMG), which came into force on 9 June 2021.

To accelerate and simplify multicenter, transnational projects in health care and health research, §287a of the Fifth Book of the German Social Code (SGB V) created regulations for the uniform application of federal law and a lead supervisory authority modeled on the General Data Protection Regulation (GDPR). Thus, if data from more than one federal state is processed, researchers can designate a lead data protection supervisory authority to take charge of the data protection review. In addition, to overcome possible regulatory differences between the federal states, Section 27 of the Federal Data Protection Act applies to cross-state projects in health care and health research (Bundesministerium für Gesundheit 2022).

4.3 Infrastructure

4.3.1 Research Data Centre Health

To provide structured and representative data for research, the Federal Ministry of Health is establishing the Research Data Centre Health at the Federal Institute for Drugs and Medical Devices. The Research Data Centre Health creates a protected and trustworthy data space to use the billing data of those with statutory health insurance for prevention and health care research and the control of the health care system. From 2023, insured persons will also have the option of voluntarily making the data stored in an Electronic Health Record (Elektronische Patientenakte (ePA) in German) available to the Health Research Data Centre in pseudonymized and encrypted form and thus also available to medical research. In addition, insured persons can also make the data in their ePA available solely on informed consent for a specific research project or specific areas of scientific research (Bundesministerium für Gesundheit 2022).

4.3.2 Electronic Health Card (eGK) and Electronic Patient Summary Record (ePKA)

Since 1 January 2015, the electronic health card (eGK) has replaced other health insurance certificates as proof of insurance when visiting a doctor or dentist. Mandatory for all insured persons, the eGK contains the administrative data of the insured person, the so-called insured person master data. The insured person's master data include, for example, name, date of birth, address, sex, and information on health insurance, such as the health insurance number and the insured status (member, family insured, or pensioner).

Since autumn 2020, insured persons can also have personal health data, such as information on drug intolerances, allergies, and chronic illnesses, knowledge of which can be necessary for treatment in an emergency, stored digitally on their eGK as emergency data. In addition, further medical information, for example, about a current pregnancy or implants, as well as contact details of treating doctors and persons who should be informed in an emergency, can also be stored in the emergency data. Another voluntary application of the eGK is the electronic medication plan (eMP).

However, no independent patient access/viewing of the data is possible. Since access to the emergency data stored on the eGK always requires using a health professional card (HBA), insured persons can only view their emergency data in a service provider environment, for example, a doctor's practice.

In further development stages of the TI, starting from 1 July 2023, the electronic emergency data will be technically developed together with the data on indications of insured persons on the existence and storage location of personal declarations into an electronic patient summary record (ePKA). The ePKA will no longer be stored on the eGK but as an online application of the TI. Insured persons can also access data in the ePKA independently—outside a service provider environment—via smartphone, tablet, or desktop computer using their ePA app. The ePA app will be made available to the patients by their health insurance fund for digital medical applications. In addition, insured persons will, in the future, also be able to provide data from their ePKA within the European Union at their request to support their treatment in other European countries. In this way, insured persons can ensure that their medical data can also be considered when they receive treatment in another EU country.

Like emergency data use, the future ePKA is voluntary for insured persons.

4.3.3 gematik: National Agency

gematik is the national agency for digital medicine in Germany. Its task is to manage the transformation of the German telematics infrastructure (Gematik GmbH n.d.).

gematik has defined six supporting pillars for the health platform. These form the basis for a more user-friendly, flexible, and dynamic digital healthcare system in Germany and are intended to ensure innovation, better care, more efficient communication, more straightforward use, and the strengthening of the autonomy of insured persons. The pillars are electronic identities (federal identity management), internet access and mobile use (universal accessibility), distributed services, structured data and standards, modern security architecture, and standard TI rules and regulations (Gematik GmbH n.d.).

gematik is taking on the following role in this context:

1. A platform for national telematics infrastructure: gematik establishes the basic functionalities and security and security measures for a common platform that can be used nationwide so that as many participants as possible can get involved.
2. A competence center and coordination office for standardization: gematik coordinates the close exchange with the standardization community, medical community, and industry. It moderates the "round table for targeted and inter-nationally compatible standardization" based on internationally recognized standards.
3. A partner for providers and users
4. A forum for future concepts in digital medicine: gematik has a broad network of contractual partners and supporters, including the central organizations of the health system as shareholders. gematik will be the forum for exchanging ideas and presenting innovative solutions for joint dialogue about the future.
5. A European partner and moderator for national cooperation: In European projects, gematik supports projects, in particular, the promotion of formats for the cross-border exchange of patient data in the EU, and works closely with other national competence centers for digital health and European authorities (Gematik GmbH 2020).

gematik's work is focused on medical services and still needs to be positioned to take on public health functions. However, many aspects of gematik are also highly relevant for public health in Germany and beyond, e.g., data security, interoperability, technical standards, and digital health literacy. The services only develop their best possible effect if they are understood, accepted, and used by their intended users.

4.4 Service and Application

The legal framework also covers the introduction of the electronic prescription (e-prescription), the creation of a new access point for digital health applications (DiGA or "app on prescription"), and the advancement of telemedicine.

As of 1 January 2021, the health insurance funds must provide insured persons with an Electronic Health Record (EHR, ePA in German) in several expansion stages.

Initially, patient data from existing applications and documentation, such as emergency data, medication plans, or doctors' letters, can be made available in the ePA.

The ePA is an insurance-managed electronic file, which is voluntary for the insured (opt-in). The insured person is the sovereign of their data. They decide from the outset which data is to be stored, who is to have access, and whether data is to be deleted again. In addition to findings, doctors' reports or X-rays, vaccination cards, maternity records, the yellow examination booklet for children, and the dental bonus booklet can also be stored in the ePA.

Sensitive health data such as findings, diagnoses, medications, or treatment reports are protected by clear rules for data protection, data security, and data protection responsibility in the telematics infrastructure. Furthermore, since 1 January 2022, insured persons can use their smartphone or tablet to individually determine who can access each document stored in the ePA (fine-grained authorization management) (Bundesministerium für Gesundheit 2022).

4.5 Standards and Interoperability

An essential prerequisite for smooth electronic communication or the exchange of information in the health sector is interoperability.

Since July 2017, the interoperability directory called "vesta" has made the standards used by the various IT systems in the health sector transparent. New electronic applications may only be financed from statutory health insurance funds if the specifications and recommendations of gematik published in the interoperability directory are considered. The directory also contains an information portal for telemedical applications and electronic applications. In addition, uniform requirements for interfaces in the information technology systems of physicians and hospitals are specified. Here, the aim is also the interoperability of different systems (Gematik GmbH 2020).

A new coordination office for interoperability in the health care system will be set up at gematik to identify needs for standardization and develop and update recommendations for using standards, profiles, and guidelines.

4.6 Summary

To summarize, in addition to legal regulations, the approaches and work of gematik to establish a uniform infrastructure and interoperability are particularly noteworthy. In general, however, there is a lack of a uniform, cross-sector strategy with an appropriate long-term financial structure, a secure, participatory inclusion of all affected segments of the population, and a fundamental discussion of what a digital health and healthcare system structure for Germany could look like, with the associated responsibilities, rights, and duties. Further, the structure and initiatives of gematik mainly cover the healthcare sector. Although one can assume effects and influences for primary prevention and the broader health system, this is not included at the moment. Germany has developed and published its digital strategy and vision, which was adopted by the federal government in August 2022. This cross-ministry, concerted effort is now publicly available as a guideline for digital policy in Germany. While the strategy represents a significant step forward, it still appears to be mainly technically driven, with limited preventive and holistic approaches. Setting clear goals and fostering multi-disciplinary collaboration remain key to addressing these gaps. For example, in 2017 Public Health England published its digital strategy, which established basic principles and foundations for accelerating digital transformation. In addition to outlining Public Health England's ambitions, it also describes the role and contributions of the digital team. The strategy sets a common approach for digital work, including guiding principles, clear responsibilities, and standards for digital development. By drawing on international best practices—such as those demonstrated by Public Health England—Germany can further enhance its digital strategy, ensuring that digital transformation is comprehensive, inclusive, and effective across all sectors of society.

Additionally, the strategy prioritizes investment to ensure that the most strategically important pieces of work are addressed first. Multi-disciplinary working, recruitment, and staff development will ensure that staff members have the right skills (Gov.uk 2017). Integrating these points of digital public health functions and operations into the German vision of a digital health system is also strongly needed. It will be an essential point for the future.

5 Outlook

Digital health has the potential to help address issues such as data and information flow, service integration, healthcare access, health trends, and prevention. Still, it exhibits many fundamental challenges faced by health systems, such as poor management, inadequate training, infrastructural limitations, diversity, equity, participation problems, and poor access to equipment and supplies. Therefore, these considerations must be addressed in addition to the specific implementation requirements introduced by digital health.

There is widespread agreement that governance is essential in digital health (Greer et al. 2019). Frameworks for analyzing governance are abundant and very diverse. However, the recommendations or improvements almost always fall into one of TAPIC's five areas (transparency, accountability, participation, integrity, and capacity).

Based on the building blocks of a national health system (leadership and governance, strategy and investment, legislation, policy and compliance, workforce, infrastructure standards and interoperability, service, and application), different aspects must be aligned, and data has to be provided to guide the transformation. Based on the national health system, national health priorities have to be discussed and decided on. The priories must align with the digital health strategy to cover all aspects of the systems. Information on the priorities, the digital strategy, and the building blocks determine the maturity of a country's digital system.

Any way of mapping a complex construct, such as the health system, is bound to be fraught with problems. This is also true of the eHealth map, which focuses on policies in the health sector and underestimates the importance of policies in other sectors. The national eHealth component map example does not address the underlying social and economic determinants of health, such as gender inequalities, education, or occupational status. In addition, it does not address the essential and dynamic linkages and interactions among the individual components. The map must be combined with good governance principles and address equity across the full range of issues to meet the needs and demands of complex health systems.

Digital public health governance involves creating and enforcing policies and regulations that promote public health while safeguarding patient privacy, security, and data. This includes establishing standards for digital health technologies, such as data security and privacy, and creating clear guidelines for using digital health services. It also includes developing mechanisms to monitor digital health services and technologies and respond to potential misuse or abuse.

Figure 3 provides a structured approach to breaking down complexity and developing indicators for evaluating digital health systems. To effectively manage digital public health, comprehensive data is required across a range of areas, including population health, health norms and values, health literacy, health service utilization, health outcomes, and healthcare costs. This data can be drawn from multiple sources, such as public health surveillance systems, administrative databases, health service and care providers, and research institutions. By focusing on these individual components, Fig. 3 helps delineate the multifaceted construct of digital public health. This approach enables the establishment of clear indicators and robust measurement strategies to monitor progress and change throughout the system transformation to digital public health. In summary, Fig. 3 not only clarifies the complexity of digital public health but also serves as a practical guide for developing evaluation frameworks and monitoring the impact of digital interventions.

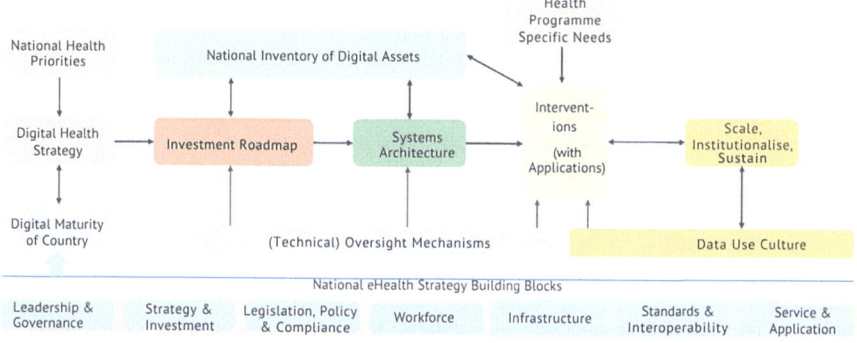

Fig. 3 System transformation to digital public health. (Source: Adapted from Mariano Junior 2020)

That information is essential, as health systems worldwide are increasingly shaped by digitalization and digital transformation. Developing and implementing robust governance structures, as outlined in this chapter, is necessary to maximize benefits and minimize errors or unintended consequences. When creating digital public health governance, a holistic approach is essential—one that considers the needs of the public, the perspectives of various stakeholders, and the potential risks and benefits associated with the adoption of digital technologies and services. This requires engaging multiple stakeholders and understanding both the regulatory and legal frameworks and the technical and social implications of digital health technologies. It is also critical to ensure that policies and regulations are clear, comprehensive, and enforceable, while paying close attention to data privacy and security. Such an approach will foster synergies among all stakeholders and align with national and European efforts to standardize digital health adoption, leverage the development of digital public health goods, and promote access to digital health services for vulnerable populations (World Health Organization Regional Committee for Europe 2022).

References

Bevir M (2013) A theory of governance. University of California Press, Berkeley, CA
Bigdeli M, Rouffy B, Lane BD, Schmets G, Soucat A (2020) Health systems governance: the missing links. BMJ Glob Health 5(8):e002533. https://doi.org/10.1136/bmjgh-2020-002533
Bundesministerium für Gesundheit (2020) Digitale Gesundheit 2020. Bundesministerium für Gesundheit, Berlin
Bundesministerium für Gesundheit (2022) E-Health—Digitalisierung im Gesundheitswesen. https://www.bundesgesundheitsministerium.de/e-health-initiative.html. Accessed 4 Aug 2022
Bundesministerium für Gesundheit (2023) Digitalisierungsstrategie. https://www.bundesgesundheitsministerium.de/themen/digitalisierung/digitalisierungsstrategie.html. Accessed 28 Mar 2023
Bundesregierung (2023) Digitalstrategie der Bundesregierung. Strategie für einen digitalen Aufbruch https://www.bundesregierung.de/breg-de/themen/digitaler-aufbruch/digitalstrategie-2072884. Accessed 28 Mar 2023
Carnicero J, Serra P (2020) Governance for digital health: the art of health systems transformation. IDB Inter-American Development Bank, Washington, DC
Darmann-Finck I, Rothgang H, Zeeb H (2020) Digitalisierung und Gesundheitswissenschaften—White Paper Digital Public Health [Digitalization and Health Sciences—White Paper Digital Public Health]. Gesundheitswesen 82(7):620–622. https://doi.org/10.1055/a-1191-4344
de Fine Licht J (2014) Transparency actually: how transparency affects public perceptions of political decision-making. Eur Polit Sci Rev 6(2):309–330. https://doi.org/10.1017/S1755773913000131
European Commission (2013) Study on corruption in the healthcare sector (Home/2011/ISEC/PR/047-A2). European Commission, Brussels
European Commission (2014) EU anti-corruption report (COM(2014) 38). European Commission, Brussels
European Commission for Democracy through Law (Venice Commission) (2011) Stocktaking on the notions of "Good Governance" and "Good Administration". Council of Europe, Strasbourg
Forest P-G, Denis J-L, Brown LD, Helms D (2015) Health reform requires policy capacity. Int J Health Policy Manag 4(5):265–266. https://doi.org/10.15171/ijhpm.2015.85
Fox DM (2010) The governance of standard-setting to improve health. Prev Chronic Dis 7:A123

Francés F, Daniel LP-C (2019) Participation as a driver of health equity. WHO, Copenhagen
Fung A (2006) Varieties of participation in complex governance. Public Adm Rev 66(s1):66–75. https://doi.org/10.1111/j.1540-6210.2006.00667.x
Gematik GmbH (2020) Arena für digitale Medizin. Whitepaper Telematikinfrastruktur 2.0 für ein föderalistisch vernetztes Gesundheitssystem. Gematik, Berlin
Gematik GmbH Gematik (n.d.). https://www.gematik.de/. Accessed 11 Aug 2022
Gov.uk (2017) Digital-first public health: Public Health England's digital strategy. Gov.uk. https://www.gov.uk/government/publications/digital-first-public-health/digital-first-public-health-public-health-englands-digital-strategy. Accessed 28 Mar 2023
Greer SL, Lillvis DF (2014) Beyond leadership: political strategies for coordination in health policies. Health Policy 116(1):12–17. https://doi.org/10.1016/j.healthpol.2014.01.019
Greer SL, Stewart EA, Wilson I, Donnelly PD (2014a) Victory for volunteerism? Scottish health board elections and participation in the welfare state. Soc Sci Med 106:221–228. https://doi.org/10.1016/j.socscimed.2014.01.053
Greer SL, Wilson I, Stewart E, Donnelly PD (2014b) 'Democratizing' public services? Representation and elections in the Scottish NHS. Public Adm 92:1090–1105
Greer SL, Wismar M, Kosinska M, World Health Organization. Regional Office for E (2015) Towards intersectoral governance: lessons learned from health system governance. Public Health Panorama 1(2):128–132
Greer SL, Wismar M, Figueras J (2016a) Introduction: strengthening governance amidst changing governance. In: Greer SL, Wismar M, Figueras J (eds) Strengthening Health System Governance. Better policies, stronger performance. European Observatory on Health Systems and Policies, Copenhagen, pp 18–41
Greer SL, Wismar M, Figueras J (2016b) Strengthening Health System Governance. Better policies, stronger performance. European Observatory on Health Systems and Policies, Copenhagen
Greer SL, Vasev N, Jarman H, Wismar M, Figueras J (2019) It's the governance, stupid! TAPIC: a governance framework to strengthen decision making and implementation. European Observatory on Health Systems and Policies, Copenhagen
Kaufmann D, Kraay A, Mastruzzi M (2009) Governance Matters. Aggregated and individual governance indicators 1996–2008. Policy Research Working Paper No. 4978. The World Bank development research group macroeconomics and growth team. Available at SSRN: https://ssrn.com/abstract=1424591
Marcelo A, Medeiros D, Ramesh K, Roth S, Wyatt P (2018) Transforming health systems through good digital health governance, vol 51. ADB Sustainable Development Working Paper Series. Asian Development Bank, Manila
Mariano Junior B (2020) Globald strategy on digital health. World Health Organization. https://commercialisation.esa.int/wp-content/uploads/2020/11/Global-Strategy-on-Digital-Health_Mariano.pdf
Meijer A, Schillemans T (2009) Fictional citizens and real effects: accountability to citizens in competitive and monopolistic markets. Public Admin Manag 14(2):254–291
Mikkelsen-Lopez I, Wyss K, de Savigny D (2011) An approach to addressing governance from a health system framework perspective. BMC Int Health Hum Rights 11(1):13. https://doi.org/10.1186/1472-698X-11-13
Odone A, Buttigieg S, Ricciardi W, Azzopardi-Muscat N, Staines A (2019) Public Health digitalization in Europe. EUPHA vision, action and role in digital public health. Eur J Pub Health 29:28–35
Peters BG (2016) Pursuing horizontal management: the politics of public sector coordination. University Press of Kansas, Lawrence
Quaglio G, Figueras J, Mantoan D, Dawood A, Karapiperis T, Costongs C, Bernal-Delgado E (2018) An overview of future EU health systems. An insight into governance, primary care, data collection and citizens' participation. J Public Health 40(4):891–898. https://doi.org/10.1093/pubmed/fdy054
Ricciardi W, Pita Barros P, Bourek A, Brouwer W, Kelsey T, Lehtonen L, Health EPoEWoIi (2019) How to govern the digital transformation of health services. Eur J Pub Health 29(Supplement_3):7–12. https://doi.org/10.1093/eurpub/ckz165

Rothstein B (2011) The quality of government: corruption, social trust and inequality in international perspective. University of Chicago Press, Chicago

Schillemans T (2008) Accountability in the shadow of hierarchy: the horizontal accountability of agencies. Public Organ Rev 8(2):175–194. https://doi.org/10.1007/s11115-008-0053-8

Seekings J (2013) Is the South 'Brazilian'? The public realm in urban Brazil through a comparative lens. Policy Polit 41(3):351–370. https://doi.org/10.1332/030557313X670118

Smith AL, Bradley RV, Bichescu BC, Tremblay MC (2013) IT governance characteristics, electronic medical records sophistication, and financial performance in U.S. hospitals: an empirical investigation. Decis Sci 44(3):483–516. https://doi.org/10.1111/deci.12019

Svallfors S (2012) Government quality, egalitarianism, and attitudes to taxes and social spending: a European comparison. Eur Polit Sci Rev 5:363–380

Tosun J, Treib O (2018) Linking policy design and implementation styles. In: Howlett M, Mukherjee I (eds) Routledge handbook of policy design. Routledge, New York, pp 316–330

Tuohy CH (2003) Agency, contract, and governance: shifting shapes of accountability in the health care arena. J Health Polit Policy Law 28(2–3):195–216. https://doi.org/10.1215/03616878-28-2-3-195

Weale A (2011) New modes of governance, political accountability and public reason. Gov Oppos 46(1):58–80. https://doi.org/10.1111/j.1477-7053.2010.01330.x

World Health Organization (2000) The World health report: 2000. Health systems: improving performance. World Health Organization, Geneva

World Health Organization (2007) Everybody's business: strengthening health systems to improve health outcomes. WHO's framework for action. World Health Organization, Geneva

World Health Organization (2016) Global diffusion of eHealth: making universal health coverage achievable: report of the third global survey on eHealth. World Health Organization, Geneva

World Health Organization (2021a) Global strategy on digital health 2020–2025. WHO, Geneva

World Health Organization (2021b) Support tool to strengthen health information systems. Guidance for health information system assessment and strategy development. WHO, Geneva

World Health Organization, International Telecommunication Union (2012) National eHealth strategy toolkit. International Telecommunication Union/World Health Organization, Geneva

World Health Organization Regional Committee for Europe (2022) Regional digital health action plan for the WHO European Region 2023–2030. WHO, Tel Aviv

Wu X, Ramesh M, Howlett M, Fritzen SA (2018) The public policy primer. Managing the policy process. Routledge, New York

Zeeb H, Pigeot I, Schüz B (2020) Digital Public Health—ein Überblick. Bundesgesundheitsblatt 63:137–144. https://doi.org/10.1007/s00103-019-03078-7

Open Access This chapter is licensed under the terms of the Creative Commons Attribution 4.0 International License (http://creativecommons.org/licenses/by/4.0/), which permits use, sharing, adaptation, distribution and reproduction in any medium or format, as long as you give appropriate credit to the original author(s) and the source, provide a link to the Creative Commons license and indicate if changes were made.

The images or other third party material in this chapter are included in the chapter's Creative Commons license, unless indicated otherwise in a credit line to the material. If material is not included in the chapter's Creative Commons license and your intended use is not permitted by statutory regulation or exceeds the permitted use, you will need to obtain permission directly from the copyright holder.

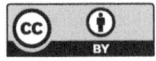

Assuring a Sufficient and Competent Public Health Workforce for Digital Public Health (EPHO 7)

Monica Georgiana Brînzac ⓘ, Rok Hrzic ⓘ, Mariam Hachem ⓘ, and Fatai Ogunlayi ⓘ

Abstract The digitalization of society is transforming health systems, presenting opportunities for using digital technologies to improve population health. *Essential Public Health Operation Seven* is about ensuring a competent public health workforce, which is crucial for delivering effective public health services. Digital public health has the potential to transform and revolutionize public health, but it also presents a set of new challenges for the public health workforce. This chapter examines the influence of digital technologies on the public health workforce and explores the challenges and opportunities for workforce development. It discusses factors needed to strengthen the public health workforce in the digital era, such as the role of competency-based education and interdisciplinary collaboration. A key component of the public health workforce is early career professionals. This chapter discusses mechanisms for engaging early career professionals in developing digital

---

M. G. Brînzac
Department of Public Health, Faculty of Political, Administrative and Communication Sciences, Babeș-Bolyai University, Cluj-Napoca, Romania

EUPHAnxt, European Public Health Association, Utrecht, Netherlands
e-mail: monica.brinzac@publichealth.ro

R. Hrzic
Department of International Health, Care and Public Health Research Institute – CAPHRI, Maastricht University, Maastricht, The Netherlands
e-mail: r.hrzic@maastrichtuniversity.nl

M. Hachem
Department of Medicine, Austin Health, Faculty of Dentistry, Medicine and Health Sciences, University of Melbourne, Heidelberg, VIC, Australia

Australian Centre for Accelerating Diabetes Innovations (ACADI), University of Melbourne, Melbourne, VIC, Australia
e-mail: mariam.hachem@unimelb.edu.au

F. Ogunlayi (✉)
Warwick Medical School, The University of Warwick, Coventry, UK

UKHSA, 10 South Colonnade, Canary Wharf, London, UK
e-mail: Fatai.ogunlayi@nhs.net

public health policies and approaches to cultivating future public health leaders in the digital era. Finally, the chapter discusses the importance of creating an ethical dimension to competency-based education for the public health workforce. This is particularly important in the digital era, given the rapid evolution of technologies and potential ethical concerns associated with digital public health.

Keywords Digital public health · Public health workforce · Competency-based education · Early career professionals

Abbreviations

ASPHER	Association of Schools of Public Health in the European Region
DiPH	Digital public health
ECP	Early Career Professional
ECR	Early Career Researcher
EMSA	European Medical Students Association
HREC	The Human Research Ethics Review Process
ICT	Information and communication technology
IRB	Institutional Review Board
mHealth	Mobile Health
OECD	Organisation for Economic Co-operation and Development
PHW	Public health workforce
REC	Research Ethics Committees
WHO	World Health Organization

1 Introduction

Health systems are fundamentally transforming in response to the digitalization of all aspects of society. Whether these transformations lead to healthier, more equitable communities in the future depends on our actions today. In particular, it depends on whether the public health workforce (PHW) is willing and able to actively shape the transformation process. In this chapter on assuring a sufficient and competent PHW (Essential Public Health Operation Seven) for digital public health (DiPH), we will examine the impact of digital technologies on the PHW, identify challenges and opportunities for workforce development that emerge, and evaluate whether the global and regional strategies for PHW development can effectively respond to the digital revolution.

DiPH stands for greater personalization, precision, automation and prediction in essential public health operations that build on improved access to health data and digital technologies. Examples include using a mobile health (mHealth) application to identify and enumerate disease occurrences (see chapter "Monitoring and Response to Health Hazards and Emergencies (EPHO2)", Kirchner et al. in this handbook), using social media platforms to increase awareness of preventive strategies (see chapter "Social Media in Digital Public Health", Sina et al. in this handbook), and constructing a data pipeline to automate disease reporting (see chapter "Public Health Data Pipelines: Moving Away from Excel to Scalable, Sustainable, Insightful, and Future-Proof Infostructure", Cilia et al. in this handbook). In contrast to digital health, DiPH focuses on the health of a population by using digital technologies to further public health objectives instead of serving individual patients (Wienert et al. 2022; Zeeb et al. 2020). However, we consider the use of digital health tools at scale, such as the widespread use of mHealth applications aimed at individuals, has significant public health implications and therefore fall within the scope of the DiPH umbrella.

Current definitions of the PHW aim to be broadly inclusive and define the PHW as everyone involved in creating a healthy environment for people (Tilson and Gebbie 2004). This includes, for example, those who work for official public health agencies at all levels of government, community-based and voluntary organizations with a health promotion focus, the public health-related staff of hospitals and health care systems, and a range of others in private industry, government, academia, and the voluntary sector (Tilson and Gebbie 2004). Defining PHW is critical because it informs how we define, measure, and improve a country's DiPH capacity. This chapter will distinguish between the *core* PHW and the *wider* PHW (Otok et al. 2018; World Health Organization 2022a). The core PHW consists of those engaged in providing public health services. This group identifies public health as the primary part of their role and has likely undergone formal training in a public health discipline and/or registration with professional bodies. Conversely, the wider PHW consist of those who contribute to one or more public health functions as part of their clinical and/or social care roles or whose work contributes to addressing the determinants of health from a wide range of other occupations and who may not have had formal public health training.

2 Evolution of Digital Public Health and Its Impact on the Public Health Workforce

Since the 1990s, the influence of information and communication technologies (ICT) in healthcare has grown. Variously termed health telematics, medical informatics, eHealth, Health 2.0, and most recently digital health (Boogerd et al. 2015; Shaw et al. 2017), this interdisciplinary field of research and practice sought out ways of improving healthcare provision through the use of technologies, ranging from electronic patient records and telemedicine to smartphones, wearable technology, and social media platforms (see chapters "Why Is It Essential to Address Digital Public Health in an Interdisciplinary Way?", Maaß et al. and "Social Media in Digital Public Health", Sina et al. in this handbook). As more of the population adopted these technologies, they also became increasingly critical for public health, particularly in the areas of population health monitoring and health promotion. This trend was amplified during the COVID-19 pandemic, during which the widespread use of digital health tools like Corona apps (Singh et al. 2020) and the emergence of social media as the dominant source of health information (Gunasekeran et al. 2022) ushered in the DiPH era.

The most significant impact of digital technologies on the PHW to date has been to expand the definition of the wider PHW to include those working in the ICT sector. Employees of social media platforms are in the pole position in the fight against health misinformation (Krishnan et al. 2021). Software developers are creating digital health interventions that official public health agencies depend on, for example applications that assist with behavioral modification and disease surveillance (Karpathakis et al. 2021). Finally, data scientists are creating data analytics products to extract insights from newly available health data while remaining conscious of the bias embedded in the available data (Xu et al. 2022). Most of these employees would likely be surprised to learn they are part of the PHW. More importantly, they may also be unaware of their impact on population health and need to be engaged to align their work with the aims of public health (see chapter "Why Is It Essential to Address Digital Public Health in an Interdisciplinary Way?", Maaß et al. in this handbook). This presents a two-fold challenge. First, their employers are typically for-profit organisations that operate in an ethical framework that does not prioritize population health. One example of this mismatch is the revelation that Meta's internal research highlighted the negative mental health impacts of Instagram use, to which the company responded by downplaying these risks (Zenone et al. 2023). Second, while examples of successful collaborations between public health professionals and the ICT industry exist, they require specific organizational models, skills, and investments that may be challenging to scale (Ford et al. 2021; Lisker et al. 2022).

The impact of digital technologies on the core PHW has been less clear. Digital technologies have sometimes created new public health subdisciplines, such as digital epidemiology (Salathé 2018). In contrast, in others, they have been used to complement existing skill sets, e.g., health promotion (Stark et al. 2022). However, by and large, there is as yet little sign of a digital transformation in the core PHW roles (Iyamu et al. 2021). The reasons for this remain unclear and may include a highly regulated working environment, many stakeholders, competing priorities, and the lack of financial and human resources, including public health professionals with relevant competencies (Benjamin and Potts 2018). Public health graduates are increasingly sought after for their data analytics skills by the for-profit sector, which may exacerbate the challenge of ensuring the right skill-mix inside public health organizations (Krasna et al. 2021a, b).

2.1 Public Health Workforce Preparedness for Digital Public Health

The digital landscape is evolving at an unprecedented pace, and public health organizations need to keep up with these advancements to effectively leverage digital tools and technologies. However, the workforce may not have the necessary skills and knowledge to navigate and utilize emerging technologies such as data analytics, artificial intelligence, telemedicine, and digital health platforms. This lack of preparedness can hinder the adoption and implementation of digital solutions in public health practice (Iyamu et al. 2022).

Among the skills for the successful adoption and implementation of DiPH is digital literacy, which refers to the ability to use digital technologies and tools effectively (UNESCO Institute for Statistics 2018). The public health workforce may have varying levels of digital literacy, with some individuals lacking basic digital skills, as described in chapter "Digital Health Literacy", Zeeb and Dratva in this handbook. Without a foundation in digital literacy, it becomes challenging to harness the full potential of digital technologies for data collection, analysis, interpretation, communication, and decision-making. This lack of preparedness hinders the ability to derive meaningful insights from the vast amounts of data available and limits evidence-based decision-making. It is crucial to address this gap and provide training and resources to enhance digital literacy across the public health workforce (Azzopardi-Muscat and Sørensen 2019; Campanozzi et al. 2023; Wong et al. 2021b).

Limited resources, including funding, infrastructure, and training opportunities, can hinder the preparedness of the public health workforce in digitalization. Investing in capacity building, providing access to training programs, and allocating resources for digital infrastructure and tools are essential to address these constraints (Organisation for Economic Co-operation and Development 2020; World Health Organization 2016).

Addressing the lack of preparedness in the public health workforce requires a multi-faceted approach. It involves investing in training and professional development programs that focus on digital literacy, data management, ethical considerations, interdisciplinary collaboration, and technology adoption. Collaboration between public health organizations, educational institutions, and technology partners is also crucial to ensure that the workforce is adequately prepared to leverage digital solutions for improved public health outcomes (Organisation for Economic Co-operation and Development 2020; Rechel and McKee 2014).

3 Approaches to Strengthening the Public Health Workforce in Digital Public Health

In the following sections, we identify four key measures for creating a PHW ready for the digital era. First, we reflect on the current efforts to professionalize the PHW and equip it with the competencies required by DiPH. Second, we examine the need for the intensification of interdisciplinary collaboration. Third, we discuss the central role early-career professionals can play in this process. Lastly, we emphasize the importance of developing a strong leadership pipeline to ensure we have a strengthened PHW in the digital era and beyond.

3.1 Professionalization and the Development of Competency-Based Education

The World Health Organization's (WHO) *Global Strategy on Human Resources for Health* (2020) highlighted that while the health workforce has a critical role in attaining the inter-related global public health objectives of sustainable development goals, ensuring the resilience of health systems and universal health coverage, there has been chronic underinvestment in appropriate training and education (World Health Organization 2020). The experience of the COVID-19 pandemic has exacerbated the challenges in health workforce development and retention (World Health Organization 2023a). Within public health, the pandemic galvanized PHW development efforts and brought a new urgency to the public health professionalization and competency development agenda (Hunter et al. 2023).

Public health professionalization is at the core of current efforts to strengthen the PHW in the digital era. Among other factors, a profession is characterized by a defined set of competencies, education that helps attain these competencies, and the recognition of achieving these competencies through certification and credentialing (Czabanowska and Middleton 2022). A recent publication by the WHO and regional professional public health associations identified essential measures for professionalizing the PHW (World Health Organization 2022b). This list includes the development of competency frameworks and competency-based education (see Table 1). However, these strategies do not explicitly address the potentially disruptive influence of digital technologies on the PHW. This is critical because harnessing the potential of DiPH will depend on its development and implementation being driven by a well-informed PHW and not solely by our increasing technological capabilities (Gómez-Ramírez et al. 2021). If the process of digitalization in public health is to realize its promise, a more deliberate approach to preparing the PHW is required.

A key lever of professionalization is the development of competency frameworks that describe the attitude, knowledge, and skills of the relevant professionals. The last decade saw a rapid expansion in developing competency frameworks for public health. They range in scope from general regional or national frameworks (Coombe et al. 2022) to topic-specific frameworks (e.g., Czabanowska et al. 2014; Toquero

Table 1 Professionalizing the PHW: measures

Measures to professionalize the public health workforce	
Policy, laws and regulations	Competency frameworks
Taxonomy, enumeration and forecasting	Job descriptions
Sustainable financing	Recruitment and retention
Accreditation	
	Competency based education and training
EPHO alignment	Licensing, certification and credentialing
Assurance of public health service delivery	Formal organization
Human resources planning and forecasting	Ethical and professional code of conduct

Source: Own table, adapted from WHO (2022b)

2023). However, as of May 2025, few competency frameworks focused on DiPH (Iyamu et al. 2025). This is important because the PHW need the right competencies to steer the digitalization process in public health more effectively and realize its potential. While necessary steps towards this objective have been made by the formation of WHO's *Digital Health Competency Framework Committee* and the development of competency frameworks adjacent to digital public health (Ahmadi et al. 2022; World Health Organization 2023b), the lack of a comprehensive and well-developed DiPH competency framework remains a critical gap. Whilst there is further work to be done to develop competency frameworks for DiPH, there is an urgent need for these frameworks to include ethics, as a core competency, to educate and build capacity of the PHW for current and future public health challenges (Wong, et al. 2021a).

3.1.1 Ethics Education and Training as a Core Competency for the Digital Public Health Workforce

The roles and responsibilities of the DiPH workforce are rapidly transforming as technology evolves and develops. The demands of the PHW continue as DiPH expands, including involvement in artificial intelligence, digital therapeutics, virtual delivery of care, user-centered and personalized technology, and eHealth or mHealth initiatives (Nazeha et al. 2020; Nebeker et al. 2019). The core ethical principles guiding public health of beneficence (doing good), non-maleficence (do no harm), justice (equal access) and autonomy (right to choose) remain as core ethical principles (Beauchamp and Childress 2001), however additional considerations need to be made for emerging digital technologies (Shaw and Donia 2021). This section will explore opportunities to embed ethics as core training for the DiPH workforce, and considerations for developing a framework for ethical decision making in DiPH to better equip the PHW.

PHW must be equipped with the competency, knowledge and skills to navigate ethical challenges raised by DiPH effectively. A key step in developing ethics competency in DiPH starts at the education and training provided to the PHW (World Health Organization 2020). A scoping review conducted in 2022 across schools of public health in the European region identified ethics training gaps in continuing professional development of PHW (Butcher et al. 2020). Whilst some schools have public health ethics modules covering a wide range of public health subjects, a notable gap in these subjects was DiPH (Butcher et al. 2020). A survey of 262 PHW in the United Kingdom identified the need for formalized training in ethics in public health to provide guidance on regularly encountered ethical issues, relying on personal reflection to resolve ethical issues, and a lack of best practice to guide ethical decision making (Viens and Vass 2020). The survey highlighted opportunities to develop resources (guidance materials, mentorship opportunities) to guide PHW (Viens and Vass 2020). Developing competency in ethical decision making may also be an opportunity to develop the diversity of the PHW for specialized roles such as ethical consultants in DiPH to guide and facilitate PHW. There is an opportunity to incorporate ethics training as part of foundational public health teaching at universities and training providers in conjunction with public health bodies. Partnering with these public health bodies can enable a curriculum that is current and responsive to the needs of the DiPH workforce. To achieve this, it is essential to incorporate competency-based education and training that address ethical dimensions of DiPH as integral components of the core curricula for public health professionals at local, national, and international level, with consideration for behavioral and cultural sensitivity (Beebeejaun and Littleford 2023). A competency framework for DiPH ethics can enable PHW to comply with a recognized standard whether it is at a local, national and or international level. This may contribute to workforce development and resilience, particularly when navigating and managing risks related to DiPH (Viens and Vass 2020). Secondly, addressing the local context in which ethics in DiPH is taught is important so that PHW are prepared adequately to serve the communities in which they live and work. To localize education, academic institutions and public health organizations may consider micro-certificates as an alternative way to upskill and educate the existing PHW in DiPH ethics.

3.1.2 Ethical Considerations for Inclusivity, Equitability and Diversity of the Digital Public Health Workforce

As the global PHW expands with greater diversity and involvement from the digital technology, economic, political, social, academic, non-for-profit and health sectors, it is imperative to ensure ethical training in DiPH that is inclusive. One of the key pillars for professionalizing the PHW is through the development of an inclusive code of ethics and professional conduct (Weeramanthri et al. 2023). Herein lies an opportunity, to develop an international code of ethics for DiPH for the PHW (Kass 2001). The first steps may be to develop an international representative body of public health professionals to address this gap. Particular attention should be given to inclusivity and diversity of voices within the DiPH workforce when formulating such codes, reflecting a cross-section of the PHW (e.g., Indigenous and First Nations people, culturally and linguistically diverse people and minority groups) (Coronado et al. 2020). Some potential ethical considerations to include in the development of frameworks may also seek to address informed consent in DiPH, including data collection procedures, privacy, accountability and inclusivity (Kass 2001).

Considerations must also be made regarding the ethical use of digital technologies by PHW particularly in low-resource settings and emergency settings. In the context of emergency and humanitarian crises the use of *mHealth* digital technologies have demonstrated effectiveness and improvements in low-resource settings such as the West African Ebola Crisis (Perakslis 2018). However, unintended consequences of DiPH must also be considered such as exacerbating health inequalities if population groups do not have access to or are not comfortable using digital technologies (Perakslis 2018). How do public health practitioners working within these environments navigate these ethical challenges of DiPH? PHW are faced with constantly evolving challenges in DiPH. Without education, training and a framework to guide us, they are left to navigate the course alone. There is an opportunity to address this gap by providing ethical frameworks and training to PHW so that the workforce is equipped to tackle future public health challenges and importantly to reduce the risk of harming those who may benefit most from DiPH (Kass 2001).

Having a PHW equipped with ethical training in DiPH will contribute to the development of a competent and ethical workforce capable of addressing the evolving challenges of DiPH and promote ethical decision-making, equipped with a deep understanding of the ethical implications of digital technologies in public health.

3.2 The Role of Interdisciplinary Collaboration and Partnerships to Enhance Workforce Competency

Public health is a complex and interconnected field that requires the involvement of diverse individuals from various backgrounds. With DiPH, as with broader public health, cross-organizational and cross-discipline collaborations and partnerships are essential in addressing up-streams societal factors impacting on health and well-being of a given population (Hunter et al. 2023). Collaboration should be done towards a mutually agreed upon aim, such as enhancing the competency of the PHW, with shared benefits and obligations. When discussing DiPH, it is essential to consider the multitude of domains that ultimately influence the health of populations. Thus, it is instrumental to acknowledge interdisciplinarity and conclusively intergenerationally planning.

In recent years, the international PHW has faced numerous adversities such as a global pandemic and regional epidemics, increasing frequency of infodemic, shortages in medication and vaccines, cost of living crises, societal unrest, and warfare. All these challenges urge a new skill set of the workforce, a new and improved approach, and competencies of the PHW and public health leadership (World Health Organization 2022a). Silos must be obliterated, and public health challenges should be tackled in a unified fashion (Czabanowska and Kuhlmann 2021). More interdisciplinary cooperation among professionals should be planned into the day-to-day activities and education of the workforce to allow them to respond to the newly emerged challenges (Griewatz et al. 2020).

As highlighted by the WHO-ASPHER *Competency Framework for the Public Health Workforce in the European Region*, collaboration and partnerships represent one of the core competencies of the public health workforce. The framework includes enabling productive collaboration, forging alliances and partnerships, fostering networking and connections, engaging in interdisciplinary and intersectoral network development, and addressing and overseeing stakeholder engagement (World Health Organization Regional Office for Europe 2020).

To better showcase the benefits of collaborations in DiPH, you can find below three examples:

1. **Public health practitioners and Epidemiologists:** Public health practitioners, such as health educators and community health workers, need to collaborate

with epidemiologists to understand disease patterns, conduct surveillance, and develop effective strategies for disease prevention and control. DiPH creates further opportunity for collaboration for example through the use of Geographical Information System surveillance, spatial analytics and adoption of algorithms to support the monitoring and management of disease outbreaks (Gamache et al. 2018). The advantages of this collaboration include better data to inform evidence-based interventions and policies; near real-time feedback and insights and a comprehensive approach to disease prevention and control, combining both population-level strategies and community-level interventions (Tsai et al. 2022; Yokomichi et al. 2021).

2. **Researchers and Public health practitioners:** Collaboration between researchers and public health practitioner facilitates the translation of research findings into practice further supported by increasing production of health data through digital applications and advances in Big Data such as genomics. This collaboration ensures that public health efforts are evidence-based and that research findings are applicable to real-world public health challenges (Nyström et al. 2018; van der Graaf et al. 2021).

3. **PHW and Advocates:** Collaboration between the PHW, health policy analysts, and advocates helps to bridge the gap between research and policy implementation. This is particularly important for DiPH where advocates can bring the voices of marginalized communities and populations to the policy-making process. This collaboration ensures that DiPH policies are grounded in evidence, consider the needs of diverse populations, and are feasible to implement (Cullerton et al. 2018; Pollack Porter et al. 2018; World Health Organization 2016).

The overall advantages of such collaborations include improved decision-making, enhanced program planning and implementation, increased effectiveness of interventions, and better health outcomes for populations. Collaboration enables the pooling of diverse expertise, resources, and perspectives, leading to more comprehensive and impactful public health initiatives (Emerson 2018; Kriegner et al. 2021; Teitelbaum et al. 2019). Public health is in a continuous transformation that prohibits a tunnel vision tactic from being sufficient for a single profession to respond to all its needs (Czabanowska and Kuhlmann 2021). Collaboration and partnership across all generations and fields is a prerequisite of public health in the twenty-first century, as mentioned in chapter "Why Is It Essential to Address Digital Public Health in an Interdisciplinary Way?", Maaß et al. in this handbook).

3.3 Significance of Engaging Early Career Professionals in Digital Public Health Workforce Development

As highlighted above, the process of digitally transforming healthcare and public health can bring about disruption. However, various technologies, including virtual care, the Internet of Things, smart wearables, artificial intelligence, big data analytics, remote monitoring, blockchain, data exchange and storage tools, as well as remote data capture tools, have demonstrated the potential to improve health outcomes by creating a continuum of care. These technologies enable advancements in DiPH interventions along with the creation of evidence-based knowledge and skills for healthcare professionals to provide support (World Health Organization 2021).

However, the European Medical Students Association (EMSA) has highlighted the shortage of skills and demanded action on promoting education and training in digital health, increasing the level of awareness and trust in digital technologies, and reframing the medical curricula to incorporate digital (public) health, while establishing platforms for faculties to share information and exchange best practices in digital (public) health education (Organisation for Economic Co-operation and Development 2019).

DiPH requires a workforce with expertise in emerging technologies, data analysis, informatics, and health communication. Engaging early career professionals allows organizations to bridge the digital skills gap by tapping into their familiarity with technology and their up-to-date knowledge of digital tools and platforms. These professionals can bring fresh perspectives, innovative ideas, and technical skills to address the digital challenges in public health (Wong, et al. 2021a). The field of digital public health is rapidly evolving with advancements in technology and data analytics. Engaging early career professionals ensures that organizations stay current with the latest trends and developments. These professionals are often more comfortable and adept at adopting and utilizing new technologies, which can accelerate the integration of digital solutions in public health practice (Martin et al. 2022; Organisation for Economic Co-operation and Development 2020).

Engaging early career professionals in digital public health builds a pipeline of talent for the future. By investing in their development, organizations ensure a sustainable workforce that can continue to drive digital transformation and innovation in public health. These professionals can assume leadership roles, mentor future generations, contribute to the ongoing growth and advancement of the field and it ensures that the workforce is equipped to tackle current and emerging public health challenges (Harper et al. 2018; Rechel and McKee 2014; Rees et al. 2023; World Health Organization 2021). By harnessing their digital skills and enthusiasm, organizations can enhance data-driven decision-making, improve health communication, and implement innovative digital interventions. Early career professionals can contribute to addressing health disparities, promoting health equity, and leveraging technology to improve population health outcomes (World Health Organization 2018).

Valuable lessons have been derived from past endeavors in implementing DiPH interventions, emphasizing the indispensable role of an informed, engaged, and proficient workforce. Consequently, it becomes imperative to support public health professionals in acquiring expertise in DiPH methodologies and foster the professional growth of those who demonstrate an interest in this domain (Robbins et al. 2020). By investing in early career professionals, organizations can build a resilient and capable workforce that drives digital transformation in public health.

3.4 Ensuring Leadership Opportunities and Career Progression for Early Career Professionals

Leadership is a craft which may be educated, cultivated, and distributed. The above-mentioned global health threats, which happened at the beginning of the 2020s, have exposed vulnerabilities within healthcare systems and underscored the necessity for our educational systems to equip health professionals for a period of rapid improvement, change management, and continuous evolution (Moore and Barnett 2021). A leadership pipeline provides opportunities for professional growth and development in DiPH. By investing in leadership development, organizations can ensure a smooth transition of leadership, minimize disruptions, and maintain institutional knowledge (Harper et al. 2018; Rechel and McKee 2014; Yphantides et al. 2015). The importance of a strong leadership pipeline has never been more evident and essential for several reasons including:

Collaboration and partnerships: Public health issues, including DiPH, often require collaboration between various stakeholders, including government agencies, community organizations, healthcare providers, and academia (Griewatz et al. 2020; Shu and Wang 2021). A leadership pipeline ensures the development of leaders with the skills to build partnerships, to foster collaboration, effectively engage with technology partners, and to align efforts towards common public health goals (Al Knawy 2021; Alanazi 2022).

Policy development and advocacy: Leaders play a crucial role in shaping policies that promote health and address social determinants of health. They need to understand public health principles, epidemiology, research methods, and policy analysis. These leaders can influence policy decisions, advocate for evidence-based practices, and work towards creating an environment that supports population health (World Health Organization Regional Office for Europe 2020).

Effective management of public health programs: Public health organizations are responsible for designing, implementing, and evaluating DiPH programs and policies to improve population health. Leaders with expertise in public health management can navigate complex challenges, allocate resources efficiently, and drive effective DiPH interventions to address public health issues (World Health Organization Regional Office for Europe 2020; Moreland-Russell et al. 2022).

Response to public health emergencies: Public health emergencies, such as disease outbreaks, natural disasters, or pandemics, require strong leadership to coordinate and mobilize resources effectively. A leadership pipeline ensures that there are capable leaders who can respond swiftly, make critical decisions, and lead interdisciplinary teams during times of crisis, communicate with the public, collaborate with other agencies, and implement emergency response strategies (Goniewicz et al. 2022; Yphantides et al. 2015).

Health equity and social justice: Whilst the benefits of DiPH are widely recognized, as discussed earlier, there is also potential for these technologies to widen inequalities. A leadership pipeline ensures that leaders are trained to recognize and address systemic barriers to health, prioritize health equity in decision-making, and work towards achieving fair and just health outcomes for all populations (Holden et al. 2016; World Health Organization Regional Office for Europe 2020).

It is imperative to cultivate new cohorts of public health professionals who can assume leadership roles to maximize the potential of DiPH and to ensure its proper integration. Comprehensive leadership development opportunities should be offered throughout the entire continuum of professional education, catering to undergraduate and postgraduate learners, trainees, and faculty members to support them (Winters et al. 2022). Thus, public health professionals must be exposed as soon as possible to leadership at all levels (World Health Organization Regional Office for Europe 2020).

Furthermore, leadership and systems thinking is one of the core competencies of public health professionals and includes the ability to

- formulate a vision, mission, and strategy,
- to lead individual task-team work,
- to lead change and innovation,
- to understand and apply the theories of complex systems in practice,
- to galvanize organizational learning and development, people development,
- and to hold emotional intelligence (World Health Organization Regional Office for Europe 2020).

Moreover, it is essential to acknowledge that DiPH is a vast domain with diverse professionals and skills. With the integration of automation and digital technologies into health services, the demand for skills in the health-sector workforce is undergoing a transformation. The successful implementation of DiPH requires a broader group of public health leaders who are skilled in ICT. These leaders must be equipped with an ample comprehension of public health practice, technology, and change management. Additionally, public health leaders should possess the skills needed to establish a team with the right group of people and coordinate their efforts so that collectively, they inhabit a fundamental digital skill. This must include a basic understanding of data collection and analysis processes, as well as how algorithms in digital tools utilize data to generate information (Organisation for Economic Co-operation and Development 2019). Programs such as fellowships, internships and mentorships, are central to ensuring a skilled leadership pipeline in health and ought to be provided throughout the entire career from beginning to end.

4 Conclusion

DiPH is transforming public health practice, presenting both challenges and opportunities for the PHW. The PHW needs to be strengthened in order to maximize the potential benefits of DiPH whilst addressing the challenges. This will require a comprehensive approach to workforce development that includes competency-based education and training that are specific to DiPH. It will also require interdisciplinary partnerships and collaborations. Engaging early career professionals is crucial for designing and implementing digital health technologies that meet population needs and for ensuring a sustainable workforce into the future. Leadership development opportunities should be provided to cultivate a skilled pipeline of leaders in DiPH. Ethical considerations must guide the use of digital technologies in public health, ensuring adherence to core ethical principles and addressing emerging ethical challenges. In order to realize the vast potential that DiPH presents, it is vital to invest into and strengthen the PHW to ensure a healthier and more equitable society in the digital era.

References

Ahmadi M, Sheikhtaheri A, Tahmasbi F et al (2022) A competency framework for Ph.D. programs in health information management. Int J Med Inform 168:104906. https://doi.org/10.1016/J.IJMEDINF.2022.104906

Al Knawy B (2021) Global data and digital public health leadership for current and future pandemic responses. Front Digit Health 3:632568. https://doi.org/10.3389/fdgth.2021.632568. PMID: 34713103; PMCID: PMC8521854

Alanazi AT (2022) Digital leadership: attributes of modern healthcare leaders. Cureus 14(2): e21969. https://doi.org/10.7759/cureus.21969. PMID: 35282530; PMCID: PMC8906562

Azzopardi-Muscat N, Sørensen K (2019) Towards an equitable digital public health era: promoting equity through a health literacy perspective. Eur J Public Health 29(Supplement_3):13–17. https://doi.org/10.1093/eurpub/ckz166. PMID: 31738443; PMCID: PMC6859513

Beauchamp TL, Childress JF (2001) Principles of biomedical ethics. Oxford University Press, Greece

Beebeejaun K, Littleford K (2023) A diverse public health workforce is more important than ever. BMJ 380:447. https://doi.org/10.1136/bmj.p447. PMID: 36828551

Benjamin K, Potts HW (2018) Digital transformation in government: lessons for digital health? Digit Health 4:205520761875916. https://doi.org/10.1177/2055207618759168

Boogerd EA, Arts T, Engelen LJ, van de Belt TH (2015) "What is eHealth": time for an update? JMIR Res Protoc 4(1):e29. https://doi.org/10.2196/RESPROT.4065

Butcher F, Schröder-Bäck P, Tahzib F (2020) Variability in public health ethics education in EUPHA and ASPHER members. Eur J Public Health 30(Supplement_5):ckaa165. 728. https://www.fph.org.uk/media/3636/fph_ethics_report_08_22-1.pdf

Campanozzi LL, Gibelli F, Bailo P, Nittari G, Sirignano A, Ricci G (2023) The role of digital literacy in achieving health equity in the third millennium society: a literature review. Front Public Health 11:1109323. https://doi.org/10.3389/fpubh.2023.1109323. PMID: 36891330; PMCID: PMC9986277

Coombe L, Severinsen CA, Robinson P (2022) Mapping competency frameworks: implications for public health curricula design. Aust N Z J Public Health 46:564–571. https://doi.org/10.1111/1753-6405.13253

Coronado F, Beck AJ, Shah G, Young JL, Sellers K, Leider JP (2020) Understanding the dynamics of diversity in the public health workforce. J Public Health Manag Pract 26(4):389–392. https://doi.org/10.1097/PHH.0000000000001075. PMID: 31688743; PMCID: PMC7190406

Cullerton K, Donnet T, Lee A, Gallegos D (2018) Effective advocacy strategies for influencing government nutrition policy: a conceptual model. Int J Behav Nutr Phys Act 15. https://doi.org/10.1186/S12966-018-0716-Y

Czabanowska K, Kuhlmann E (2021) Public health competences through the lens of the COVID-19 pandemic: what matters for health workforce preparedness for global health emergencies. Int J Health Plann Manage 36:14–19. https://doi.org/10.1002/HPM.3131

Czabanowska K, Middleton J (2022) Professionalism of the public health workforce—how to make it happen? J Public Health (Oxf) 44:i54–i59. https://doi.org/10.1093/PUBMED/FDAC091

Czabanowska K, Smith T, Könings KD et al (2014) In search for a public health leadership competency framework to support leadership curriculum—a consensus study. Eur J Public Health 24:850–856. https://doi.org/10.1093/EURPUB/CKT158

Emerson K (2018) Collaborative governance of public health in low- and middle-income countries: lessons from research in public administration. BMJ Glob Health 3:e000381. https://doi.org/10.1136/BMJGH-2017-000381

Ford KL, Portz JD, Zhou S et al (2021) Benefits, facilitators, and recommendations for digital health academic-industry collaboration: a mini review. Front Digit Health 3:616278. https://doi.org/10.3389/FDGTH.2021.616278

Gamache R, Kharrazi H, Weiner JP (2018) Public and population health informatics: the bridging of big data to benefit communities. Yearb Med Inform 27(1):199–206. https://doi.org/10.1055/s-0038-1667081. Epub 2018 Aug 29. PMID: 30157524; PMCID: PMC6115205

Gómez-Ramírez O, Iyamu I, Ablona A, Watt S, Xu AXT, Chang HJ, Gilbert M (2021) On the imperative of thinking through the ethical, health equity, and social justice possibilities and limits of digital technologies in public health. Can J Public Health 112(3):412–416. https://doi.org/10.17269/s41997-021-00487-7. Epub 2021 Mar 16. PMID: 33725332; PMCID: PMC7962628

Goniewicz K, Burkle FM, Hall TF, Goniewicz M, Khorram-Manesh A (2022) Global public health leadership: the vital element in managing global health crises. J Glob Health 12:03003. https://doi.org/10.7189/jogh.12.03003. PMID: 35136593; PMCID: PMC8818292

Griewatz J, Yousef A, Rothdiener M et al (2020) Are we preparing for collaboration, advocacy and leadership? Targeted multi-site analysis of collaborative intrinsic roles implementation in medical undergraduate curricula. BMC Med Educ 20:35. https://doi.org/10.1186/s12909-020-1940-0

Gunasekeran DV, Chew A, Chandrasekar EK et al (2022) The impact and applications of social media platforms for public health responses before and during the COVID-19 pandemic: systematic literature review. J Med Internet Res 24(4):e33680. https://doi.org/10.2196/33680

Harper E, Leider JP, Coronado F, Beck AJ (2018) Succession planning in state health agencies in the United States: a brief report. J Public Health Manag Pract 24:473. https://doi.org/10.1097/PHH.0000000000000700

Holden K, Akintobi T, Hopkins J et al (2016) Community engaged leadership to advance health equity and build healthier communities. Soc Sci (Basel) 5. https://doi.org/10.3390/SOCSCI5010002

Hunter MB, Ogunlayi F, Middleton J, Squires N (2023) Strengthening capacity through competency-based education and training to deliver the essential public health functions: reflection on roadmap to build public health workforce. BMJ Glob Health 8:e011310. https://doi.org/10.1136/BMJGH-2022-011310

Iyamu I, Xu AXT, Gómez-Ramírez O et al (2021) Defining digital public health and the role of digitization, digitalization, and digital transformation: scoping review. JMIR Public Health Surveill 7:e30399. https://doi.org/10.2196/30399

Iyamu I, Gómez-Ramírez O, Xu AX, Chang HJ, Watt S, Mckee G, Gilbert M (2022) Challenges in the development of digital public health interventions and mapped solutions: findings from a scoping review. Digit Health 8:20552076221102255. https://doi.org/10.1177/20552076221102255. PMID: 35656283; PMCID: PMC9152201

Iyamu I, Ramachandran S, Chang HJ, Kushniruk A, Ibáñez-Carrasco F, Worthington C, Davies H, McKee G, Brown A, Gilbert M (2025) Considerations for adapting digital competencies and training approaches to the public health workforce: an interpretive description of practitioners' perspectives in Canada. BMC Public Health 25(1):122. https://doi.org/10.1186/s12889-024-21089-1. PMID: 39794767; PMCID: PMC11720584

Karpathakis K, Libow G, Potts HWW et al (2021) An evaluation service for digital public health interventions: user-centered design approach. J Med Internet Res 23(9):e28356

Kass NE (2001) An ethics framework for public health. Am J Public Health 91(11):1776–1782. https://doi.org/10.2105/ajph.91.11.1776. PMID: 11684600; PMCID: PMC1446875

Krasna H, Czabanowska K, Beck A et al (2021a) Labour market competition for public health graduates in the United States: a comparison of workforce taxonomies with job postings before and during the COVID-19 pandemic. Int J Health Plann Manage 36:151–167. https://doi.org/10.1002/HPM.3128

Krasna H, Kornfeld J, Cushman L et al (2021b) The new public health workforce: employment outcomes of public health graduate students. J Public Health Manag Pract 27:12–19. https://doi.org/10.1097/PHH.0000000000000976

Kriegner S, Ottersen T, Røttingen JA, Gopinathan U (2021) Promoting intersectoral collaboration through the evaluations of public health interventions: insights from key informants in 6 European countries. Int J Health Policy Manag 10(2):67–76. https://doi.org/10.34172/ijhpm.2020.19. PMID: 32610746; PMCID: PMC7947666

Krishnan N, Gu J, Tromble R et al (2021) Research note: examining how various social media platforms have responded to COVID-19 misinformation. Harv Kennedy Sch Misinform Rev 2. https://doi.org/10.37016/MR-2020-85

Lisker S, Sarkar U, Aguilera A, Lyles CR (2022) Operationalizing academic-industry partnerships to advance digital health equity: lessons learned. J Health Care Poor Underserved 33:152–172. https://doi.org/10.1353/HPU.2022.0164

Martin LT, Chandra A, Nelson C et al (2022) Technology and data implications for the public health workforce. Big Data 10:S25. https://doi.org/10.1089/BIG.2022.0208

Moore BA, Barnett JE (2021) Leadership in public health. In: Case studies in clinical psychological science: bridging the gap from science to practice, pp 1–7. https://doi.org/10.1093/MED/9780198816805.003.0017

Moreland-Russell S, Saliba LF, Weno ER, Smith R, Padek M, Brownson RC (2022) Leading the way: competencies of leadership to prevent misimplementation of public health programs. Health Educ Res 37(5):279–291. https://doi.org/10.1093/her/cyac021

Nazeha N, Pavagadhi D, Kyaw BM, Car J, Jimenez G, Tudor Car L (2020) A digitally competent health workforce: scoping review of educational frameworks. J Med Internet Res 22(11):e22706. https://doi.org/10.2196/22706

Nebeker C, Torous J, Bartlett Ellis RJ (2019) Building the case for actionable ethics in digital health research supported by artificial intelligence. BMC Med 17:1–7. https://doi.org/10.1186/S12916-019-1377-7/TABLES/1

Nyström ME, Karltun J, Keller C et al (2018) Collaborative and partnership research for improvement of health and social services: researcher's experiences from 20 projects. Health Res Policy Sys 16:46. https://doi.org/10.1186/s12961-018-0322-0

Organisation for Economic Co-operation and Development (2020) Empowering the health workforce

Organisation for Economic Co-operation and Development Health Policy Studies (2019) Engaging and transforming the health workforce. In: Health in the 21st century: putting data to work for stronger health systems. OECD Publishing

Otok R, Richardson E, Czabanowska K, Middleton J (2018) The public health workforce. In: Rechel B, Jakubowski E, McKee M et al (eds) Organization and financing of public health services in Europe [Internet]. (Health Policy Series, No. 50). European Observatory on Health Systems and Policies, Copenhagen

Perakslis ED (2018) Using digital health to enable ethical health research in conflict and other humanitarian settings Chesmal Siriwardhana and Donal O'mathuna. Confl Health 12:1–8. https://doi.org/10.1186/S13031-018-0163-Z/TABLES/2

Pollack Porter KM, Rutkow L, McGinty EE (2018) The importance of policy change for addressing public health problems. Public Health Rep 133(1_suppl):9S–14S. https://doi.org/10.1177/0033354918788880. PMID: 30426876; PMCID: PMC6243447

Rechel B, McKee M (2014) Facets of public health in Europe. Open University Press

Rees GH, James R, Samadashvili L, Scotter C (2023) Are sustainable health workforces possible? Issues and a possible remedy. Sustainability 15:3596. https://doi.org/10.3390/SU15043596

Robbins T, Zucker K, Abdulhussein H, Chaplin V, Maguire J, Arvanitis TN (2020) Supporting early clinical careers in digital health: nurturing the next generation. Digit Health 6:2055207619899798. https://doi.org/10.1177/2055207619899798. PMID: 32010451; PMCID: PMC6971955

Salathé M (2018) Digital epidemiology: what is it, and where is it going? Life Sci Soc Policy 14:1. https://doi.org/10.1186/S40504-017-0065-7

Shaw JA, Donia J (2021) The sociotechnical ethics of digital health: a critique and extension of approaches from bioethics. Front Digit Health 3:725088. https://doi.org/10.3389/FDGTH.2021.725088

Shaw T, McGregor D, Brunner M et al (2017) What is eHealth (6)? Development of a conceptual model for eHealth: qualitative study with key informants. J Med Internet Res 19(10):e324. https://doi.org/10.2196/JMIR.8106

Shu Q, Wang Y (2021) Collaborative leadership, collective action, and community governance against public health crises under uncertainty: a case study of the Quanjingwan community in China. Int J Environ Res Public Health 18:1–12. https://doi.org/10.3390/IJERPH18020598

Singh HJL, Couch D, Yap K (2020) Mobile health apps that help with COVID-19 management: scoping review. JMIR Nurs 3(1):e20596. https://doi.org/10.2196/20596

Stark AL, Geukes C, Dockweiler C (2022) Digital health promotion and prevention in settings: scoping review. J Med Internet Res 24(1):e21063. https://doi.org/10.2196/21063

Teitelbaum JB, Theiss J, Boufides CH (2019) Striving for health equity through medical, public health, and legal collaboration. J Law Med Ethics 47(2_suppl):104–107. https://doi.org/10.1177/1073110519857330. PMID: 31298128

Tilson H, Gebbie KM (2004) The public health workforce. Annu Rev Public Health 25:341–356. https://doi.org/10.1146/ANNUREV.PUBLHEALTH.25.102802.124357

Toquero CMD (2023) Addressing infodemic through the comprehensive competency framework of media and information literacy. Thai J Public Health 45:e132–e133. https://doi.org/10.1093/PUBMED/FDAB412

Tsai E, Allen P, Saliba LF, Brownson RC (2022) The power of partnerships: state public health department multisector collaborations in major chronic disease programme areas in the United States. Health Res Policy Syst 20(1):80. https://doi.org/10.1186/s12961-021-00765-3. PMID: 35804420; PMCID: PMC9264297

van der Graaf P, Cheetham M, Redgate S et al (2021) Co-production in local government: process, codification and capacity building of new knowledge in collective reflection spaces. Workshops findings from a UK mixed methods study. Health Res Policy Syst 19:12. https://doi.org/10.1186/s12961-021-00677-2

Viens AM, Vass C (2020) Frameworks and guidance to support ethical public health practice. J Public Health (Oxf) 42(1):203–207. https://doi.org/10.1093/pubmed/fdz007. PMID: 31271205

Weeramanthri T, Tahzib F, Thomas J, Czabanowska K, Coombe L, Robinson P (2023) Public health ethics in the education and training of our public health workforce. Popul Med 5(Supplement):A744. https://doi.org/10.18332/popmed/164347

Wienert J, Jahnel T, Maaß L (2022) What are digital public health interventions? First steps toward a definition and an intervention classification framework. J Med Internet Res 24(6):e31921. https://doi.org/10.2196/31921

Winters RC, Chen R, Lal S, Chan TM (2022) Six principles for developing leadership training ecosystems in health care. Acad Med 97(6):793–796. https://doi.org/10.1097/ACM.0000000000004640. Epub 2022 Feb 22. PMID: 35703908

Wong BLH, Khurana MP, Smith RD et al (2021a) Harnessing the digital potential of the next generation of health professionals. Hum Resour Health 19:50. https://doi.org/10.1186/s12960-021-00591-2

Wong BLH, Siepmann I, Chen TT et al (2021b) Rebuilding to shape a better future: the role of young professionals in the public health workforce. Hum Resour Health 19:82. https://doi.org/10.1186/S12960-021-00627-7

World Health Organization (2016) Global strategy on human resources for health: Workforce 2030. World Health Organization, Geneva

World Health Organization (2018) Engaging young people for health and sustainable development: strategic opportunities for the World Health Organization and partners. WHO, Geneva

World Health Organization (2020) Global strategy on human resources for health: workforce 2030. WHO, Geneva. https://www.who.int/publications/i/item/9789241511131

World Health Organization (2021) Global strategy on digital health 2020–2025

World Health Organization (2022a) National workforce capacity to implement the essential public health functions including a focus on emergency preparedness and response. World Health Organization, Geneva

World Health Organization (2022b) Roadmap to professionalizing the public health workforce in the European Region. World Health Organization, Copenhagen

World Health Organization (2023a) What the COVID-19 pandemic has exposed: the findings of five global health workforce professions. World Health Organization, Geneva

World Health Organization (2023b) Open call for experts to serve as members of the Digital Health Competency Framework Committee. https://www.who.int/news-room/articles-detail/open-call-for-experts-to-serve-as-members-of-the-digital-health-competency-framework-committee. Accessed 6 Jun 2023

World Health Organization Regional Office for Europe (2020) WHO-ASPHER competency framework for the public health workforce. World Health Organization Regional Office for Europe, Copenhagen

Xu J, Xiao Y, Wang WH et al (2022) Algorithmic fairness in computational medicine. EBioMedicine 84:104250. https://doi.org/10.1016/J.EBIOM.2022.104250

Yokomichi H, Mochizuki M, Yamagata Z (2021) Encouraging cross-disciplinary collaboration and innovation in epidemiology in Japan. Front Public Health 9:641882. https://doi.org/10.3389/fpubh.2021.641882. PMID: 33869131; PMCID: PMC8044351

Yphantides N, Escoboza S, Macchione N (2015) Leadership in public health: new competencies for the future. Front Public Health 3:24. https://doi.org/10.3389/fpubh.2015.00024. PMID: 25767792; PMCID: PMC4341427

Zeeb H, Pigeot I, Schüz B (2020) Digital public health—an overview. Bundesgesundheitsblatt Gesundheitsforschung Gesundheitsschutz 63:137–144. https://doi.org/10.1007/S00103-019-03078-7/TABLES/1

Zenone M, Kenworthy N, Maani N (2023) The social media industry as a commercial determinant of health. Int J Health Policy Manag 12:1–4. https://doi.org/10.34172/IJHPM.2022.6840

Open Access This chapter is licensed under the terms of the Creative Commons Attribution 4.0 International License (http://creativecommons.org/licenses/by/4.0/), which permits use, sharing, adaptation, distribution and reproduction in any medium or format, as long as you give appropriate credit to the original author(s) and the source, provide a link to the Creative Commons license and indicate if changes were made.

The images or other third party material in this chapter are included in the chapter's Creative Commons license, unless indicated otherwise in a credit line to the material. If material is not included in the chapter's Creative Commons license and your intended use is not permitted by statutory regulation or exceeds the permitted use, you will need to obtain permission directly from the copyright holder.

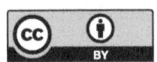

Assuring Sustainable Organizational Structures and Financing for Digital Public Health (EPHO 8)

Oliver Lange and Wolf Rogowski

Abstract Essential Public Health Operation (EPHO) 8 requires the assurance of sustainable financing to provide efficient, effective, and responsive services. Pursuing this purpose requires evidence on how a digital public health (DiPH) intervention impacts health, the environment, and scarce public health resources. Health economic evaluation provides a set of standards to generate this evidence. Based on the Consolidated Health Economic Evaluation Reporting Standards (CHEERS), this chapter discusses points to consider when evaluating (preventive) DiPH interventions. Specific issues arise, for example, from rapid technological change and the potential for long-term effects beyond the technological life cycle of single interventions. Also, which benefits and harms are to be considered in the economic evaluation depends on the decision maker, and there can be large differences between the decision makers who may acquire DiPH technologies (e.g., private households, health systems, other public payers, and companies). As interventions may have an intersectoral impact, a broader perspective may be necessary. There is also a growing need to account for the planetary boundaries of ecologically sustainable healthcare and public health. These issues can influence the results of an economic evaluation. Therefore it is particularly important for those making decisions on DiPH interventions to reflect on their assumptions and justify which areas may be affected beyond health.

Keywords Economic evaluation · Cost-utility · Cost-effectiveness · Cost-benefit · Digital health · Digital public health · Climate change · Life-cycle analysis

---

O. Lange (✉) · W. Rogowski
Institute of Public Health and Nursing Research (IPP), University of Bremen, Bremen, Germany

Leibniz Science Campus Digital Public Health Bremen, Bremen, Germany
e-mail: olange@uni-bremen.de; rogowski@uni-bremen.de

Abbreviations

CHEERS	Consolidated Health Economic Evaluation Reporting Standards
CO_2	Carbon Dioxide
DHI	Digital Health Intervention
DiPH	Digital Public Health
EEIO-LCA	Environmentally Extended Input-Output Life-Cycle Assessment
eHealth	Electronic Health
EPHO	Essential Health Operation
GHG	Greenhouse Gas Emissions
HEAP	Health Economic Analysis Plan
ISO	International Organization for Standardization
LCA	Life Cycle Assessment
mERA	Mobile Health Evidence Reporting and Assessment Checklist
mHealth	Mobile Health
NICE	National Institute for Health and Care Excellence
QALYs	Quality-Adjusted-Life-Years
RCT	Randomized Controlled Trials
SMS	Short Message Service
TIDieR	Template for the Intervention Description and Replication
TIDieR-telehealth	Template for the Intervention Description and Replication for Telehealth Intervention
WHO	World Health Organization

1 Introduction

Like any other public activity, public health operations have to account for limited resources. The purpose of EPHO 8 "is to ensure sustainable organizations and financing for public health to provide efficient, effective and responsive services. This entails developing services that are integrated, have minimal environmental impact with maximal health gain, and have sufficient funding for long-term planning. Sustainability in public health services will ensure that health is protected and promoted today and in the future" (WHO Regional Office for Europe 2022). Pursuing this purpose requires evidence of a service's impact on health, the environment, and limited public health budgets. This is our focus in the current chapter.

1.1 Generating Evidence of Sustainable Financing for Digital Public Health

In the policy debate, the financial[1] sustainability of health systems is frequently understood as a goal in its own right: to ensure a balance between entitlements granted to the covered population and available funds (Thomson et al. 2009). However, this may lead to policy focus on achieving fiscal balance, ignoring the possible impact of cost containment policies on other health systems goals like efficiency and equity (Thomson et al. 2009). We, therefore, follow Thomson et al. (2009) by viewing financial sustainability as a constraint to be respected rather than a goal in its own right.

Analyzing how to make (rational) decisions in the face of resource constraints can be seen as the definition of economics (Rogowski and Elsner 2021). Generally, there are always more decision options that could be pursued than resources available, which would be necessary to realize them. For example, in public health, there are always individuals that could benefit from more promotion of physical activity, dietary counseling, or different genetic or other screening programs if more programs were offered or more efforts were made to promote programs tailor them to individual preferences. Besides medical, epidemiological, legal, or ethical considerations, one unavoidable question for wisely spending health resources is how to invest a given budget in such a way as to obtain as much benefit as possible or how to obtain some amount of benefit with as low cost as possible.

To meet health system objectives in the face of increasing costs and resource constraints, policymakers have three options: increase the amount of funding, contain costs by reducing services, and increase efficiency by achieving more with existing resources (Thomson et al. 2009).

This chapter focuses on the third goal because digital technologies are associated with various promises to increase the effectiveness and efficiency of health services. For example, they may help to overcome spatial and temporal distances in monitoring health status and delivering health services, thereby reducing unnecessary transport, double diagnoses, avoidable diseases, and hospitalizations (see: Leppert and Greiner 2016).

This topic is timely as reimbursement agencies are currently handling various novel digital interventions. In Germany, for example, digital prevention courses are made available at the cost or with co-payments from sickness funds, which have to provide verification of effectiveness from the "Prüfstelle Prävention" (Prevention Testing Center). Also, since the Digital Healthcare Act came into force in 2019, digital interventions such as weight-loss apps for patients with obesity can be covered by statutory health insurance (Lantzsch et al. 2022).

Generally, "digital intervention" and "digital technology" are very broad terms. Similarly, "digital public health" (DiPH) can be understood broadly as the

---
[1] For organizational issues related to digital technologies, please see the chapter on EPHO 6 (Assuring Governance for Health and Wellbeing, Forberger) in this handbook.

digitalization of vertical public health functions encompassing all aspects of public health, such as health protection, health promotion, disease prevention, healthcare and preparedness for public health (WHO 2018). However, the broader one's concept of DiPH, the more difficult it is to make specific statements on its contribution to the efficiency of health resource spending. Therefore, we follow the view of DiPH presented by Zeeb et al. (2020), who focus on population, health promotion, disease prevention, and public health topics such as equity. In this view, DiPH contrasts with other concepts like eHealth, mHealth, digital health, and telemedicine, which all focus on medicine and medical treatment. Although this chapter draws on some literature regarding those concepts, our focus is on (preventive) DiPH interventions such as smartphone and wearable interventions targeting weight loss.

To assess whether investing in new DiPH interventions is an efficient use of health systems' scarce resources, evidence of their cost-effectiveness is needed. This evidence can be generated by health economic evaluations. Depending on the type of evaluation, DiPH interventions can be compared to conventional alternatives in terms of costs per clinical health outcome (cost-effectiveness analysis); cost per generic health outcome, such as quality-adjusted life years (QALYs; cost-utility analysis); cost per disaggregated set of outcomes (cost-consequences analysis); or in net monetary benefit comparing costs to benefits measured in monetary values (cost-benefit analysis) (Drummond et al. 2015). Chapter "Evaluation of Digital Public Health Interventions", Lange et al. in this handbook briefly summarizes evidence of the effectiveness and cost-effectiveness of DiPH interventions. In this chapter, we focus on the methods of assessing their cost-effectiveness.

DiPH interventions impact not only the scarce financial resources of health systems but also the scarce environmental resources used as inputs and the limited capacities to absorb emissions from health systems. These impacts may be desirable if, for example, a digital program for promoting physical activity reduces the number of individuals commuting by car to sports facilities or the number of hospital admissions and their associated carbon footprints (cf. Lange et al. 2022). However, the impacts may also be detrimental to the environment. For example, owing to the rebound effect, increases in material or energy efficiency of digital devices may be more than offset by the direct and embedded energy and material use of the growing number of devices and applications (Court and Sorrell 2020; Galvin 2015; Zhou et al. 2019). Therefore, we cover how to account for environmental impact in the economic assessment of DiPH efficiency.

1.2 Existing Knowledge and Targeted Gaps

Various articles describe methodological challenges in the economic evaluation of digital healthcare. However, they focus on digital health (e.g., Gomes et al. 2022; Kwee et al. 2022), digital mental health (e.g., Jankovic et al. 2020), or telemedicine (e.g., Bergmo 2012; Dávalos et al. 2009; Rojas and Gagnon 2008). To our knowledge, there is no systematized account of methodological challenges in the economic evaluation of (preventive) DiPH interventions. According to Weatherly et al. (2009), standard techniques are limited for preventive interventions. The authors cite four reasons: first, costs and benefits are connected to populations instead of individuals; second, as costs and benefits are typically wider for public health, an intersectoral approach may be needed to comprehensively identify them; third, commonly used approaches for measuring and valuing health benefits (e.g., QALYs) may fail to capture the intended effects; and fourth, standard methods of health economic evaluation may not sufficiently account for health inequalities, which are a particular feature of many public health interventions (Weatherly et al. 2009).

Therefore, this chapter aims to discuss relevant aspects for the economic evaluation of (preventive) DiPH interventions, considering both issues of digitalization and the specific challenges of assessing interventions for prevention and health promotion.

A central reference on how to conduct health economic evaluations transparently is the Consolidated Health Economic Evaluation Reporting Standards (CHEERS) (Husereau et al. 2022a). CHEERS aims to ensure that all types of economic evaluation are interpretable and useful for decision-making by specifying which details should be included (Husereau et al. 2022a). We use CHEERS for structuring methodological challenges in the economic evaluation of DiPH interventions. Following this structure, Sect. 1.2 will elaborate on the primary public health challenges regarding economic evaluation and then address points to consider in evaluation.

In environmental evaluations of digital technologies, it is necessary to capture not only the environmental impacts associated with the technology's use—e.g., energy use and associated carbon dioxide (CO_2) emissions—but also those associated with its resource use, production, transport, and disposal. In short, a life-cycle perspective is required.

Broadly, two methodological approaches serve this purpose. First, process-based life-cycle assessments (LCAs) require the identification of all processes and systems used to generate the intended outcome of a product throughout its life cycle. Data on all relevant material and energy flows within these processes is collected in a life-cycle inventory and used to build a life-cycle model. Subsequently, the environmental impacts of these flows are analyzed, usually based on approved models such as ReCiPe or TRACI. The final phase of process-based LCAs is the interpretation of results, including sensitivity analyses and discussion of limitations. Methodological standards for conducting process-based LCAs are provided by the International Organization of Standardization's (ISO) norms 14,040 and 14,044 (Matthews et al. 2018).

Second, environmentally extended input-output life-cycle assessments (EEIO-LCAs) estimate environmental impacts based on a top-down approach, in contrast to the bottom-up approach of a process-based LCA. The environmental impacts of an economy are allocated to its different industry sectors through input-output tables documenting the material and product exchanges between industry sectors. Extending these accounts of product flows in monetary values by environmental satellite accounts allows the calculation of emission factors per end product of the economy's industries—i.e., estimates of environmental impacts like CO_2 emissions per euro spent on products from a given industry. Multi-regional EEIO models allow for the inclusion of environmental impacts caused by production processes outside a national economy (Huang et al. 2009; Minx et al. 2009). While the estimates of environmental impacts from EEIO-LCA are less accurate than process-based LCA, they are easier to obtain. This is because health sector accounting frameworks provide standards for reporting costs per cost type. Frequently, these cost types (e.g., drugs or food) can be associated with industries (e.g., pharmaceutical or food industry) for which emission factors are available. Thus, environmental impacts like carbon footprint can be estimated by multiplying costs from bookkeeping data with readily available emission factors (see, e.g., Zhang et al. 2022).

While standards for conducting process-based or EEIO-LCA are available, the reporting standards are far less developed than those for other methods relevant to public health, such as health economic evaluations (for an example dedicated to carbon footprint, see: Lange et al. 2022). Additionally, there is an open question regarding whether and how the assessment of environmental scarcities by LCA can be integrated into health economic evaluations of DiPH. Environmental goals could be included on the effect side of economic evaluations by developing some aggregate measure of benefit that includes environmental benefit. Alternatively, environmental costs could be included on the cost side, extending the perspective of costs to environmental ones. In addition to reporting points to consider in evaluating DiPH interventions using standard health economic methods, the following section will elaborate on how environmental impacts might be integrated into the analysis.

2 Assuring Sustainable Financing and Considering Environmental Impacts

CHEERS provides a benchmark for transparency in its guidance on what to report in health economic evaluations. Its 28 items can also be used as a transparency checklist in systematic reviews of health economic evaluations (Lange 2022a). The following discusses methodological challenges concerning each item sequentially.

2.1 Title, Abstract, and Introduction

CHEERS requires that the title identifies the study as an economic evaluation and specifies the interventions being compared (item #1). Next, the abstract should describe the interventions (item #2), and the introduction should present the study question and its relevance for policy practice (item #3) (Husereau et al. 2022a). These criteria may appear rather generic for evaluations of DiPH interventions. It should be kept in mind, however, that reviews tracking the evidence in this field typically rely on information in the titles and abstracts to decide whether to include a study. Therefore, to ensure proper evidence synthesis, it is important to explicitly state the digital component early in the study report.

While standardized definitions of various digital health applications have been proposed, there is still a lack of standardized terminology for digital health interventions (DHI) (Burrell et al. 2022). Until such a generally agreed-upon terminology has been developed, it would be desirable if the aim of the intervention is stated alongside a description of the technology by which it is delivered (for example, A cost-effectiveness analysis of a weight-loss intervention delivered by mobile app and wearables vs. face-to-face meetings).

2.2 Health Economic Analysis Plan

CHEERS item #4 requires an indication of whether a health economic analysis plan (HEAP) was developed (Husereau et al. 2022a). HEAPs are used as study protocols and describe trials, parameters, and assumptions before an economic evaluation is conducted. Standardization of HEAPs is a new requirement for health economic evaluations. For trial-based economic evaluations, the authors of CHEERS (Husereau et al. 2022b) referred to a recent Delphi study and determined that 58 items should be included (Thorn et al. 2021), clustered into the following subsections: administrative information, trial introduction & background, economic approach/overview, financial data collection & management, economic data analyses, modeling, reporting/publishing, and appendixes.

However, as chapter "Evaluation of Digital Public Health Interventions", Lange et al. in this handbook explains, standard randomized controlled trials (RCTs) may not be the best approach for establishing evidence on the effectiveness of DiPH interventions. Decision-analytic modeling is a more flexible approach that can integrate different types of evidence; however, it is still unclear how HEAPs should be designed for model-based health economic evaluations. Additionally, study protocols are common practice in study-based economic evaluations (e.g., describing an RCT) but not for model-based economic evaluations. Generally, it appears possible to state the research question, justify the choice of perspective and the included effects and costs, and scientifically discuss a decision-analytic model before the analysis is conducted. However, decision-analytic models should incorporate the best available evidence, and new evidence may be published during the modeling work, especially in the dynamic field of DiPH.

2.3 Study Population and Setting

The choice of a study population to which a DiPH intervention is offered typically has various effects on effectiveness and cost-effectiveness. Thus, CHEERS requires a detailed description of the characteristics of the study population (item #5).

Preventive public health interventions, in particular, may use a heterogeneous target population (Haddix et al. 2002). Therefore, besides the study population, relevant subgroups should be identified. CHEERS also requires the provision of contextual information on setting and location that may impact the results (item #6 in Husereau et al. 2022a).

The selection of a study population and subgroups always depends on the decision problem and other parameters (e.g., setting and location). It should be noted that the study population does not always correspond to the target population. For example, a weight-loss app may be considered very effective based on study results obtained from individuals with obesity, but this result may not be transferable to the general population. This difference in effects may relate not only to absolute effects (e.g., if a cardiovascular drug prevents more myocardial infarctions in high-risk than low-risk patients) but also relative effects like risk reduction if perception, understanding, and reaction to the digital stimulus differ across subgroups (e.g., if diagnosed patients feel more affected by their disease than undiagnosed persons and thus are more adherent to prevention (Jankovic et al. 2020)). Unlike specific clinical interventions like bowel cancer screenings, DiPH interventions like smartphone apps are available to all. For a smartphone app aiming to help the user lose weight (and reduce their risk of chronic diseases), the effect could be higher in a group of obese or overweight persons. Additionally, the use of a DiPH intervention may mutually complement another treatment; for example, if a physician gives a diabetes patient detailed instructions on how to use a nutrition app, whereas an individual user in the general population lacks access to this information.

2.4 Comparators

CHEERS item #7 ("Comparator") requires a study to cautiously report the interventions or strategies being compared (Husereau et al. 2022a). Given the complexity of digital technologies, it is not easy to describe a DiPH intervention in a standardized manner. Different frameworks offer guidance on effectively describing an intervention or comparator.

For example, for the Template for the Intervention Description and Replication (TIDieR), a specific variant was developed to improve the reporting of research and ultimately maximize the potential for reproducing and implementing telehealth interventions (TIDieR-telehealth) (Rhon et al. 2022). TIDieR-telehealth requires reporting of the intervention name, rationale, used materials (e.g., software), procedures (e.g., remote delivery), intervention provider, type of location, number of times the intervention was delivered and over what period, details of any personalization or modification, and various other details.

While TIDieR-telehealth is a generic framework for telehealth interventions only, the mobile health evidence reporting and assessment (mERA) checklist (Agarwal et al. 2016) provides reporting guidance for mHealth interventions that could be adapted to describe digital aspects of the intervention and comparator in more detail. For example, mERA distinguishes between intervention delivery (e.g., SMS or face-to-face) and intervention content. Further, it requires the reporting of available infrastructure (electricity or connectivity), technology platforms (soft- and hardware), and interoperability (integration with existing health information systems). These technical aspects could be further investigated in environmental analyses by considering how many additional resources are necessary to implement the evaluated intervention.

Another framework is CONSORT-EHEALTH, a list of items for reporting web-based and mobile health interventions (Eysenbach 2011). It was developed specifically for use in publishing RCTs and contains 17 subitems deemed essential and 35 subitems considered to be highly recommended. Especially in DiPH, with countless apps available, these frameworks for describing an intervention can increase reproducibility.

While several frameworks are available to support detailed descriptions of interventions, the question remains of what constitutes the DiPH intervention's comparator. For non-digital public health interventions, examples of comparators are no program, standard care, or best alternative therapy (Haddix et al. 2002). Kolasa and Kozinski (2020) recommend that the value of a digital intervention should be expressed in comparison to the current standard of care. However, any comparator group is exposed to the multitude of other available digital interventions, making it unclear what constitutes "standard (digital) care" or "best alternative therapy." In particular, if a smartphone app intervention is compared to business as usual, various other apps are potentially freely available. The difference in effect between doing nothing and the intervention might be much larger than that between the intervention and business as usual. Also, clinical-trial participants in the "business as usual" group can access numerous other digital interventions (Murray et al. 2016). Therefore, the comparator choice may need to be specific to digital interventions.

Gomes et al. (2022) propose considering "digital and non-digital comparators and whether DHI replaces or complements existing technology" (Gomes et al. 2022). "For mHealth solutions without a comparator, a model-based full economic evaluation may be possible, drawing on primary data on the program's implementation costs" (LeFevre et al. 2017). Moreover, Gomes et al. (2022) propose a comparator for interventions in an area where other digital interventions are implemented and dominate digital care. First, the intervention could be compared to an alternative way of implementing the same DHI (Gomes et al. 2022). For example, Jones et al. (2022), Mizdrak et al. (2020), and Cleghorn et al. (2019) conduct model-based economic evaluations and evaluate the promotion of various existing apps. Second, the intervention could be compared to a competing DiPH (Gomes et al. 2022). For weight-loss interventions, many manufacturers of wearables or apps offer a similar function so that economic evaluation could compare against competing alternatives. Third, an appropriate comparator might be an "existing technology that the DHI is replacing" (Gomes et al. 2022). For instance, a physical activity and weight-loss intervention may involve a new sensor that gives feedback on user behavior by measuring the pulse, replacing generic feedback.

However, given the rapidity of technological development, effectiveness data may be lacking for some comparators. Therefore, model-based economic evaluation may need to use a comparator with the best available evidence rather than the most appropriate comparator.

Also, the distinction between digital and non-digital comparators can pose difficulties, as the digital aspects can only be considered one part of the intervention. This is further illustrated by the fact that McNamee et al. (2016) related digital interventions to the concept of complex interventions. Finally, there are various intermediate stages en route to a full digital intervention.

2.5 *Perspective*

CHEERS item #8 requires that the perspective is stated, i.e., the viewpoint from which the analysis is conducted. This viewpoint is the basis for determining which costs and benefits should be included (Haddix et al. 2002).

As indicated in chapters "A Framework to Develop and Evaluate Digital Public Health", Pan et al. (Domain "Costs and Economics") and "Evaluation of digital public health interventions", Lange et al. (Section "Evaluation of Cost-Effectiveness") in this handbook, stating the perspective is more complex for DiPH than for standard healthcare interventions. Suppose the aim is to evaluate a new device tracking physical activity, which is intended to improve the user's pleasure and performance when engaging in physical exercise like running, with the ultimate aims of improving their health status and lowering their risk of diabetes, stroke, and cardiovascular diseases. When evaluating a medical intervention like a new cancer drug, adopting a healthcare-payer perspective is straightforward. However, various perspectives may be relevant for (preventive) DiPH interventions:

- First, a private individual perspective might be appropriate because DiPH interventions (e.g., apps promoting physical activity) are frequently offered to individuals for free, and devices (e.g., activity trackers) are frequently acquired by individuals based on their preferences. Therefore, evaluations could plausibly include costs to private budgets and benefits of satisfying individual preferences.
- Second, DiPH interventions (sometimes even the same ones offered to private customers) may be covered by healthcare payers. In this case, a payer perspective would likely be considered appropriate, focused on health benefits and healthcare costs.
- Third, DiPH interventions may also be covered by other public payers like federal, state, or local governments as part of a digitalization strategy. In such cases, measuring both costs and benefits in monetary units might frequently be most appropriate to enable a cost-effectiveness comparison against the different alternative uses of scarce public budgets beyond the health system.

- Fourth, DiPH interventions may also be funded by companies for their employees. In such cases, an economic evaluation will likely be conducted regarding return on investment from a company perspective.

Formal health economic evaluations are generally conducted by healthcare and public health payers. Consequently, health outcomes are likely to be a key focus when evaluating DiPH interventions. Nevertheless, it appears important not to restrict the cost perspective to the narrow health(care) payer perspective but to incorporate a societal viewpoint. One reason is that a societal perspective has been explicitly recommended for preventive interventions (Haddix et al. 2002), which is an important aspect of our concept of DiPH. There have also been calls to include a societal perspective in digital health frameworks so as to account for costs outside the healthcare sector (Gomes et al. 2022). Especially for preventive DiPH interventions, spillover effects within households (particularly behavioral changes) could be better captured through a societal perspective (McNamee et al. 2016), as could productivity losses (see, e.g., Cobos-Campos et al. 2021; Song and Kanaoka 2018).

2.6 Time Horizon

CHEERS item #9 requires the study's time horizon to be stated and justified. A distinction needs to be made between the time horizon of the intervention, the effectiveness studies, and the analytical time horizon. For example, a digital weight-loss intervention with a duration of three months could be assessed in a follow-up study that estimates the effects after one year. This follow-up may conclude that the digital intervention decreases the risk of developing diabetes or heart disease, which are potentially long-term chronic diseases. Therefore, even if the intervention lasted only a few months, it seems reasonable to choose a broader analytical time horizon.

Particularly for preventive interventions, a lifelong time horizon typically appears ideal because present costs and future benefits are involved (Crowley et al. 2018). If the chosen time horizon were too short, the results would be distorted by missing not only relevant effects but also, especially for DiPH, the expected costs to maintain an intervention. For example, a digital food diary needs updates to remain functional as operating systems change on the used device.

This call for long time horizons contrasts with the short technology cycles of DiPH interventions. Rapid technological progress constantly renews the ways interventions are offered. For example, while web-based applications were more common a few years ago, they have now been largely replaced by smartphone applications. Individuals get used to digital devices, so constant innovation may even be required for a digital prevention program to maintain users' adherence. Given the rapid technological development of DiPH interventions, there is a lack of data for respective technologies over longer time periods. Consequently, it is unclear how long-term adherence and effectiveness can be achieved and should be modeled in economic evaluation. Assumptions must likely be made that need validation or testing in sensitivity analyses (Jankovic et al. 2020).

2.7 Discount Rate

Related to the choice of time horizon, CHEERS item #10 requires reporting the discount rate, which is only relevant for time horizons longer than one year.

The concept of time preference describes the extent to which an equal amount of benefit is valued more in the present than in the future. It is typically assumed that individuals prefer health benefits received today over future health benefits (Haddix et al. 2002). Consequently, economic evaluation discounts interventions' costs and benefits. Given that the effects of preventive public health interventions potentially occur over a long time horizon, the choice of discount rate can be expected to have a significant impact as higher discount rates diminish future costs and effects in the cost-effectiveness estimate (Crowley et al. 2018).

However, the last few years have seen remarkably rapid technological development in sensors, smartphones, and other tech through which digital health services are delivered. This leads to a conundrum: While time preference suggests that an investment should be made now rather than in the future, technology dynamics suggest that the same amount (in real terms) would generate significantly more effects if invested in the future rather than now. Thus, there may be a trade-off between accounting for time preference and accounting for rapid technological change.

2.8 Selection, Measurement, and Valuation of Outcomes

CHEERS items #10, #11, and #12, respectively, require a description of which outcomes are used, how they are used, and how there are valued. Depending on the intervention purpose, various outcomes could be considered. As pointed out in the section on perspective (see Sect. 2.5), relevant outcomes can include what individuals value (for whatever reason), standard health outcomes used in health economic evaluation, or outcomes that matter to other payers, such as workplace health effects for employers.

Even within health systems, DiPH interventions may be used for various purposes. The NICE Evidence Standards Framework for digital health and care technologies (Unsworth et al. 2021) contains ten functional categories on three levels (tier A: System impact; tier B: Understanding and communicating; and tier C: Interventions). These categories describe the purposes of digital health technologies most frequently funded by the health system. Many are also relevant for DiPH as conceptualized in this chapter—e.g., in tier A, system services like the COVID-19 warning app for preventive behavior; in tier B, health diaries using fitness wearables for general health monitoring; or in tier C, preventive behavior change. Following the framework, each tier is associated with specific evidence standards, with higher evidence requirements for tier C. For digital health technologies in tier C, only those in the functional categories of treatment, active monitoring, calculating, or diagnosing require evidence of effectiveness from RCTs with clinical outcomes. The effectiveness of preventive-behavior or self-management interventions should be established by experimental or quasi-experimental comparative studies, preferably with patient-reported or other relevant outcomes using validated tools but possibly also with outcomes like physiological measures (i.e., user satisfaction and engagement) or care process indicators (i.e., admissions and appointments). For other functions, the framework requires evidence of aspects such as user acceptability or credibility with health and social care professionals without the need to conduct RCTs (Unsworth et al. 2021).

For economic analysis, NICE recommends cost-utility analysis following the institute's standard methodology. If the benefit cannot be estimated in terms of QALYs, cost-consequence analysis is recommended, also following NICE standards. In addition, budget impact analysis is recommended (Unsworth et al. 2021).

There are several value-assessment guidelines for digital health interventions; they typically incorporate different aspects like organizational impact, data security, or technical considerations (Kolasa and Kozinski 2020). NICE recommends aggregating all relevant outcomes in terms of QALYs or reporting them in a disaggregated manner as part of a cost-consequences analysis. By contrast, Kolasa and Kozinski (2020) recommend establishing a multi-criteria score representing the clinical, organizational, behavioral, and technical performance of a digital health solution in the context of its implementation (Kolasa and Kozinski 2020).

Given the requirement of EPHO 8 to account for ecological sustainability, environmental effects could be integrated into the outcomes when economically evaluating DiPH interventions, either by listing them among the effects in cost-consequences analysis or by integrating them into some new multi-attribute value or utility score. However, because EPHO 8 requires minimizing environmental impacts, it might be more straightforward to integrate them among the costs. This approach would recognize that the environment represents scarce ecological resources used for providing the benefits of DiPH. The following section elaborates further.

2.9 Resources and Costs

CHEERS item #14 ("Measurement and valuation of resources and costs") requires a description of how costs were valued. Relatedly, item #15 stipulates that the currency, price date, and conversion method should be reported.

Besides the typical categories of costs and cost savings of public health programs (Haddix et al. 2002), which can be cross-sectoral (Weatherly et al. 2009), various other types of costs might need to be considered in the economic evaluation of DiPH interventions. These costs can broadly be structured by whether they accrue for intervention content or delivery and whether they accrue before or during and after the intervention (see Fig. 1).

One cost feature of DiPH interventions is the need for frequent updates, whether to adapt design and manageability, maintain compatibility with operating systems, or implement new features (Gomes et al. 2022). As McNamee et al. (2016) point out, digital interventions that are not updated cease to function.

Following Gomes et al. (2022), digital interventions are also characterized by high fixed and low variable costs because the incremental costs for additional users are close to zero. Consequently, studies with small sample sizes would result in an overestimation of mean costs per user (Gomes et al. 2022). A counter-balancing assumption is that DiPH interventions are typically more effective if recipients receive human support to ensure they apply the digital technology as intended (Gomes et al. 2022; Yardley et al. 2016). Any associated personnel costs need to be taken into account. However, this needs to be seen in the context of rapid technological change. Digital interventions have already evolved from mere advice on websites to individualized feedback using sensors. The fast pace of technological change and the time required to evaluate health services, in general, may result in studies being outdated and effectiveness underestimated, and new technologies may successfully substitute for human input.

The mERA checklist (Agarwal et al. 2016) includes various single components that can play a role in digital interventions. For example, if interoperability is

	Interventions' content	
	• Evidence assessment regarding the target condition (causes, treatments) • Evidence assessment regarding interventions suitable for digitalization (e.g. by means of individualized content or behavior change techniques) • Research about user preferences • Costs of developing content (McNamee et al. 2016)	• Staff time to deliver the intervention (Jankovic et al. 2020) • Human input/staff time for user involvement (Gomes et al. 2022) • Updates for the look, feel, navigation, and rewards for use (Gomes et al. 2022) • Modifying features of the content as far as warranted given new evidence (Gomes et al. 2022)
Pre-intervention		*During & post-intervention*
	• Equipment costs (Jankovic et al. 2020) • Capital costs (Jankovic et al. 2020) • Patient recruitment or technology dissemination (Jankovic et al. 2020) • Infrastructure costs to adopt programs (Crowley et al. 2018) • Costs of developing and implementing design (navigation menus, graphical elements) (McNamee et al. 2016) • Costs of developing and testing software and user experience (McNamee et al. 2016)	• Costs of infrastructure to sustain DiPH interventions over time (Crowley et al. 2018) • Website maintenance and hosting (Jankovic et al. 2020) • Software updates to ensure sustained compatibility with users' operating systems or web browsers (Gomes et al. 2022) • Updates of features promised to be up-to-date (e.g., information, content, navigation menus, graphical elements) (Gomes et al. 2022)
	Interventions' delivery (technology & infrastructure)	

Fig. 1 Potentially relevant costs specific for DiPH interventions. (Source: Own figure based on McNamee et al. 2016; Gomes et al. 2022; Jankovic et al. 2020; Crowley et al. 2018)

emphasized, additional costs may be incurred, and additional standards may need to be set by health legislation. Also, data security may have a high impact on costs. These and other requirements, such as ethical concerns, should be considered to investigate whether meeting them impacts the costs of DiPH interventions.

Increasingly visible ecological scarcities may necessitate accounting for resource constraints set by planetary boundaries (Rockstroem et al. 2009) and include environmental issues. One increasingly important concept that aims to bridge health and environmental considerations is "planetary health," summarized by Whitmee et al. (2015) as "the health of human civilisation and the state of the natural systems on which it depends." DiPH interventions consume not only scarce financial resources of health systems but also scarce natural resources like the planetary capacity to absorb greenhouse gas (GHG) emissions. There are different methodological links between cost analysis in health economic evaluation and environmental assessment. The need to report quantities and prices of resources separately was more prominent in early guidelines for reporting economic evaluations (Drummond and Jefferson 1996) but is still required by CHEERS (Husereau et al. 2022a, b). If all resources used are transparently listed and quantified in both physical units and prices, this provides a highly valuable starting point for LCAs. In particular, lists by cost type (e.g., server infrastructure or electrical energy) can be easily translated into lists of respective environmental impacts if the costs can be linked to industry sectors for which cost-based emission factors are available from EEIO-LCA databases (for an example of carbon footprint in hospital care, see: Zhang et al. 2022).

Where environmental impacts are not adequately priced (which is often the case), they constitute external costs that ought to be included in the analysis. However, further specification is needed on which environmental impacts should be included and whether and how they should be aggregated, converted into monetary terms, and reported. Until such guidance is issued on health economic evaluation in general or for DiPH in particular, one approach could be to select some core impacts, such as GHG emissions, and list them in a disaggregated manner in addition to the intervention's monetary costs.

2.10 Model, Analytics, Heterogeneity, and Uncertainty

For model-based economic evaluations, CHEERS item #16 requires the report to describe which model is used. This is supplemented by item #17, which requires a description of all methods for analyzing, transforming, extrapolating, and validating the model. CHEERS item #18 additionally requires transparency on the methods used to analyze differences between subgroups, while item #20 calls for clarity on any sources of uncertainty.

For evaluating DiPH interventions, model-based economic evaluation, and, consequently, CHEERS item #16 appear particularly relevant because modeling does have advantages (Briggs et al. 2006) which apply to DiPH. First, decision-analytic modeling allows estimation of long-term effects and cost-effectiveness, which would otherwise only be possible through costly long-term studies (and, in contrast to pharmaceutical companies, is unlikely to be financially feasible for digital technology manufacturers). Second, model-based analyses can more easily integrate different types of data, such as effectiveness data from N-of-1 trials and other new trial designs unsuitable for the cost questionnaires used in standard RCTs. Third, modeling studies make it easier to account for technology dynamics by integrating data on the most recent versions of DiPH interventions or modeling respective scenarios (given that, after a long-time study, the DiPH technology used is very likely to be outdated).

Model-based economic evaluations of DiPH interventions must also cope with particularly high structural uncertainty, given that rapid development may change technologies and care patterns. It is also difficult to account for parameter uncertainty: DiPH studies may, in fact, assess quite different interventions, so pooled estimates may be misleading because variance is due to technological differences, not the uncertainty of outcomes. Therefore, there is a particular need for transparency about the modeling methods—ideally, open-source models are required to allow early estimation of the cost-effectiveness of new DiPH interventions.

As for other highly dynamic technologies for which cost-effectiveness cannot be easily estimated before market entry, new forms of coverage with evidence development and evidence generation alongside use in public health practice (Brandes et al. 2016; Rogowski et al. 2016) could be important complements to decision-analytic modeling of DiPH. This is because model-based cost-effectiveness estimates need validation to ensure the efficient use of scarce resources funding a DiPH intervention compared to other available digital and analog public health interventions.

As individualized interventions are possible in DiPH, the role of heterogeneity and the need to establish evidence about ever smaller subgroups assume high importance (theoretically up to an n = 1 level of heterogeneity). However, this area needs further research.

2.11 Distributional Effects and Stakeholder Engagement

CHEERS item #19 requires describing the distribution of impacts across different individuals or how priority populations are accounted for, which is especially important for evaluating DiPH interventions. These considerations may also have a bearing on CHEERS item #21, which requires transparency about the involvement of patients or any other affected stakeholders in the study design.

Generally, for prevention interventions, the determinants of health and disease are critical, as addressing them may be necessary to prevent ill health. As far as these determinants are distributed unequally across socioeconomic groups (and thus interacting with them becomes a matter of chance, not individual choice), resulting health inequalities give rise to equity concerns that ought to be accounted for in the design and (economic) evaluation of DiPH interventions.

A widely used framework for understanding determinants of health and health inequalities is the socioecological "rainbow" model. In this model, Dahlgren and Whitehead (2007) organize these determinants on five hierarchical levels: (a) general socioeconomic, cultural, and environmental conditions; (b) living and working conditions; (c) social and community networks; (d) individual lifestyle factors; and (e) the individual-level stable characteristics like age and sex (Dahlgren and Whitehead 2007: 20).

In the economic evaluation of DiPH interventions, it is important to consider that these five layers are permeated by digital technologies and that health inequalities increasingly depend on digital determinants (Jahnel et al. 2022). Generally, the probability of individuals adhering to behavioral advice in prevention or screening programs strongly influences a program's effectiveness and cost-effectiveness (for an example of secondary prevention, see: Rogowski 2009; Rogowski et al. 2012). When assessing DiPH interventions, it should be considered that factors like adherence can be influenced by relevant developments in these five layers. For example, inequalities in the sustained use of a wearable device and smartphone app to promote physical activity can be influenced by lower internet bandwidth in deprived areas (living and working conditions level), differential exposure to online misinformation (social and community networks level), or unequal distribution of digitally mediated sedentary behavior (individual lifestyle factors level) (see: Jahnel et al. 2022, Fig. 1).

There are different methodological approaches to incorporate equity concerns into health economic evaluation (Cookson et al. 2017). In circumstances as complex as described in the previous paragraph, equity impact analysis may be particularly relevant as it allows assessing costs and effects using equity-relevant variables—e.g., by assessing the additional costs and effects of providing some digital infrastructure or device not typically available in a deprived group to equalize adherence to the digital intervention.

The move to involve patients, the public, and other stakeholders in designing economic evaluations is still in its infancy but represents a potentially important step toward enhancing the quality and acceptance of health economic research (Husereau et al. 2022b). Particularly for evaluating DiPH interventions, the need to appropriately account for the complexity of distributional effects may justify exploring new ways of involving relevant stakeholder groups in evaluation design.

2.12 Results and Discussion

Under the heading "Results," CHEERS items #22–25 require the presentation of information on all analytical input parameters, a summary of key results (such as the uncertainty of analytical values, discount rate, or time horizon), and details of the effect of engagement with patients or stakeholders. The same points discussed in the sections above must be considered for the economic evaluation of DiPH interventions.

Next, item #26 ("Discussion") requires a critical assessment of the limitations, any ethical or equity considerations not captured, and what effects these may have on patients, policy, or practice. Given the points to consider presented above, limitations are likely an essential aspect of the economic evaluation of DiPH interventions. Even with the ambition to provide comprehensive analysis, it is unlikely that every type of cost or outcome can be captured: there may be limited available data on all nuances of costs and benefits or insufficient room to address all possible sources of equity concerns. It may be neither possible nor necessary to incorporate all relevant aspects in estimating average costs per health outcome.

Finally, items #27 and #28, respectively, require the reporting of funding sources and conflicts of interest (Husereau et al. 2022a). As for other (public) health interventions, sufficient public funding must be allocated to evaluation to ensure unbiased estimates of the relative merits of different DiPH options currently available to health systems.

2.13 Accounting for Planetary Boundaries

While CHEERS provides valuable guidelines on points to consider in the economic evaluation of DiPH interventions, it naturally omits the reporting of items not yet standard in health economic evaluations—in particular, how to account for constraints set by the planetary boundaries.

Properly reporting results from process-based or EEIO-LCAs requires more than merely presenting emission factors for cost types and the results of multiplying them with cost values. LCA should be explicit about reasons for excluding certain processes from the analysis (e.g., the negligible additional energy consumption of a smartphone during use in a DiPH intervention); the temporal, geographical, and technological representativeness of data used in the analysis (e.g., assessing whether the GHG emission factors assumed for electrical energy consumption correspond with the energy mix in the intervention region); or ideally report environmental impacts per life-cycle phase (e.g., to estimate what proportions of GHG emissions arise during the program itself, the production phase of its components such as activity trackers, or the phase of their disposal) (Keil et al. 2023; Lange et al. 2022). No guidance currently exists on which of these LCA items can appropriately be identified alongside CHEERS items and which may need to be reported separately to provide a transparent assessment from a planetary benefits or costs perspective. Further research is necessary to fill this research gap.

3 Conclusion

DiPH is a field characterized by highly dynamic technologies. While web-based and browser-based applications were once considered innovative, DiPH interventions today entail smartphone applications, wearables, and mobile devices. Therefore, economic evaluations have to cope with the fact that available effectiveness studies frequently incorporate yesterday's technologies.

The perspective of an evaluation appears particularly important in the economic evaluation of DiPH interventions, which can incur private benefits, health effects relevant to healthcare and public health payers, or effects relevant to companies. Which costs and benefits are applicable, and consequently which evaluation method is most appropriate, needs to be determined more explicitly than is necessary, for example, in the economic evaluation of pharmaceuticals.

Specific issues in the cost assessment of DiPH interventions include the need for continuous updates to maintain compatibility with computer or smartphone operating systems. Economic evaluation might consider updated costs and the restricted time horizon of intervention effects. Another key issue is that high fixed costs may be incurred during development, particularly for software-based interventions, but the incremental costs of including additional users are close to zero.

In the face of climate change, how might economic evaluations of DiPH interventions account for the planetary boundaries of ecologically sustainable public health? Besides listing points to consider in evaluating DiPH interventions using standard methods of economic evaluation, this chapter has offered initial thoughts on incorporating planetary scarcities which requires expanding the evaluation methods to create a complete picture of economic impact.

Note: An earlier version of this chapter was reproduced and made available within the doctoral thesis of Oliver Lange (2022b).

References

Agarwal S, LeFevre AE, Lee J, L'Engle K, Mehl G, Sinha C, Labrique A (2016) Guidelines for reporting of health interventions using mobile phones: mobile health (mHealth) evidence reporting and assessment (mERA) checklist. BMJ 352:i1174. https://doi.org/10.1136/bmj.i1174

Bergmo TS (2012) Approaches to economic evaluation in telemedicine. J Telemed Telecare 18(4):181–184. https://doi.org/10.1258/jtt.2012.111112

Brandes A, Schwarzkopf L, Rogowski WH (2016) Using claims data for evidence generation in managed entry agreements. Int J Technol Assess Health Care 32(1–2):69–77. https://doi.org/10.1017/S0266462316000131

Briggs A, Sculpher M, Claxton K (2006) Decision modelling for health economic evaluation. Oxford Univ. Press, Oxford

Burrell A, Zrubka Z, Champion A, Zah V, Vinuesa L, Holtorf AP, Di Bidino R et al (2022) How useful are digital health terms for outcomes research? An ISPOR special interest group report. Value Health 25(9):1469–1479

Cleghorn C, Wilson N, Nair N, Kvizhinadze G, Nghiem N, McLeod M, Blakely T (2019) Health benefits and cost-effectiveness from promoting smartphone apps for weight loss: multistate life table modeling. JMIR mHealth and uHealth 7(1):13. https://doi.org/10.2196/11118

Cobos-Campos R, Mar J, Apinaniz A, de Lafuente AS, Parraza N, Aizpuru F, Orive G (2021) Cost-effectiveness analysis of text messaging to support health advice for smoking cessation. Cost Eff Resour Alloc 19(1):9. https://doi.org/10.1186/s12962-021-00262-y

Cookson R, Mirelman AJ, Griffin S, Asaria M, Dawkins B, Norheim OF, Verguet S, Culyer AJ (2017) Using cost-effectiveness analysis to address health equity concerns. Value Health 20(2):206–212

Court V, Sorrell S (2020) Digitalisation of goods: a systematic review of the determinants and magnitude of the impacts on energy consumption. Environ Res Lett 15(4):3001. https://doi.org/10.1088/1748-9326/Ab6788

Crowley DM, Dodge KA, Barnett WS, Corso P, Duffy S, Graham P, Greenberg M et al (2018) Standards of evidence for conducting and reporting economic evaluations in prevention science. Prev Sci 19(3):366–390. https://doi.org/10.1007/s11121-017-0858-1

Dahlgren G, Whitehead M (2007) European strategies for tackling social inequalities in health: levelling up part 2. WHO Regional Office for Europe, Copenhagen, DK

Dávalos ME, French MT, Burdick AE, Simmons SC (2009) Economic evaluation of telemedicine: review of the literature and research guidelines for benefit-cost analysis. Telemed J E Health 15(10):933–948. https://doi.org/10.1089/tmj.2009.0067

Drummond MF, Jefferson TO (1996) Guidelines for authors and peer reviewers of economic submissions to the BMJ. The BMJ Economic Evaluation Working Party. BMJ 313(7052):275–283

Drummond MF, Sculpher MJ, Claxton K, Stoddart GL, Torrance GW (2015) Methods for the economic evaluation of health care programmes. Oxford University Press, Oxford

Eysenbach G (2011) CONSORT-EHEALTH: improving and standardizing evaluation reports of web-based and mobile health interventions. J Med Internet Res 13(4):e126

Galvin R (2015) The ICT/electronics question: structural change and the rebound effect. Ecol Econ 120:23–31. https://doi.org/10.1016/j.ecolecon.2015.08.020

Gomes M, Murray E, Raftery J (2022) Economic evaluation of digital health interventions: methodological issues and recommendations for practice. PharmacoEconomics 40(4):367–378. https://doi.org/10.1007/s40273-022-01130-0

Haddix AC, Teutsch SM, Corso PS (2002) Prevention effectiveness: a guide to decision analysis and economic evaluation. Oxford University Press, Oxford

Huang YA, Lenzen M, Weber CL, Murray J, Matthews HS (2009) The role of input–output analysis for the screening of corporate carbon footprints. Econ Syst Res 21(3):217–242

Husereau D, Drummond M, Augustovski F, de Bekker-Grob E, Briggs AH, Carswell C, Caulley L et al (2022a) Consolidated Health Economic Evaluation Reporting Standards 2022 (CHEERS 2022) statement: updated reporting guidance for health economic evaluations. BMJ 376:e067975. https://doi.org/10.1136/bmj-2021-067975

Husereau D, Drummond M, Augustovski F, de Bekker-Grob E, Briggs AH, Carswell C, Caulley L et al (2022b) Consolidated Health Economic Evaluation Reporting Standards (CHEERS) 2022 explanation and elaboration: a report of the ISPOR CHEERS II Good Practices Task Force. Value Health 25(1):10–31

Jahnel T, Dassow HH, Gerhardus A, Schuz B (2022) The digital rainbow: digital determinants of health inequities. Digit Health 8:20552076221129093

Jankovic D, Bojke L, Marshall D, Saramago Goncalves P, Churchill R, Melton H, Brabyn S, Gega L (2020) Systematic review and critique of methods for economic evaluation of digital mental health interventions. Appl Health Econ Health Policy 19(1):17–27. https://doi.org/10.1007/s40258-020-00607-3

Jones AC, Grout L, Wilson N, Nghiem N, Cleghorn C (2022) The cost-effectiveness of a mass media campaign to promote smartphone apps for weight loss: updated modeling study. JMIR Form Res 6(4):e29291. https://doi.org/10.2196/29291

Keil M, Viere T, Helms K, Rogowski W (2023) The impact of switching from single-use to reusable healthcare products: a transparency checklist and systematic review of life-cycle assessments. Eur J Pub Health 33(1):56–63. https://doi.org/10.1093/eurpub/ckac174

Kolasa K, Kozinski G (2020) How to value digital health interventions? A systematic literature review. Int J Environ Res Public Health 17(6):2119

Kwee A, Teo ZL, Ting DSW (2022) Digital health in medicine: Important considerations in evaluating health economic analysis. Lancet Reg Health Western Pac 23:100476. https://doi.org/10.1016/j.lanwpc.2022.100476

Lange O (2022a) Health economic evaluation of preventive digital public health interventions using decision-analytic modelling: a systematized review. BMC Health Serv Res 23:268. https://doi.org/10.1186/s12913-023-09280-3

Lange O (2022b) Economic evaluation of digital public health. Dissertation, Fachbereich 11: Human- und Gesundheitswissenschaften der Universität Bremen, Bremen. https://doi.org/10.26092/elib/2187

Lange O, Plath J, Dziggel TF, Karpa DF, Keil M, Becker T, Rogowski WH (2022) A transparency checklist for carbon footprint calculations applied within a systematic review of virtual care interventions. Int J Environ Res Public Health 19(7474):1–14

Lantzsch H, Eckhardt H, Campione A, Busse R, Henschke C (2022) Digital health applications and the fast-track pathway to public health coverage in Germany: challenges and opportunities based on first results. BMC Health Serv Res 22(1):1182

LeFevre AE, Shillcutt SD, Broomhead S, Labrique AB, Jones T (2017) Defining a staged-based process for economic and financial evaluations of mHealth programs. Cost Effect Resour Alloc 15(1):5. https://doi.org/10.1186/s12962-017-0067-6

Leppert F, Greiner W (2016) Finanzierung und Evaluation von eHealth-Anwendungen (Funding and evaluation of ehealth applications). In: Fischer F, Krämer A (eds) eHealth in Deutschland. Anforderungen und Potenziale innovativer Versorgungsstrukturen (ehealth in Germany. Requirements and potential of innovative structures of care). Springer-Verlag GmbH, Berlin

Matthews HSH, Chris T, Matthews DH (2018) Life cycle assessment: quantitative approaches for decisions that matter. www.lcatextbook.com

McNamee P, Murray E, Kelly MP, Bojke L, Chilcott J, Fischer A, West R, Yardley L (2016) Designing and undertaking a health economics study of digital health interventions. Am J Prev Med 51(5):852–860. https://doi.org/10.1016/j.amepre.2016.05.007

Minx JC, Wiedmann T, Wood R, Peters GP, Lenzen M, Owen A, Scott K et al (2009) Input–output analysis and carbon footprinting: an overview of applications. Econ Syst Res 21(3):187–216

Mizdrak A, Telfer K, Direito A, Cobiac LJ, Blakely T, Cleghorn CL, Wilson N (2020) Health gain, cost impacts, and cost-effectiveness of a mass media campaign to promote smartphone apps for physical activity: modeling study. J Med Internet Res 22(6):e18014. https://doi.org/10.2196/18014

Murray E, Hekler EB, Andersson G, Collins LM, Doherty A, Hollis C, Rivera DE et al (2016) Evaluating digital health interventions: key questions and approaches. Am J Prev Med 51(5):843–851. https://doi.org/10.1016/j.amepre.2016.06.008

Rhon DI, Fritz JM, Kerns RD, McGeary DD, Coleman BC, Farrokhi S, Burgess DJ et al (2022) TIDieR-telehealth: precision in reporting of telehealth interventions used in clinical trials—unique considerations for the Template for the Intervention Description and Replication (TIDieR) checklist. BMC Med Res Methodol 22(1):161. https://doi.org/10.1186/s12874-022-01640-7

Rockstroem J, Steffen W et al (2009) A safe operating space for humanity. Nature 461(7263):472–475

Rogowski WH (2009) The cost-effectiveness of screening for hereditary hemochromatosis in Germany: a remodeling study. Med Decis Mak 29(2):224–238. https://doi.org/10.1177/0272989X08327112

Rogowski WH, Elsner W (2021) How economics can help mitigate climate change—a critical review and conceptual analysis. In: Bremen Papers on Economics & Innovation, p 2106. https://ideas.repec.org/p/atv/wpaper/2106.html

Rogowski WH, Grosse SD, Meyer E, John J, Palmer S (2012) Die Nutzung von Informationswertanalysen in Entscheidungen über angewandte Forschung. Der Fall des genetischen Screenings auf Hämochromatose in Deutschland. Bundesgesundheitsblatt Gesundheitsforschung Gesundheitsschutz 55(5):700–709

Rogowski W, John J, Ijzerman M (2016) Translational health economics. In: Scheffler RM (ed) World scientific handbook of global health economics and public policy, vol 3. World Scientific

Rojas SV, Gagnon MP (2008) A systematic review of the key indicators for assessing telehomecare cost-effectiveness. Telemed J E Health 14(9):896–904. https://doi.org/10.1089/tmj.2008.0009

Song M, Kanaoka H (2018) Effectiveness of mobile application for menstrual management of working women in Japan: randomized controlled trial and medical economic evaluation. J Med Econ 21(11):1131–1138. https://doi.org/10.1080/13696998.2018.1515082

Thomson S, Foubister T, Figueras J, Kutzin J, Permanand G, Bryndová L (2009) Addressing financial sustainability in health systems. Policy summary prepared for the Czech European Union Presidency Ministerial Conference on the Financial Sustainability of Health Systems in Europe. https://apps.who.int/iris/handle/10665/107966

Thorn JC, Davies CF, Brookes ST, Noble SM, Dritsaki M, Gray E, Hughes DA et al (2021) Content of Health Economics Analysis Plans (HEAPs) for trial-based economic evaluations: expert Delphi consensus survey. Value Health 24(4):539–547. https://doi.org/10.1016/j.jval.2020.10.002

Unsworth H, Dillon B, Collinson L, Powell H, Salmon M, Oladapo T, Ayiku L et al (2021) The NICE Evidence Standards Framework for digital health and care technologies—developing and maintaining an innovative evidence framework with global impact. Digit Health 7:20552076211018617. https://doi.org/10.1177/20552076211018617

Weatherly H, Drummond M, Claxton K, Cookson R, Ferguson B, Godfrey C, Rice N et al (2009) Methods for assessing the cost-effectiveness of public health interventions: key challenges and recommendations. Health Policy 93(2):85–92. https://doi.org/10.1016/j.healthpol.2009.07.012

Whitmee S, Haines A, Beyrer C, Boltz F, Capon AG, de Souza Dias BF, Ezeh A et al (2015) Safeguarding human health in the Anthropocene epoch: report of The Rockefeller Foundation-Lancet Commission on planetary health. Lancet 386(10007):1973–2028

WHO (2018) Essential public health functions, health systems and health security: developing conceptual clarity and a WHO roadmap for action. World Health Organization, Geneva

WHO Regional Office for Europe (2022) EPHO8: Assuring sustainable organisational structures and financing. https://www.euro.who.int/en/health-topics/Health-systems/public-health-services/policy/the-10-essential-public-health-operations/epho8-assuring-sustainable-organisational-structures-and-financing. Accessed 7 May 2022

Yardley L, Spring BJ, Riper H, Morrison LG, Crane DH, Curtis K, Merchant GC et al (2016) Understanding and promoting effective engagement with digital behavior change interventions. Am J Prev Med 51(5):833–842. https://doi.gov/10.1016/j.amepre.2016.06.015

Zeeb H, Pigeot I, Schüz B (2020) Leibniz-WissenschaftsCampus Digital Public Health B [Digital public health-an overview]. Bundesgesundheitsbl Gesundheitsforsch Gesundheitsschutz 63(2):137–144. https://doi.org/10.1007/s00103-019-03078-7

Zhang X, Albrecht K, Herget-Rosenthal S, Rogowski W (2022) Estimation of carbon footprints for hospital care based on routine G-DRG accounting data in Germany: an application to acute decompensated heart failure. J Ind Ecol 26(3)

Zhou XY, Zhou DQ, Wang QW, Su B (2019) How information and communication technology drives carbon emissions: a sector-level analysis for China. Energy Econ 81:380–392. https://doi.org/10.1016/j.eneco.2019.04.014

Open Access This chapter is licensed under the terms of the Creative Commons Attribution 4.0 International License (http://creativecommons.org/licenses/by/4.0/), which permits use, sharing, adaptation, distribution and reproduction in any medium or format, as long as you give appropriate credit to the original author(s) and the source, provide a link to the Creative Commons license and indicate if changes were made.

The images or other third party material in this chapter are included in the chapter's Creative Commons license, unless indicated otherwise in a credit line to the material. If material is not included in the chapter's Creative Commons license and your intended use is not permitted by statutory regulation or exceeds the permitted use, you will need to obtain permission directly from the copyright holder.

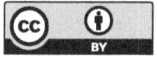

Advocacy, Communication, and Social Mobilization for Health (EPHO 9)

Rasmus Cloes, Christopher Jones, Hajo Zeeb, and Benjamin Schüz

Abstract In this chapter, we discuss the potential and challenges of digital communication in advocacy and social mobilization for public health. Digitalization has significantly impacted the flow of information, both positive and negative, emphasizing the need for evidence-based communication to counter misinformation and speculation. Using the COVID-19 infodemic as an example, we highlight how social mobilization through social networks can influence public health. Digital communication poses both increased opportunities for advocacy and social mobilization and increased risks through complex digital environments and disparities in digital health literacy among different population groups. In order to be effective for advocacy and social mobilization, digital health communication needs to be timely, transparent, accurate, and appropriate. We use three examples to exemplify the potential and risks of digital communication for social mobilization and advocacy: (1) the German Competence Network Public Health COVID-19, which utilized digital technology to compile and disseminate evidence to policymakers, (2) the adverse impact of misinformation and the strategies employed by "super sharers" on social media to spread misleading health-related information, and (3) how digital communication enables grassroots digital tactics in planetary health activism.

We highlight important processes and preconditions to find effective solutions to communicate and inform efficiently and independently in the digital space while

R. Cloes (✉) · H. Zeeb
Leibniz-Institute for Prevention Research and Epidemiology-BIPS, Bremen, Germany
e-mail: cloes@leibniz-bips.de; zeeb@leibniz-bips.de

C. Jones
Institute for Public Health and Nursing Research (IPP), University of Bremen, Bremen, Germany

Center for Preventive Medicine and Digital Health (CPD), Mannheim Medical Faculty of Heidelberg University, Mannheim, Germany
e-mail: christopher.jones@medma.uni-heidelberg.de

B. Schüz
Institute for Public Health and Nursing Research (IPP), University of Bremen, Bremen, Germany
e-mail: benjamin.schuez@uni-bremen.de

addressing the dynamics of the attention economy and the influence of major digital corporations.

Keywords Digital communication · Advocacy · Infodemics · Social mobilization

1 Introduction

Advocacy for public health entails a broad range of activities, and with communication and interaction heavily digitalized, many new opportunities and additional features have arisen. Compared to the origins of the use of "advocacy" for health promotion in the Ottawa Charter (1986), the flow of information between and within different stakeholder groups has taken on new dimensions in terms of amount, speed, breadth, and diversity. This explicitly includes misinformation and speculation critical of evidence-based communication to support public health aims and concepts, such as the avalanche of misinformation spread during the COVID-19 pandemic. The infodemic[1] exemplified the power of—in this case, adverse—social mobilization for health through social networks.

On the other hand, opportunities for advocacy and social mobilization for public health have increased substantially through digital technologies, as many chapters of this handbook attest. Overall, the topic of digital communication and advocacy is closely linked to (digital) health literacy in the population as well as among major public stakeholders—those who find it easier to access, interpret and act upon health-related information are both more likely to engage in more health-related activities, but also to engage with and publicly discuss health-related topics. At the same time, levels of (digital) health literacy differ substantially between population groups and are often correlated with educational attainment (Van Der Vaart and Drossaert 2017). Digital health communication and advocacy also include science communication in public health. Here, the goal is to support the decision-making of individuals and policy actors, as recently highlighted during the COVID-19 pandemic, but also with respect to longer-term endeavors such as evidence-based communication about tobacco, alcohol, and other chronic disease risk factors. Today's health communication is largely digital or builds on cross-media approaches that include digital as well as traditional tools. Timeliness, transparency, accuracy, a non-manipulative approach, and appropriateness for the respective target group are central aspects of good health communication (Oxman et al. 2022) that remain highly relevant for digital health communication. Participation and empowerment are further central cornerstones

---

[1] According to the WHO, the term infodemic describes the rapid spread and amplification of information, both true and false, through various communication channels, including social media, websites, news, and word of mouth. The term highlights the challenge of navigating a vast sea of information to identify accurate and reliable sources, which is critical in times when access to reliable information is crucial (Zielinski 2021).

with major importance for social mobilization, although these are not sufficiently considered and supported in (digital and other) health communication concepts.

The following sections discuss three examples of digital communication for social mobilization and advocacy to highlight how digital technology can serve this Essential Public Health Operation (EPHO). The first example, the German Competence Network Public Health COVID-19, highlights how digital technology can facilitate effective communication among public health stakeholders to communicate health-related evidence to policymakers. The second case, health-related misinformation and social mobilization through social media, highlights how this EPHO must also target maladaptive health communication and social mobilization. In contrast, the third example, planetary health activism, highlights grassroots digital tactics and processes that support social mobilization through interwoven links with the analog space. Table 1 provides an overview of goals, methods, and digital tools to explain how we conceptualized the examples in this chapter.

Table 1 Goal-related concepts of EPHO 9 linking the examples in this chapter

EPHO goal	Target	Methods	Digital tools	Example
Advocacy	Policymakers	Policy briefs	Production: group coordination tools (e.g., Slack) Dissemination: websites, mailing, social media	German COVID-19 Competence Network
		Public briefings	Livestreams (e.g., YouTube)	Independent SAGE
Communication	Individuals	Behavior change communication	Social Media campaigns	COVID-19 vaccination information
		Prevention of sharing misinformation	Interventions in social media	Super sharer prevention
		Prevention of believing in misinformation	Pre- or debunking misinformation	Misinformation flags in social media
Social Mobilisation	Individuals	Group alignment and identification	Social media: personal expression of celebrities	Linking celebrity testimonials to #hashtags
	Local groups	Linking local action to global movements	Publishing activism on social media: hashtags	Linking activities to #hashtags
	Individuals	Engagement in political processes	Digital platforms	Local digital platforms for participation in local legislation

Source: Own table

2 Digitally Compiling and Disseminating Evidence: The Example of the German Competence Network Public Health COVID-19

Right at the beginning of the COVID-19 pandemic in April 2020, the German Competence Network Public Health COVID-19 was established as an ad hoc consortium of more than 25 scientific societies and organizations that are active in the field of public health, representing disciplines such as epidemiology, statistics, social sciences, demography, and medicine. 15 interdisciplinary working groups collected, identified, and responded to critical areas of concern in the COVID-19 pandemic, such as modeling, ethics, or risk communication. The objective was to quickly and flexibly provide coordinated expertise on COVID-19 for the then-current discussions and decision-making. Outputs of the Competence Network were mainly rapid review-based policy briefs but also included statements, video events, and other formats. The target groups for the information were stakeholders and multipliers such as politicians, journalists, or physicians.

The strong influence of digitization was already evident in the knowledge generation stage. Web-based instant messaging services, such as Slack, enabled teams to work together efficiently and exchange content on a time-shifted and geographically separated basis, an essential requirement in an infectious disease pandemic (Amankwah-Amoah et al. 2021). Digital collaboration on joint manuscripts was swiftly established through similar channels. This collaboration, made possible by digitization, helped to counteract the emerging infodemic to some extent: through digital collaboration, the societies avoided the appearance of numerous comparable but uncoordinated statements on the same topic, e.g., on the efficacy of face masks to mitigate COVID-19, on the role of indoor settings for the spread of the virus or the importance of school closures.

Without such coordination, every scientific society or organization might have worked on its own statement or rapid review—possibly with varying outcomes and potentially conflicting messaging—as has happened in the past (Zielinski 2021).

Once the present evidence on a topic was summarized and a final paper was available, the goal was to disseminate it to the appropriate stakeholders and multipliers. For this purpose, reports were first made freely available on the main website of the Competence Network. A summary on the respective report provided a quick overview of the key messages as decision-makers request concise information during pandemics (Cloes et al. 2015). The information about a new policy brief was then disseminated via the Twitter account (today: X; however, since the network was called Twitter at the time the examples were used, this name should be used in this text) of the Competence Network, press releases, and informal channels of the scientists involved. Direct contact with the main authors was also offered.

The results of this work were often judged as mixed by the participants (Seidler et al. 2021; Evers et al. 2021). On the one hand, it was considered positive that national media picked up numerous reports and that some recommendations were considered the basis for legislation at the time. On the other hand, the Competence Network members criticized politicians' lack of interest in some of the policy briefs.

A critical look at the dissemination channels used and successes achieved can help classify these assessments. At the time, Twitter was used as the primary social network for disseminating information, as it was the most suitable network in German-speaking countries for reaching journalists and politicians (Nuernbergk 2020). At times, more than 1000 people followed the Competence Network on Twitter, representing small followership at best—and in particular compared to the 177,000 followers of Independent SAGE, a similar informal group of scientists in the UK with the explicit goal of informing policy. However, these 1000 followers included numerous journalists from relevant media, such as the major daily Süddeutsche Zeitung, or other essential stakeholders like politicians, their consultants, or decision-makers from, for example, health-related institutions. Here, the posts often achieved reasonable interaction rates and reached a correspondingly large audience.

The webpage views of the various individual publications provide a cautious indication of how much interest the individual topics generated. It should be noted that multiple hits or other factors may distort these figures. The fact sheets, statements, and policy briefs achieved between 17,000 and 31,000 page views—good statistics, considering the stakeholder orientation of the statements. Overall, these numbers are relatively homogeneous compared with other websites. However, the situation is different for media mentions. Here, a classic picture of the society of singularities emerges (Reckwitz 2018), rewarding pointed theses with attention and punishing balanced assessments with disregard. If the Competence Network's assessments had clear, simple messages, they made it to numerous media outlets and thus to the public more often. If, however, the assessments were more cautious and deliberative, their dissemination was sluggish. This shows that the communication of public health topics is subject to the same dynamics of the attention economy as all other issues in our society.

Ultimately, it remains positive to note that the opportunity for digital collaboration in creating harmonized policy briefs and statements might have counteracted the infodemic to a certain extent. Even though this claim lacks concrete numbers, this remains a relevant proposition that should be considered for future comparable situations. What persists is the fundamental problem of digital communication, which strongly depends on intensification to make a message heard. Here, public health must continue to look for appropriate solutions to communicate and inform efficiently in the digital space.

3 Adverse Mobilization Against Public Health Goals: The Impact and Strategies of "Super Sharers" of Dis- and Misinformation on Social Media

While digital communication of health topics can potentially achieve quicker policy influence, there are specific risks to the online discourse around health information and misinformation.

Nearly three out of four US adults regularly look for health information online, and this number will likely increase as users increasingly rely on social media. It is estimated that 5% of all internet searches are health-related, not counting the amount of information presented automatically in users' feeds and through advertisements (Swire-Thompson and Lazer 2020). Despite this overall shift towards democratizing and making health information accessible to all, including those previously disadvantaged due to age, education, or income, it has also added new risks for individuals and public health. It remains essential to recognize that laypeople are not health experts, and the freedom to research one's ailments or specific health interests in such an information-rich environment can come at a cost.

Disinformation (information created with malicious intent to deceive) and misinformation (created or shared without clear deceptive intent) are introduced by various sources and through different channels. The vastness of the internet makes it challenging to separate fact from fiction, even for those highly motivated (Lazer et al. 2018; Pennycook and Rand 2021). Studies show that false information diffuses significantly farther, faster, deeper, and more broadly than true information (Vosoughi et al. 2018. This is due to the novelty of the content and the strong emotions it elicits, such as disgust, fear, and surprise (Vosoughi et al. 2018). Furthermore, engagement with fake news is very much concentrated: only 1% of individuals see 80% of the false information, and just 0.1% of individuals share 80% of this misleading content (Grinberg et al. 2019).

However, contrary to the widespread assumption, large-scale virality, where information rapidly spreads from person to person, is rare. Content often becomes popular because influential accounts share it with their audiences (Goel et al. 2012). Hence, individuals and corporations with large social media audiences have a greater responsibility to ensure the accuracy of the health information they share. Predictably, however, influential social media figures have instead assumed the role of "super sharers" of misleading health-related information by disseminating sensational and emotionally charged messages tailored to their followers' ideologies and expectations and manipulating scientific uncertainty (Allchin 2023). The resulting broad and far-reaching spread and public endorsement of such misleading content can create false legitimacy and suggest a fake balance with current scientific knowledge. In a similar vein, suggestions by "super sharers" given to topic experts to "debate" them on topics such as the effectiveness of vaccines undermine a factually clear evidence base.

We illustrate this with a case study of Joe Rogan podcasts: Joe Rogan is a popular right-leaning US podcast host with an estimated following of more than 17 million users. On his podcast, he has repeatedly expressed vaccine-critical views. Consequently, Rogan's platform has become a hub for vaccine dis- and misinformation both by himself and through comments on the website and in the podcast. As a result, a study found that only 27% of his followers planned on getting vaccinated against COVID-19 (Rathje et al. 2022). For example, a 2023 podcast episode featured a conversation with US politician Robert F. Kennedy Jr., a then known anti-vax activist and now the 26th United States Secretary of Health and Human Services. Multiple factually incorrect pieces of vaccine disinformation were published unchecked during the episode, and known conspiracy theories about vaccinations were peddled. This disinformation found strong support within Rogan's networks on social media and widespread criticism outside of these circles. Peter Hotez, Professor of Pediatrics and Molecular Virology & Microbiology at Baylor College of Medicine, took to Twitter to substantially criticize Rogan and Kennedy. Rogan replied by inviting Hotez to a "debate" during one of his upcoming podcasts, but as Hotez declined, offering a one-on-one conversation instead, Rogan (and like-minded Elon Musk) started aiming personal attacks at Hotez, questioning his morals, undermining his professional qualifications while suggesting he would be receiving personal benefits for his support of "big pharma."

This episode showcases a variety of strategies and mechanisms contributing to the proliferation of health-related dis- and misinformation through such super sharers. One such strategy is using sensational, novel, and emotionally charged content. This capitalizes on how social media platforms are built: their algorithms prioritize content that generates high levels of engagement through strong emotional reactions indicated by, for example, likes, shares, and comments. Specifically, disinformation is often presented through empowering narratives (e.g., the emphasis on examining the, unfortunately, pre-selected and biased evidence by oneself), presents over-simplified solutions to complex health issues, or advocates for personal freedom against suggested control by others (e.g., the federal government or medical experts; Swire-Thompson and Lazer 2020). These narratives resonate with individuals' emotions and desire for autonomy and control over health-related decisions, thus increasing appeal and reach (Berger and Milkman 2012; Peters et al. 2009).

A second strategy is the manipulation of scientific uncertainty. Health-related information is often surrounded by a degree of uncertainty as scientists continue to work on understanding the issue. Super sharers exploit this uncertainty by presenting disinformation embedded into alternative, easy-to-follow narratives that challenge the current scientific consensus (if there already is one) and offer a much simpler solution without uncertainty. This strategy can then help create a false equivalence or balance between rigorous scientific knowledge and unfounded theories, with social media users having been shown to engage less with high-quality information if the low-quality information is easier to understand or more engaging (Loeb et al. 2019).

As a third strategy, super sharers leverage their popularity and perceived authority, lending credibility to the misleading content they propagate. They are often seen as trustworthy sources by their audience, especially if they have a large following supporting their views through, e.g., likes and shares. In this case, the resulting changes to social norms lend additional support to the shared content and strengthen the overall impetus to believe and share (Ecker et al. 2022).

Furthermore, super sharers tap into their followers' expectations and ideologies. They frame their narratives in ways that appeal to their audience's pre-existing beliefs, morals, and values, thereby increasing the likelihood of acceptance and sharing (Ecker et al. 2022; Swire-Thompson and Lazer 2020). For example, they may align their disinformation with political ideologies or sentiments opposing conventional medicine, as seen in the rise of the QAnon movement in the US or the Querdenker ("lateral thinker") in Germany (Kutscher 2022; Rathje et al. 2022). The rise of these groups shows how disinformation can have a real-world impact as it shapes public perceptions, prompts societal unrest, and creates mistrust in scientific expertise and public health measures. During the COVID-19 pandemic, such protests disrupted social cohesion, hindered an effective public health response, and pressured policymakers (Bridgman et al. 2020; Kim et al. 2022; Roozenbeek et al. 2019).

Finally, super sharers often engage in public disputes with reputable sources, as in the case of Joe Rogan challenging an expert in the respective field to a debate on his show. These public feuds increase the visibility and reach of the misleading content and undermine the credibility of reliable sources by presenting them as unwilling to engage in open discussion or following personal interests. This strategy thus further entrenches disinformation, making it more difficult to counteract.

In conclusion, the strategies employed by super sharers of health dis- and misinformation are sophisticated, focused on creating content that spreads far through their network and heavily targeted towards their specific audience. They exploit the features of social media platforms, manipulate scientific uncertainty, leverage their influence, tap into existing biases, and engage in public disputes to spread false content. Countering these strategies and the spread of misleading health-related content, in general, is crucial and requires concerted and systematic efforts from public health experts, social media platform providers, and the public alike to promote accurate information and support health-related decision-making for all (Wang et al. 2019). Such strategies need to include both thorough fact-checking to debunk currently widespread mis- and disinformation (Whitehead et al. 2023) and, if possible, prebunking efforts, during which audiences are prepared that they will be exposed to misinformation together with correct information and strategies to identify misinformation (e.g., Roozenbeek et al. 2022). In addition, measures within social media networks to limit further sharing posts by super sharers, such as misinformation flags and behavioral interventions (e.g., Jones et al. 2023), can help limit super sharers' impact. Ironically, there might be something to be learned from super sharers on how such efforts could look.

4 Digital Social Mobilization in Young Target Groups: Planetary Health and Climate Activism

Besides mis- and disinformation, there are also adaptive examples of extensive social mobilization through a concerted effort weaving together online digital communication and analog protest action (which is recorded, streamed, and multiplied digitally). Online mediated movements for planetary health through climate activism—hereafter broadly summarized under *#FridaysforFuture*—would not have been possible without the current state of digital communication and mobilization through social media.

One key defining feature of such digitally mediated movements—in contrast to, e.g., environmental activism in the 1970s and 1980s—is that rapid digital communication between members and local groups linked to the movement allows faster connections between members and mobilization through a more personalized expression of opinions and direct personal appeal to members and others, such as the press, at the same time. It has been hypothesized that, in contrast to previous movements, which required explicit joining of groups and centralized action, social media-mediated movements allow large-scale voluntary personal expression, leading to connection and identification with the movement ("connective action"; Bennett and Segerberg 2013). These processes can be facilitated if celebrities or social media multipliers with many followers support a cause through personal expression. In this vein, using social media also allows linking previously isolated and potentially inconsequential events to a larger, global cause and movement, thus amplifying the content of these actions (Boulianne et al. 2020). Whether this truly reflects a reinvigorated interest in democratic processes, as some optimistic observers claim (Pickard 2022), remains to be seen—similar processes underlie mobilization for non-democratic and maladaptive activism causes (see previous example).

Online conversation within and with the movement (e.g., through comments to posts by particularly prominent actors such as Swedish activist Greta Thunberg) is supposed to negotiate and reinforce positions within activist movements (Oliveira et al. 2023). While this notion also holds true for communication within more traditional offline movements, the fluid and unorganized nature of online conversations on social media allows linking personal experiences or local actions (see above) within a broader global stream of communication through markers such as hashtags (e.g., #fridaysforfuture) or mentions (e.g., @GretaThunberg), thus increasing the reach of such otherwise isolated utterances.

The COVID-19 pandemic further increased the digital component of climate activism, as previous public activities, such as school strikes on Fridays, became increasingly difficult under pandemic restrictions. At the same time, the co-occurrence of the COVID-19 pandemic with the ongoing climate crisis led to the common discussion of pandemic-related topics and climate topics, ranging from discussing a nexus between the causes of a zoonotic pandemic and climate change to solidarity among activists, compliance with pandemic regulations, and creative approaches to new digital forms of protesting (Sorce and Dumitrica 2023).

From a science communication perspective (Soßdorf and Burgi 2022), it has been noted that, in particular, the climate activist movement has self-appropriated a role as science communicators and employed "following the science" as a key identity feature and potentially as a moral resource to legitimize both claims and activism. At the same time, the study by Soßdorf and Burgi (2022) suggests that this moral aspect of science as a resource leads activists to reject the idea of using science as a strategic communication tool—i.e., strategically cherry-picking those scientific findings that best match an agenda, a key feature that differentiates climate activists from, e.g., creators and disseminators of health-related disinformation on social media. This notion of science as a resource could also (potentially) explain the markedly strong compliance with pandemic control measures such as masking and vaccinations among climate activists.

While this case study of climate activism highlights the grassroots and fluid as well as disruptive character of the processes that lead to social mobilization for health-related issues, attempts to systematically encourage digital participation of younger citizens using digital platforms can be effective—particularly so if they are linked to concrete local matters such as participation in urban spatial planning or local policy agenda setting (Ambrosino et al. 2023).

5 Conclusion

The examples highlight that digital tools already play a crucial role in mobilizing and advocating health-related issues. Digitalization in this field was substantially advanced through the COVID-19 pandemic and crisis-related grassroots mobilization actions. Learnings from this critical period are likely to shape the future digital health communication and advocacy landscape as health information and communication, as well as the exchange and interaction among health professionals, continue to move into the digital space. Critical processes of digital advocacy seem to be identified through connection, amplification through celebrities and key figures, moral resources, integration of other ongoing issues, and mobilization through local topics of concern. If these are either proactively addressed or organically developed through the online discourse, digital tools have substantial potential to support and sustain adaptive change for better health. However, as shown earlier, similar processes underlie the proliferation of dis- and misinformation and can significantly hinder public health efforts. Thus, digital health communication and advocacy must be taken very seriously by public health agencies, institutions, and professionals to actively shape health information and social mobilization for the health agenda.

References

Allchin D (2023) Ten competencies for the science misinformation crisis. Sci Educ 107(2):261–274. https://doi.org/10.1002/sce.21746

Amankwah-Amoah J, Khan Z, Wood G, Knight G (2021) COVID-19 and digitalization: the great acceleration. J Bus Res 136:602–611. https://doi.org/10.1016/j.jbusres.2021.08.011

Ambrosino A et al (2023) Youth and democracy: digital opportunities for the future of participation. In: Rouet G, Côme T (eds) Participatory and digital democracy at the local level. Contributions to political science. Springer, Cham. https://doi.org/10.1007/978-3-031-20943-7_5

Bennett WL, Segerberg A (2013) The logic of connective action. Cambridge University Press, Cambridge

Berger J, Milkman KL (2012) What makes online content viral? J Mark Res 49(2):192–205. https://doi.org/10.1509/jmr.10.0353

Boulianne S, Lalancette M, Ilkiw D (2020) "School strike 4 climate": social media and the international youth protest on climate change. Media Commun 8(2):208–218. https://doi.org/10.17645/mac.v8i2.2768

Bridgman A, Merkley E, Loewen PJ, Owen T, Ruths D, Teichmann L, Zhilin O (2020) The causes and consequences of COVID-19 misperceptions: understanding the role of news and social media. Harv Kennedy Sch Misinform Rev 1(3):10.37016/mr-2020-028

Cloes R, Ahmad A, Reintjes R (2015) Risk communication during the 2009 influenza A (H1N1) pandemic: stakeholder experiences from eight European countries. Disaster Med Public Health Prep 9(2):127–133. https://doi.org/10.1017/dmp.2014.124

Ecker UKH, Lewandowsky S, Cook J, Schmid P, Fazio LK, Brashier N, Kendeou P, Vraga EK, Amazeen MA (2022) The psychological drivers of misinformation belief and its resistance to correction. Nat Rev Psychol 1(1):13–29. https://doi.org/10.1038/s44159-021-00006-y

Evers S, Zeeb H, Gerhardus A (2021) "Wissen generieren: Das" Kompetenznetz Public Health zu COVID-19. Public Health Forum 29(1):15–18. https://doi.org/10.1515/pubhef-2020-0131

Goel S, Watts DJ, Goldstein DG (2012) The structure of online diffusion networks. In: Proceedings of the 13th ACM conference on electronic commerce. ACM, Valencia, Spain, pp 623–638

Grinberg N, Joseph K, Friedland L, Swire-Thompson B, Lazer D (2019) Fake news on Twitter during the 2016 U.S. presidential election. Science 363(6425):374–378. https://doi.org/10.1126/science.aau2706

Jones CM, Diethei D, Schoning J, Shrestha R, Jahnel T, Schuz B (2023). Impact of Social Reference Cues on Misinformation Sharing on Social Media: Series of Experimental Studies. J Med Internet Res. 25:e45583 https://doi.org/10.2196/45583

Kim S, Capasso A, Ali SH, Headley T, DiClemente RJ, Tozan Y (2022) What predicts people's adherence to COVID-19 misinformation? A retrospective study using a nationwide online survey among adults residing in the United States. BMC Public Health 22(1):2114. https://doi.org/10.1186/s12889-022-14431

Kutscher S (2022) Fake news and the illusion of truth: the influence of media on German political discourse in the wake of COVID-19. Sortuz: Oñati J Emerg Socio-Legal Stud 11(2):142–169

Lazer DMJ, Baum MA, Benkler Y, Berinsky AJ, Greenhill KM, Menczer F, Metzger MJ, Nyhan B, Pennycook G, Rothschild D, Schudson M, Sloman SA, Sunstein CR, Thorson EA, Watts DJ, Zittrain JL (2018) The science of fake news. Science 359(6380):1094–1096. https://doi.org/10.1126/science.aao2998

Loeb S, Sengupta S, Butaney M, Macaluso JN, Czarniecki SW, Robbins R, Braithwaite RS, Gao L, Byrne N, Walter D, Langford A (2019) Dissemination of misinformative and biased information about prostate cancer on YouTube. Eur Urol 75(4):564–567. https://doi.org/10.1016/j.eururo.2018.10.056

Nuernbergk C (2020) Das Publikum von Politikjournalisten als Interaktionspartner auf Twitter: Interaktionsstruktur, Motive und Erfahrungen anschreibender Nutzer. Z Polit 30:241–259. https://doi.org/10.1007/s41358-020-00219-2

Oliveira E, Rodriguez-Amat JR, Isabel Ruiz-Mora I, Zeler I (2023) The fluid and disruptive shape of activism: strategic communication in #fridaysforfuture. Int J Strateg Commun 17(4):301–324. https://doi.org/10.1080/1553118X.2023.2204299

Oxman AD, Fretheim A, Lewin S et al (2022) Health communication in and out of public health emergencies: to persuade or to inform? Health Res Policy Syst 20:28. https://doi.org/10.1186/s12961-022-00828-z

Pennycook G, Rand DG (2021) The psychology of fake news. Trends Cogn Sci 25(5):388–402. https://doi.org/10.1016/j.tics.2021.02.007

Peters K, Kashima Y, Clark A (2009) Talking about others: emotionality and the dissemination of social information. Eur J Soc Psychol 39(2):207–222. https://doi.org/10.1002/ejsp.523

Pickard S (2022) Young environmental activists and Do-It-Ourselves (DIO) politics: collective engagement, generational agency, efficacy, belonging and hope. J Youth Stud 25(6):730–750. https://doi.org/10.1080/13676261.2022.2046258

Rathje S, He JK, Roozenbeek J, Van Bavel JJ, van der Linden S (2022) Social media behavior is associated with vaccine hesitancy. PNAS Nexus 1(4):pgac207. https://doi.org/10.1093/pnasnexus/pgac207

Reckwitz A (2018) Die Gesellschaft der Singularitäten. Zum Strukturwandel der Moderne, Berlin, Suhrkamp

Roozenbeek J, Schneider CR, Dryhurst S, Kerr J, Freeman ALJ, Recchia G, van der Bles AM, van der Linden S (2019) Susceptibility to misinformation about COVID-19 around the world. R Soc Open Sci 7(10):201199. https://doi.org/10.1098/rsos.201199

Roozenbeek J, van der Linden S, Goldberg B, Rathje S, Lewandowsky S (2022) Psychological inoculation improves resilience against misinformation on social media. Sci Adv 8(34):eabo6254. https://doi.org/10.1126/sciadv.abo6254

Seidler A, Nußbaumer-Streit B, Apfelbacher C, Zeeb H (2021) Rapid Reviews in Zeiten von Covid-19—Erfahrungen im Zuge des Kompetenznetzes Public Health zu Covid-19 und Vorschlag eines standardisierten Vorgehens. Das Gesundheitswes 83(3):173–179. https://doi.org/10.1055/a-1380-0926

Sorce G, Dumitrica D (2023) #fighteverycrisis: pandemic shifts in Fridays for future's protest communication frames. Environ Commun 17(3):263–275. https://doi.org/10.1080/17524032.2021.1948435

Soßdorf A, Burgi V (2022) "Listen to the science!"—the role of scientific knowledge for the Fridays for Future movement. Front Commun 7:983929. https://doi.org/10.3389/fcomm.2022.983929

Swire-Thompson B, Lazer D (2020) Public health and online misinformation: challenges and recommendations. Annu Rev Public Health 41(1):433–451. https://doi.org/10.1146/annurev-publhealth-040119-094127

Van Der Vaart R, Drossaert C (2017) Development of the digital health literacy instrument: measuring a broad spectrum of health 1.0 and health 2.0 skills. J Med Internet Res 19(1):e27

Vosoughi S, Roy D, Aral S (2018) The spread of true and false news online. Science 359(6380):1146–1151. https://doi.org/10.1126/science.aap9559

Wang Y, McKee M, Torbica A, Stuckler D (2019) Systematic literature review on the spread of health-related misinformation on social media. Soc Sci Med 240:112552. https://doi.org/10.1016/j.socscimed.2019.112552

Whitehead HS, French CE, Caldwell DM, Letley L, Mounier-Jack S (2023) A systematic review of communication interventions for countering vaccine misinformation. Vaccine 41(5):1018–1034. https://doi.org/10.1016/j.vaccine.2022.12.059

World Health Organization. Regional Office for Europe. (1986). Ottawa Charter for Health Promotion, 1986. https://iris.who.int/handle/10665/349652

Zielinski C (2021) Infodemics and infodemiology: a short history, a long future. Rev Panam Salud Publica 45:e40. https://doi.org/10.26633/RPSP.2021.40

Open Access This chapter is licensed under the terms of the Creative Commons Attribution 4.0 International License (http://creativecommons.org/licenses/by/4.0/), which permits use, sharing, adaptation, distribution and reproduction in any medium or format, as long as you give appropriate credit to the original author(s) and the source, provide a link to the Creative Commons license and indicate if changes were made.

The images or other third party material in this chapter are included in the chapter's Creative Commons license, unless indicated otherwise in a credit line to the material. If material is not included in the chapter's Creative Commons license and your intended use is not permitted by statutory regulation or exceeds the permitted use, you will need to obtain permission directly from the copyright holder.

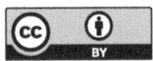

Advancing Public Health Research to Inform Policy and Practice (EPHO 10)

H. Zeeb and S. Forberger

Abstract This chapter outlines the potential of digital technology to advance public health research and inform evidence-based policies and practices. A substantial increase in research output in digital public health, mainly since about 2010, attests to the growing importance and dynamic of the field. Rather than discussing individual research methods or a specific research agenda, the chapter uses a concrete example to discuss relevant principles: a novel digital public health platform incorporating citizen science, participatory health research, and systems science concepts. The SMART framework is a platform to combine community-based participatory research, citizen science, and systems science, combining mobile phones and sensor technology with qualitative data collection. It is a starting point for a holistic human-centered digital public health research approach. Further overarching aspects illustrated in the chapter comprise Artificial Intelligence, advanced visualization and analytics, ethical issues, and data management. Digital public health research has to be conducted in interdisciplinary teams, and there is an increasing number of networks and centers that enhance these collaborations. The chapter stresses the need for continued investment in digital public health research and innovation to harness technology's transformative potential.

Keywords Public health · Policy · Complexity · Data science · Citizen science · Systems science · Evidence

---

H. Zeeb (✉)
Leibniz Institute for Prevention Research and Epidemiology—BIPS, Bremen, Germany

Health Sciences Bremen, University of Bremen, Bremen, Germany

Leibniz ScienceCampus Digital Public Health Bremen, Bremen, Germany
e-mail: zeeb@leibniz-bips.de

S. Forberger
Leibniz Institute for Prevention Research and Epidemiology—BIPS, Bremen, Germany
e-mail: forberger@leibniz-bips.de

1 Introduction

Public health research is crucial in informing evidence-based policies and practices that promote population health and well-being. Digitalization, notably the development and application of information and communication technology (ICT), offers unprecedented opportunities to advance public health research by facilitating data collection, analysis, and dissemination (Boulos et al. 2014; Kamel Boulos and Al-Shorbaji 2014; United Nations Educational Scientific Cultural Organization 2012). The boundaries are being pushed further as Artificial Intelligence becomes more widely used in public health research.

The essential public health operation 10 (EPHO10) deals with advancing public health research to inform public health policy and services. This operation can be supported in several ways, all of which may be more or less strongly affected by digitalization. Developing new descriptive, analytical, and experimental research methods, technologies, or systemic solutions for public health problems lies at the core of this function and is strongly influenced by digital transformation. Through the establishment of public health as an applied academic research discipline, the field has grown substantially over the past decades. In addition, alliances and partnerships for public health research are essential for EPHO10. It encompasses the development of public health research priorities and practice, strengthening institutional capacities and financing of public health research and knowledge brokering, and the operational linkage between research institutions and policymakers to optimize the translation of research findings to policy. One example is the Portuguese National Programme for the Promotion of Healthy Eating (PNPAS). PNPAS was created to improve the population's nutritional status, stimulate the physical and economic availability of healthy foods and create conditions so that the population can value, appreciate, and integrate them into their daily routines. However, an important challenge for food and nutrition policies is the targeting of other sectors when the health sector mainly promotes and executes a policy. This challenge is related to the necessity of a broad multi-sectoral approach, establishing alliances and partnerships among the different government sectors to create healthy food environments. Based on the evidence, in 2016, the Portuguese government created a workgroup to develop an inter-ministerial strategy for promoting healthy eating. After one year of intense work, the Integrated Strategy for the Promotion of Healthy Eating (EIPAS) was initiated by Order n.° 11,418/2017 on December 29, 2017 (Graça et al. 2018). Further, public health policy research, such as in the European Policy Evaluation Network (PEN), has been added to this operation (Ahrens et al. 2022). The current chapter will touch on the first two aspects and highlight select initiatives and partnerships that foster digital public health research.

Research on eHealth, mHealth, and digital (public) health has increased substantially since 2010. While large publication databases such as PubMed only listed about 1000 or fewer topical publications annually before 2010, the early 2020s saw this number increase ten-fold to roughly 10,000 published papers each year. The research questions and approaches are highly diverse and elude any overall characterization. Regarding empirical research methods, surveys, monitoring, and other descriptive approaches outnumber randomized trials, cohorts, or case-control studies. Just below 10% of all publications mention qualitative or mixed methods research.

Given the policy orientation that digital public health research eventually aspires to, looking at phases of the policy-making process provides a first insight into the research potential in this context. Policies are ideally constructed based on supporting scientific evidence. Large-scale data collections, generally framed as Big Data, can substantially influence all phases of the policy cycle. During the agenda-setting phase, the use of digital technologies can increase the accuracy, efficiency, speed, and legitimacy of the formulated policies through, for example, advanced analytics, allowing for a variety of sources to be researched and analyzed to understand the policy landscape (Loftis and Mortensen 2020; Nowlin 2016). Technology has a strong potential to help identify problems and conceptualize solutions more accurately and in greater detail, thereby supplementing traditional research techniques and approaches. During the other phases of the cycle, digital technologies can also advance policymaking by supporting cost-savings, real-time evaluations, better and potentially more targeted services, or fraud reduction (Pencheva et al. 2020).

However, harnessing the potential of Big Data is highly complex. The challenges range from technical and application risks and governance to moral and ethical issues, particularly concerning aspects of the digital divide (see chapter "Digital Health Inequality", Brand et al. in this handbook). Many other critical aspects have been identified, such as insufficient data and information sharing, inadequate funding and resources, and issues associated with (lack of) interdisciplinary collaboration (Brownson et al. 2006; Minkler and Wallerstein 2008).

Our working hypothesis for this chapter is that current evidence-informed public health policy is best supported by research insights that address real-world, often complex, population health problems. Digital technologies can be instrumental in collecting large amounts of data for this objective. Ideally, the population affected by the public health problem is part and parcel of the research processes.

Therefore, the current chapter does not aim to provide an overview of the many topics, methodological approaches, and applications that shape digital public health research, as many of the other chapters in this handbook discuss research in various ways. Here, we present and discuss an exemplary, integrative research approach that may provide food for thought for digital public health researchers, policymakers, and other stakeholders.

2 Modern Integrated Digital Public Health Research

The view that a better understanding of individual determinants of population health leads to interventions and policies that effectively tackle poor health outcomes at the population level is contrasted by a perspective that acknowledges the complexity of many population health issues and calls for appropriate solutions in light of this complexity. While there are undoubted successes of targeted population health policies building on evidence about individual health determinants (e.g., in the field of cancer prevention or infection control), current public health problems may often benefit from a systems science approach that takes complex contexts, time-dependent dynamics in risks and resources, and other population aspects, into account (Carey et al. 2015).

Digitalization can be a crucial driver of integrating information from diverse contexts, existing and newly set-up databases, and different sectors into a system that yields policy-relevant insights into complex health problems. It can enhance speed, differentiation, timeliness, and availability of data for decisions, as shortly alluded to in the introduction. A fascinating development in this respect is that a large and still increasing part of the population globally now possesses or has access to devices that can generate, store, and communicate research data—their mobile phones (International Telecommunication Union 2022). This wide distribution can, at best, strengthen equity while providing vast amounts of data that can be used to inform policy. Involving citizens as partners in research is the hallmark of citizen science (Den Broeder et al. 2018). If applied to digital technologies and their use in public health research, these approaches might address and minimize the risk of widening existing health disparities if heterogeneous population groups, particularly the disenfranchised, can be engaged in research (King et al. 2019). This is also important to reduce bias and conduct high-quality digital public health research. For example, using mobile phone data in epidemics to monitor population movements and contact frequencies requires an equity-oriented public health research approach to avoid drawing conclusions from skewed data that do not consider socio-economic (digital) disparities. Equity and a human-centered approach remain cornerstones of modern public health, acknowledging that social determinants are key drivers of population health that need to be addressed by research and policy (Israel et al. 2010). But to address them, social determinants must be recognized and considered in the modeling, as well as the explanatory contextual and structural conditions that lead to their emergence and consolidation. Further, as described in this handbook's chapter (Digital health literacy, Zeeb and Dratva), there remain significant differences in digital skills between population groups that may also pose obstacles to digital public health research.

Mobile phones are a vital part of the day-to-day life of many people and are the primary one-stop communication device at home, work, and while moving about (Katapally et al. 2018). Further, they are a way to integrate citizen science into the research process and to foster collaboration between citizens and researchers to triangulate critical data. This collaboration can take many forms, such as qualitative perceptions via audio, video, photo-enabled, and just-in-time ecological momentary assessments; traditional and novel quantitative data via the deployment of surveys in real-time; and objective data sensed via in-built smartphone sensors (e.g., accelerometers, pedometers, global positioning system, or more invasive approaches like glucose monitoring; Katapally et al. 2018). Further mobile phone interaction data, app use, and individual consumer data can also be collected. Initiatives such as the SMART Platform aim to integrate citizen science, community-based participatory research, and systems science in studying population health monitoring, integrated knowledge translation, and policy interventions explicated through digital technologies, primarily mobile phones (Katapally 2019).

2.1 A Multi-Pronged Digital Methodological Research Framework

Katapally (2019) describes the evolution of the SMART (an acronym for *Saskatchewan, let's move and map our activity*) study into a digital methodologic platform and toolkit for population health research. The evidence-based SMART framework supports population health surveillance, knowledge integration, and implementation and evaluation of subsequent interventions. It draws its conceptual roots from the pillars described earlier: citizen and systems science and community-based participatory health research practices (Katapally 2019). As a platform, it caters to different study designs. It engages with citizens who collect data via mobile phones, for example, using the various sensors integrated into most modern smartphones. Surveys and ecologic momentary assessments (Shiffman et al. 2008) are means of data acquisition, and the platform allows the linking of these population-generated data with administrative and policy data and healthcare utilization data. Data from these different levels and sources can then be used to inform policymakers and other stakeholders.

The citizen science aspect of SMART is taken care of by the joint development of research questions, data collection, and results returned to the citizens. For example, in a recent study on smartphone use, weight status, and self-rated health, adolescents and young adults, contacted through school engagement sessions, acted as citizen scientists to record data on their mobile phones (Brodersen et al. 2023). Qualitative systems mapping and problem structuring are core approaches integrated into the digital platform. This is intended to lead to repeated and differentiated data collection by engaged citizen scientists using mixed-methods approaches. The data generated can subsequently support dynamic modeling, the results of which are back-translated to all stakeholders, again via mobile phones used for data collection and other means. Those points are important as they increase research capacity, incorporate community perspectives on problems and solutions, and improve public awareness and acceptance of actions to improve health.

Figure 1 provides a conceptual overview of the research framework, highlighting the intended integration of community-based participatory research, citizen science, and systems science via ubiquitous tools. While some similarities exist with the cyclical nature of the public health action cycle, the SMART framework explicitly includes the different contributors, stakeholders, levels of data processes, and stakeholder engagement in (digital) public health research.

The technological versatility, viability, and applicability of the specific SMART approach and platform are of little interest to the current chapter. However, it is

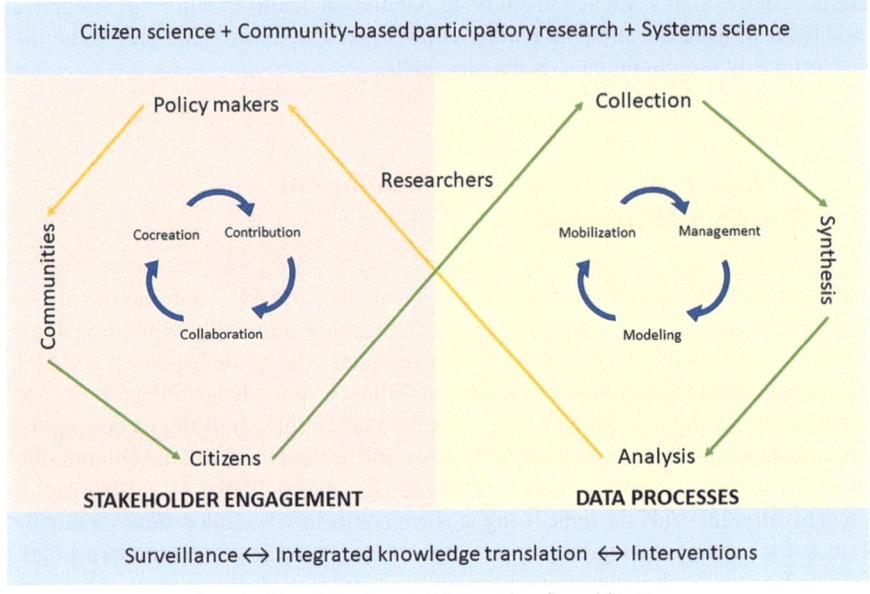

Fig. 1 SMART framework. (Source: Own figure, adapted from Katapally 2019)

noted that several projects in Canada and India have been based on this approach. The research principles and concepts, i.e., citizen and systems science and participatory health research, are essential for digital public health research to inform policy and practice. While there is a strong focus on equity and the use of digital tools available to the populations affected by specific public health problems, the envisaged integration with data sources from different levels, including other digitally collected data, offers a flexible and context-responsive approach to research-based management of public health problems.

3 Some Further Issues in Integrated Digital Public Health Research

3.1 The Emerging Generative Artificial Intelligence Toolkit

While SMART offers a platform to link community-based participatory research, citizen and systems science, mobile phones, and sensor technology provide opportunities to work with large amounts of data, which will increasingly be analyzed with the help of generative Artificial Intelligence.

The rise of generative Artificial Intelligence (AI) offers new opportunities to advance public health research by automating tasks, enhancing data analysis, and generating novel insights (Topol 2019) (see also chapter "AI Meets Digital Public Health", Steinert et al. in this handbook). Generative AI, which includes techniques such as Deep Learning, Natural Language Processing, and reinforcement learning, can be used to analyze large datasets, identify patterns and trends, and generate predictions or recommendations (Ching et al. 2018). In public health research, generative AI can revolutionize disease surveillance, risk prediction, and personalized medicine by providing more accurate and timely information to inform decision-making and resource allocation (Ioannidis and Khoury 2018). It should be noted, however, that without the analytical advances inherent to AI, the data revolution can only be seen as a shift in the amount of data available rather than a fundamental change to research methods and generated insights (Pencheva et al. 2020).

The application of AI in prevention is wide-ranging, in principle. AI methodology is used, for example, for water quality monitoring and Legionella protection by simulating conditions that can prevent legionellosis outbreaks in a water system (Sinčak et al. 2014). Another example is the utilization of AI applications to enhance adult weight loss. A scoping review by Chew et al. (2021) reviewed 66 studies about Artificial Intelligence enhancing adult weight loss, encompassing some 2000 participants. Three domains of self-regulation were identified: self-monitoring, optimizing goal setting, and self-control. The main AI applications were: (a) a machine perception that focused on food recognition, eating behavior, physical activity, and energy balance estimation; (b) predictive analytics covering predicting weight loss, intervention fidelity, dietary lapses, and emotional eating; and (c) real-time analytics with personalized micro-interventions capturing behavioral data instantaneously, optimized predictive models for behavioral deviance, and improved behavioral self-control through adaptive and personalized nudges/prompts (Chew et al. 2021). AI applications may tend to focus on personalization and individualization, as in this example. Still, other research and application areas, e.g., health promotion, are also likely to benefit from advances in AI development. Pandemic preparedness and control are areas where AI has already had an impact that will likely grow in the coming years.

From a governance perspective, findings from a review of 250 cases across the European Union show that different AI technologies and applications might be used for different governance functions. This may include addressing common governmental problems in resource allocation, gaining insights from large databases and handling diverse data, and leveraging digital technology to reduce the human workload, including many repetitive procedural tasks (Van Noordt and Misuraca 2022). For example, data-driven precision governance can enhance hazard preparedness and response efforts (Hondula et al. 2018) or supervise policies' implementation processes by detecting irregularities (Maciejewski 2017).

As the AI toolkit evolves, public health researchers must stay informed about emerging technologies, their strengths, and associated pitfalls by, for example, integrating this expert knowledge into education and university training programs. Through collaboration with experts in AI and data science, the full potential of generative AI in shaping evidence-based policies and practices can be brought to use. At the same time, interdisciplinary approaches help to ensure that limitations, risks, and ethical considerations are taken care of (see chapters "AI Meets Digital Public Health", Steinert et al. and "Ethical Implications of User Autonomy in Digital Public Health", Dassow and Mildner, in this handbook). A research agenda on achieving and advancing the idea of "staying informed," ideally with a vital component of shaping AI methodologies for public health, would be an essential task for digital public health research in the coming years.

3.2 Harnessing Visualization Techniques and Advanced Analytics

Big Data analytics offers a powerful tool for generating insights from diverse and large-scale datasets generated through primary data collection by researchers or citizens or from secondary data sources, which can inform public health policy and strategy (Raghupathi and Raghupathi 2014). For example, Electronic Health Records, social media data, and mobile health applications can provide valuable information on population health trends and the determinants of health (Bates et al. 2014). Data visualization techniques, such as geographic information systems (GIS) and interactive dashboards, can be very helpful in communicating research findings to policymakers, practitioners, and the public. For example, during the COVID-19 pandemic, many public health agencies and universities developed interactive dashboards presenting frequent updates of case numbers and other relevant data and reached broad audiences. These tools can help to make complex data more accessible and understandable, ultimately facilitating evidence-based decision-making in public health (Kamel Boulos et al. 2019) by strengthening geographical approaches and displaying regional differences. However, research gaps exist, for example, regarding user-friendliness, user information needs, and the role of users as information contributors to dashboards.

4 Research Ethics

Public health professionals are expected to navigate a range of ethical considerations in their research, policy development, and implementation efforts (Bayer and Fairchild 2016). Using digital technologies further challenges this critical area (see chapter "Ethical Implications of User Autonomy in Digital Public Health", Dassow and Mildner, in this handbook). Balancing individual rights and privacy concerns with the broader public health goals can be challenging, particularly in infectious disease control or surveillance activities (Childress et al. 2002) but also concerning health data collected via social media, personal sensors, etc. Ethical considerations for health research data access, sharing, and use include aspects of confidentiality and privacy, violations of data reuse expectations and approvals, valid consent to safeguard research participants' rights, and the potential impact of sharing on public trust (Maseme 2022). Digital technology and AI development have typically been in the hand of a select group of engineers, scientists, programmers, and platform architects. In many cases, aspects of ethnic, cultural, gender, age, geographic, or economic diversity of human life have either not been considered at all or have not been sufficiently considered.

Addressing the many ethical challenges of AI and digital technology for public health requires a solid commitment to ethical principles and frameworks, as well as ongoing training and capacity building for public health professionals to ensure that policies and interventions are designed and implemented in ways that respect individual rights and promote social justice (Lee 2012). This also calls for an appropriate overview of and attention to the constantly evolving digital technology opportunities and potential health-related applications. This monitoring task needs to be shouldered by networks or institutions with sufficient capacity.

4.1 Research Data Management

The increasing digitalization of public health research is inherently linked to modern requirements and approaches to research data management. Like other research fields, digital public health research must implement FAIR principles. The data are so large that those who create them can only manage to analyze a fraction of the entire dataset. FAIR principles stand for making data findable, accessible, interoperable, and reusable (FAIR) by humans and but even more importantly, by machines. With a focus on digital technology and increasingly large and complex data in public health research, this topic may pose particular challenges as privacy requirements feature much more highly in human health data than in other research fields.

Goldsmith et al. (2021) define public health data science as "the study of formulating and rigorously answering questions to advance health and well-being using a data-centric process that emphasizes clarity, reproducibility, effective communication, and ethical practices" (Goldsmith et al. 2021). This definition encompasses the increasing reliance on computational technologies in public health research and aspects of communication and ethics that are highly relevant to public health research and the policy information process. Strengthening the data-centric process associated with public health data science also requires more collaboration between "traditional" public health researchers, bioinformaticians, engineers, and other quantitative disciplines. At the same time, ethics, social science research, and other fields already closely aligned with public health remain important. Research data management is essential for the digital preservation, reusability, and archiving of scientific data. This encompasses the entire research data lifecycle: from project planning to generating and storing data, metadata description and documentation to data archiving and post-archiving use. This also includes the conscious decision as to which data from the research process should be preserved in the long term. Digital public health research, as with other research fields, must implement research data management models that are transparent and accessible to team members and external audiences.

4.2 Networking and Interaction

The interdisciplinary requirements and challenges of digital public health research have been discussed in chapter "Why Is It Essential to Address Digital Public Health in an Interdisciplinary Way?" Maaß et al. in this handbook on interdisciplinarity. One way to organize these collaborations is through dedicated networks that actively integrate various disciplines under a joint research agenda. The Leibniz ScienceCampus Digital Public Health in Bremen, Germany, represents such an endeavor, bringing together scientists from ICT, epidemiology, law, public health, philosophy, and other disciplines under a common umbrella. Other related activities, partly motivated by particular structural challenges such as low population density and demographic change in the respective region, have been launched elsewhere in Germany, including in the Lausitz region in Brandenburg (Lausitz Center for Digital Public Health—LauZeDiPH) or at the University of Siegen (Digital model region healthcare tripoint) and internationally, for example at the Center for Global Digital Health Innovation at Johns Hopkins Bloomberg School of Public Health. These centers can be well suited to coordinate different research streams, provide joint data infrastructures and arrange for a lively research development environment that attracts early career researchers, experienced scientists, and policymakers alike.

5 Conclusion

Advancing public health research to inform policy and practice requires various tools and resources, with digital technologies gaining increasing leverage in data collection, management, interaction, and communication. Public health problems are often complex, and applying digital tools systematically and sensibly may hold significant promises for advancing public health research and its potential to support policy development and inform public health practice. As the digital landscape continues to evolve, interdisciplinary collaboration, open access to information, and investment in digital public health research and innovation are critical to unlocking the full potential of digital technology in public health. Moreover, it appears vital to finance not-for-profit research in digital public health, as it might not be a financially viable business model to develop or evaluate applications on ethical and legal merits—or to develop frameworks that can do that. This is where publicly funded research is needed to drive, inform, and perhaps reign in commercial research and development activities.

By harnessing these opportunities, public health researchers and professionals, together with members of the population participating in research, can be empowered to generate insights, support informed decision-making, and implement and evaluate digital interventions that improve population health and well-being.

We thank Brian Wong and Stephan Buttigieg for input into earlier versions of the chapter.

References

Ahrens W, Brenner H, Flechtner-Mors M, Harrington JM, Hebestreit A, Kamphuis CBM, Kelly L, Laxy M, Luszczynska A, Mazzocchi M, Murrin C, Poelman MP, Steenhuis I, Roos G, Steinacker JM, Van Lenthe F, Zeeb H, Zukowska J, Lakerveld J, Woods CB (2022) Dietary behaviour and physical activity policies in Europe: learnings from the Policy Evaluation Network (PEN). Eur J Pub Health 32:iv114–iv125

Bates D, Saria S, Ohno-Machado L, Shah A (2014) Big data in health care: using analytics to identify and manage high-risk and high-cost patients. Health Aff 33:1123–1131

Bayer R, Fairchild AL (2016) Means, ends and the ethics of fear-based public health campaigns. J Med Ethics 42:391–396

Boulos MN, Brewer AC, Karimkhani C, Buller DB, Dellavalle RP (2014) Mobile medical and health apps: state of the art, concerns, regulatory control and certification. Online J Public Health Inform 5:229

Brodersen K, Hammami N, Katapally TR (2023) Is excessive smartphone use associated with weight status and self-rated health among youth? A smart platform study. BMC Public Health 23:234

Brownson RC, Kreuter MW, Arrington BA, True WR (2006) Translating scientific discoveries into public health action: how can schools of public health move us forward? Public Health Rep 121:97–103

Carey G, Malbon E, Carey N, Joyce A, Crammond B, Carey A (2015) Systems science and systems thinking for public health: a systematic review of the field. BMJ Open 5:e009002

Chew HSJ, Ang WHD, Lau Y (2021) The potential of artificial intelligence in enhancing adult weight loss: a scoping review. Public Health Nutr 24:1993–2020

Childress JF, Faden RR, Gaare RD, Gostin LO, Kahn J, Bonnie RJ, Kass NE, Mastroianni AC, Moreno JD, Nieburg P (2002) Public health ethics: mapping the terrain. J Law Med Ethics 30:170–178

Ching T, Himmelstein DS, Beaulieu-Jones BK, Kalinin AA, Do BT, Way GP, Ferrero E, Agapow P-M, Zietz M, Hoffman MM, Xie W, Rosen GL, Lengerich BJ, Israeli J, Lanchantin J, Woloszynek S, Carpenter AE, Shrikumar A, Xu J, Cofer EM, Lavender CA, Turaga SC, Alexandari AM, Lu Z, Harris DJ, Decaprio D, Qi Y, Kundaje A, Peng Y, Wiley LK, Segler MHS, Boca SM, Swamidass SJ, Huang A, Gitter A, Greene CS (2018) Opportunities and obstacles for deep learning in biology and medicine. J R Soc Interface 15:20170387

Den Broeder L, Devilee J, Van Oers H, Schuit AJ, Wagemakers A (2018) Citizen science for public health. Health Promot Int 33:505–514

Goldsmith J, Sun Y, Fried LP, Wing J, Miller GW, Berhane K (2021) The emergence and future of public health data science. Public Health Rev 42:1604023

Graça P, Gregório MJ, De Sousa SM, Brás S, Penedo T, Carvalho T, Bandarra NM, Lima RM, Simão AP, Goiana-Da-Silva F, Freitas MG, Araújo FF (2018) A new interministerial strategy for the promotion of healthy eating in Portugal: implementation and initial results. Health Res Policy Syst 16:102

Hondula DM, Kuras ER, Longo J, Johnston EW (2018) Toward precision governance: infusing data into public management of environmental hazards. Public Manag Rev 20:746–765

International Telecommunication Union (2022) Mobile phone ownership [Online]. https://www.itu.int/itu-d/reports/statistics/2022/11/24/ff22-mobile-phone-ownership/ Accessed Jul 2023

Ioannidis JPA, Khoury MJ (2018) Evidence-based medicine and big genomic data. Hum Mol Genet 27:R2–R7

Israel BA, Coombe CM, Cheezum RR, Schulz AJ, Mcgranaghan RJ, Lichtenstein R, Reyes AG, Clement J, Burris A (2010) Community-based participatory research: a capacity-building approach for policy advocacy aimed at eliminating health disparities. Am J Public Health 100:2094–2102

Kamel Boulos MN, Al-Shorbaji NM (2014) On the Internet of Things, smart cities and the who healthy cities. Int J Health Geogr 13:10

Kamel Boulos MN, Peng G, Vopham T (2019) An overview of GeoAI applications in health and healthcare. Int J Health Geogr 18:7

Katapally TR (2019) The SMART framework: integration of citizen science, community-based participatory research, and systems science for population health science in the digital age. JMIR mHealth uHealth 7:e14056

Katapally TR, Bhawra J, Leatherdale ST, Ferguson L, Longo J, Rainham D, Larouche R, Osgood N (2018) The SMART study, a mobile health and citizen science methodological platform for active living surveillance, integrated knowledge translation, and policy interventions: longitudinal study. JMIR Public Health Surveill 4:e31

King AC, Winter SJ, Chrisinger BW, Hua J, Banchoff AW (2019) Maximizing the promise of citizen science to advance health and prevent disease. Prev Med 119:44–47

Lee LM (2012) Public health ethics theory: review and path to convergence. J Law Med Ethics 40:85–98

Loftis MW, Mortensen PB (2020) Collaborating with the machines: a hybrid method for classifying policy documents. Policy Stud J 48:184–206

Maciejewski M (2017) To do more, better, faster and more cheaply: using big data in public administration. Int Rev Adm Sci 83:120–135

Maseme M (2022) Ethical considerations for health research data governance. In: Kumar BS (ed) Data integrity and data governance. IntechOpen, Rijeka

Minkler M, Wallerstein N (2008) Community-based participatory research for health: from process to outcomes. Wiley, San Francisco

Nowlin MC (2016) Modeling issue definitions using quantitative text analysis. Policy Stud J 44:309–331

Pencheva I, Esteve M, Mikhaylov SJ (2020) Big data and AI—a transformational shift for government: so, what next for research? Public Policy Admin 35:24–44

Raghupathi W, Raghupathi V (2014) Big data analytics in healthcare: promise and potential. Health Inform Sci Syst 2:3

Shiffman S, Stone AA, Hufford MR (2008) Ecological momentary assessment. Annu Rev Clin Psychol 4:1–32

Sinčak P, Ondo J, Kaposztasova D, Virčikova M, Vranayova Z, Sabol J (2014) Artificial intelligence in public health prevention of legionelosis in drinking water systems. Int J Environ Res Public Health 11:8597–8611

Topol EJ (2019) High-performance medicine: the convergence of human and artificial intelligence. Nat Med 25:44–56

United Nations Educational Scientific Cultural Organization (2012) Policy guidelines for the development and promotion of open access. UNESCO, Paris

Van Noordt C, Misuraca G (2022) Artificial intelligence for the public sector: results of landscaping the use of AI in government across the European Union. Gov Inf Q 39:101714

Open Access This chapter is licensed under the terms of the Creative Commons Attribution 4.0 International License (http://creativecommons.org/licenses/by/4.0/), which permits use, sharing, adaptation, distribution and reproduction in any medium or format, as long as you give appropriate credit to the original author(s) and the source, provide a link to the Creative Commons license and indicate if changes were made.

The images or other third party material in this chapter are included in the chapter's Creative Commons license, unless indicated otherwise in a credit line to the material. If material is not included in the chapter's Creative Commons license and your intended use is not permitted by statutory regulation or exceeds the permitted use, you will need to obtain permission directly from the copyright holder.

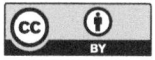

Engineering Digital Public Health

From Smartwatches to Research Tools: Unlocking the Potential of Modern Health Monitoring Technology

Anke V. Reinschluessel, Bastian Dänekas, Thomas Eßmeyer, Katharina Hasenlust, and Rainer Malaka

Abstract A broad range of sensing technologies, devices, and platforms allow interested users or physicians to observe various health-related aspects of the user's health. This chapter discusses what modern devices can measure and how users can access and interpret recorded data. Many commercially available devices are capable of measuring data such as heart rate and heart rate variability, sleep cycles, walking steadiness, or electrocardiograms using only a smartwatch and a smartphone. In this chapter, we provide a brief overview these technologies and tools, how they are used for research purposes and highlight potential avenues for future work and upcoming challenges.

Keywords Sensors · User-generated data · Health · Consumer technologies · Health data · Medical devices

Abbreviations

AI Artificial intelligence
API Application programming interface
CGM Continuous glucose monitoring
ECG Electrocardiography

Anke V. Reinschluessel, Bastian Dänekas, Thomas Mildner and Katharina Hasenlust contributed equally with all other contributors.

A. V. Reinschluessel (✉)
Digital Media Lab, University of Bremen, Bremen, Germany

HCI Group, University of Konstanz, Konstanz, Germany
e-mail: anke.reinschluessel@uni-konstanz.de

B. Dänekas · T. Eßmeyer · K. Hasenlust · R. Malaka (✉)
Digital Media Lab, University of Bremen, Bremen, Germany
e-mail: daenekba@uni-bremen.de; mildner@uni-bremen.de; kahasenl@uni-bremen.de; malaka@tzi.de

HCI   Human-computer interaction
IMU   Inertial measurement unit
PPG   Photoplethysmography

1 Introduction

The wide range of available sensing technologies, devices, and platforms presents exciting opportunities for digital public health (DiPH). Some solutions have been specifically designed for health applications (e.g., health wristbands), while others are based on off-the-shelf technologies adapted for DiPH applications. Ambient data recordings through our everyday technical devices, such as smartphones or smartwatches, allow for numerous advantages when compared to sporadic diagnostic measurements of the past, for instance, when visiting a doctor. Digital infrastructures allow healthcare and medical professionals and automated services to gain deep insights into their patients' medical history, leading to highly personalized treatment (Cancela et al. 2021). Personal devices offer their users increased insight into and control of health-related issues in their daily lives, enabling them to be more autonomous with regard to their own health, both mentally and physically.

What a suitable technology or platform for DiPH can be is not clearly defined, nor is what it might entail. This chapter will, therefore, offer an overview of available technology and a few exemplary interfaces to access the collected data and their use in research. The wide availability of technologies including the high pace at which they are developed and introduced to potential users, poses the risk that this chapter will be quickly outdated. To maintain relevance, we take a human-centered perspective focusing on the current state-of-the-art while employing examples that can be generalized. This chapter begins by explaining how data are collected in the first place, highlighting common technologies used for recording health-related data and describe how these data are stored and processed. We will also provide a general overview of the benefits when users are empowered to self-monitor aspects of their health. Here, an important factor is the availability and accessibility of mobile applications to translate the data into an easily comprehensible format using natural language and assisting visuals. As these data further open avenues for interesting research fields, we will outline current work building on related technologies to illuminate potential future impacts.

2 Sensors

Today, health data and health conditions can be easily monitored by a plethora of sensors that are integrated into the devices that serve as our daily companions. Smartwatches, for instance, are able to detect and count steps taken throughout the day, calculate heart rate and its variability, and even track our sleep quality.

Looking closer at our heart rate, one of the most commonly recorded health data, there are two ways to measure it. The first option is to record the heart's electrical activity through electrocardiography (ECG) (Feather et al. 2020). The device detects small electrical pulses and changes during the cardiac cycle via electrodes placed on a person's skin. ECGs are commonly used in professional medical devices but can also be found in chest straps at an affordable price. Chest straps are often used in professional sports and can send data through Bluetooth to another device (Lapinski et al. 2009). However, these chest straps are sometimes uncomfortable to wear and can cause skin abrasion. Furthermore, the use of ECGs can also be found in some smartwatches. With the benefit of being ubiquitous compared to chest traps, the accuracy of smartwatches is worse than other professional devices.

The second method of measuring heart rate is by using the process of photoplethysmography (PPG). This measurement method uses optical sensors built into smartwatches or other wearable devices. By sending light from small LEDs through the skin, the sensor detects the volume of blood flowing through the body. This information is then used to derive a heart rate (Castaneda et al. 2018). Unfortunately, optical sensors are prone to optical noise. Since the sensor sends light through the skin, dirt, water, motion, and other disruptive factors can lower the accuracy of the calculated heart rate throughout the measuring process Singh et al. (2018). Conclusively, PPGs have been shown to be less exact compared to ECGs (Singh et al. 2018). However, some smartwatches are able to detect the heart rate with a 96% accuracy compared to ECGs (Pasadyn et al. 2019).

Next to measuring the heart rate, most smartwatches are also able to calculate the heart rate variability. This value is defined by the time between two heartbeats. Heart rate variability is a value that describes how adaptable the body is in a certain situation to either mental or physical stress. The higher the heart rate variability of the person, the more variance the time intervals between two heartbeats have. Therefore, if stress occurs, the body is able to react to that stress by increasing the heart rate and getting more oxygen sent through our blood into our body to get more energy for that situation. A low heart rate variability correlates to higher mortality, being easily exhausted, and having decreased cognition (Dekker et al. 2000; Shaffer and Venner 2013). The heart rate variability also reflects how recovered an athlete is (Makivić et al. 2013). Also, a sudden lower heart rate variability indicate a high amount of stress which increases the chances of getting sick (Shaffer and Ginsberg 2017).

Another sensor combination commonly used in smartwatches or smartphones is an inertial measurement unit (IMU). An IMU consists of a three-axis accelerometer (measuring acceleration), a three-axis gyroscope (measuring rotation), and a three-axis magnetometer (measuring magnetic fields). Initially used in ships or airplanes for navigation, these units can detect specific motion patterns. Especially in combination with GPS, IMUs can detect steps taken during the day, the speed of running, or the distance walked. IMUs have also been shown to detect exercise execution in athletes. Furthermore, IMUs are also used in systems for fall detection for older adults. Cameras can also be used for motion detection. Similar to IMUs, high-resolution cameras are built into modern smartphones. With the help of software libraries like OpenCV,[1] skeletal movement can be derived and used for further motion analysis.

Sensors can also be used to help people cope with chronic health conditions like diabetes. Through continuous glucose monitoring (CGM), affected persons can monitor their insulin level and react to it accordingly. CGM can be done with either real-time-CGM (rtCGM) or intermittent scanning CGM (iscCGM). rtCGM systems have three parts: a sensor, a transmitter, and a receiver. The sensor is either placed directly under the skin of the arm by professional medical staff or on the skin of the belly. The sensors measure the glucose level in the tissue fluid every five minutes and send the data to the receiver, which can display all the information. If there is a risk of hyperglycemia or hypoglycemia, the receiver triggers an acoustic or vibration alarm so that countermeasures can be taken.

iscCGM systems consist of just a sensor and an app. The sensor is placed at the back of the upper arm. Compared to rtCGM systems, the glucose level is not sent every 5 min to the app but has to be scanned by the user. However, like the rtCGM systems, an alarm is triggered if glucose levels are too high or too low. To stop the alarm, the user must scan the sensor and let the application read out the glucose levels.

This only describes a few possibilities for using sensors in lightweight mobile devices. There are numerous other sensors to scan for temperature, environmental data, like pollution or weather conditions, and more. They offer a vast spectrum of patient and context-specific data that can help us cope with everyday health issues and chronic diseases, monitor daily routines, and help us evaluate our fitness and health levels. In most applications, these sensor data are incorporated into platforms that aggregate information and provide insights gathered by the sensors and summarize the current health status of an individual. Examples of how these platforms work and can be divided into categories are presented in the next section.

3 From Sensor Data to Usable Data

The abundance of sensors available on the market that are already built into commercially available wearable devices, such as smartwatches, fitness trackers, or medical devices, allow for extensive data recording for an interested user, e.g., health-conscious persons or athletes, or patients in a medical context. Another user group is researchers, who can use the devices to easily record additional physiological data for a specific context or work on expanding the potential of the wearable devices (see Sect. 4 for examples). In the medical context, Lu et al. (2020) categorized the application of wearables into four areas: health and safety monitoring, chronic disease management, disease diagnosis and treatment, and rehabilitation. Although, based on the description given by them (based on the reviewed

---

[1] https://opencv.org/, accessed 12th July 2023.

literature), the use of an interested person would come within the category "health and safety monitoring" as it generally describes the everyday application areas of wearable devices, especially more complex devices like smartwatches. In the following paragraphs, we will describe how users can access their data and present a few exemplary applications aggregating the recorded data. Furthermore, as not all health data are recorded by wearables equipped with sensors, we briefly highlight the usage of user-generated data and provide an application example in the context of "chronic disease management." Lastly, we briefly discuss potential problems with the current data presentation.

One challenge originating from the vast amount of data is to provide the information in a usable and understandable way to the owners of these devices. Most modern wearables have the tracking hardware conveniently integrated, and they either have a pre-installed interface, such as the Apple Health App (see Fig. 1) or apps or web interfaces that are available to view the data. The Apple Health App aggregates data from two central sources: the iPhone and the Apple watch, a smartwatch integrated with a fitness tracker. Additionally, other apps can feed their data into the

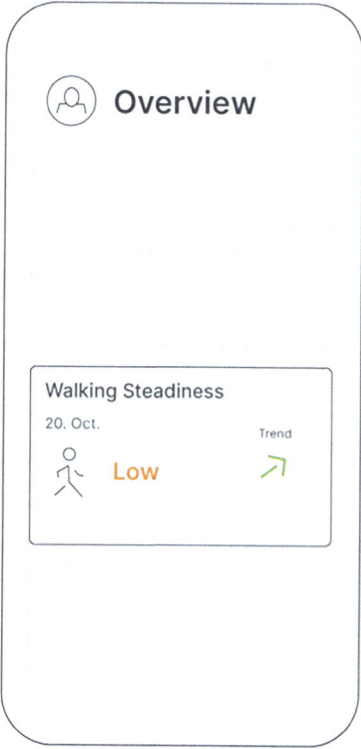

Fig. 1 An overview of the current walking steadiness of a person. (Source: Own figure)

Fig. 2 An overview of the Cardio Fitness level of a person. (Source: Own figure)

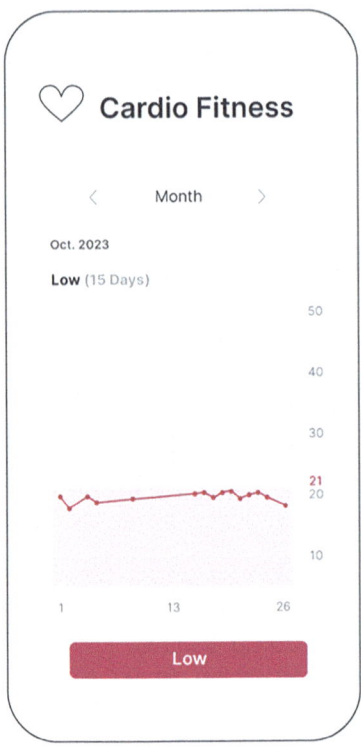

Health App, such as Fitbit,[2] Komoot,[3] Nike training,[4] One Drop Diabetes Management,[5] and many more. Thus, the Health App provides an overview of various health-related data—mainly focusing on health and safety monitoring but also providing limited chronic disease management. Additionally, it already provides an interpretation, e.g., how the cardio fitness level is based on the information available (see Fig. 2). While these data are presented to the user on a mobile device, other brands also provide web interfaces to view the data (cf. Fitbit Dashboard Fig. 3).

Where these applications primarily target the general public and athletes, there are also apps and measuring devices certified as medical devices. They visualize the data for their users allowing doctors to monitor their patients better. One example would be KardiaPro[6] device that can record an ECG and relay the data to the attending cardiologist. In Germany, doctors can even prescribe apps and medical devices to support tracking certain diseases. As diabetes is a widespread illness, monitoring one's blood sugar values is essential and of interest to the attending physician. Apps

---

[2] https://www.fitbit.com/global/us/home, accessed 12th July 2023.
[3] https://www.komoot.com/, accessed 12th July 2023.
[4] https://www.nike.com/de/ntc-app, accessed 12th July 2023.
[5] https://onedrop.today/, accessed 12th July 2023.
[6] https://clinicians.alivecor.com/, accessed 12th July 2023.

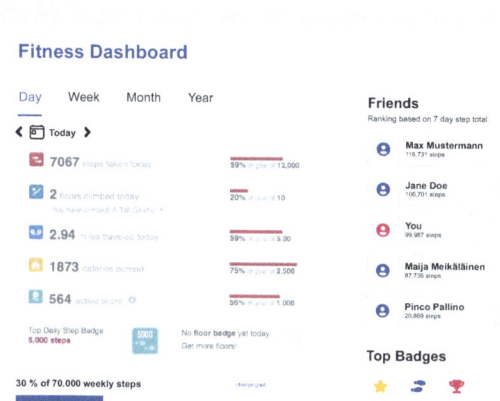

Fig. 3 An exemplary dashboard giving an overview of aggregated data. (Source: Own figure)

like FreeStyle Libre[7] are designed for people with diabetes who wear a sensor measuring their blood sugar values. The app provides real-time feedback on the condition, and the user can also share this information externally.

All the presented applications are similar in that they rely on data measured by dedicated sensors and hardware, e.g., a fitness tracker, a blood sugar sensor, or an ECG-capable device. For data derived from the sensors listed in Sect. 2, the processing and interpretation of the data are especially critical, as the raw values measured are often very noisy and rarely readable to an untrained eye much the same as a standard ECG. It is particularly helpful for users to see their data put into context; for example, see the sketch based on commercially available tools in Fig. 1, which tells the user their walking steadiness is okay. A similar perspective is given in the sketch in Fig. 2, which shows a more raw value, but the interpretation is provided on the bottom in the form of the text stating "low". Most often, the information is presented in a graph that allows the user to compare their performance and their individual goals over a period of a week or month, and even compared to others, as seen in Fig. 3.

Apps can also provide an overview of health-related data entered by the users and not automatically tracked by specific hardware. Several apps visualize and interpret data that the user consciously created. One commonly known example is digital food diaries to keep an overview of the number of calories, fiber, nutrients, etc., digested (e.g., MyFitnessPal[8]) or to examine the relationship between food and health issues (e.g., Nutrimizer[9]). But diseases can also be tracked using digital means. One example is the DMKG-App (DMKG = Deutsche Migräne- und

---

[7] https://www.freestylelibre.de/produkte/freestylelibre-apps.html, accessed 12th July 2023.
[8] https://www.myfitnesspal.com/, accessed 12th July 2023.
[9] https://nutrimizer-app.com/Nutrimizer/, accessed 12th July 2023.

Kopfschmerzgesellschaft, in English: German Migraine and Headache Society), which is accompanied by a web interface that allows for entering further information that can be shared with the attending neurologist. The app prompts the users daily to enter data about their day—whether they had a migraine or headache. If they experienced either, the app asks if and what medication they took and if additional symptoms like dizziness or a migraine aura appeared. The system then provides an overview of the data, for example, the average duration of the headache (see Fig. 4 top graph) and the reported pain level (see Fig. 4 bottom graph). It is an excellent example of how modern health technology can support chronic disease management by facilitating documentation of disease activity by the patient and sharing of this documentation with the treating physician.

Overall, one of the main features of these applications is to present aggregated data—either automatically tracked by dedicated devices or manually entered by the

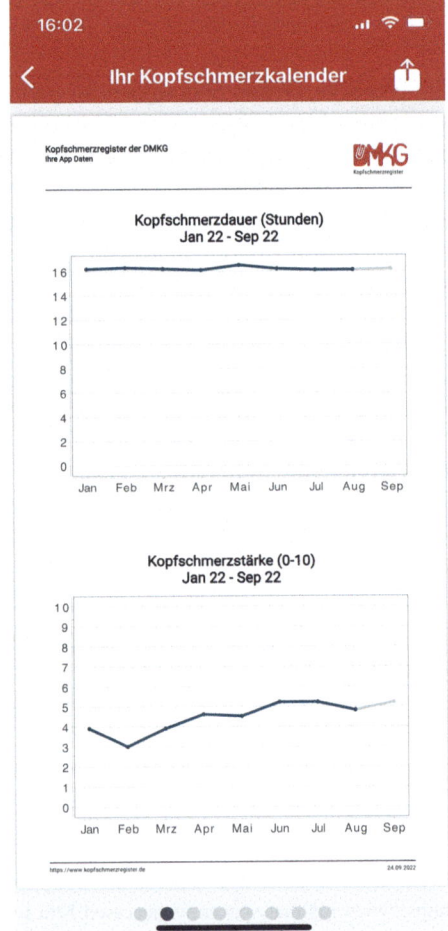

Fig. 4 One overview of user-entered data for a migraine and headache tracking app. Top graph: average duration of the headache; bottom graph: the reported pain level. (Source: DMKG-App, German Migraine and Headache Society)

user—understandable for users without medical training. Often the designers rely on some form of graphs that might be enriched with numbers. Based on the interface snippets of this section, the designers seemed to be aware of color blindness aspects, as they avoided obvious red-green contrasts to make it readable for everyone, including those with the most common forms of color blindness. Nevertheless, as the data are presented primarily in a visually appealing way, the question of accessibility arises. Most designs are "premised on implicit assumptions about the reader's sensory, cognitive, and motor abilities" (Marriott et al. 2021). Therefore, everyone without these abilities does not have access to the benefits of data visualization and have only limited access to the underlying information. There are diverse solutions that allow blind or visually impaired people to access the data, such as alt texts, sonification, or tactile graphics (Marriott et al. 2021). But with continuously generated graphs based on the latest input, these solutions do not work. There is some rudimentary support from the accessibility features of different devices. For example, Apple has a "VoiceOver" feature[10] that reads out the chosen data point when the user selects specific parts on the graph. But this is far away from creating access to the benefits of visualization. Therefore, we look forward to the technical advancements of the future, making the data accessible to everyone in an easily usable, insightful, and unrestricted way and also providing a well-designed user experience for everyone.

4 Smart Devices as Research Tools

Besides the various opportunities for end consumers mentioned in the previous section, another field of application for smart devices is becoming increasingly important: research. One prominent use case is equipping test persons of drug trials with wearables measuring physiological data both to achieve higher safety through continuous monitoring and to get deeper insights into the medication's effects (Izmailova et al. 2017). Additionally, there are plenty of examples to be found in psychological research, such as Triantafillou et al. (2019), who used smartphone-based ecological momentary assessments[11] and activity recognition provided by the respective Android API[12] in order to explore the relationship between sleep quality and mood. In the context of a study examining the physical and mental health of college students during the COVID-19 pandemic, Gilley et al. (2022) provided their participants with Fitbit[13] wristbands hoping to get additional information from other fitness indicators, e.g., based on daily steps. Another example is the study of Faust et al.

---

[10] https://support.apple.com/guide/iphone/turn-on-and-practice-voiceover-iph3e2e415f/ios, accessed 12th July 2023.
[11] https://www.gov.uk/guidance/ecological-momentary-assessment, accessed 12th July 2023.
[12] https://developer.android.com/guide/topics/location/transitions, accessed 12th July 2023.
[13] https://www.fitbit.com/global/eu/home, accessed 12th July 2023.

(2021) whose objective "was to quantify how an individual's physical health changes in response to negative life events by testing for deviations in their physiological and behavioral state (PB State)." The PB State comprised resting heart rate, physical activity, and sleep duration measured by Garmin[14] Vivosmart-3. Using fitness trackers instead of users self-reporting data through surveys was reasoned by recall bias. In general, other benefits of using consumer devices as research instruments might be lower costs and effort both for participants and researchers (Izmailova et al. 2017), unexpected insights resulting in new hypotheses (Chromik et al. 2022) and undistorted observations of participants in their everyday lives (Chromik et al. 2022). Nevertheless, several challenges remain, such as data security and privacy or lack of competence in handling the vast amounts of generated data on the researchers' part (Izmailova et al. 2017).

5 Future Directions and Chances

The previous sections presented a broad range of application scenarios for health monitoring technology. However, there is still great potential to be fulfilled in the future. In our view, both end consumers and researchers will profit from three particularly noteworthy trends:

1. **Higher-level information thanks to Artificial Intelligence (AI):** Going beyond the use of devices as a tool for recording mere physiological data, researchers are trying to feed more and more sophisticated AI models with the help of health monitoring technology: For example, the approach of wearable-based detection of COVID-19 infections is—among other research groups all over the world—pursued by Risch et al. (2022) with the name "COVI-GAPP." A cohort from Lichtenstein was equipped with Ava fertility trackers and asked to wear them at night so that respiratory rate, heart rate, heart rate variability, skin temperature, and skin perfusion measurements could be performed. Besides this, the participants were tested for COVID-19 on fixed dates as well as in case of symptoms within the duration of the study. The collected data were used to train a Recurrent Neural Network to predict a COVID-19 infection during the presymptomatic phase. The project's overall aim is to give people an easily accessible tool that informs about a possible COVID-19 infection at an early stage and thus limits the risk of virus spread. Furthermore, wearable-generated data are not only useful concerning the analysis of a person's physical condition but also in terms of health-related behavior. For instance, Kappattanavr et al. (2022) examined the performance of a random forest classifier trained on wrist motion data to recognize food intake gestures. The researchers addressed an application scenario where people get automatic smartphone notifications directly after meals reminding them to keep their food

---

[14] https://www.garmin.com/en-US/, accessed 12th July 2023.

diaries. Their idea was to ensure adherence to a healthy diet, which might prevent the onset of diabetes in the long term. As these technologies require significant amounts of user-generated health data to achieve high performance, privacy issues arise. One approach is Federated Learning[15] which provides that model training is performed on the user's device itself so that only model updates are sent to a central server coordinating the training process. However, there are still some pitfalls regarding data security, e.g., attackers trying to reconstruct the original data from the updates. In order to defend against these "reconstruction attacks"[16] a possible solution could be utilizing Differential Privacy[17] i.e., adding a certain amount of noise to the data before sending it to the central server. Islam et al. (2022) demonstrated this procedure using the example of model training on genomic data.

2. **Further and newly developed sensor technology:** As existing sensors are improved, and new types of sensors are developed, the number of possibilities in terms of health-related applications for (wearable) devices also increases. One exciting field is that of flexible and/or textile sensors. They promise to be much more comfortable compared to common sensors made from rigid materials, offer improved sensitivity due to better fit onto the skin (Zazoum et al. 2022), and allow the performance of new kinds of measurements, e.g., bending movements of the trunk (Patiño et al. 2020). However, several issues regarding, for example, energy supply and efficiency, washability, and regulatory framework for safety (Tat et al. 2022) still need to be solved.

3. **Embedding in larger systems:** Although, as discussed in (1), even a single fitness tracker may address many health challenges, combining different sensor technologies or integrating them into larger systems allows to create value for health in more complex contexts. An example of this might be medical emergencies. Haghi et al. (2021) presented a communication platform for information exchange between an alerting system (e.g., smart home, wearable), a responding system (e.g., ambulance), and curing system (e.g., hospital). A scenario could be the fall of a person in their home detected by a wearable and/or smart home device: n available ambulance gets both alerted and provided with detailed information (e.g., the person's exact position in the building and his medical condition based on previous illnesses and current physiological data) automatically. Finally, the person is brought to a suitable hospital in the surrounding area (Paul L. Reichertz Institute 2020).

---

[15] https://en.wikipedia.org/wiki/Federated_learning, accessed 12th July 2023.
[16] https://en.wikipedia.org/wiki/Reconstruction_attack, accessed 12th July 2023.
[17] https://de.wikipedia.org/wiki/Differential_Privacy, accessed 12th July 2023.

6 Discussion and Conclusion

Digital technology for public health is a trend that is here to stay. As outlined in this chapter, we already have access to a great variety of sensors, applications, and devices that are established on the market and used by a broad user population.

The benefits of these techniques range from individual health tracking and feedback for individual adaptations of, for instance, user behavior or medication to epidemiologic health research with large cohorts of users. Yet, many issues need to be addressed. This chapter has discussed some of them, along with current solutions and future developments in this chapter. Along the pipeline from data acquisition to aggregation and presentation are various challenges that need engineering, AI, and HCI solutions.

On the one hand, these technologies bear the potential to increase public health significantly on an individual and cohort level. They can help identify/diagnose problems, provide long-term data, give feedback, and support prevention, cure, and rehabilitation for many current health threats such as obesity, diabetes, mental health, infectious diseases, and more.

But next to this bright future, there are still big challenges that must be solved. In particular, data privacy and security issues become susceptible to exploitation when large amounts of highly sensitive health data are collected from users over long periods of time and aggregated on individual mobile or centralized servers.

More technical issues arise from the multi-device and multi-platform infrastructure that is also extremely dynamic. If health data are to be collected reliably over a long time span, compatibility issues need to be resolved.

For future development, however, the focus must not be distracted from technical questions but should be guided by a human-centered approach, as the goal of all these developments should be a sustainable improvement of the users' health.

References

Cancela J, Charlafti I, Colloud S et al (2021) Chapter 2—Digital health in the era of personalized healthcare: opportunities and challenges for bringing research and patient care to a new level. In: Syed-Abdul S, Zhu X, Fernandez-Luque L (eds) Digital health. Elsevier, pp 7–31. https://doi.org/10.1016/B978-0-12-820077-3.00002-X

Castaneda D, Esparza A, Ghamari M et al (2018) A review on wearable photoplethysmography sensors and their potential future applications in health care. Int J Biosens Bioelectron 4(4):195. https://doi.org/10.15406/ijbsbe.2018.04.00125

Chromik J, Kirsten K, Herdick A et al (2022) Sensorhub: multimodal sensing in real-life enables home-based studies. Sensors 22:408. https://doi.org/10.3390/s22010408

Dekker JM, Crow RS, Folsom AR et al (2000) Low heart rate variability in a 2-minute rhythm strip predicts risk of coronary heart disease and mortality from several causes: the ARIC study. Circulation 102(11):1239–1244. https://doi.org/10.1161/01.CIR.102.11.1239

Faust L, Feldman K, Lin S et al (2021) Examining response to negative life events through fitness tracker data. Front Digit Health 3:659088. https://doi.org/10.3389/fdgth.2021.659088

Feather A, Randall D, Waterhouse M (2020) Kumar and Clark's clinical medicine E-Book. Elsevier Health Sciences

Gilley KN, Baroudi L, Yu M et al (2022) Risk factors for COVID-19 in college students identified by physical, mental, and social health reported during the fall 2020 semester: observational study using the roadmap app and fitbit wearable sensors, vol 9. JMIR Publications, Toronto, p e34645

Haghi M, Barakat R, Spicher N et al (2021) Automatic information exchange in the early rescue chain using the International Standard Accident Number (ISAN). Healthcare 9:996. https://doi.org/10.3390/healthcare9080996

Islam T, Ghasemi R, Mohammed N (2022) Privacy-preserving federated learning model for healthcare data. In: 2022 IEEE 12th Annual Computing and Communication Workshop and Conference (CCWC). IEEE, pp 0281–0287. https://doi.org/10.1109/CCWC54503.2022.9720752

Izmailova E, Wagner J, Perakslis E (2017) Wearable devices in clinical trials: hype and hypothesis. Clin Pharmacol Ther 104:42–52. https://doi.org/10.1002/cpt.966

Kappattanavr A, Kremser M, Arnrich B (2022) Have your cake and log it too: a pilot study leveraging imu sensors for real-time food journaling notifications. In: HEALTHINF. https://doi.org/10.5220/0010845500003123

Lapinski M, Berkson E, Gill T et al (2009) A distributed wearable, wireless sensor system for evaluating professional baseball pitchers and batters. In: 2009 International symposium on wearable computers. IEEE, pp 131–138. https://doi.org/10.1109/ISWC.2009.27

Lu L, Zhang J, Xie Y et al (2020) Wearable health devices in health care: narrative systematic review. JMIR mHealth uHealth 8(11):e18,907

Makivić B, Djordjević Nikić M, Willis MS (2013) Heart rate variability (HRV) as a tool for diagnostic and monitoring performance in sport and physical activities. J Exerc Physiol Online 16(3):103–131

Marriott K, Lee B, Butler M et al (2021) Inclusive data visualization for people with disabilities: a call to action. Interactions 28(3):47–51. https://doi.org/10.1145/3457875

Pasadyn SR, Soudan M, Gillinov M et al (2019) Accuracy of commercially available heart rate monitors in athletes: a prospective study. Cardiovasc Diagn Ther 9(4):379. https://doi.org/10.21037/cdt.2019.06.05

Patiño AG, Khoshnam M, Menon C (2020) Wearable device to monitor back movements using an inductive textile sensor. Sensors 20:905. https://doi.org/10.3390/s20030905

Paul L. Reichertz Institute (2020) ISAN: International Standard Accident Number. https://www.youtube.com/watch?v=PEwHyKCvnhU. Accessed 18 Oct 2022

Risch M, Grossmann K, Aeschbacher S et al (2022) Investigation of the use of a sensor bracelet for the presymptomatic detection of changes in physiological parameters related to COVID-19: an interim analysis of a prospective cohort study (COVI-GAPP). BMJ Open 12:e058274. https://doi.org/10.1136/bmjopen-2021-058274

Shaffer F, Ginsberg JP (2017) An overview of heart rate variability metrics and norms. Front Public Health 5:258. https://doi.org/10.3389/fpubh.2017.00258

Shaffer F, Venner J (2013) Heart rate variability anatomy and physiology. Biofeedback 41:13–25. https://doi.org/10.5298/1081-5937-41.1.05

Singh N, Moneghetti KJ, Christle JW et al (2018) Heart rate variability: an old metric with new meaning in the era of using mHealth technologies for health and exercise training guidance. part two: prognosis and training. Arrhythmia Electrophysiol Rev 7(4):247. https://doi.org/10.15420/aer.2018.30.2

Tat T, Chen G, Zhao X et al (2022) Smart textiles for healthcare and sustainability. ACS Nano 16:13301–13313. https://doi.org/10.1021/acsnano.2c06287

Triantafillou S, Saeb S, Lattie EG et al (2019) Relationship between sleep quality and mood: Ecological momentary assessment study. JMIR Ment Health 6(3):e12613. https://doi.org/10.2196/12613

Zazoum B, Batoo K, Khan M (2022) Recent advances in flexible sensors and their applications. Sensors (Basel, Switzerland) 22:4653. https://doi.org/10.3390/s22124653

Open Access This chapter is licensed under the terms of the Creative Commons Attribution 4.0 International License (http://creativecommons.org/licenses/by/4.0/), which permits use, sharing, adaptation, distribution and reproduction in any medium or format, as long as you give appropriate credit to the original author(s) and the source, provide a link to the Creative Commons license and indicate if changes were made.

The images or other third party material in this chapter are included in the chapter's Creative Commons license, unless indicated otherwise in a credit line to the material. If material is not included in the chapter's Creative Commons license and your intended use is not permitted by statutory regulation or exceeds the permitted use, you will need to obtain permission directly from the copyright holder.

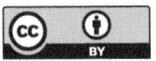

AI Meets Digital Public Health

Lars Steinert, Daniel Diethei, Viktoria Hoel, Horst K. Hahn, Karin Wolf-Ostermann, Marvin N. Wright, and Tanja Schultz

Abstract While Artificial Intelligence (AI) has already brought disruptive changes to public health (PH), the effective deployment of AI technologies requires an interdisciplinary approach to address ethical, legal, societal, and security challenges. This chapter aims to provide PH experts with a common understanding of AI and the terminology to facilitate interdisciplinary collaborations. Furthermore, this chapter highlights the potential of AI for the field of PH, particularly the emerging field of digital public health (DiPH). For this purpose, the chapter briefly introduces the concepts of AI and its applications through actual examples from DiPH. Thereafter, a critical perspective is presented on ensuring AI deployment in DiPH while adhering to ethical regulations. To demonstrate how an AI intervention can be responsibly implemented, a tablet-based activation system for people with dementia is used as an example.

Lars Steinert, Daniel Diethei and Viktoria Hoel contributed equally with all other contributors.

L. Steinert · T. Schultz (✉)
Cognitive Systems Lab, University of Bremen, Bremen, Germany
e-mail: lars.steinert@uni-bremen.de; tanja.schultz@uni-bremen.de

D. Diethei
Human-Computer Interaction, University of Bremen, Bremen, Germany
e-mail: diethei@uni-bremen.de

V. Hoel · K. Wolf-Ostermann
Department of Nursing Science Research, University of Bremen, Bremen, Germany
e-mail: hoel@uni-bremen.de; wolf-ostermann@uni-bremen.de

H. K. Hahn
Fraunhofer Institute for Digital Medicine MEVIS, Bremen, Germany
e-mail: horst.hahn@mevis.fraunhofer.de

M. N. Wright
Leibniz Institute for Prevention Research and Epidemiology—BIPS, Bremen, Germany
e-mail: wright@leibniz-bips.de

Keywords Artificial Intelligence · Computer science · Digital public health · Machine Learning · Human-Computer Interaction · AI applications · Cognitive systems · Technical assistance systems · Recommender systems · Ethical design

Abbreviations

AI	Artificial Intelligence
CBF	Content-based filtering
CF	Collaborative filtering
DiPH	Digital public health
DL	Deep Learning
EHR	Electronic Health Records
FACS	Facial Action Coding System
FDA	US Food and Drug Administration
IEEE	Institute of Electrical and Electronics Engineers
ML	Machine Learning
NLP	Natural Language Processing
PH	Public health
PLWD	People living with dementia
RS	Recommender system
WHO	World Health Organization

1 Introduction

Major advances in algorithms, computational power, and the increasing availability of data have led to a rise in Artificial Intelligence (AI) applications in many domains, including digital public health (DiPH). This is unsurprising given the potential individual and societal benefits of improving public health (PH) outcomes, e.g., quality of life for individuals and cost reductions for health systems. Machine Learning (ML)—a subfield of AI—could help to shed more light on the causes of poor health, e.g., unhealthy diets leading to obesity or diabetes. Based on such findings, AI could also be used to develop target-oriented and individualized interventions, for example, by providing at-risk individuals with food recommendations to decrease their risk of cardiovascular diseases. AI might even outperform human experts for some restricted tasks, as it has been shown for image-based cancer detection in mammography (Wu et al. 2020).

Due to the high potential of AI technologies in PH, there has been an increasing amount of scientific literature on "AI in PH." Accordingly, the number of publications focusing on this topic more than doubled between 2017 and 2020, peaked in 2021 and has since reached over 100,000 publications per year (see Fig. 1).

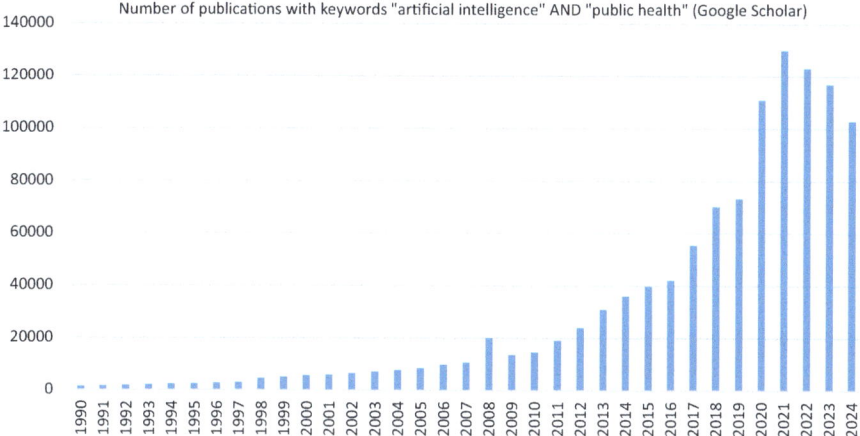

Fig. 1 Bar chart showing the number of publications with the keywords "artificial intelligence" AND "public health" on Google Scholar over 35 years. The chart indicates that publications doubled between 2017 and 2020, peaked in 2021, and has since reached over 100,000 publications per year (Source: Own figure)

Lately, AI has become a strategic focus area in public health both on international and national levels, driven by its potential to improve prevention, diagnostics, surveillance, and personalized care. Research and investment in AI for public health have surged after the COVID-19 pandemic, and are expected to rapidly grow and diversify with substantial funding from both public and private sectors. However, the promises associated with these advancements have not yet been fully implemented at the "frontlines of clinical practice" (Panch et al. 2019). The National Academy of Medicine even warns of another AI winter due to disillusionment by patients (Matheny et al. 2019). Andrew Ng, one of the pioneers of Deep Learning (DL), remarks: "It turns out that just because someone publishes a paper showing AI performs at a level similar or maybe superior to a certified clinician, there remains much work to take into production. All AI, and not just in healthcare, have a proof-of-concept to the production gap" (Goled 2021). This missing clinical impact of AI technologies is partly due to a lack of robust evaluation studies that include quality of care and patient outcomes. Furthermore, the comparability of different AI approaches across studies remains challenging due to varying methodologies and metrics. Also, the black box phenomenon of artificial neural networks is an issue, i.e., the difficulty of linking the network weights to the approximated function and thereby interpreting what the network learned. Lastly, algorithmic bias, namely, the discrimination of already disadvantaged groups due to gender, race, and socio-economic status, raises ethical issues (Kelly et al. 2019).

Emerging AI technologies rely on the expertise of diverse domains, such as PH, computer science, medicine, and Human-Computer Interaction. Interdisciplinarity is required to develop and integrate solutions into the clinical world successfully. While computer scientists might not always select datasets representative of the patient population, clinicians might not have the required understanding of how AI technologies work and, therefore, might distrust AI at large (Nebeker et al. 2019). For a more in-depth discussion about interdisciplinarity in PH, refer to chapter "Why Is It Essential to Address Digital Public Health in an Interdisciplinary Way?", Maaß et al. in this handbook. To guide the design and implementation of responsible AI systems, organizations such as the Institute of Electrical and Electronics Engineers (IEEE) and the World Health Organization (WHO) developed ethics principles (Shahriari and Shahriari 2017). Adherence to these frameworks is supposed to contribute to fairer, more transparent, and more effective AI systems.

In this chapter, we briefly introduce the field of AI, present applications of AI systems in PH, discuss principles of ethical design, and, lastly, give a specific use case for an AI PH technology in dementia care.

2 Artificial Intelligence in Public Health

Over the past decade, AI has become ubiquitous in many research fields due to the increased data volumes generated by humans and machines, improvements in computer power and data storage capacities, and advances in algorithms and sensors. While this progress can be observed in various PH areas such as health promotion (Kreps and Neuhauser 2013), disease prevention (Vaishya et al. 2020), or early disease diagnosis (Behrens et al. 2007), the potential of AI does not seem to have been exhausted yet. Instead, AI technologies will probably become more accurate and reliable in the future and therefore have an even more significant impact on our everyday lives. Despite the major role of AI in current and future PH applications, no universally agreed-upon definition of AI currently exists. One suggestion by Kaplan and Haenlein (2019) defines AI as "a system's ability to interpret external data correctly, to learn from such data, and to use those learnings to achieve specific goals and tasks through flexible adaptation." This broad definition shows that AI is a rather generic term for a wide range of data-driven subfields, including ML (Sect. 2.1) or recommender systems (Sect. 2.2). The corresponding approaches usually require large amounts of data, or even Big Data, to accurately and reliably solve their dedicated tasks. The term "Big Data" is generally referred to when data display some or all of the following five characteristics (Benke 2017; Deiner et al. 2016):

1. Volume (massive datasets)
2. Variability (lack of structure, consistency, and context)
3. Variety (includes different sources, i.e., image, audio, numerical, and text data)
4. Velocity (real-time processing and very high speed of transmission)
5. Veracity (accuracy, noise, and data uncertainty).

Typical data sources for PH could be, for example, Electronic Health Records (EHR), participatory surveillance systems (e.g., crowdsourcing or mapping), patient monitoring devices (e.g., smartwatches or glucometers), social media, online data, geographical data, or consumption data (Gall and Suzuki 2019). Combining different data sources including biosignals allows for a more holistic view of individual patients or populations, and enables the design of biosignal-adaptive AI systems (Schultz and Mädche, 2023). While numerous studies have provided evidence for the benefits of linking different data sources to target PH (Chen et al. 2015a; Predić et al. 2013), it should be kept in mind that data may be affected by certain biases caused by data selection, confounding variables, or a lack of generalizability (Khoury and Ioannidis 2014).

2.1 Machine Learning

Machine Learning (ML) is a part of AI, defined by Arthur Samuel (1959) as the "field of study that gives computers the ability to learn without being explicitly programmed." ML refers to computational methods which combine fundamental concepts from computer science with ideas from statistics, probability, and optimization (Mohri et al. 2018). These algorithms use data to solve predefined tasks such as recognizing patterns or making predictions (Mohri et al. 2018). The quality and the amount of data are crucial factors for the ML algorithm's success (Mohri et al. 2018). Traditionally, data are preprocessed using domain expertise and converted into a representation ("Feature," "Predictor," or "Independent Variable") based on which ML algorithms could recognize patterns (LeCun et al. 2015). A special area of ML that has raised attention in the last decade is Deep Learning (DL). DL algorithms do not require any manual feature extraction process but can be fed with raw data, e.g., whole Computed Tomography images (Chlebus et al. 2018), and automatically extract a representation suitable for the task at hand (LeCun et al. 2015). However, these algorithms usually require more data than traditional ML approaches. In general, ML algorithms are categorized into supervised (Sect. 2.1.1) and unsupervised learning (Sect. 2.1.2).

2.1.1 Supervised Learning

Supervised learning algorithms use labeled training data, i.e., data samples with a corresponding class assignment, which serve as targets for the desired output (ground truth). Thus, a function can be learned that maps the input to an output based on the provided input-target examples (Mohri et al. 2018). An optimal mapping function allows the algorithm to correctly classify the output for inputs that were not a part of the training data and, thus, have not been seen by the model (Mohri et al. 2018). The input, or training data, consists of training examples ("samples") which are pairs of an "individual measurable property or characteristic of a phenomenon" ("Feature," "Predictor," or "Independent Variable") or raw data such as images, and the associated label (or "Dependent Variable") (Mohri et al. 2018). Depending on the label scaling, supervised ML approaches can be divided into classification (nominal or ordinal scale) and regression (interval or ratio scale) tasks.

Classification tasks can aim for the discrimination of at least two classes. An example of a classification task is the dementia disease diagnosis with the aim of classifying participants into those who have developed dementia (class 1) and those who have not (class 0). Features could be extracted from an individual's speech data (Weiner et al. 2019). Typical classification algorithms are decision trees, support vector machines, or neural networks. A corresponding regression task could be the prediction of the continuous outcome of the processing time for a Mini-Mental-State Exam (which usually takes 30 min) to test for cognitive functioning among older people based on the same features. Regression types range from simple linear regression, which models a linear relationship between a scalar response and one explanatory variable, to nonlinear regression with universal approximators, e.g., neural networks or radial basis functions. Other practical examples of supervised learning problems in PH include cancer (Behrens et al. 2007) or diabetes (Kavakiotis et al. 2017) screening.

2.1.2 Unsupervised Learning

In contrast to supervised learning, the data in unsupervised learning are not labeled. Instead, unsupervised learning algorithms analyze and identify (hidden) patterns or structures in data without knowing the ground truth. In the absence of labeled test data, it is difficult to measure the performance of these algorithms (Mohri et al. 2018). Unsupervised learning algorithms can be utilized for three main tasks: (1) clustering, (2) association, and (3) dimensionality reduction (IBM 2022).

1. Clustering defines the partitioning of a dataset into homogeneous subsets ("clusters") using algorithms. Samples belonging to the same cluster have similar features, while samples from different clusters are dissimilar. Typical clustering algorithms are K-means or Gaussian mixture models.
2. Association defines a rule-based method for finding relationships between features in a given dataset to determine samples that often occur together (IBM 2022).
3. Dimensionality reduction defines the transformation of an initial data structure into a lower-dimensional representation (Bishop 2006). Typical algorithms are principal component analysis (PCA) or autoencoders based on neural networks.

2.2 Recommender Systems

Recommender systems (RS) have successfully been used in many research areas and applications (Aggarwal 2016; Park et al. 2012). RS algorithms aim to support users in finding relevant items (objects the RS recommends to users) in large item catalogs, which can, otherwise, be a challenging task that can lead to unhappiness ("Paradox of Choice"; Schwartz and Schwartz 2004). In the context of PH, these item recommendations could, for example, be scientific papers on public health for researchers (Chen et al. 2015b), healthy meals for people who are searching for food recipes (Trattner and Elsweiler 2018), decision support for medical diagnoses (Thong 2015), or engaging activation contents for people living with dementia (PLWD) and their (in)formal caregivers (Schultz et al. 2021) (see Sect. 5). A basic RS requires two kinds of data (Aggarwal 2016), namely user-item interactions, such as ratings of the PLWD for a specific activation content, and attribute information about the user and the item, such as textual profiles or keywords which describe an activation content. Traditionally, RS approaches can be differentiated based on which information they use to generate recommendations. These are called (1) content-based and (2) collaborative filtering approaches.

1. Content-based filtering (CBF) approaches aim to recommend items similar to those a user has liked in the past. This liking can be provided implicitly or explicitly by the user (Ricci et al. 2015). The attributes of previously liked items, e.g., the keywords ('tags') describing an individual activation content, are added to the user profile, which, as a result, outlines the user's interests. The RS can then compare the user profile and the remaining (unseen) items and recommend items that are similar to the user profile. Accordingly, the resulting model is user-dependent, i.e., user profiles are solely built based on the information provided by the given user (Ricci et al. 2015). This is favorable when dealing with a limited number of users or if the user group is particularly heterogeneous in their interests. The latter could be the case when aiming to provide activation content recommendations to PLWD (Schultz et al. 2021). One disadvantage of these approaches is that recommendations are only based on the users' existing interests and lack the ability to explore new interest areas (Google for Developers 2022a).

2. Collaborative filtering (CF) approaches consider not only similarities between items (as in CBF) but also between users (Google for Developers 2022a). In particular, CF approaches identify users whose preferences are similar to that of a reference used to recommend items that the reference user rated positively (Ricci et al. 2015). This means that an item can be recommended to user A based on the interests of user B (Google for Developers 2022a). CF can therefore overcome some of the limitations of CBF approaches. As recommendations are based not only on a given user's interests but on a group of similar users, CF approaches can support users in discovering new interests (Google for Developers 2022b). CF approaches are not suitable for small and heterogeneous user groups.

3 AI Applications in Public Health

In this section, we provide a brief overview that illustrates to which public health domains AI has already made important contributions and in which directions it might develop.

3.1 Health Promotion

Health promotion is "the process of enabling people to increase control over their health and its determinants, and thereby improve their health" (WHO 1986). An essential prerequisite for providing useful digital services in health promotion is the efficient and casual identification of populations that indicate "high-risk" behavior. AI-based methods deployed on smart devices like smartphones and smartwatches are very suitable since they allow for a fully automated around the clock identification and screening of large numbers of people at low cost. Furthermore, an always-available natural communication with users is required to provide advice and feedback on health-related issues. A logical choice is AI-enabled chatbots that support users in their daily life, provide feedback, and prompt users with questions on what went well or poorly (Aggarwal 2016; Park et al. 2012).

3.2 Disease Prevention

Disease and disability are affected by environmental factors, genetic predisposition, disease agents, and lifestyle choices and are dynamic processes that begin before individuals realize they are affected. Disease prevention relies on anticipatory actions, which, in addition to health promotion, are a part of essential PH functions, as defined by the WHO (2018). According to their definition, disease prevention can be categorized as primary (prevention prior to the occurrence of injury or disease), secondary (prevention by reducing the impact of disease or injury after its occurrence), and tertiary prevention (prevention through improved quality of life by, for example, rehabilitation; Wienert et al. 2022).

AI-based services have much to offer in this field of application, e.g., by continuously tracking common environmental risks, such as air pollution, sun exposure, and weather conditions, or by keeping track of individual "high-risk" habits, such as smoking or using drugs. The accumulation of such data allows AI-enabled methods to identify underlying causes of poor health and to provide personalized information and prevention strategies. Some examples are mental health applications for day-to-day tracking, which give advice and provide feedback to individuals seeking advice (Baclic et al. 2020). However, communicating with individuals on such sensitive topics requires tact and empathy. AI-enabled chatbots or avatars have not been able to deliver these two skills to date.

3.3 Surveillance and Outbreak Response

PH surveillance is "the ongoing, systematic collection, analysis, and interpretation of health-related data essential to planning, implementing, and evaluating PH practice" (Teutsch and Thacker 1995). PH surveillance benefits from AI through mathematical models to support decision-making. Besides traditional PH data, digital traces—data collected from sources such as blogs, video reports, and internet searches—become increasingly important in informing PH surveillance. One example is online content analysis for real-time critical event detection and mitigation. AI is already being used to predict, model, and slow the spread of disease in epidemic situations worldwide, for instance, to fight Dengue fever in resource-poor settings. Dengue fever is a vector-borne disease that has spread rapidly around the globe in recent years. About half of the world's population is currently at risk. Researchers have developed an ML tool to identify weather and land-use patterns associated with Dengue fever transmission in Manila. The ML algorithm has learned over many iterations how to fine-tune its model to predict Dengue occurrence with increasing accuracy (Wahl et al. 2018).

In their systematic review, Adadi et al. (2021) show that (1) the most prevalent AI applications are related to the health response; (2) DL models are dominating the landscape of AI solutions devoted to COVID-19; and (3) reviews with a synthesis aim and anticipation vision are scarce in the explored literature. The knowledge gathered from Adadi et al.'s umbrella review was used to conduct a foresight exercise for the post-pandemic period, with results predicting that the next AI generation will exhibit the properties of efficiency, sustainability, openness, autonomy, creativity, responsibility, and precision/personalization (Adadi et al. 2021).

3.4 Early Diagnosis of Diseases

AI helps clinicians make earlier, faster, and more accurate diagnoses, e.g., in radiology or dermatology. Current AI technology outperforms humans in specific tasks, such as classifying early lung or breast cancer (Svoboda 2020). Lung cancer is one of the deadliest forms of cancer—about 75% of those affected die within five years of diagnosis. However, when cancers are detected early, the prognosis improves drastically. In 2019, a team of researchers at Northwestern University reported that their system correctly identified the early stages of lung cancer 94% of the time, outperforming a panel of 6 veteran radiologists (Svoboda 2020).

Today, early diagnosis can be achieved for many conditions by improving the extraction of clinical insight and feeding such insight into a well-trained and validated system (Jiang et al. 2017). For instance, the US Food and Drug Administration (FDA) permitted diagnosis software designed to detect wrist fractures in adult patients (FDA 2018). Several studies examined the potential of AI in the timely and precise diagnosis of disease. Supervised methods effectively capture nonlinear relationships for complex and multifactorial disease classification. In a cohort study of 260 patients, Abedi et al. (2017) found that their model could diagnose acute cerebral ischemia better than trained emergency medical respondents. Although noisy data and experimental limitations reduce the clinical utility of the models, DL methods can address these limitations by reducing the dimensionality of the data through layered auto-encoding analyses. Examples include the analysis of more than 1400 images from 308 histopathology regions of the skin to detect basal cell carcinoma and differentiate malignant from benign lesions, achieving a diagnostic accuracy of >90%; or examination of more than 41,000 digital-screening breast mammograms for identifying dense or non-dense breast tissue, where the interpreting radiologist accepted 94% of the 10,763 DL assessments (Cruz-Roa et al. 2013). Another example of early diagnosis is the prediction of Alzheimer's dementia up to 12 years prior to diagnosis through analysis of conversational speech (Weiner et al. 2019).

3.5 AI Systems for Healthcare

For health systems, AI can support personnel in complex tasks or decision-making, e.g., scheduling patients. Moreover, Natural Language Processing (NLP) is used to analyze unstructured text in medical literature and electronic medical records to support clinical decision-making or track population health behavior. Using data from the web, for example, NLP has been applied to a wide range of PH challenges, from improving treatment protocols to tracking health disparities (Wahl et al. 2018).

3.6 Search and Retrieval of Health-Related Research

For health research, AI can, for example, conduct an automated systematic review and analysis of the information in scientific publications and unpublished data. AI systems have the potential to "read" and triage all of the approximately 1.3 million research articles indexed by PubMed each year and can, therefore, drastically reduce human resources allocated for such tasks (Baclic et al. 2020).

3.7 Digital Twins in Health-Related Research

Another example of AI in health research is using "in silico" data that describe the numerical methods used in drug development by modeling biological systems in clinical trial studies and hospital databases. This approach gives the researchers the ability to partially replace animals or humans in a clinical trial and generates virtual patients with specific characteristics to enhance the outcome of such studies. These methods are especially helpful for pediatric or orphan disease trials and can be applied in pharmacokinetics and pharmacodynamics from the preclinical phase to post-marketing (Harnisch et al. 2013). A large "in silico" randomized, placebo-controlled Phase III clinical trial study enabled investigators to use virtual treatments on synthetic patients with Crohn's disease. Results showed a positive correlation between the initial disease activity score and the drop in the disease activity score associated with different medications' efficacy (Abedi et al. 2016). In silico clinical trials can have considerable potential in the design and discovery phases of biomedical products, biomarker identification, dosing optimization, or the duration of the proposed intervention (Noorbakhsh-Sabet et al. 2019).

3.8 Robots and AI

To address the shortage of healthcare staff, robots are increasingly used to take over human caregiver tasks. Becker (2018) classifies robots in healthcare into three categories: (1) exercise devices and tools, (2) telepresence robotics and assistive devices, and (3) social-interactive robotics. Typical tasks include lifting, suturing, delivering goods, and assisting with mobility (Kerr et al. 2017). More than in other AI fields, socio-technical factors will determine the patients' and practitioners' acceptance.

4 Ethical Design of AI in Public Health

Despite the major contributions of AI in DiPH, applications constitute significant ethical challenges. This section shortly outlines key aspects of the ethical design of AI in DiPH, utilizing the eight imperatives postulated by the IEEE in their Global initiative's *Ethically Aligned Design* (Shahriari and Shahriari 2017). These eight imperatives have been adapted to the DiPH context by merging them with WHO's six "Key ethical principles for the use of artificial intelligence for health" in their *Guidance on Ethics & Governance of Artificial Intelligence for Health* (WHO 2021). The merging of the eight imperatives of IEEE and WHO's six key principles and contextualization to the field of DiPH resulted in four fundamental principles of ethically designed AI in DiPH, outlined below.

4.1 Transparency and Explainability

Algorithms on which AI systems in DiPH are based should be transparent and explainable to the greatest extent possible according to the capacity of relevant assessors, including, but not limited to, patients, (in)formal caregivers, healthcare providers, and decision-makers. Accordingly, how and why a system arrived at a particular recommendation should be transparent to ensure it meets safety and efficacy standards. Transparency also includes accurate information about assumptions and limitations of AI technologies, which should be available before their design and deployment and be regularly updated. This requires measurable performance indicators following safety and efficacy standards that can be robustly tested by independent controllers. Information on these performance indicators must be adjusted and accessible to the greatest extent possible to the impacted population.

4.2 Inclusiveness and Equity

AI funders, developers, and users should first strive to maximize PH and well-being on a population level while minimizing the risk of misuse and bias. This requires AI to be inclusive, available, and effective for all individuals, irrespective of their racial/ethnic background, gender, age, income, ability, and more. AI systems should be developed based on identified PH needs in the population, necessitating the active participation of those affected by the systems' decisions to ensure that all stakeholders—not only the technology companies—benefit from its use. The potential disproportionate effects of AI technologies on specific population groups must be monitored and evaluated to avoid bias and discrimination.

4.3 Human Rights, Autonomy, and Data Agency

Rigorous and comprehensive data protection laws are required to safeguard individuals' privacy and confidentiality while enabling individuals to provide informed, valid consent. Individuals must be able to specify who can process what personal data for what purpose. The legal frameworks must also ensure the empowerment of individuals to access, share and control their own personal data. Finally, such frameworks are required to ensure that the employment of AI in PH never, under any circumstances, undermines the autonomy of individuals and communities in remaining in control of medical decisions and healthcare systems. To ensure that empowerment and autonomy are upheld, interdisciplinary efforts are required to translate technical consideration with existing and forthcoming legal obligations into informed policy.

4.4 Responsibility and Accountability

AI deployment in PH efforts must be based on clear and verifiable objectives in promoting PH. Furthermore, clear responsibility, culpability, accountability, and liability must be distinguished for all funding, development, and implementation phases in PH efforts. A system for registration and record-keeping is needed to ensure adherence to these obligations and to minimize the risk of misuse through a methodical and transparent examination of rights and obligations in every decision-making process.

5 Example: a Digital Intervention for People Living with Dementia (I-CARE)

5.1 Dementia

Dementia is an overarching term describing a group of symptoms caused by disease, impacting memory, behavior, thinking, and social abilities (Dröes et al. 2017). These symptoms severely interfere with the activities of daily living and social autonomy of people living with dementia (PLWD), as well as adversely impacting the health and well-being of the people who provide care (Gauthier et al. 2021). Caregivers of PLWD are exposed to the highest degree of stress and burden compared to any other caregiving group (Prince et al. 2009), soliciting spearheaded PH efforts to mitigate the adverse outcomes for caregivers and care recipients. There are currently more than 55 million PLWD worldwide, an astounding number expected to increase beyond 130 million by 2050 (WHO 2017). The need for health promotion as well as primary and secondary prevention for this population is imminent. However, as there is no known cure for dementia to this date, prevention at the tertiary level must not be trivialized. Consequently, tertiary disease prevention efforts in dementia focus increasingly on psychosocial interventions, where there is growing evidence to suggest that technology-driven psychosocial interventions can enhance the well-being of PLWD and their caregivers (Beard et al. 2009; Brodaty and Donkin 2009; Hoel et al. 2021; Jang et al. 2004). Tertiary prevention in dementia aims to positively affect the quality of life of PLWD and caregivers by mitigating the negative impacts of the symptoms of the disease. The use of AI methods and systems in dementia care might create opportunities to reduce the global burden of dementia and enable novel technologies to improve the lives of PLWD and their caregivers (Ienca et al. 2018). The following subsections will present an example of tertiary prevention for PLWD and their caregivers using AI in a tablet-based activation system called I-CARE (Schultz et al. 2018, 2021; Steinert et al. 2020).

5.2 Activation System I-CARE

I-CARE is a tablet-based activation system that provides stimuli of different types that aim for general maintenance or enhancement of the cognitive and social functioning of PLWD. To address the latter, the system is designed to be jointly used by PLWD and their (in)formal caregivers. I-CARE provides a pool of 346 activation contents (stimuli) of different types, i.e., image galleries, videos, audios, quizzes, games, phrases, and texts. By that, the system provides activities that demand different levels of cognitive processing (active and passive contents). Individual activation contents cover various everyday-life topics, e.g., gardening, sports, or baking, specifically designed or selected for this user group. I-CARE collects multimodal data by using the tablet's camera and microphone to capture video and audio signals,

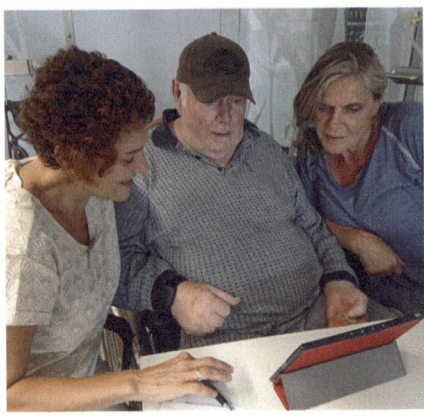 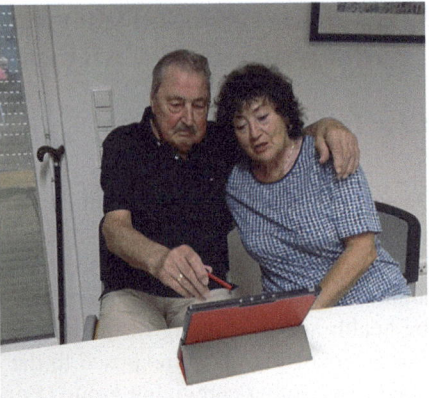

Fig. 2 Two photos side by side showing people interacting with the I-CARE system: in the left image, three people are gathered around the I-CARE tablet on a table, with, one instructor explaining the use of the I-CARE system to two participants. In the right image, a couple engages in an activation session using the I-CARE system together. © AWO Karlsruhe. (Source: AWO Karlsruhe, reprinted with permission)

using the graphical user interface to log the interaction events, and an E4 wristband (Empatica 2022) to record physiological responses from the user. After each activation content, the system asks the PLWD for a rating of how well they liked the activation ("Did you enjoy the content?") on a smiley rating scale (positive, neutral, negative). Figure 2 shows two exemplary situations from the activation sessions.

5.3 AI in I-CARE

The I-CARE system includes several applications of AI in the form of intelligent services. Intelligent services provide information about individual activation sessions in the form of user actions and reactions and context information (Schultz et al. 2021).

5.3.1 User Modeling and Recommender System

The RS in I-CARE is designed to support the user in finding potentially likable activation content to aim for long-term well-being and motivation. For this, the system uses a content-based filtering approach. Each activation item is described with multiple tags, while the user profile contains the tags of the positively rated items by the user. An item is considered positive if its rating is greater than or equal to the user's rating average.

For the individual activation of users who have never interacted with I-CARE before, a new user profile is initialized based on biographical information

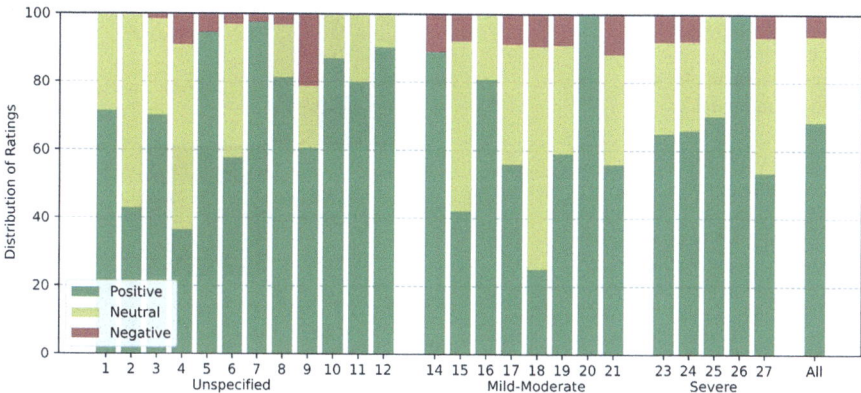

Fig. 3 Stacked bar chart showing the distribution of ratings in percentage across individual participants (1 to 27) grouped according to their diagnosed dementia stage (unknown, mild-moderate, severe). Each bar is divided into segments representing Positive (green), Neutral (yellow), and Negative (red) ratings. Positive ratings significantly outweigh neutral and negative ratings. (Source: Own figure)

(e.g., on occupation and hobbies), which is entered during the first sessions. Individualization also excludes specific content that might be considered inappropriate or potentially traumatic. Once biographical information is provided, I-CARE recommends cohort-specific activation content. As the system usage increases, user profiles become more tailored to observed individual preferences.

Recommendations are generated based on the similarities of a user profile to all possible activation items for the user. The similarity is based on the minimal distance between the tags inside the ConceptNet (Speer et al. 2016). A recommendation list is generated as a list of items sorted in descending order according to the similarities of the user profile to each item. Negatively rated items are removed from the list and appended to the end. For each new rating, the rating average of the user profile is re-calculated, and the ratings are re-divided into positive and negative. Since the set of tags in a user profile can change, the similarities between the user profile and the items are recalculated. Providing the participants with activation content based on their previous likings has proved to be very successful, as shown in Fig. 3. It can be seen that activations with the I-CARE system were mostly perceived positively. Positive activations may improve the participant's mood (Cohen-Mansfield 2018).

5.3.2 Automatic Engagement Recognition

While research suggests that cognitive stimulation, social integration, and physical activity are modifiable factors to reduce dementia prevalence (Livingston et al. 2020), these factors are still important after the onset of the disease. Engaging PLWD in meaningful activities is a pivotal cornerstone of secondary therapy, which

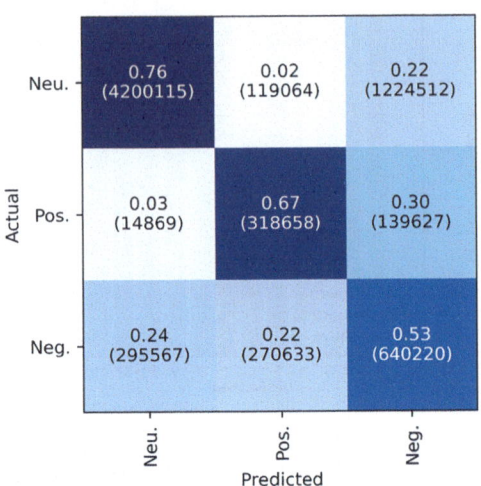

Fig. 4 Confusion matrix heatmap showing classification results for the automatic emotional engagement recognition. Rows represent actual classes: Neutral (Neu.), Positive (Pos.), and Negative (Neg.). Columns represent predicted classes (Source: Own figure)

can improve well-being and quality of life (Cohen-Mansfield et al. 2009), and reduce agitation (Cohen-Mansfield et al. 1992). Accordingly, activation sessions must be engaging to trigger these positive effects. While asking participants for explicit feedback can be intrusive and interrupt the activation flow, ML approaches such as neural networks enable the system to automatically recognize participants' level of engagement based on different biosignals from facial expressions, speech, head and body pose as well as eye gaze. Combining different behavioral channels seems especially important as dementia can lead to aphasia (Cummings et al. 1985) or blunted affect (Jones et al. 2015; Kumfor and Piguet 2012), which may impair or disable certain human communication channels.

Using ML to automatically recognize the emotional engagement of PLWD during their interaction with the I-CARE system can, for example, improve the activation content recommendations provided by the system, i.e., the RS can recommend content similar to those that have been engaging in the past. Figure 4 shows the recognition results of such a system. This system can recognize neutral, positive, and negative emotional expressions of PLWD on a video-frame basis.

5.3.3 Facial Analysis and Emotion Recognition

The I-CARE system offers an intelligent service for facial analysis based on video data (Gehrig et al. 2015; Stiefelhagen 2011). During the activation sessions, the facial analysis service estimates real-time head posture and facial expressions from volunteering users' camera data. To recognize users by their faces, a model is trained at the beginning of the first session with the I-CARE tablet. During training, features are extracted and collected as long as a face can be detected in the video and landmarks can be identified. After successful training, the model is stored in the associated user profile and reloaded for the next activation session in which this person re-appears. Based on an analysis of facial expressions, three concepts for emotion recognition were implemented: the identification of prototypical emotional categories (Richter et al. 2012), the estimation of continuous emotion dimensions, and the Facial Action Coding System (FACS; Ekman and Friesen 1978) based facial expressions analysis without interpretation of emotions. The employed algorithms are based on Machine Learning; thus, the facial analysis accuracy will benefit as larger amounts of data become available.

5.3.4 Biosignal Analysis Based on Interactions, Psychophysiological Indicators, and Voice

The system learns users' content preferences from explicit assessments and implicit feedback based on the recorded interactions (touch screen, microphone, and camera) as well as from physical and psychological indicators derived from biosignals. In addition to the tablet, users were offered an Empatica E4 wristband (Empatica 2022) that measures biosignals related to movement, electrodermal activity, and heart rate based on the integrated sensors. The former refers to the user's physical activity, while the latter two signals are used to assess physical and psychological parameters (e.g., stress, attention, emotions, enthusiasm). In addition, the facial analysis provides information on facial reactions to activation content (e.g., smiles, astonishment), while the analysis of voice recordings allows quantitative statements about whether the activation encourages interpersonal communication.

5.4 *Ethical Considerations for the AI System I-CARE*

Lacking or inadequate translation of ethical considerations to specific settings are major obstacles to successfully adopting AI technologies in a dementia care context (Ienca et al. 2017). As a part of providing an automatic RS, the I-CARE system acquires biographic information and various biosignals. Information such as age, (previous) occupation, and interests are recorded in each user's individual profile. Biosignals derived from speech, facial expressions, and physiological processes are collected through audio and video recordings as well as via the sensor-wristband Empatica E4, measuring physiological responses such as pulse and skin moisture, which can provide information about reactions and the degree to which a person is engaged in the activation. Due to the intimate nature of such data, ethical considerations need to be at the forefront in the development and implementation phase. Therefore, the use case of I-CARE is concluded with setting-specific ethical considerations, following the four fundamental ethical considerations for AI in DiPH, outlined in Sect. 4.

Transparency in I-CARE refers to the availability of comprehensible information to anyone implementing or using the I-CARE system, including managers/organizational leaders, caregivers in supportive roles, or PLWD as users. All stakeholders involved in implementing I-CARE have access to information about the nature and purpose of all data collected, as well as how these data are utilized to generate recommended activation contents. Information on complex issues requires particular considerations when adapting it to people with cognitive impairments. In developing and evaluating I-CARE, this information has been adapted to the dementia context, as PLWD have the right to receive information about things that affect them, presented in a way that is as easy to understand as possible (DEEP 2015). The I-CARE system's objectives, functions, and, more importantly, (biosignal) data recording from individuals are thus explained to the extent possible according to the capacity of PLWD and their caregivers (Schultz et al. 2021). This includes adaptations of the language, style, length, and format of the information contained within and around the I-CARE system. Finally, all information is also provided verbally to PLWD and their caregivers in debriefing meetings.

To ensure *inclusiveness*, the risk of systematic bias in the automatic engagement recognition necessitates algorithms that can recognize participants' engagement irrespective of participants' characteristics that influence their facial features, such as age and skin color. The dataset used for training an engagement recognition system for I-CARE consisted of elderly PLWD, an often underrepresented group in similar tasks. At this point, however, the system can be considered biased due to the dataset upon which the engagement recognition system is trained consisting only of a Caucasian sample. A larger dataset including people with different ethnicities and nationalities is still needed to meet the principle of inclusiveness.

The *equity* considerations when using AI technologies such as I-CARE in dementia care are concerned with enabling users with equal conditions to use the technology. This includes striving to maximize access and consequent adoption for all socioeconomic classes (Ienca et al. 2018). Although this is a goal that cannot be achieved in the short-term due to the novelty of AI applications in public health efforts, AI systems such as the one encompassed in I-CARE should be deeply integrated into digital devices and services to ensure the availability for everyone entering and living in the digitalized world.

In order to *safeguard human rights, autonomy, and data agency*, the recorded biosignals and biographical data are processed and archived in pseudonymized form. Personal autonomy is maximized when end users are not passive objects of top-down designs but when the AI technology is adapted to their needs (Ienca et al. 2018). As such, I-CARE has been developed in close collaboration with PLWD, formal and informal caregivers, in designing and selecting the I-CARE activation content and piloting the system (Schultz et al. 2021). Furthermore, individuals can specify their user profile by providing personal and biographical information, for example, their previous profession, based on which the I-CARE system can recommend appropriate activation content. This information is stored on a highly secured IT system to best protect an individual's privacy and confidentiality.

By providing engaging activation content, the I-CARE system serves PH aims, namely tertiary disease prevention. Multiple outcome measures can be examined to evaluate this approach's success, such as the level of engagement as a mediating variable for the activation success or standardized cognitive ability tests. *Clear responsibility and accountability* for the system to serve these aims can be attributed to the study team who developed and implemented the system. As such, a rigorous process to establish ethical guidelines and guiding principles in the development phase of I-CARE was conducted to guide all actors involved in the interdisciplinary consortium ranging from geriatricians, gerontologists, psychologists, healthcare scientists, and nurses to engineers and computer scientists (Schultz et al. 2021).

6 Conclusion and Outlook

In this chapter, we illustrated current and future developments of AI in PH and discussed the challenges of sustainable and responsible AI algorithms and their implementations for DiPH applications. We highlighted that AI has the potential to make healthcare more affordable, effective, and accessible in almost all health domains, compensating for issues of traditional health systems.

We suggested that the discussion about AI technologies should not only focus on what is technologically feasible but also address ethical considerations. AI developers are responsible for ensuring that no individual or group is disadvantaged due to their race, gender, age, religion, or socioeconomic status, to name a few. We presented a set of principles to guide designers and developers of AI systems for PH to ensure ethical design in their applications. Furthermore, we noted that AI is not yet broadly implemented in clinical practice despite several algorithms outperforming clinicians in specific tasks such as diagnosing cancer from CT scans. We argued that the community might experience another AI winter unless future evaluation studies are robust and include health outcomes. The future will show whether the "hype" of AI in PH will live up to its high expectations.

Finally, we are convinced that AI and Big Data will shape the future of public health. AI will leverage Big Data to either inform clinicians or even make decisions autonomously. As digital health researchers and practitioners, it is our shared responsibility to safeguard the design, development, and implementation of AI algorithms as well as their applications. As the European Patients' Forum states: "Medical breakthroughs of the future will be increasingly defined by our ability to collect, share and understand health-relevant data in vast quantities" (European Patients Forum 2018).

References

Abedi V, Lu P, Hontecillas R et al (2016) Chapter 28—Phase III placebo-controlled, randomized clinical trial with synthetic Crohn's disease patients to evaluate treatment response. In: Emerging trends applications and infrastructures for computational biology, bioinformatics, and systems biology, pp 411–427. https://doi.org/10.1016/B978-0-12-804203-8.00028-6

Abedi V, Goyal N, Tsivgoulis G et al (2017) Novel screening tool for stroke using artificial neural network. Stroke 48:1678–1681

Adadi A, Lahmer M, Nasiri S (2021) Artificial Intelligence and covid-19: a systematic umbrella review and roads ahead. J King Saud Univ Comput Inform Sci 34:5898–5920

Aggarwal CC (2016) Recommender systems. Springer, Cham

Baclic O, Tunis M, Young K et al (2020) Challenges and opportunities for public health made possible by advances in natural language processing. Can Commun Dis Rep 46:161–168

Beard RL, Knauss J, Moyer D (2009) Managing disability and enjoying life: how we reframe dementia through personal narratives. J Aging Stud 23:227–235

Becker H (2018) Robotik in der Gesundheitsversorgung: Hoffnungen, Befürchtungen und Akzeptanz aus Sicht der Nutzerinnen und Nutzer. In: Pflegeroboter. Springer Gabler, Wiesbaden, pp 229–248

Behrens S, Laue H, Althaus M et al (2007) Computer assistance for MR based diagnosis of breast cancer: present and future challenges. Comput Med Imaging Graph 31:236–247

Benke KK (2017) Uncertainties in big data when using internet surveillance tools and social media for determination of patterns in disease incidence. JAMA Ophthalmol 135:402

Bishop CM (2006) Pattern recognition. Springer, New York

Brodaty H, Donkin M (2009) Family caregivers of people with dementia. Dialogues Clin Neurosci 11:217–228

Chen H-H, Ororbia II AG, Giles CL (2015a) ExpertSeer: a keyphrase based expert recommender for digital libraries. https://doi.org/10.48550/arXiv.1511.02058

Chen M, Zhang Y, Li Y et al (2015b) AIWAC: affective interaction through wearable computing and cloud technology. IEEE Wirel Commun 22:20–27

Chlebus G, Schenk A, Moltz JH et al (2018) Automatic liver tumor segmentation in CT with fully convolutional neural networks and object-based postprocessing. Sci Rep 8:1–7

Cohen-Mansfield J (2018) Do reports on personal preferences of persons with dementia predict their responses to group activities? Dement Geriatr Cogn Disord 46:100–108

Cohen-Mansfield J, Marx MS, Werner P (1992) Observational data on time use and behavior problems in the nursing home. J Appl Gerontol 11:111–121

Cohen-Mansfield J, Dakheel-Ali M, Marx MS (2009) Engagement in persons with dementia: the concept and its measurement. Am J Geriatr Psychiatry 17:299–307

Speer R, Chin J, Havasi C (2016) Conceptnet 5.5: An open multilingual graph of general knowledge. https://arxiv.org/abs/1612.03975

Cruz-Roa AA, Arevalo Ovalle JE, Madabhushi A, González Osorio FA (2013) A deep learning architecture for image representation, visual interpretability and automated basal-cell carcinoma cancer detection. Med Image Comput Comput Interv 16:403–410. https://doi.org/10.1007/978-3-642-40763-5_50

Cummings JL, Benson DF, Hill MA, Read S (1985) Aphasia in dementia of the Alzheimer type. Neurology 35:394–394

D.E.E.P. (2015) Involving people with dementia in creating dementia friendly communities. https://dementiavoices.org.uk/wp-content/uploads/2013/11/DEEP-Guide-Involving-people-with-dementia-in-Dementia-Friendly-Communities.pdf. Accessed Jul 2023

Deiner MS, Lietman TM, McLeod D et al (2016) Surveillance tools emerging from search engines and social media data for determining eye disease patterns. JAMA Ophthalmol 134:1024–1029

Dröes RM, Chattat R, Diaz A et al (2017) Social health and dementia: a European consensus on the operationalization of the concept and directions for research and practice. Aging Ment Health 21:4–17

Ekman P, Friesen WV (1978) Manual for the facial action coding system. Consulting Psychologists Press, Palo Alto

Empatica (2022) E4 Wristband I real-time physiological signals I wearable PPG, EDA, temperature, motion sensors. https://www.empatica.com/research/e4. Accessed 22 Jun 2023

European Patients Forum (2018) Data saves lives. https://www.eu-patient.eu/. Accessed Jul 2023

Food US, Administration D (2018) FDA permits marketing of artificial intelligence algorithm for aiding providers in detecting wrist fractures. https://www.fda.gov/newsevents/newsroom/pressannouncements/ucm608833.htm. Accessed Jul 2023

Gall C, Suzuki E (2019) 5 Big data: a new dawn for public health? https://www.oecd-ilibrary.org/sites/f24cb567-en/index.html?itemId=/content/component/f24cb567-en

Gauthier S, Rosa-Neto P, Morais J, Webster C (2021) World Alzheimer Report 2021: journey through the diagnosis of dementia. Alzheimer's Disease International, London

Gehrig T, Al-Halah Z, Ekenel HK, Stiefelhagen R (2015) Action unit intensity estimation using hierarchical partial least squares. In: Proceedings of the 2015 11th IEEE international conference and workshops on automatic face and gesture recognition, Ljubljana, Slovenia, pp 1–6. Accessed Jul 2023

Goled S (2021) Real-world application of AI in healthcare is still a challenge. In: Analytics India Magazine. https://analyticsindiamag.com/real-world-application-of-ai-in-healthcare-is-still-a-challenge/. Accesses Jun 2023

Google Developers (2022a) Content-based filtering advantages & disadvantages—machine learning. https://developers.google.com/machine-learning/recommendation/content-based/summary. Accessed Jul 2023

Google Developers (2022b) Google for developers. Collaborative filtering—machine learning. https://developers.google.com/machine-learning/recommendation/collaborative/basics. Accessed Jul 2023

Harnisch L, Shepard T, Pons G, Della Pasqua O (2013) Modeling and simulation as a tool to bridge efficacy and safety data in special populations. CPT Pharmacometrics Syst Pharmacol 27:28. https://doi.org/10.1038/psp.2013.6

Hoel V, Feunou CM, Wolf-Ostermann K (2021) Technology-driven solutions to prompt conversation, aid communication and support interaction for people with dementia and their caregivers: a systematic literature review. BMC Geriatr 21:157

IBM (2022) What is unsupervised learning? https://www.ibm.com/topics/unsupervised-learning. Accessed 22 Jun 2023

Ienca M, Fabrice J, Elger B et al (2017) Intelligent assistive technology for Alzheimer's disease and other dementias: a systematic review. J Alzheimers Dis 56:1301–1340

Ienca M, Wangmo T, Jotterand F et al (2018) Ethical design of intelligent assistive technologies for dementia: a descriptive review. Sci Eng Ethics 24:1035–1055

Jang Y, Mortimer JA, Haley WE, Graves ARB (2004) The role of social engagement in life satisfaction: its significance among older individuals with disease and disability. J Appl Gerontol 23:266–278

Jiang F, Jiang Y, Zhi H et al (2017) Artificial intelligence in healthcare: past, present and future. Stroke Vasc Neurol 2:230–243

Jones C, Sung B, Moyle W (2015) Assessing engagement in people with dementia: a new approach to assessment using video analysis. Arch Psychiatr Nurs 29:377–382

Kaplan AM, Haenlein M (2019) Siri, Siri, in my hand: who's the fairest in the land? On the interpretations, illustrations, and implications of artificial intelligence. Bus Horiz 62:15–25

Kavakiotis I, Tsave O, Salifoglou A et al (2017) Machine learning and data mining methods in diabetes research. Comput Struct Biotechnol J 15:104–116

Kelly CJ, Karthikesalingam A, Suleyman M (2019) Key challenges for delivering clinical impact with artificial intelligence. BMC Med 17:195

Kerr I, Millar J, Corriveau N (2017) Robots and artificial intelligence in health care. In: Erdman J, Gruben V, Erin Nelson E (eds) Canadian health law and policy, 5th edn, LexisNexis, Toronto, p 257. https://doi.org/10.2139/ssrn.3395890

Khoury MJ, Ioannidis JP (2014) Big data meets public health. Science 346:1054–1055

Kreps GL, Neuhauser L (2013) Artificial intelligence and immediacy: designing health communication to personally engage consumers and providers. Patient Educ Couns 92:205–210

Kumfor F, Piguet O (2012) Disturbance of emotion processing in frontotemporal dementia: a synthesis of cognitive and neuroimaging findings. Neuropsychol Rev 22:280–297

LeCun Y, Bengio Y, Hinton G (2015) Deep learning. Nature 521:436–444

Livingston G, Huntley J, Sommerlad A et al (2020) Dementia prevention, intervention, and care: 2020 report of the Lancet Commission. Lancet 396:413–446

Matheny M, Israni ST, Ahmed M, Whicher D (2019) Artificial intelligence in health care: the hope, the hype, the promise, the peril. National Academy of Medicine, Washington, DC

Mohri M, Rostamizadeh A, Talwalkar A (2018) Foundations of machine learning. MIT Press, Cambridge

Nebeker C, Torous J, Bartlett Ellis RJ (2019) Building the case for actionable ethics in digital health research supported by artificial intelligence. BMC Med 17:137

Noorbakhsh-Sabet N, Zand R, Zhang Y, Abedi V (2019) Artificial intelligence transforms the future of health care. Am J Med 132:795–801

Panch T, Mattie H, Celi LA (2019) The "inconvenient truth" about AI in healthcare. NPJ Digit Med 2:77

Park DH, Kim HK, Choi IY, Kim JK (2012) A literature review and classification of recommender systems research. Expert Syst Appl 39:10059–10072

Predić B, Yan Z, Eberle J et al (2013) Exposuresense: integrating daily activities with air quality using mobile participatory sensing. In: 2013 IEEE international conference on pervasive computing and communications workshops. PERCOM workshops. IEEE, San Diego, CA, pp 303–305. https://doi.org/10.1109/PerComW.2013.6529500

Prince M, Jackson MJ, Ferri DCP et al (2009) World Alzheimer Report 2009. Alzheimer's Disease International, London

Ricci F, Rokach L, Shapira B (2015) Recommender systems: introduction and challenges. In: Recommender systems handbook. Springer, Boston, MA, pp 1–34

Richter M, Gehrig T, Ekenel HK (2012) Facial expression classification on web images. In: Proceedings of the 21st international conference on pattern recognition, Tsukuba Japan, 11–15 November 2012, pp 3517–3520

Arthur Samuel AL (1959) Some studies in machine learning using the game of checkers. IBM Journal of research and development, 3(3), 210–229.

Schultz T, Putze F, Schulze T et al (2018) I-Care—Ein Mensch-Technik Interaktionssystem zur individuellen Aktivierung von Menschen mit Demenz. Tagungsband der Clusterkonferenz. https://www.pflegeinnovationszentrum.de/wp-content/uploads/2018/12/18.-I-CARE-Ein-Mensch-Technik-Interaktionssystem-zur-Individuellen-Aktivierung-von-Menschen-mit-Demenz.pdf. Accessed Jul 2023

Schultz T, Putze F, Steinert L et al (2021) I-CARE-an interaction system for the individual activation of people with dementia. Geriatrics 6(2):51. https://doi.org/10.3390/geriatrics6020051

Schwartz B, Schwartz B (2004) The paradox of choice: why more is less. ECCO, New York

Schultz T, Maedche A (2023) Biosignals meet Adaptive Systems. SN Appl. Sci. 5, 234. https://doi.org/10.1007/s42452-023-05412-w

Shahriari K, Shahriari M (2017) IEEE standard review—ethically aligned design: a vision for prioritizing human wellbeing with artificial intelligence and autonomous systems. In: 2017 IEEE Canada International Humanitarian Technology Conference, Toronto, Canada, 21–22 July 2017

Steinert L, Putze F, Küster D, Schultz T (2020) Towards engagement recognition of people with dementia in care settings. In: Proceedings of the 2020 international conference on multimodal interaction (ICMI'20), New York, NY, 22 October 2020, pp 558–565

Stiefelhagen R, Fischer M, Ekenel HK (2011) Person re-identification in TV series using robust face recognition and user feedback. Multimed Tools Appl 55:83–104. https://doi.org/10.1007/s11042-010-0603-2

Svoboda E (2020) Artificial intelligence is improving the detection of lung cancer. Nature 587:20–20

Teutsch SM, Thacker SB (1995) Planning a public health surveillance system. Epidemiological Bulletin: Pan American Health Organization. 16:1–6

Thong NT (2015) HIFCF: an effective hybrid model between picture fuzzy clustering and intuitionistic fuzzy recommender systems for medical diagnosis. Expert Syst Appl 42:3682–3701

Trattner C, and Elsweiler D (2018) Chapter 20: Food Recommendations, Collaborative Recommendations, pp. 653–685. https://doi.org/10.1142/9789813275355_0020

Vaishya R, Javaid M, Khan IH, Haleem A (2020) Artificial intelligence (AI) applications for COVID-19 pandemic. Diabetes Metab Syndr Clin Res Rev 14:337–339

Wahl B, Cossy-Gantner A, Germann S, Schwalbe NR (2018) Artificial intelligence (AI) and global health: how can AI contribute to health in resource-poor settings? BMJ Glob Health 3:e000798. https://doi.org/10.1136/bmjgh-2018-000798

Weiner J, Frankenberg C, Schröder J, Schultz T (2019) Speech reveals future risk of developing dementia: predictive dementia screening from biographic interviews. In: 2019 IEEE automatic speech recognition and understanding workshop (ASRU), pp 674–681

Wienert J, Jahnel T, Maaß L (2022) What are digital public health interventions? First steps toward a definition and an intervention classification framework. J Med Internet Res 24:e31921. https://doi.org/10.2196/31921

World Health Organization (1986) Ottawa Charter for Health Promotion first international conference on health promotion. https://www.afro.who.int/publications/ottawa-charter-health-promotion-first-international-conference-health-promotion. Accessed 22 Jun 2023

World Health Organization (2017) Global action plan on the public health response to dementia 2017–2025. WHO, Geneva

World Health Organization (2018) Essential public health functions, health systems and health security: developing conceptual clarity and a WHO roadmap for action. https://www.who.int/publications/i/item/9789241514088. Accessed 22 Jun 2023

World Health Organization (2021) Ethics and governance of artificial intelligence for health: WHO guidance. https://www.who.int/publications/i/item/9789240029200. Accessed Jul 2023

Wu N, Phang J, Park J et al (2020) Deep neural networks improve radiologists' performance in breast cancer screening. IEEE Trans Med Imaging 39:1184–1194

Open Access This chapter is licensed under the terms of the Creative Commons Attribution 4.0 International License (http://creativecommons.org/licenses/by/4.0/), which permits use, sharing, adaptation, distribution and reproduction in any medium or format, as long as you give appropriate credit to the original author(s) and the source, provide a link to the Creative Commons license and indicate if changes were made.

The images or other third party material in this chapter are included in the chapter's Creative Commons license, unless indicated otherwise in a credit line to the material. If material is not included in the chapter's Creative Commons license and your intended use is not permitted by statutory regulation or exceeds the permitted use, you will need to obtain permission directly from the copyright holder.

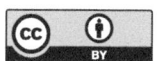

Use of Secondary and Registry Data for Digital Public Health

Timm Intemann, Ulrike Haug, and Iris Pigeot

Abstract Digitalization has changed virtually every aspect of the health sector. Enormous amounts of health data are now generated almost by default and stored continuously by various organizations and institutions, which can be very useful for health research. In addition, the sharing and re-use of data is playing an ever-increasing role in science, which is also evident in the recognition of the FAIR principles. These state that scientifically usable data should be FAIR (**f**indable, **a**ccessible, **i**nteroperable, and **r**eusable). Although some secondary and registry data sources are findable and accessible, full implementation of the FAIR principles requires more effort. At the same time, the international landscape of such data is very diverse and difficult to survey. Moreover, the advantages and potential of using these data have not yet been fully exploited. In this chapter, we will give an overview of important secondary data sources and registries available in Germany, Europe, and worldwide, highlight the advantages of using secondary and registry data for public health research, and provide an overview of methodological requirements and possibilities using record linkage. Finally, we provide perspectives on the use of secondary and registry data for digital public health to enable a widespread FAIRification of health data.

Keywords Accessibility · FAIRification of research data · Findability · Record linkage · Register data

---

T. Intemann
Leibniz Institute for Prevention Research and Epidemiology—BIPS, Bremen, Germany
e-mail: intemann@leibniz-bips.de

U. Haug
Leibniz Institute for Prevention Research and Epidemiology—BIPS, Bremen, Germany

Faculty of Human and Health Sciences, University of Bremen, Bremen, Germany
e-mail: haug@leibniz-bips.de

I. Pigeot (✉)
Leibniz Institute for Prevention Research and Epidemiology—BIPS, Bremen, Germany

Faculty of Mathematics and Computer Science, University of Bremen, Bremen, Germany
e-mail: pigeot@leibniz-bips.de

Abbreviations

CPRD	Clinical Practice Research Datalink (database)
DFG	Deutsche Forschungsgemeinschaft, German Research Foundation
DOI	Digital Object Identifier
EHIF	Estonian Health Insurance Fund
EMA	European Medicines Agency
FAIR	Findable, accessible, interoperable, and reusable (principles)
GePaRD	German Pharmacoepidemiological Research Database
GP	General practitioner
NAKO	NAKO Gesundheitsstudie, German National Cohort
NDB	National Insurance Claims Database
NFDI	National Research Data Infrastructure
NFDI4Health	National Research Data Infrastructure for Personal Health Data
RfII	Rat für Informationsinfrastrukturen, German Council for Scientific Information Infrastructures
SEER	Surveillance, Epidemiology and End Results (program)
SNDS	Sytème Nationale des Données de Santé
SNIIRAM	Système National d'Informations Inter-Régimes de l'Assurance Maladie
ZfKD	Zentrum für Krebsregisterdaten, German Centre for Cancer Registry Data

1 Introduction

Historically, data collection often occurred at the beginning of a research project and was an essential but costly part. Researchers had to recruit participants, develop measurement methods, carry out surveys, and/or conduct experiments and examinations, among other things. Although purpose-generated primary data remain a key aspect of public health research, the increasing digitalization of the health sector now also offers the opportunity to answer research questions using readily available secondary data. Vast amounts of health data are now generated and stored continuously by different institutions and organizations for various purposes, e.g., for billing purposes with health insurance funds or the documentation of procedures in hospitals and in the practices of general and specialist practitioners. From a research perspective, this type of data is referred to as secondary data, as the use in research is not the primary purpose but only the secondary one (Swart et al. 2015). For this reason, secondary data must be carefully prepared before they can be used in research (Swart et al. 2015). The term secondary data may be distinguished from the term registry data. Registries usually focus on one topic and one population, e.g., disease registries on one specific disease in one country or region (Porta 2008; Sund et al. 2014). The European Medicines Agency (EMA) defines patient-centric registries, so-called patient registries, as "organised systems that use observational methods to collect uniform data on a population defined by a particular disease, condition or exposure, and that is followed over time" (European Medicines Agency 2023). Although registries usually depend on secondary data sources, such as notifications by doctors, the aim of their work is usually also research, e.g., research on disease etiology or evaluation of therapeutic measures. To achieve their aims, registries combine health information from different sources, systematically prepare it and ideally make it available to the scientific community. Digitalization has led to an increasing number of such registries and secondary data sources worldwide, which are extremely valuable for public health research.

If we understand digital public health as the application of information and communication technologies for public health (Zeeb et al. 2020), then using secondary and registry data in health research can be regarded as an elementary component of digital public health. Without the development in information and communication technologies, i.e., developments of powerful computers, storage media, database systems, fast internet connections, analysis software, and analysis methods, the complex tasks of collection, storage, maintenance, provision, real-time updates, and analysis of these data at the current high level could not be conceivable.

This shows that the metaphor "data are the oil of the digital era" (The Economist 2017) is, in particular, applicable to secondary and registry data: similar to oil in the ground or under the seabed, secondary and registry data are already there, but direct use is not always possible. As with oil wells, data sources must first be found, developed, and made accessible, and the oil or data must be processed before they can be put to good use. Unlike oil, however, data do not lose their value when used, but their use rather underlines the value of the data in the first place or even increases the value.

Reusing data should therefore be in the interest of the general public and the data creator. These aspects are considered with the so-called FAIR principles introduced by Wilkinson et al. (2016). They argue that scientific data should be FAIR (**f**indable, **a**ccessible, **i**nteroperable, and **r**eusable) to promote "knowledge discovery and innovation." These requirements can also be applied to secondary and registry data enabling digital public health to maximize population health benefits. In the absence of a comprehensive catalog of all secondary and registry data sources in most countries, let alone at the global level, FAIRification of secondary and registry data is far from being achieved.

Providing such a catalog is also beyond the scope of this chapter. However, we will provide an overview and insights into important person-related secondary data sources and registries available in Germany, Europe, and worldwide and document findability and accessibility (Sect. 2). Second, we will highlight the potential and benefits of secondary and registry data for public health research (Sect. 3). Third, we will take a closer look at the approach of record linkage to further increase the benefits of secondary and registry data and open up even more new possibilities for digital public health. Finally, we will provide requirements for and perspectives on the use of secondary and registry data for digital public health.

2 Findability and Accessibility of Secondary and Registry Data

The landscape of secondary data sources and registries is very heterogenous and differs by country. This depends, among others, on the following:

- Data protection regulations, which may or may not be research-friendly, e.g., in Estonia, notifying medical registries was briefly prohibited in 1998, and linking death and cancer registry databases was prohibited from 2001 to 2007, which subsequently has changed, allowing researchers again to access and link comprehensive medical registry data (Rahu et al. 2020; Rahu and McKee 2008),
- Political structure (e.g., degree of centralization),
- Organization of the healthcare sector (e.g., with one universal national health service or multiple health insurance providers),
- Efforts made to establish secondary and registry data sources, e.g., when scientists tried to reconstruct the cause of death information for the cancer registry for the period when linkage to the death registry was not allowed (Rahu et al. 2020) and
- The respective country's culture, e.g., Denmark is recognized as "a society which has already moved far in the direction of Big Data," including the widespread use of a personal identification number (Holm and Ploug 2017).

Especially in the Nordic countries (Denmark, Iceland, Finland, Norway, and Sweden), many different health registries are available which are based on a legal foundation and whose funding is secured (Sund et al. 2014). Further efforts have been and are being made at the national and international levels in order to obtain an overview of these data sources and make the corresponding data findable and accessible. On the national level, the Nordic countries certainly represent excellent examples in this regard. Numerous papers (Laugesen et al. 2021; Maret-Ouda et al. 2017; Sund et al. 2014) and well-structured internet platforms (Danish Health Data Authority 2023; Norwegian Institute of Public Health 2020) provide overviews of the data sources accessible for health research in these countries. Ideally, such platforms use the benefits of digitalization for the FAIRification of their data. This includes the publication of necessary metadata (e.g., data descriptions and dictionaries), tools for interactive non-disclosive database queries, and a transparent non-discriminatory online application process for scientific use files. Such platforms or catalogs also exist or are being developed in other countries. For example, in Germany, an expert report compiled all (known) health registries in Germany (Niemeyer et al. 2021), and the consortium NFDI4Health, as part of the National Research Data Infrastructure (NFDI) initiative, is in the process of establishing such a catalog for all personal health data including secondary and registry data in Germany (Fluck et al. 2021).

In addition to such national initiatives, there are also international initiatives and publications that primarily focus on specific topics, e.g., the European cancer registries (European Network of Cancer Registries 2023), neuromuscular diseases registries (TREAT-NMD 2023), or databases on pharmacoepidemiology (Sturkenboom and Schink 2021) and pharmacovigilance (European Network of Centres for Pharmacoepidemiology and Pharmacovigilance 2023). In the following subsections, we present different secondary and registry data sources important for digital public health and shed light on them with regard to findability and accessibility. A rough overview of global examples of secondary and registry data sources by country is provided in Fig. 1. Tables 1 and 2 systematically summarize the information on data sources and initiatives from this chapter.

2.1 Disease Registries

A disease/condition registry falls under the term of a patient registry according to the EMA definition (see introduction). The oldest and most widespread examples of such registries are cancer registries. The first such registries were established on a regional level in Hamburg in 1926 (Arndt et al. 2020) and on a country level in Denmark in 1943 (Storm 1988). Today, in many European countries, cancer registration is regulated by law and ensures full coverage of all cancer cases in the adult population (Forsea 2016). The International Association of Cancer Registries and the International Agency of Research on Cancer provide international standards for cancer registration. Usually, cancer registries collect information on personal identification (personal identification numbers or names), date of birth, sex, place of residence, diagnoses, topography, morphology/histology, stage, and vital status and provide anonymized analysis data sets for health research. Cancer registries provide detailed information on the number of cancer cases and their development over time as well as used therapy methods and their influence on survival. Furthermore, if cancer registry data are linked with other study data, the variables on cancer and survival can serve as outcomes in association analyses, e.g., for the evaluation of cancer screening programs. In the best sense of accessibility, some cancer registries, such as the German Centre for Cancer Registry Data (ZfKD), also provide data dictionaries, a web tool for interactive non-disclosive database queries, and a transparent application process for scientific use files (German Centre for Cancer Registry Data 2023).

In addition to cancer registries, there is a large number of other disease registries. For example, in Germany alone, there are at least 199 additional registries (Niemeyer et al. 2021), particularly for chronic or rare diseases (Workman 2013). However, typically, no special laws apply to these registries, and a similar nationwide coverage of the population as in cancer registries cannot be achieved. A notable exception is the Estonian Tuberculosis Registry which officially registers all diagnosed tuberculosis cases in Estonia and also offers non-disclosive database queries, contact details for data access, and further metadata (Tervise Arengu Instituut 2015). Other registries often depend on the commitment of clinics and patients. Examples are the German Stroke Registry (German Stroke Registry 2023) and the North American Multiple Sclerosis Registry (Maelstrom 2021).

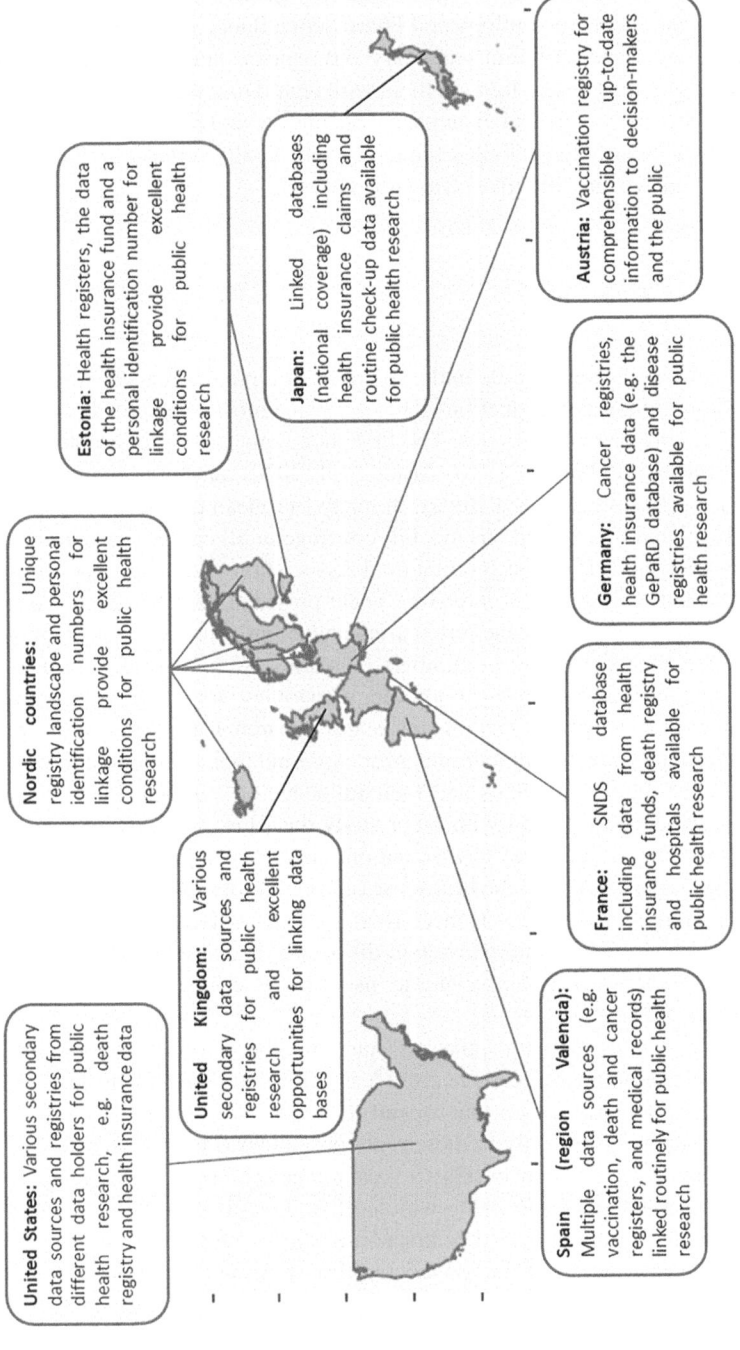

Fig. 1 Worldwide examples of secondary and registry data sources for public health. (Source: Own figure)

Table 1 Overview of example initiatives, reviews, and platforms

Title/name	Country/countries	Source
Reviews		
Databases for pharmacoepidemiological research	International	Sturkenboom and Schink (2021)
Cancer registries in Europe—going forward is the only option	Europe	Forsea (2016)
Nordic registry-based cohort studies: possibilities and pitfalls when combining Nordic registry data	Nordic countries	Maret-Ouda et al. (2017)
Nordic health registry-based research: a review of healthcare systems and key registries	Nordic countries	Laugesen et al. (2021)
The Nordic medical birth registers--a potential goldmine for clinical research	Nordic countries	Langhoff-Roos et al. (2014)
Use of health registers	Nordic countries	Sund et al. (2014)
Gutachten zur Weiterentwicklung medizinischer Register zur Verbesserung der Dateneinspeisung und-anschlussfähigkcit [Expert opinion on the further development of medical registers to improve data integration and interoperability]	Germany	Niemeyer et al. (2021)
Initiatives and networks for findability		
Neuromuscular diseases registries	International	https://treat-nmd.org/
Maelstrom Research	International	https://www.maelstrom-research.org/page/catalogue
European Network of Cancer Registries	Europe	https://www.encr.eu/
European Network of Centres for Pharmacoepidemiology and Pharmacovigilance	Europe	https://www.encepp.eu/
NFDI4Health	Germany	www.nfdi4health.de
Data owners offering platforms for data access of multiple sources		
Danish Health Data Authority: eSundhed	Denmark	https://www.esundhed.dk/
Norwegian Institute of Public Health: Health registries	Norway	https://www.fhi.no/en/hn/health-registries/
National Institute for Health Development of Estonia: Registers	Estonia	https://en.tai.ee/en/r-and-d/registers/

Source: Own table

Table 2 Overview of single example data sources for scientific use (which are not covered in the reviews or data owner platforms in Table 1)

Data source	Country	Source
Disease registries		
German Centre for Cancer Registry Data	Germany	https://www.krebsdaten.de/Krebs/EN/
German Stroke Registry	Germany	https://www.german-stroke-registry.de/
Health product and health service registries		
German screening colonoscopy registry	Germany	Adler et al. (2013)
Prescription registries (see Table 1, Sund et al. 2014)		
Medical birth registries		
Congenital Anomaly Register and Information Service and Annual District Birth Extracts	Wales	Schlüter et al. (2019)
Causes of death registry		
National Death Index	United States	https://www.cdc.gov/nchs/ndi/about.htm
Medical care databases and health records		
Clinical Practice Research Datalink	United Kingdom	Gallagher et al. (2021); https://cprd.com/
Health insurance data		
Medicare and Medicaid	United States	https://resdac.org/
Estonian Health Insurance Fund	Estonia	Puksand and Lätt (2021)
SNIIRAM database	France	Moore et al. (2021)
German Pharmacoepidemiological Research Database	Germany	Haug and Schink (2021)
Social data		
Finnish registers on pensions, social benefits, social assistance or child welfare	Finland	Gissler and Haukka (2004)
Danish registers on personal income and transfer payments	Denmark	Baadsgaard and Quitzau (2011)
Danish Population Education Register	Denmark	Jensen and Rasmussen (2011)
German pension insurance and unemployment insurance	Germany	https://www.konsortswd.de/en/datacentres/all-datacentres/fdz-rv/ https://fdz.iab.de/

Data source	Country	Source
Linkage databases		
National Insurance Claims Database (NDB)	Japan	Sato and Ohe (2021)
SEER-Medicare database	United States	https://healthcaredelivery.cancer.gov/seermedicare/overview/
Sytème Nationale des Données de Santé (SNDS) database	France	Moore et al. (2021)
Valencia health system integrated database	Spain	García-Sempere et al. (2020)
Further (specific) data sources		
German National Dose Register	Germany	https://www.bfs.de/EN/topics/ion/radiation-protection/occupation/register/register_node.html
Danish Twin Registry	Denmark	Skytthe et al. (2011)
Registry on sudden deaths in soccer	Worldwide	https://www.uni-saarland.de/fakultaet-hw/fifa/en.html
Iceland's genealogical database	Iceland	https://www.decode.com/research; https://www.islendingabok.is/english

Source: Own table

2.2 Health Product and Health Service Registries

Health product and health service registries are patient registries similar to disease registries regarding structure and content not focusing on a specific disease but on a health product (e.g., specific drugs, vaccines, and medical devices) or health service (e.g., coloscopy screening (Adler et al. 2013)). These registries can be used to determine the incidence of the use of health products and services and to track their development over time. They can also be used to verify the safety of treatments.

Throughout the course of the COVID-19 vaccination campaigns, vaccination or immunization registries have become the focus of public attention, e.g., to inform individuals about their vaccination status and to enable individuals to prove their status as with the Wisconsin Immunization Registry (Wisconsin Department of Health Services 2023). The Council of the European Union called for the improvement of vaccination registries for monitoring vaccination programs even before the COVID-19 pandemic (Council of the European Union 2018). In addition to countries with a high degree of health data registration as the Nordic countries, Austria, for example, established a central vaccination registry in 2012 (Paul et al. 2021). This enables service functions for individuals but can also be used for statistical purposes and provides comprehensible up-to-date information to decision-makers and the public (Federal Ministry of Social Affairs 2023).

2.3 Prescription Registries

Prescription registries collect information on the prescriptions of persons in a specific population. For example, they can be used to track prescription frequencies and compare them between regions. They are particularly important for monitoring drugs after market approval (as described in Sect. 3 of this chapter). This type of registry is especially well established in the Nordic countries, where these registries cover the entire population (Furu et al. 2010; Sund et al. 2014). Such databases contain information on patients, prescribers, prescribed drugs, and prescribing pharmacies (Furu et al. 2010). Useful metadata and information on data access for the Norwegian Prescription Database can be found on the website of the Norwegian Institute of Public Health (Norwegian Institute of Public Health 2016). A web tool for interactive non-disclosive database queries is also provided to create statistical reports on the numbers of prescriptions by drug, sex, year, age, and region (Norwegian Institute of Public Health 2021).

2.4 Medical Birth Registries

Birth registration is a human right and necessary for newborns to exercise their legal rights as citizens. Worldwide, the vast majority of children are registered by the age of five (Unicef 2019). Nevertheless, scientifically accessible medical birth registries are only available in a few countries. Such registries systematically collect and provide information on all births in one country. This can include information about the mother (e.g., diagnoses), the course of pregnancy, the delivery, and the newborn (e.g., birthweight and diagnoses). Medical birth registries, like those in the Nordic countries, can be used to study risk factors for adverse events and diseases in mothers and newborns (Langhoff-Roos et al. 2014). While Germany lacks a nationwide medical birth registry (Bundesärztekammer 2022), such registries exist not only in the Nordic countries but also, for example, in Estonia (where the platform of the National Institute for Health Development offers the same services as for the tuberculosis registry) (Tervise Arengu Instituut 2015) and Wales (Schlüter et al. 2019).

2.5 Causes of Death Registries

This type of registry is also known as national death index, death or mortality registry, and contains information on all cases of death in a country and for all citizens, including information on personal demographics and the causes of death. The issued death certificates are usually the basis for a death registry. Such registries are widespread and can be found, in the United States (Center for Disease Control and Prevention 2021), Estonia (Tervise Arengu Instituut 2015), or the Nordic countries (Sund et al. 2014), to name a few. In Germany, a nationwide cause-of-death registry for scientific research does not exist, although it has been demanded for a long time (German Data Forum 2011; Luttmann et al. 2019).

2.6 Medical Care Databases and Health Records

General practitioners (GPs), medical specialists, hospitals, and other healthcare facilities routinely produce, process, and store patient-related health data for medical care that have high scientific value. These institutions' medical databases do not only include information regarding one disease, product, prescription, or event but also health records covering the whole course of treatment. For example, hospitals collect diagnostic, service, and clinical data, among others, pertaining to the patient's stay. In many countries, these institution-related data in the form of an electronic patient record are not only shared for medical care across different facilities but also used for scientific purposes or to provide transparency for patients.

Denmark certainly represents an outstanding example in this regard. As early as 2003, the Danish eHealth Portal was established: A communication platform for sharing healthcare data between healthcare providers and giving patients access to their personal health data (e.g., diagnosis and treatment information) (sundhed.dk 2016). The platform also provides a number of service functions, such as appointment booking.

The scientifically useable databases of medical care usually include information on patient demographics, diagnoses, and treatments (Gallagher et al. 2021; Sund et al. 2014). Some databases also include information on prescriptions, medication, or results of laboratory and medical tests, and even lifestyle factors (Gallagher et al. 2021). Comparing data sources across countries is often difficult due to different medical care strategies (e.g., varying national guidelines for the treatment of diseases or medical responsibilities) and because, typically, different institutions feed the databases. In the Nordic countries, such databases are called hospital discharges, inpatient care, outpatient hospital, or ambulatory care registries. They cover nearly the entire population of the respective countries, and the oldest dates back to 1967 (Sund et al. 2014).

In the absence of a complete official registration, valuable health research databases can be created when health institutions join forces, as in the UK, where health data have been collected by GPs (currently more than 1750) to form the so-called Clinical Practice Research Datalink (CPRD) database. This database covers 24% of the population and forms the basis for more than 3000 peer-reviewed publications since 1988 (Gallagher et al. 2021; Medicines and Healthcare products Regulatory Agency 2023a). The patients of the participating GPs have the opportunity to opt-out if they do not want to share their data for scientific purposes. The CPRD platform (Medicines and Healthcare products Regulatory Agency 2023b) informs the public, scientists, and doctors about completed and planned studies, data protection, data access, linkage with other data sources, and pricing. In addition, important metadata information is provided. Two services of the platform should be emphasized: first, a Digital Object Identifier (DOI) is assigned to each available data set version to ensure reproducibility and citability. Second, the platform offers synthetic data sets, e.g., for training purposes.

2.7 Health Insurance Data

If one of the aforementioned databases is not available or the required data are not accessible for research questions on diseases, treatments, prescriptions, or mortality, claims data from health insurance companies can be a very useful alternative data source. Since the data are primarily used for administrative purposes, in particular, databases of private health insurance companies might vary considerably due to different insurance conditions. In contrast, databases of statutory health insurance providers are often highly standardized. Data from both private and statutory health insurance companies must be maintained and harmonized before they can be used for scientific purposes. Usually, for every insured person, there is data on sex and age, diagnoses, drug dispensations, services, and procedures, i.e., information that overlaps with information from medical care data, health records, and prescription registries. Such data can be used for research. For example, in the United States, data from the public health insurance funds for older persons, persons with disabilities, and low incomes (Medicare and Medicaid) (Research Data Assistance Center 2023) are provided for research; in Estonia, data from the Estonian Health Insurance Fund covering 95% of the Estonian population (EHIF database) (Puksand and Lätt 2021) are available. In France, data from the three main health insurance funds covering 95% of the French population (SNIIRAM database) (Moore et al. 2021) can be used for research purposes; and in Germany, data from four statutory health insurance providers covering 20% of the German population (GePaRD database) are used mainly for research in drug safety (Haug and Schink 2021).

2.8 Social Data

Individual educational attainment, occupation, unemployment, and other socioeconomic factors have a significant impact on health. This implies that databases with information on these factors play an increasingly important role in public health research, e.g., the Finnish registers on pensions, social benefits, social assistance, or child welfare (Gissler and Haukka 2004) and the Danish registers on personal income and transfer payments (Baadsgaard and Quitzau 2011). This is also reflected in social and occupational epidemiology, where studies are conducted on social inequality or health risks of occupations, e.g., when differences in post-infarction drug treatment between groups of different educational backgrounds are investigated (Ringbäck Weitoft et al. 2008). In addition, in many studies, socio-economic factors have to be accounted for as potential confounders (Platzbecker et al. 2022a). For this reason, databases including individual social information unfold their usefulness for public health by linking or enriching other data sources with this information (see Sect. 4 of this chapter). For example, individual data from the German National Cohort (NAKO) have been linked to information on employment history and pension status obtained from German pension insurance and unemployment insurance (Schipf et al. 2020). In the Nordic countries, information regarding education, income, and occupation can also be retrieved from various registries and linked with health registers for public health research (Furu et al. 2010), e.g., the Danish Population Education Register (Jensen and Rasmussen 2011).

2.9 Linkage Databases

In some countries, health databases are routinely generated by linking two or more of the aforementioned types of databases providing another important source for public health research. Such linkage databases acknowledge the need for enriched information for frequently conducted analyses. Examples of such linkage databases can be found:

- In Japan, where insurance claims data are routinely linked with health data from routine check-ups with nationwide coverage (e.g., including results of medical and laboratory tests and lifestyle information) (Sato and Ohe 2021),
- In the United States, where insurance claims data from the Medicare program are routinely linked with data from cancer registries (SEER-Medicare database) (National Cancer Institute 2023),
- In France, where data from health insurance companies, the death registry, and the national hospital discharge database are linked to form the Sytème Nationale des Données de Santé (SNDS) database (Moore et al. 2021) and
- In Spain, where in the region of Valencia, data from multiple sources, including the mortality registry, population information system, cancer registry, vaccination registry, and medical records, are linked to form the Valencia health system integrated database (García-Sempere et al. 2020).

2.10 Further (Specific) Registries and Secondary Data Sources

In addition to the registries and secondary data sources already mentioned, there is a vast number of other databases from governmental and non-governmental institutions, some of which are very specific. As early as 2000, Denmark alone had nearly 200 registries (Frank 2000), and in Sweden today, there are 108 so-called quality registers alone, which aim at ensuring the quality of healthcare services (Biobank Sweden 2023). Examples of further registries demonstrating the variety of available data sources are the German National Dose Register, which registers occupational radiation exposure operated by the Federal Office for Radiation Protection (Federal Office for Radiation Protection 2023), the Danish Twin Registry, which registers all twin pairs in Denmark since 1870 (Skytthe et al. 2011), a worldwide registry on sudden deaths in soccer initiated by the International Soccer Association (Universität des Saarlands 2023), and Iceland's genealogical database, which is held by a private company (deCODE genetics 2023; Íslendingabók 2023).

3 Potential of Secondary and Registry Data

The benefits of using secondary and registry data for public health research are manifold. As the existing databases are typically made available for research without informed consent (but only under strict data protection rules and with the approval of the regulatory authorities), the data are free of non-responder bias and thus reflect the real-world setting. This is of utmost importance in public health research, given that underserved and vulnerable populations, which are often underrepresented in primary data studies, are important target groups for public health monitoring and interventions. In addition, secondary and registry data are free of recall bias, which reduces misclassification. Even though potential misclassification still requires consideration, for example, due to incorrect recording of diagnoses, this limitation can often be overcome. The development and validation of algorithms that use the full spectrum of information available in the database (e.g., cancer treatment in addition to cancer diagnosis codes) is a valuable approach in this regard.

Concrete examples can best illustrate the benefits of secondary and registry data for public health research. One example is the monitoring and evaluation of cancer screening programs. Many countries offer population-based programs for the early detection of breast, colorectal, and cervical cancer, but only a few countries have screening registries with the information required to monitor and evaluate these programs. Given that screening tests are typically reimbursed by health insurance companies, health claims data contain information on screening tests. They facilitate the description of adherence to these programs overall as well as by age, sex, regional factors, comorbidity, and—depending on the database—also by socio-economic status. As health claims data contain not only information on screening tests but also on other diagnostic procedures, they can even provide a more comprehensive picture as compared to screening registries. For example, the German screening colonoscopy registry reported that only 20% of the eligible age groups utilize this screening offer (Kretschmann et al. 2021). A recent analysis of German claims data investigating the utilization of both screening and diagnostic colonoscopies in Germany showed that the overall uptake of colonoscopy in these age groups is 45–50% (Hornschuch et al. 2022). Thus, the analysis of secondary data revealed that screening colonoscopy provides only a part of the picture of colonoscopy use in Germany, i.e., it is essential to consider both types of colonoscopy when interpreting colorectal cancer trends in Germany. If secondary data have valid information on cancer outcomes, they may also be a valuable data source to investigate the effectiveness of screening. Unlike data from screening registries, they have information beyond age and sex, rendering it possible to adjust for potential confounders. Furthermore, they typically offer a larger sample size than primary data, which is crucial for screening evaluation, and they have information on the exact data of screening examinations enabling analyses that avoid time-related biases. Recent examples of such evaluations include studies on the effectiveness of screening colonoscopy and mammography screening based on U.S. Medicare data

(García-Albéniz et al. 2017; García-Albéniz et al. 2020) and a study on site-specific effectiveness of screening colonoscopy based on German claims data (Braitmaier et al. 2022).

Pharmacoepidemiology is another public-health-relevant topic for which secondary data such as health claims or medical record data play an important or even crucial role. Even though the effectiveness and safety of drugs are carefully investigated before market approval based on clinical trials, these studies leave several questions on drug safety unanswered. Clinical trials are mostly not large enough to detect rare side effects, and their follow-up is not long enough to detect late side effects. Moreover, older and comorbid patients, as well as pregnant women and children, are typically underrepresented or excluded from these trials, and the drugs are administered under controlled conditions, which may differ from their utilization in a real-world setting. To close these gaps, observational data are needed, but primary data studies are too small and selected for this purpose. Secondary data sources used in pharmacoepidemiology mostly cover data from millions of unselected persons. However, for rare drug exposures or specific subgroups, even single secondary data sources may be too small. As a consequence, there is often collaboration between databases from various countries. Post-approval safety studies requested by health authorities, for example, are typically conducted by such international consortia. Even though this poses challenges in terms of data harmonization, several strategies to conduct these multi-database studies have been developed (Gini et al. 2020). There are also networks of databases to support international studies on drug safety in specific populations, such as pregnant women (Thurin et al. 2022).

Pharmacoepidemiological studies based on secondary data investigate the risk of drugs or their utilization. To investigate risks, an analytical study design aiming for causal interpretation is required, and it always has to be considered carefully whether secondary data contain sufficient information to adjust for relevant confounders. For example, many post-approval safety studies requested by health authorities are expected to investigate, amongst other endpoints, whether the drug exposure leads to an increase in cancer risk. Most secondary data, however, lack information on smoking, which is the main risk factor for lung cancer and also increases the risk of many other cancers. There are several options to address such limitations, such as quantitative bias analysis, the use of proxy variables, or—if a subsample is linked to primary data—two-phase designs. Still, it should be kept in mind that secondary data may not be suitable to give valid answers to all open questions on the risk of drugs in a real-world setting. Drug utilization studies are less challenging and can provide valuable answers to the question of whether recommendations to minimize risks are followed by practitioners. For example, there are teratogenic drugs, i.e., drugs with reproductive toxicity, that must not be prescribed to pregnant women or women planning to become pregnant. Secondary data sources containing information on pregnancies facilitate monitoring of drug use before and during pregnancy. Recent analyses based on German claims data showed that there is a relevant number of children with malformations who were exposed to teratogenic drugs during early pregnancy because treatment was stopped too late before pregnancy, suggesting that prescribers were not aware of the elimination half-life of these drugs (Platzbecker et al. 2022b; Wentzell et al. 2023). The results of such drug utilization studies can directly inform health authorities to improve risk minimization measures. Drug utilization studies are also useful for monitoring public health-relevant trends such as the prescribing of antibiotics (Scholle et al. 2022), which is of high importance given the fight against antibiotic resistance.

In summary, these examples illustrate the tremendous potential of using secondary and registry data for public health research. In several situations, they are even the only option and thus fill important gaps in this field. They also have limitations, many of which can be overcome by measures that ensure data quality and minimize misclassification, as well as by careful planning of studies, including bias analyses.

4 Record Linkage

Record linkage refers to the merging of data on the same person from different databases, i.e., the database resulting from record linkage contains information from all considered databases, and the obtained information is assigned to the corresponding person (Christen et al. 2020). For example, if a cancer register and a death register are linked, the resulting data set contains information on the cancer and the cause of death.

The technical challenge is to assign data from a particular person in the first database to the data from the same person in the second database. Different record linkage methods exist, e.g., probabilistic and deterministic record linkage (Fellegi and Sunter 1969; Kollhorst et al. 2022). These methods use personally identifiable information—variables called identifiers. If one variable enables a unique assignment to a person, it is called a unique identifier (Christen et al. 2020), as the personal identification numbers of the Nordic countries, which makes record linkage simple. If a unique identifier is unavailable, multiple person-related variables, so-called quasi-identifiers, are used in combination. Together they can lead to a useful assignment, e.g., if the variables name, birth date, place of residence, and disease are used together. However, without a unique identifier, record linkage is usually not error-free, and the resulting data set is usually subject to errors. Analyses based on such a data set could lead to biased results and limited scientific generalizability (Kollhorst et al. 2022). In addition to the technical challenges, data privacy concerns may impede record linkage of databases or even make it impossible, e.g., if a database must not be linked, if a unique identifier or an appropriate quasi-identifier is not available, or if the approval process is overly complex (Kollhorst et al. 2022; Pigeot et al. 2021). However, privacy concerns must be weighed against the opportunities that record linkage opens for population health—not to mention that there are appropriate measures at hand to maximize data privacy (encryption, pseudonymization/anonymization, trusted third party, separation of medical and identifying data, and access restrictions).

In many countries, e.g., the Nordic countries, the UK, or Estonia, record linkage of databases is common practice. This is facilitated by unique identifiers and promoted by service platforms that inform researchers about accessible databases, central application processes, linkage opportunities, the legal basis, and costs. Furthermore, the value of record linkage is well known, as expressed by Sund et al. (2014):

> *Anonymous data and statistical information have some value especially for descriptive epidemiological purposes, but the real value of register-based information systems depends on the possibility for record linkages.*

This means, for example, with a vaccination or cancer registry alone, vaccinated persons or cancer cases can be counted, and prevalences and incidences can be calculated, which is undoubtedly relevant. However, linking information allows researchers to investigate associations in order to discover causes of diseases and side effects and make predictions. In a review by Furu et al. (2010), drug utilization studies and studies on drug effects using the prescription databases linked with cancer, cause of death, central population, education, hospital, medical birth, patient and/or road accident registries are listed to demonstrate the impact of these studies for national decision-making regarding drug prescriptions. The following two example studies used record linkage of secondary and registry data and illustrate the outstanding potential for health research in countries with possibilities for extensive record linkage:

- In Denmark, a tool has been developed based on the analysis of linked data from civil registration, education, income, prescription, patient, care, and mortality registries of more than 1.3 million people over 55 years of age to assess the risk of an older person needing healthcare and to enable more intelligent management of care provision (Wright et al. 2021).
- In England, linking data from GPs, testing laboratories, hospitals, and mortality registries of almost four million adolescents demonstrated the benefit of SARS-CoV-2 vaccination for this group already in September 2021 (Gurdasani et al. 2021).

This shows that complex linkage studies cannot only be conducted quickly and cost-effectively with an impressive sample size but also have a direct impact on the level of information in the service of public health.

5 Conclusion

Digitalization has led to a steadily increasing stock of health data that are more or less automatically generated and should be made available to the research community for the benefit of the general public. The overview given above has shown the wide variety of disease/health registries and secondary health databases that would allow the fast generation of results to improve public health without the time-consuming and cost-intensive collection of primary data. This was shown, for instance, when exploiting the administrative databases of statutory health insurance companies to improve public health by checking adherence to certain treatment guidelines (see chapter "Surveillance of Population Health and Well-Being", by Ahrens and Pigeot in this handbook, where, among others, the use of electronic healthcare records for surveillance purposes is described).

However, the reuse of these data is still hindered for several reasons. The findability of these data is usually limited since no common metadata schema for health data is available that would facilitate a structured search for adequate data sets to answer a specific research question. But even if appropriate data can be identified, access is typically restricted since such person-related data are highly sensitive, and their use has to adhere to existing data protection regulations and comply with ethical requirements. Here, we would need a unified, preferably semi-automated approach to check user requests, whether they are, e.g., in line with the existing data protection and ethical regulations or with the informed consent given by study participants. The value of existing data would be further increased if the various sources could be linked to create a full picture of all factors causing a certain disease. Thus, adequate prevention measures can be developed and implemented for the general public. This would, however, not only require a change in the legal framework of possibilities for record linkage in Germany comparable to other European countries (see Sect. 4 of this chapter) but also an improved interoperability of different databases by, for example, a unified coding system. Interoperability of the various databases would also facilitate the easy reuse of these data because no new data structures have to be learned, and different coding systems have to be applied.

A cultural change is needed besides these more technical and legal requirements. On the one hand, researchers need to be willing to share their data with other researchers to enable the entire community to derive the maximum benefit from the data. On the other hand, sharing research data with others requires significant efforts with respect to the documentation and management of such data, which must also be scientifically recognized and should lead to an increase in scientific reputation. It is to be expected that such a cultural change will take time, but it is worth the effort since data are an invaluable resource that must be harnessed to the benefit of the wider public. To put it in a nutshell:

There is a strong argument to be made that leaving data unshared is an impediment to the scientists of the future. (Nat Commun 2018)

Beyond impeding future scientists, leaving data unshared would be a missed opportunity for the improvement of the health status of the general public. Denying access to health data would lead to essential knowledge gaps. Closing such gaps is crucial to obtain as much information as possible for understanding the etiology of a disease in order to set up targeted interventions and provide optimized treatments.

All these requests call for the establishment of a research data infrastructure that supports the FAIRification of research data across the various disciplines in Germany—an endeavor that has been taken up by an initiative of the German Federal and State governments (German Joint Science Conference) based on recommendations of the German Council for Scientific Information Infrastructures (RfII). The aims of such a National Research Data Infrastructure (NFDI) are (1) to systematically manage scientific and research data; (2) to provide long-term data storage, backup, and accessibility; (3) to network data both nationally and internationally; and (4) to bring multiple stakeholders together via a coordinated network of consortia providing science-driven data services (German Research Foundation 2022).

As a member of this network, the consortium National Research Data Infrastructure for Personal Health Data (NFDI4Health) (NFDI4Health 2023) is devoted to the FAIRification of individual health data. NFDI4Health was among the first nine consortia funded and started in October 2020. It will set up an infrastructure that (1) enables the findability of and access to structured health data from registries, administrative health databases, clinical trials, epidemiological studies, and public health surveillance; (2) allows a centralized search for and access to existing decentralized epidemiological and clinical data infrastructures; (3) facilitates record linkage of different data sources, harmonized data quality assessments, federated analyses of personal health data, and the generation of synthetic data sets while complying with privacy regulations and ethical requirements; (4) develops new machine-processable consent mechanisms and innovative data access services; (5) to support cooperation between clinical trial research, epidemiological and public health communities; and that (6) fosters the interoperability of currently fragmented IT solutions.

A successful implementation of an overarching research data infrastructure through the close cooperation of the various NFDI consortia will even improve the impact of data sharing on public health since it will offer the unique opportunity of linking health data with environmental, social, or occupational data. This will allow researchers to create a more holistic view to understand the etiology of common, widespread diseases.

This perspective can even be widened by also considering other types of secondary data as they are, e.g., generated by wearables. Linking these data to health data would be extremely valuable to also better understand the role of lifestyle behaviors regarding the development of a certain disease. Of course, record linkage and data sharing of these sensitive data must always be based on secure technical solutions that comply with current data protection regulations and consider potential ethical concerns.

In addition, this German initiative is embedded in a wider European perspective as, e.g., the European Open Science Cloud (European Commission 2022b) and with respect to health data in the set-up of a European Health Data Space. The latter should (1) "facilitate access to non-identifiable health data for researchers and innovators, "(2) "assist policy makers and regulators in accessing relevant non-identifiable health data," (3) "enable health professionals to have access to relevant health data" and (4) "empower individuals to have control over their health data" where the ultimate goals are "better diagnosis and treatment, improved patient safety, continuity of care and improved healthcare efficiency" as well as "better health policy" and "greater opportunities for research and innovation" (European

Commission 2022a). For this purpose, access to healthcare records, health data from apps and medical devices, and health data in registries should be made possible for the benefit of public health.

Acknowledgements This work was done as part of the NFDI4Health Consortium (www.nfdi4health.de). We gratefully acknowledge the financial support of the Deutsche Forschungsgemeinschaft (DFG, German Research Foundation)—project number 442326535.

References

Adler A, Lieberman D, Aminalai A, Aschenbeck J, Drossel R, Mayr M, Mroß M et al (2013) Data quality of the German screening colonoscopy registry. Endoscopy 45(10):813–818. https://doi.org/10.1055/s-0033-1344583

Arndt V, Holleczek B, Kajüter H, Luttmann S, Nennecke A, Zeissig SR, Kraywinkel K, Katalinic A (2020) Data from population-based cancer registration for secondary data analysis: methodological challenges and perspectives. Gesundheitswesen 82(Suppl 1):S62–S71. https://doi.org/10.1055/a-1009-6466

Baadsgaard M, Quitzau J (2011) Danish registers on personal income and transfer payments. Scand J Public Health 39(7 Suppl):103–105. https://doi.org/10.1177/1403494811405098

Biobank Sweden (2023) National registers and quality registers. https://biobanksverige.se/en/research/national-registers-and-quality-registers/. Accessed 6 Jan 2023.

Braitmaier M, Schwarz S, Kollhorst B, Senore C, Didelez V, Haug U (2022) Screening colonoscopy similarly prevented distal and proximal colorectal cancer: a prospective study among 55–69-year-olds. J Clin Epidemiol 149:118–126. https://doi.org/10.1016/j.jclinepi.2022.05.024

Bundesärztekammer (2022) Beschluss der Bundesärztekammer über die Stellungnahme "Erhebung von Fehlbildungen bei Neugeborenen". Dtsch Arztebl Int 119(47):1–9. https://doi.org/10.3238/arztebl.2022.Stellungnahme_Fehlbildungen2022

Center for Disease Control and Prevention (2021) About the NDI. https://www.cdc.gov/nchs/ndi/about.htm. Accessed 6 Jan 2023.

Christen P, Ranbaduge T, Schnell R (2020) Linking sensitive data. Springer, Heidelberg

Council of the European Union (2018) Council recommendation of 7 December 2018 on strengthened cooperation against vaccine-preventable diseases. Off J Eur Union 466:1–7

Danish Health Data Authority (2023) eSundhed. https://www.esundhed.dk/. Accessed 6 Jan 2023.

Data sharing and the future of science (2018) Nat Commun 9(1):2817. https://doi.org/10.1038/s41467-018-05227-z

deCODE genetics (2023) Unrivaled capabilities. https://www.decode.com/research/. Accessed 6 Jan 2023.

European Commission (2022a) European Health Data Space. https://ec.europa.eu/commission/presscorner/detail/en/fs_22_2713. Accessed 6 Jan 2023.

European Commission (2022b) European Open Science Cloud (EOSC). https://research-and-innovation.ec.europa.eu/strategy/strategy-2020-2024/our-digital-future/open-science/european-open-science-cloud-eosc_en. Accessed 6 Jan 2023.

European Medicines Agency (2023) Patient registries. https://www.ema.europa.eu/en/human-regulatory/post-authorisation/patient-registries. Accessed 6 Jan 2023.

European Network of Cancer Registries (2023) Welcome to ENCR. https://www.encr.eu/. Accessed 6 Jan 2023.

European Network of Centres for Pharmacoepidemiology and Pharmacovigilance (2023) About ENCePP. https://www.encepp.eu/. Accessed 6 Jan 2023.

Federal Ministry of Social Affairs, Health, Care and Consumer Protection (2023) COVID-19 in Austria. https://info.gesundheitsministerium.gv.at. Accessed 6 Jan 2023.

Federal Office for Radiation Protection (2023) National dose register (SSR). https://www.bfs.de/EN/topics/ion/radiation-protection/occupation/register/register_node.html. Accessed 6 Jan 2023.

Fellegi IP, Sunter AB (1969) A theory for record linkage. J Am Stat Assoc 64(328):1183–1210. https://doi.org/10.1080/01621459.1969.10501049

Fluck J, Lindstädt B, Ahrens W, Beyan O, Buchner B, Darms J, Depping R et al (2021) NFDI4Health—Nationale Forschungsdateninfrastruktur für personenbezogene Gesundheitsdaten. Bausteine Forschungsdatenmanagement 2:72–85. https://doi.org/10.17192/bfdm.2021.2.8331

Forsea A-M (2016) Cancer registries in Europe—going forward is the only option. Ecancermedicalscience 10:641. https://doi.org/10.3332/ecancer.2016.641

Frank L (2000) When an entire country is a cohort. Science 287(5462):2398–2399. https://doi.org/10.1126/science.287.5462.2398

Furu K, Wettermark B, Andersen M, Martikainen JE, Almarsdottir AB, Sørensen HT (2010) The Nordic countries as a cohort for pharmacoepidemiological research. Basic Clin Pharmacol Toxicol 106(2):86–94. https://doi.org/10.1111/j.1742-7843.2009.00494.x

Gallagher AM, Kousoulis AA, Williams T, Valentine J, Myles P (2021) Clinical Practice Research Datalink (CPRD). In: Sturkenboom M, Schink T (eds) Databases for pharmacoepidemiological research, 1st edn. Springer, Cham, pp 57–65

García-Albéniz X, Hsu J, Bretthauer M, Hernán MA (2017) Screening colonoscopy to prevent colorectal cancer among medicare beneficiaries aged 70 to 79 years. Ann Intern Med 166(10):758–759. https://doi.org/10.7326/l17-0138

García-Albéniz X, Hernán MA, Hsu J (2020) Continuation of annual screening mammography and breast cancer mortality in women older than 70 years. Ann Intern Med 173(3):247. https://doi.org/10.7326/l20-0827

García-Sempere A, Orrico-Sánchez A, Muñoz-Quiles C, Hurtado I, Peiró S, Sanfélix-Gimeno G, Diez-Domingo J (2020) Data resource profile: the valencia health system integrated database (VID). Int J Epidemiol 49(3):740–741e. https://doi.org/10.1093/ije/dyz266

German Centre for Cancer Registry Data (2023) Database query. https://www.krebsdaten.de/Krebs/EN/Database/databasequery_step1_node.html. Accessed 6 Jan 2023.

German Data Forum (2011) Ein Nationales Mortalitätsregister für Deutschland: Bericht der Arbeitsgruppe und Empfehlung des Rates für Sozial- und Wirtschaftsdaten (RatSWD). https://www.konsortswd.de/wp-content/uploads/Bericht_Empfehlung_Mortalitaetsregister.pdf. Accessed 3 Jan 2023.

German Research Foundation (2022) National Research Data Infrastructure. https://www.dfg.de/en/research_funding/programmes/nfdi/index.html. Accessed 6 Jan 2023.

German Stroke Registry (2023) German Stroke Registry. https://www.german-stroke-registry.de/. Accessed 6 Jan 2023.

Gini R, Sturkenboom MCJ, Sultana J, Cave A, Landi A, Pacurariu A, Roberto G et al (2020) Different strategies to execute multi-database studies for medicines surveillance in real-world setting: a reflection on the European model. Clin Pharmacol Ther 108(2):228–235. https://doi.org/10.1002/cpt.1833

Gissler M, Haukka J (2004) Finnish health and social welfare registers in epidemiological research. Nor Epidemiol 14:113–120

Gurdasani D, Bhatt S, Costello A, Denaxas S, Flaxman S, Greenhalgh T, Griffin S et al (2021) Vaccinating adolescents against SARS-CoV-2 in England: a risk-benefit analysis. J R Soc Med 114(11):513–524. https://doi.org/10.1177/01410768211052589

Haug U, Schink T (2021) German Pharmacoepidemiological Research Database (GePaRD). In: Sturkenboom M, Schink T (eds) Databases for pharmacoepidemiological research, 1st edn. Springer, Cham, pp 119–124

Holm S, Ploug T (2017) Big data and health research—the governance challenges in a mixed data economy. J Bioeth Inq 14(4):515–525. https://doi.org/10.1007/s11673-017-9810-0

Hornschuch M, Schwarz S, Haug U (2022) 10-year prevalence of diagnostic and screening colonoscopy use in Germany: a claims data analysis. Eur J Cancer Prev 31(6):497–504. https://doi.org/10.1097/cej.0000000000000736

Íslendingabók (2023) English summary. https://www.islendingabok.is/english. Accessed 6 Jan 2023.

Jensen VM, Rasmussen AW (2011) Danish education registers. Scand J Public Health 39(Suppl 7):91–94. https://doi.org/10.1177/1403494810394715

Kollhorst B, Reinders T, Grill S, Eberle A, Intemann T, Kieschke J, Meyer M et al (2022) Record linkage of claims and cancer registries data—evaluation of a deterministic linkage approach based on indirect personal identifiers. Pharmacoepidemiol Drug Saf 31:1287–1293. https://doi.org/10.1002/pds.5545

Kretschmann J, El Mahi C, Lichtner F, Hagen B (2021) Früherkennungskoloskopie Jahresbericht 2019. In: Zentralinstitut für die kassenärztliche Versorgung in Deutschland. https://www.zi.de/fileadmin/images/content/PDFs_alle/Koloskopie-Jahresbericht_2019.pdf. Accessed 7 Feb 2023

Langhoff-Roos J, Krebs L, Klungsøyr K, Bjarnadottir RI, Källén K, Tapper AM, Jakobsson M et al (2014) The Nordic medical birth registers—a potential goldmine for clinical research. Acta Obstet Gynecol Scand 93(2):132–137. https://doi.org/10.1111/aogs.12302

Laugesen K, Ludvigsson JF, Schmidt M, Gissler M, Valdimarsdottir UA, Lunde A, Sørensen HT (2021) Nordic health registry-based research: a review of health care systems and key registries. Clin Epidemiol 13:533–554. https://doi.org/10.2147/clep.S314959

Luttmann S, Eberle A, Kibele E, Ahrens W (2019) Perspektiven für ein bundesweites Mortalitätsregister: Erfahrungen mit dem Bremer Mortalitätsindex. Bundesgesundheitsblatt Gesundheitsforschung Gesundheitsschutz 62(12):1500–1509. https://doi.org/10.1007/s00103-019-03049-y

Maelstrom (2021) North American Research Committee on Multiple Sclerosis Registry. https://www.maelstrom-research.org/study/narcoms. Accessed 6 Jan 2023.

Maret-Ouda J, Tao W, Wahlin K, Lagergren J (2017) Nordic registry-based cohort studies: possibilities and pitfalls when combining Nordic registry data. Scand J Public Health 45(Suppl 17):14–19. https://doi.org/10.1177/1403494817702336

Medicines & Healthcare products Regulatory Agency (2023a) Bibliography. https://cprd.com/bibliography. Accessed 6 Jan 2023.

Medicines & Healthcare products Regulatory Agency (2023b) Clinical Practice Research Datalink. https://cprd.com/. Accessed 6 Jan 2023.

Moore N, Blin P, Lassalle R, Thurin N, Bosco-Levy P, Droz C (2021) National Health Insurance Claims Database in France (SNIRAM), Système Nationale des Données de Santé (SNDS) and Health Data Hub (HDH). In: Sturkenboom M, Schink T (eds) Databases for pharmacoepidemiological research, 1st edn. Springer, Cham, pp 131–140

National Cancer Institute (2023) SEER-Medicare: brief description of the SEER-Medicare Database. https://healthcaredelivery.cancer.gov/seermedicare/overview/. Accessed 6 Jan 2023.

NFDI4Health (2023) National Research Data Infrastructure for Personal Health Data. https://www.nfdi4health.de/en/. Accessed 6 Jan 2023.

Niemeyer A, Semler SC, Veit C, Hoffmann W, van den Berg N, Röhring R (2021) Gutachten zur Weiterentwicklung medizinischer Register zur Verbesserung der Dateneinspeisung und-anschlussfähigkeit. https://www.bundesgesundheitsministerium.de/fileadmin/Dateien/5_Publikationen/Gesundheit/Berichte/REG-GUT-2021_Registergutachten_BQS-TMF-Gutachtenteam_2021-10-29.pdf. Accessed 16 Jan 2023.

Norwegian Institute of Public Health (2016) Norwegian Prescription Database. https://www.fhi.no/en/hn/health-registries/norpd/norwegian-prescription-database. Accessed 6 Jan 2023.

Norwegian Institute of Public Health (2020) Health registries. https://www.fhi.no/en/hn/health-registries. Accessed 6 Jan 2023.

Norwegian Institute of Public Health (2021) Welcome to the Norwegian Prescription Database. https://www.norpd.no/. Accessed 6 Jan 2023.

Paul KT, Janny A, Riesinger K (2021) Austria's digital vaccination registry: stakeholder views and implications for governance. Vaccines 9(12):1495. https://doi.org/10.3390/vaccines9121495

Pigeot I, Bongaerts B, Eberle A, Katalinic A, Kieschke J, Luttmann S, Meyer M et al (2021) Verknüpfung von Abrechnungsdaten gesetzlicher Krankenkassen mit Daten epidemiologischer Krebsregister: länderspezifische Möglichkeiten und Limitationen. Bundesgesundheitsblatt Gesundheitsforschung Gesundheitsschutz 65:615–623. https://doi.org/10.1007/s00103-021-03475-x

Platzbecker K, Schäfer W, Haug U, Asendorf M, Reinold J, Schink T, Kollhorst B, Haux R (2022a) Does the socioeconomic status differ between users of potentially NDMA-contaminated generic valsartan and users of brand-name valsartan in Germany? MIBE 18(1):Doc03. https://doi.org/10.3205/mibe000236

Platzbecker K, Wentzell N, Kollhorst B, Haug U (2022b) Fingolimod, teriflunomide and cladribine for the treatment of multiple sclerosis in women of childbearing age: description of drug utilization and exposed pregnancies in Germany. Mult Scler Relat Disord 67:104184. https://doi.org/10.1016/j.msard.2022.104184

Porta M (2008) A dictionary of epidemiology. Oxford University Press, New York

Puksand H, Lätt S (2021) Estonian Health Insurance Fund (EHIF) database. In: Sturkenboom M, Schink T (eds) Databases for pharmacoepidemiological research, 1st edn. Springer, Cham, pp 199–203

Rahu M, McKee M (2008) Epidemiological research labelled as a violation of privacy: the case of Estonia. Int J Epidemiol 37(3):678–682. https://doi.org/10.1093/ije/dyn022

Rahu K, McKee M, Mägi M, Rahu M (2020) The fall and rise of cancer registration in Estonia: the dangers of overzealous application of data protection. Cancer Epidemiol 66:101708. https://doi.org/10.1016/j.canep.2020.101708

Research Data Assistance Center (2023) Find, request and use CMS data. https://resdac.org/. Accessed 6 Jan 2023.

Ringbäck Weitoft G, Ericsson Ö, Löfroth E, Rosén M (2008) Equal access to treatment? Population-based follow-up of drugs dispensed to patients after acute myocardial infarction in Sweden. Eur J Clin Pharmacol 64(4):417–424. https://doi.org/10.1007/s00228-007-0425-y

Sato D, Ohe K (2021) Japan—National Insurance Claims Database (NDB). In: Sturkenboom M, Schink T (eds) Databases for pharmacoepidemiological research, 1st edn. Springer, Cham, pp 267–274

Schipf S, Schöne G, Schmidt B, Günther K, Stübs G, Greiser KH, Bamberg F et al (2020) Die Basiserhebung der NAKO Gesundheitsstudie: Teilnahme an den Untersuchungsmodulen, Qualitätssicherung und Nutzung von Sekundärdaten. Bundesgesundheitsbl 63(3):254–266. https://doi.org/10.1007/s00103-020-03093-z

Schlüter DK, Griffiths R, Adam A, Akbari A, Heaven ML, Paranjothy S, Nybo Andersen AM et al (2019) Impact of cystic fibrosis on birthweight: a population based study of children in Denmark and Wales. Thorax 74(5):447–454. https://doi.org/10.1136/thoraxjnl-2018-211706

Scholle O, Asendorf M, Buck C, Grill S, Jones C, Kollhorst B, Riedel O et al (2022) Regional variations in outpatient antibiotic prescribing in Germany: a small area analysis based on claims data. Antibiotics 11(7):836. https://doi.org/10.3390/antibiotics11070836

Skytthe A, Kyvik KO, Holm NV, Christensen K (2011) The Danish Twin Registry. Scand J Public Health 39(Suppl 7):75–78. https://doi.org/10.1177/1403494810387966

Storm HH (1988) Completeness of cancer registration in Denmark 1943–1966 and efficacy of record linkage procedures. Int J Epidemiol 17(1):44–49. https://doi.org/10.1093/ije/17.1.44

Sturkenboom M, Schink T (eds) (2021) Databases for pharmacoepidemiological research. Springer, Cham

Sund R, Gissler M, Hakulinen T, Rosén M (2014) Use of health registers. In: Ahrens W, Pigeot I (eds) Handbook of epidemiology, 2nd edn. Springer, New York, pp 707–730

sundhed.dk (2016) Background. https://www.sundhed.dk/borger/service/om-sundheddk/om-organisationen/ehealth-in-denmark/background/. Accessed 6 Jan 2023.

Swart E, Gothe H, Geyer S, Jaunzeme J, Maier B, Grobe TG, Ihle P (2015) Gute Praxis Sekundärdatenanalyse (GPS): Leitlinien und Empfehlungen. Gesundheitswesen 77(2):120–126. https://doi.org/10.1055/s-0034-1396815

Tervise Arengu Instituut (2015) Registers. https://en.tai.ee/en/r-and-d/registers/. Accessed 6 Jan 2023.

The Economist (2017) The world's most valuable resource is no longer oil, but data. https://www.economist.com/leaders/2017/05/06/the-worlds-most-valuable-resource-is-no-longer-oil-but-data. Accessed 2 Feb 2022.

Thurin NH, Pajouheshnia R, Roberto G, Dodd C, Hyeraci G, Bartolini C, Paoletti O et al (2022) From inception to ConcePTION: genesis of a network to support better monitoring and communication of medication safety during pregnancy and breastfeeding. Clin Pharmacol Ther 111(1):321–331. https://doi.org/10.1002/cpt.2476

TREAT-NMD (2023) List of registries by disease. https://treat-nmd.org/resources-support/patient-registries/list-of-registries-by-disease. Accessed 6 Jan 2023.

Unicef (2019) What is birth registration and why does it matter?. https://www.unicef.org/stories/what-birth-registration-and-why-does-it-matter. Accessed 6 Jan 2023.

Universität des Saarlands (2023) Sudden death in football. https://www.uni-saarland.de/fakultaet-hw/fifa/en.html. Accessed 6 Jan 2023.

Wentzell N, Kollhorst B, Reinold J, Haug U (2023) Use of methotrexate in girls and women of childbearing age, occurrence of methotrexate-exposed pregnancies and their outcomes in Germany: a claims data analysis. Clin Drug Investig 43(2):109–117. https://doi.org/10.1007/s40261-022-01227-6

Wilkinson MD, Dumontier M, Aalbersberg IJ, Appleton G, Axton M, Baak A, Blomberg N et al (2016) The FAIR guiding principles for scientific data management and stewardship. Sci Data 3(1):1–9. https://doi.org/10.1038/sdata.2016.18

Wisconsin Department of Health Services (2023) Immunizations: Wisconsin Immunization Registry. https://www.dhs.wisconsin.gov/immunization/wir.htm. Accessed 6 Jan 2023.

Workman TA (2013) Engaging patients in information sharing and data collection: the role of patient-powered registries and research networks. Agency for Healthcare Research and Quality (US). https://www.ncbi.nlm.nih.gov/books/NBK164513/pdf/Bookshelf_NBK164513.pdf. Accessed 23 Dec 2023

Wright MN, Kusumastuti S, Mortensen LH, Westendorp RGJ, Gerds TA (2021) Personalised need of care in an ageing society: the making of a prediction tool based on register data. J R Stat Soc Ser A Stat Soc 184(4):1199–1219. https://doi.org/10.1111/rssa.12644

Zeeb H, Pigeot I, Schüz B (2020) Digital public health—ein Überblick. Bundesgesundheitsbl 63(2):137–144. https://doi.org/10.1007/s00103-019-03078-7

Open Access This chapter is licensed under the terms of the Creative Commons Attribution 4.0 International License (http://creativecommons.org/licenses/by/4.0/), which permits use, sharing, adaptation, distribution and reproduction in any medium or format, as long as you give appropriate credit to the original author(s) and the source, provide a link to the Creative Commons license and indicate if changes were made.

The images or other third party material in this chapter are included in the chapter's Creative Commons license, unless indicated otherwise in a credit line to the material. If material is not included in the chapter's Creative Commons license and your intended use is not permitted by statutory regulation or exceeds the permitted use, you will need to obtain permission directly from the copyright holder.

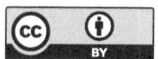

Ethical Implications of User Autonomy in Digital Public Health

Hans-Henrik Dassow and Thomas Eßmeyer

Abstract This chapter explores the landscape of ethical frameworks and design concepts in digital public health. Our primary focus lies on the concept of autonomy in relation to users, with a particular focus on health data. We begin by discussing autonomy concepts from the domain of Human-Computer Interaction (HCI), which we carry over to the context of health data, including Big Data practices. We then consider the perspective of ethical autonomy frameworks relevant to (un)ethical design practices. As research in HCI has noticed malicious and deceptive practices, we follow up on the current discourse on dark patterns. Trying to find answers for practitioners to develop ethical systems, we offer an overview of user-empowering frameworks protecting their autonomy. Lastly, we discuss the ethical implications of user autonomy in health-related domains showing possible directions for future works pursuing empowering designs.

Keywords User autonomy · Ethical design · Health data · Big Data practices · Health application

---

H.-H. Dassow (✉)
Institute for Philosophy, University of Bremen, Bremen, Germany

Faculty of Mathematics and Informatics, University of Bremen, Bremen, Germany

Juniorprofessorship for Medical Ethics with a focus on Digitization, Faculty for Health Sciences Brandenburg, University of Potsdam, Potsdam, Germany
e-mail: dassow@uni-potsdam.de

T. Eßmeyer
Leibniz ScienceCampus Digital Public Health Bremen, Bremen, Germany

Faculty of Mathematics and Informatics, University of Bremen, Bremen, Germany
e-mail: mildner@uni-bremen.de

1 Introduction

The increasing popularity of free-to-use medical health applications for mobile devices directly impacts people's awareness of their personal health and their usage of assisting technologies. Wearables, such as Fitbits or the Apple Watch, offer their users real-time overviews of their current fitness as well as potentially deeper-seated health issues. This presents novel opportunities within public health sectors by enabling the monitoring of patients more precisely, improved disease management, personalized therapy, as well as better health education (Heidel and Hagist 2020). Moreover, as the industry pushes for technological development, a problematic phenomenon known as "cultural lag" (Andalibi and Buss 2020) arises. This phenomenon refers to an increased gap in which technological advances occur in such rapid intervals that society lags behind in reflecting on possible outcomes before their employment. Being on the back foot as researchers poses an ethical problem, where we often do not understand potential harm before it is too late. In the context of sensible health data, often generated and handled without a clear understanding of mobile device users, Peraklis and Coravos (2019) have questioned how such data should be dealt with. They suggest that health data should be handled with equal diligence to blood in healthcare, shifting the attention towards the intimacy that is connected to this particular kind of data:

> *We propose that health-care data records are digital specimens and should be treated with the same rigor, care, and caution afforded to physical medical specimens*—(Peraklis and Coravos 2019)

Although doctors usually explain to their patients the need to take blood samples for specific tests, app developers rarely present their users with a precise overview of how their data will be used. This leads to many users not understanding what exact data is stored and how it is later used by the developers. Concealment of when data is collected and how it is handled poses ethical and legal concerns regarding the failed protection of users' privacy. These concerns have further been acknowledged by scholars who analyzed possible exploitation of users' data based on a large data set of health applications (Tangari et al. 2021). Unfortunately, the user interfaces of those apps may further amplify this transparency issue instead of empowering users to make well-informed decisions when selecting preferred options in privacy-related settings.

Through a Human-Computer Interaction lens, techniques to design persuasive interfaces are well-known and researched. For instance, Thaler and Sunstein's concept of "nudges" describe the practice, as the term suggests, to "nudge" users into carrying out or inhibiting specific actions (Thaler and Sunstein 2008). Thus, practitioners have a tool to steer users' decisions toward a predefined goal that may grant them certain benefits. Although the practice shows how persuasive design can push users to beneficial behaviors (Grassl et al. 2020), others use these techniques more maliciously by tricking users into taking actions that are often to their disadvantage. Prior research has investigated these unethical design practices resulting in comprehensive taxonomies for so-called "dark patterns," coined by Brignull (2010), who defined them as tricks used by designers to harm users while gaining an advantage.

In this chapter, we begin by looking at the design of collecting health data through an ethically motivated lens. We then draw connections from ethical conflicts and frameworks, including the exceptionally ethical relevance of users' health data to research on unethical design practices, which we discuss in the context of dark patterns. In doing so, we provide guidance on how ethical data collection in the era of Big Data branches out with the ethical design of app interfaces. Central to this ethically aligned design approach is the ethical concept of autonomy, which is implicitly or explicitly reflected in all following considerations.

2 (Un-)Autonomous Design

Any object or interface communicates its affordances through *design* as if to steer users to undertake predefined actions. Although this poses a provocative claim, it also applies to everyday objects. If we consider a mug, no inscriptions are necessary to tell us how to use it. Once filled with a hot beverage, its users will be happy to find some form of handle that allows them to hold it without potentially burning their fingers. Many product designs aim to be easily accessible while communicating their functionalities non-verbally. In a sense, the aim of designers is to create products that guide users into using them in a particular way. Within the HCI community, this presents a common understanding of how users engage with designs, prominently addressed in Norman's popular book "The Design of Everyday Things" (Norman 1990).

Recognizing the potential impact ubiquitous technologies have on society, Friedman and Nissenbaum (1997) established their concept of user autonomy to keep agency with the individual and not the device. They define autonomous individuals as people who can formulate, plan, and follow personal goals and take actions that will, in their beliefs, bring them closer to said goals. In this sense, ubiquitous technologies, such as today's smartphones, should offer users desired options to achieve their aims. Or, in a contrary setting: A health application that counts users' daily steps measuring them against pre-set achievements but denies users from setting personal goals takes away a sense of agency that would allow users to acknowledge control over their own actions (Synofzik et al. 2008). Instead, the authors would argue that the app should be designed to empower users to use it to their liking. However, a step-tracking app that allows custom achievements to be set to zero may limit any potential positive impact on its users' physical health. Here, developers have the difficult task of considering both user autonomy (i.e., enabling them to establish their own goals and values and possess the ability to plan and act accordingly to achieve their goals and uphold their values (Friedman and Nissenbaum 1997)), self-determination (i.e., the theory on how factors influence people's ability to uphold basic psychological needs such as competence, relatedness, and autonomy (Ryan and Deci 2018)), and fitness motivations to help users improve their health.

Although developed within an economic environment, the aforementioned concept of "nudges" (Thaler and Sunstein 2008) became a well-known concept in HCI research. Thaler and Sunstein define nudges as interventions designed to change people's decision-making processes in predictable ways. Nudges can thus be used to guide users' focus in any preset direction. This is because they exploit our cognitive biases to lead our decisions (Sunstein 2017).

An often-referenced and known example in the public health domain can be observed in the national differences in organ donations (Molina-Pérez et al. 2019; Sharif and Moorlock 2018). While some countries, such as Germany, require citizens to actively choose to donate their organs, citizens of other countries, like Austria or France, are forced to opt out if they do not desire to donate willingly. Comparison data of different nations and their donating strategies paint an interesting picture that shows significantly more potential donors in those countries who follow the opt-out strategy. While this particular case of nudging is often perceived as a positive and beneficial take in healthcare environments, nudges also yield the potential to be used in unethical ways. In a similar vein, but with contrary results, Munson et al. (2015) showed that nudges can also have negative effects. Studying people's commitment to personal goals in the form of health-increasing walking activities, the authors found that publicly sharing personal goals leads to people making fewer commitments to avoid criticism. After all, nudges are powerful tools to create pervasive interactions, but they must be implemented with care as their outcomes can contradict original aims.

3 Special Ethical Attention Toward Health Data in the Age of Big Data Practices

Intuitively, one would expect a definition of health data and Big Data practices at the beginning of this section or at least a comparison of different definitions from different disciplines. In the case of Big Data practices, various definitions can be found due to the relevance of Big Data for different scientific disciplines (Favaretto et al. 2020). We follow (Gudivada et al. 2015) and define Big Data practices as practices that rely on computing infrastructures that capture, process, and analyze large and complex data sets characterized by volume, velocity, variety, veracity, and value. In contrast, a literature search on the term "health data" did not produce satisfactory results that meet interdisciplinary demands with a focus on ethical challenges. Furthermore, no suitable definitions can be found on the WHO homepage,[1] although many other central terms from public health are defined by the WHO (e.g., health

---

[1] WHO homepage: https://www.who.int/

equity, health promotion). Consequently, recourse to legal texts and academic literature from the field of law is not only appropriate but necessary.

The fact that the term "health data" does not appear explicitly is not due to any oversight. Legislation here deliberately refers to health-related data in order to achieve better coverage of legal grey areas: "Legal commentary considers the concept of data concerning health in the General Data Protection Regulation (GDPR) to leave grey areas in its scope. The concept is constructed either wide or narrow. The narrow construction of the concept defines that data concerning health only includes such data that is processed for purposes pertaining to the health of the user. This simplification of the scope of data concerning health is motivated by the desire to clarify the grey areas of the application of the concept. However, this simplification ultimately results in high risks for users" (Schäfke-Zell 2022). The cumbersome term "data concerning health" refers not only to legal challenges of interpretation but also to ethical challenges. A legal interpretation of "data concerning health" that is too narrow may be legally justifiable but can also pose major conflicts from an ethical perspective: First, we will discuss significant risks from an ethical perspective. In particular, the focus will be on ethical risks arising from Big Data practices. When implementing Big Data practices, ethical conflicts arise in balancing these risks with the benefits and opportunities for individuals, groups, and entire health systems.

3.1 Risks, Opportunities, and Duties

One of the most prominent ethical risks relates to data linking and data evaluation procedures and is summarized under the keywords of de- and recon-textualization. From an ethical perspective concerning health, two central issues are of interest (German Ethics Council 2018): First, pseudonymization and anonymization of collected data are accepted methods to protect users from misuse and abuse of their data and to increase willingness to share or donate data. The use of algorithms in the context of Big Data practices repeatedly succeeds in undoing supposedly secure pseudonymization and anonymization and uniquely identifying users (Acar et al. 2014). From an ethical point of view, the problem arises from the fact that against the background of technical developments, users can no longer be assured that their data do not permit identification (Metcalf and Crawford 2016). The second central aspect does not concern the identity of the users but the quality of the data, pointing again to the problem of a narrow definition of data concerning health. Communicating the purposes when collecting data is a central principle of data ethics. It is common to use data only for specific purposes, for example, consumer data for marketing purposes or data on academic achievements for job applications. However, the technical state of Big Data practices no longer allows us to determine the exact purpose of data. For example, seemingly insensitive data relating to shopping behavior can suddenly become essential data for health insurers, as patterns in consumer behavior could indicate different health conditions. If the data falls into the wrong hands, considerable damage can result for those users acting in good faith. Big Data practices are therefore characterized by the fact that they also raise relevant questions about privacy, data security, and data misuse (Kupwade Patil and Seshadri 2014). At this point, we come full circle regarding an overly narrow interpretation of data concerning health, which leads to a high risk for users who are often unaware at the time of data collection whether they are presenting companies with health-related data according to the GDPR.

A one-sided pessimistic view on using Big Data practices in the context of data concerning health would not objectively highlight the ethical conflicts. Positive aspects are likewise of ethical relevance. In particular, Big Data-driven medicine, which is also reflected in precision medicine and personalized medicine, holds great promise for medical advances: Big Data practices could significantly improve early cancer detection (Ngiam and Khor 2019), for instance, helping to identify lung metastases at an early predictive stage (Li et al. 2022). Similarly, promising findings are evident from studies in psychiatric treatments (Češková and Šilhán 2021) and the development and improvement of medications (Chakravarty et al. 2021). Many other applications have yet to be considered while promising exciting findings.

All these considerations ultimately point to the ethical conflict through which policy-makers, researchers, and healthcare providers are entitled—or even obliged—to promote the implementation of Big Data practices in order to provide people with the best possible therapies without neglecting the privacy of individuals and population groups. Although the collection and use of data pose many risks to individuals, there are also aspects of solidarity, including the commitment to donate "data for the sake of the good" (Hummel and Braun 2020). Given these considerations, it is reasonable to consider the ethical implications of sharing data for scientific purposes in specific cases of digital epidemiology to assess whether individuals may be obliged to share their data (Mittelstadt et al. 2018).

4 An Ethical Framework for Autonomy

The ethical conflicts described above cannot be resolved using a universal remedy. There are good reasons to both promote and oppose the promotion of Big Data practices in digital public health. It is the challenge of politics, science, and society as a whole to address these risks adequately. On the one hand, ethical standards are an effective means to this end. On the other hand, economic opportunities are leading particularly private-sector players to adopt Big Data practices. Ethical standards tend to find less approval in the private sector, as they often contradict the profit orientation of companies. Privatizing Big (health) Data can therefore be considered ethically risky for good reasons. In the long term, this could promote health injustices and inequities rather than reduce them (Wilbanks and Topol 2016). To respond to this risk, everyone affected by the usage of digital devices must retain the possibility of determining the use of their own data, regardless of whether these data are health-related or not. Here, the concept of autonomy comes into play. It is also reflected in the concepts of user autonomy and data sovereignty, which we would like to present as purposeful for the self-determination of an autonomous individual in the digital age later in this chapter. The concept of the data subject, which is of central importance in the GDPR, is also an expression of the view that users and other producers of data should be able to decide autonomously about their own data, thus becoming the subjects of their own data again.

The etymological analysis of the word autonomy already indicates that autonomy describes the possibility of a subject of agency to prescribe laws and rules for itself and to act according to them (autonomy: from Greek: autos "self," nomos "rule" or "law"). On this basis, there are different views on what constitutes autonomy, to what extent the underlying theories are ideal or non-ideal, and the practical implications that follow from these different views (Dworkin 1981). The influential "Principles of Biomedical Ethics" by Tom Beauchamp and James F. Childress (Beauchamp and Childress 2019) take the approach of a non-ideal theory of autonomy, which implies that total autonomy remains an unattainable ideal. From an ethical point of view, it does not follow this circumstance to restrict autonomy arbitrarily. The approximation to the ideal of autonomy remains an ethical obligation. That is why they name one of their four core ethical principles "Respect for Autonomy" instead of "Autonomy."

Underlying the ethical principle of respect for autonomy is the non-ideal three-condition theory of autonomy: "We analyze autonomous action in terms of normal choosers who act (1) intentionally, (2) with understanding, and (3) without controlling influences that determine their action. This uncomplicated account is designed to be coherent with the premise that the everyday choices of generally competent persons are autonomous and to be sufficient as an account of autonomy [.]" (Beauchamp and Childress 2019). In this paper we propose the non-ideal theory of autonomy and its three conditions of autonomous action as the core principles of user autonomy in digital public health. To elaborate on these principles, we will illustrate in our own words how Beauchamp and Childress define the three conditions of autonomous action and add a short example from the domain of Digital Public Health to highlight the significance of autonomy in Digital Public Health.

According to the authors, (1) intentional actions require mental representations of the planned sequence of actions. The intentionality of an action is determined by the correspondence between its execution and an agent's prior conception, even though the outcome may differ from the plan. An agent can be any person who performs an action in everyday life. Actions that the agent performs reluctantly can still be classified as intentional. The presence of conflicting motivations and preferences does not diminish the intentional or autonomous nature of an action. Even anticipated but undesirable consequences can be part of a coherent intentional plan of action (Beauchamp and Childress 2019). To illustrate this point, we propose a scenario from the domain of Digital Public Health: A technoskeptical person deliberately uses a digital contact tracing app during a pandemic, having formed a clear mental plan to use it to protect themselves and others, even though they have concerns about privacy and data security. Their autonomous action is a deliberate decision qualified by the intention to protect people's health, despite not being fully convinced of the benefits of this technology.

Furthermore, autonomous action should be accompanied by (2) an understanding of an action. The capacity to understand may be limited by various factors such as illness, irrationality or lack of maturity. Deficiencies in communication processes can also negatively impact understanding. However, autonomous action requires only substantial rather than complete understanding. Demanding fully autonomous decision-making from patients and research participants would deprive their actions of practical significance, since human action, in reality, is rarely completely autonomous (Beauchamp and Childress 2019). Returning to our example, the technoskeptikal person can improve their understanding of the pandemic as well as benefits and risks of technological interventions. To do so, they can collect additional information to make an informed decision by weighing the benefits and concerns of using the app—even if they cannot be sure to have obtained all available information.

Otherwise, misinformation and manipulation may influence understanding as a condition for autonomous action, which segues to the third condition of autonomous action within non-ideal theory: the (3) absence of control by external or internal factors that limit individual self-determination. Central to this analysis is the distinction between influence and controlling influence, since not all forms of influence qualify as control. In examining non-control and voluntariness, coercion and manipulation emerge as key categories of influence. While the focus often lies on external controlling influences—typically of an interpersonal nature—internal factors such as mental illness are equally relevant for autonomy (Beauchamp and Childress 2019).

In terms of a non-ideal theory, the ethical framework of autonomy outlined above applies to our endeavour for several reasons. First, Beauchamp and Childress' framework is not only suitable for applied ethics in general, but was explicitly developed for health issues. Secondly, this autonomy framework has proven its practicality and effectiveness in the context of public health ethics, and there are no apparent reasons not to apply this framework to digital public health in general (Marckmann 2020). Third, this autonomy framework can be applied to ethical design in digital public health because it requires developers and designers to strive for an ideal of autonomy, even if it cannot be fully achieved.

5 A Brief Overview of the Landscape of Deceptive Design Practices

In digital contexts, the autonomy of users can be undermined through various malicious and deceptive tricks. A growing interest among HCI researchers highlights negative implications, further driven by noticing exploitative practices developed to steer users' actions with potentially harmful consequences (Gray et al. 2018; Mathur et al. 2021). When Brignull introduced the concept of dark patterns over a decade ago, he introduced them as harmful interface tricks, often identified in online shopping websites, that are designed to steer users into taking undesired and unfavored actions beneficial to the operator (Brignull 2010). In past years, related research has extended this work, primarily focusing on e-commerce (Mathur et al. 2019). Others, however, have started to investigate domains, such as games (Zagal et al. 2013), social media (Mildner and Savino 2021; Mildner et al. 2023a, b), or studied dark patterns in mobile applications (Di Geronimo et al. 2020).

In the following paragraphs, we will outline, to the best of our knowledge, essential findings from dark pattern research while discussing the potential impact on public health sectors. Here, certain difficulties stem from the varying approaches of prior work when describing dark patterns. Whereas some work proposes more general *strategies* (Gray et al. 2018) or *techniques* (Conti and Sobiesk 2010), some consider domain-specific *types* (Brignull 2010). For simplification and understandability, we will look at all dark patterns alongside. Table 1 offers an overview of the

Table 1 Table listing dark patterns from eight works

Brignull (2010)	Conti and Sobiesk (2010)	Zagal et al. (2013)	Greenberg et al. (2014)
• Trick Questions • Sneak into Basket • Roach Motel • Privacy Zuckering (1) • Confirmshaming • Disguised Ads • Price Comparison Prevention • Misdirection • Hidden Costs • Bait and Switch (1) • Forced Continuity • Friendly Spam	• Coercion • Distraction • Forced Work • Manipulating Navigation • Restricting Functionality • Trick • Confusion • Exploiting Errors • Interruption • Obfuscation • Shock	• Grinding • Impersonation • Monetized Rivalries • Pay to Skip • Playing by Appointment • Pre-Delivered Content • Social Pyramid Schemes	• Attention Graber • Bait and Switch (2) • The Social Network Of Proxemic Contracts Or Unintended Relationships • Captive Audience • We Never Forget • Disguised Data Collection • Making Personal Information Public • The Milk Factor
Bösch et al. (2016)	Gray et al. (2018)	Gray et al. (2020)	Mathur et al. (2019)
• Privacy Zuckering (2) • Hidden Legalese Stipulations • Shadow User Profiles • Bad Defaults • Immortal Accounts • Information Milking • Forced Registration • Address Book Leeching	• Nagging • Obstruction • Sneaking • Interface Interference • Forced Action	• Automating the User • Two-Faced • Controlling • Entrapping • Nickling-and-Diming • Misrepresenting	• Countdown Timers • Limited-time Messages • High-demand Messages • Activity Notifications • Testimonials of Uncertain Origins • Hard to Cancel • Visual Interference • Low-stock Messages • Hidden Subscriptions • Pressured Selling • Forced Enrollment

Sources: Own figure based on Brignull (2010), Conti and Sobiesk (2010), Zagal et al. (2013), Greenberg et al. (2014), Bösch et al. (2016), Gray et al. (2018, 2020), and Mathur et al. (2019)

68 dark patterns considered here, based on a comprehensive literature review by Mathur et al. (2021). Note that although some dark patterns share the same name, they yield distinct descriptions. We, therefore, consider them independently.

As previously stated, Bringull initiated the search for dark patterns describing a first set of twelve. Soon after, various streams of research continued to establish a maturing taxonomy. Thereby identified and described, dark patterns vary quite a bit in how they govern people's decision-making. For the simplicity of this section, we will only discuss dark patterns impacting public health sectors and limit the scope based on their manifestation. Therefore, we propose three dimensions: (1) Graphic; (2) Linguistic; and (3) Procedural. While these high-level dimensions help to sort most dark patterns based on specific situations, the different levels of abstractions used to describe them hinder some from being assigned to a single dimension.

5.1 The Graphic Dimension

Dark patterns that work on a *graphic* dimension use visual design strategies to deceive users. For instance, Brignull's "Disguised Ads" (Brignull 2010) dark pattern aims to hide advertisements behind inconspicuous designs creating false expectations. Both "Visual Interference" (Mathur et al. 2019) and "Interface Interference" (Gray et al. 2018) describe instances where colorization or positioning of elements is used in order to visually place specific elements above others to steer their users' focus away from unwanted interactions and toward the designer's goal. A well-understood example has been noticed in consent banners across the web. Here, different types of dark patterns often work together, overcomplicating interactions and coercing decisions. Such interfaces are designed to enforce consent for collecting personal data and sharing them with third parties. Whereas a consent button is highlighted in prominent colors or shades, an opposite option is usually colored in low-contrast grey scales or nested deep in the banner's settings. However, this type of behavior is not limited to consent banners but can also be found in mobile Health (mHealth) apps that contain sensitive personal health data. Manipulating users into unwillingly sharing personal data leads to the ethical problems discussed earlier. It can be further enhanced further graphics-based dark patterns such as Bösch et al.'s "Bad Defaults" (Bösch et al. 2016) that utilize strategies similar to Brignull's "Privacy Zuckering" dark pattern. Figs. 1 and 2 illustrate two cases of dark patterns employing visual design strategies to deceive users.

Inspired by Facebook's default setup to collect more data than most users would willingly provide, many applications follow a similar path by having settings switches set to share such data when installed, forcing the user into a cumbersome task to manually go through them and toggle them into a more desired state.

Fig. 1 Example of the 'Bad Default' dark pattern. The visibility of the users' profile is set to public by default. (Source: Own figure)

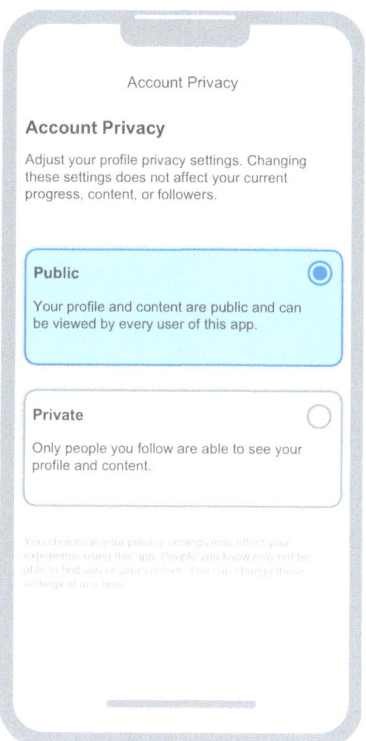

5.2 The Linguistic Dimension

Staying with the example of mHealth apps, some dark pattern types restrict user agency on a *linguistic* dimension. The "Confirmshaming" dark pattern (Brignull 2010) belongs to this category by semantically confusing users or targeting their emotions by shaming them into specific actions, thus decreasing their autonomy. Regarding mHealth apps, we can imagine a scenario where an app could use "Confirmshaming" when users try to end their subscription to the service, similar to those offered by many fitness apps. It could prompt the user with a shameful message before allowing them to leave for good. A sentence such as *"Are you sure you want to quit your membership and risk losing all your fitness progress by not having access to our great programs anymore?"* could push users into staying with a service keeping a potential financial and data-driven burden. "Trick Questions" (Brignull 2010), "Limited-time Messages" (Mathur et al. 2019), and "High-demand Messages" (Mathur et al. 2019) work similarly by pressuring users to make decisions that are mainly beneficial for the service provider.

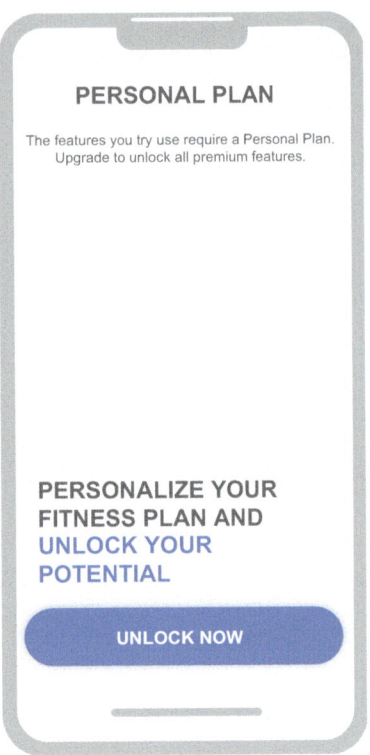

Fig. 2 Example of the 'Forced Action' dark pattern in a "free-to-use" workout application, limiting access to certain functionalities. (Source: Own figure)

5.3 The Procedural Dimension

If a user is still motivated to end their subscription with the service, they will often face dark patterns that work on a *procedural* level by creating unnecessary steps to obscure the deactivation of their account. Described as "Roach Motel" by Brignull and "Hard to Cancel" by Mathur et al., these dark patterns envelop interaction sequences to hinder the user from following through with their goal by obscuring, delaying, or hiding necessary information. First, the option to delete an account or end a current subscription could be nested deeply in an app's settings menu, making it difficult to find. When activated, the process often contains walls of text that may overwhelm a user through additional dark patterns from the linguistic dimension, finally leading them to give up. Unnecessary actions could be required, defined as "Forced Actions" by Gray et al. (2018), demanding the user to enter a password or solve small tasks (i.e., Captcha's) to confirm a user's authenticity, even if they are already logged in to the service. Once these steps are successfully completed, certain services may force the user again to wait 30 days until their cancellation is processed. A ridiculous time compared to the mere minutes needed to create a new account. This example highlights how the different dimensions overlap, resulting in complex situations for users to navigate.

5.4 Dark Patterns as a Continuum

The examples mentioned above highlight the complexity in which dark patterns occur. Moreover, it becomes evident that one dark pattern rarely exists alone. It is challenging to assign dark patterns distinct dimensions. More often than not, they will check multiple boxes. They can be found on single interfaces as graphic elements or overt messages but could also describe a sequence of steps leading to unwanted actions. To offer some level of overview, Fig. 3 is our attempt to place the dark patterns discussed in this section in the three dimensions. Placing all 69 dark patterns would have resulted in an incomprehensible graphic; thus, we have limited it to those mentioned in the previous sections. Fig. 4 illustrates the differences between two dark pattern strategies with regard to the three dimensions.

Despite their differences, dark patterns have one thing in common: They take away people's autonomy to create harmful disadvantages. Unlike nudges that also alter people's decision space, dark patterns have been repeatedly shown to be too difficult for users to avoid (Bongard-Blanchy et al. 2021; Di Geronimo et al. 2020). Meanwhile, the gap between novel technologies and research understanding of their impact widens. While highlighting the necessity to continue this research and understand the risks of unethical designs in places where users are often most vulnerable, regulations need to address these concerns in order to protect users (see chapter "Social Media in Digital Public Health", Sina et al. in this handbook).

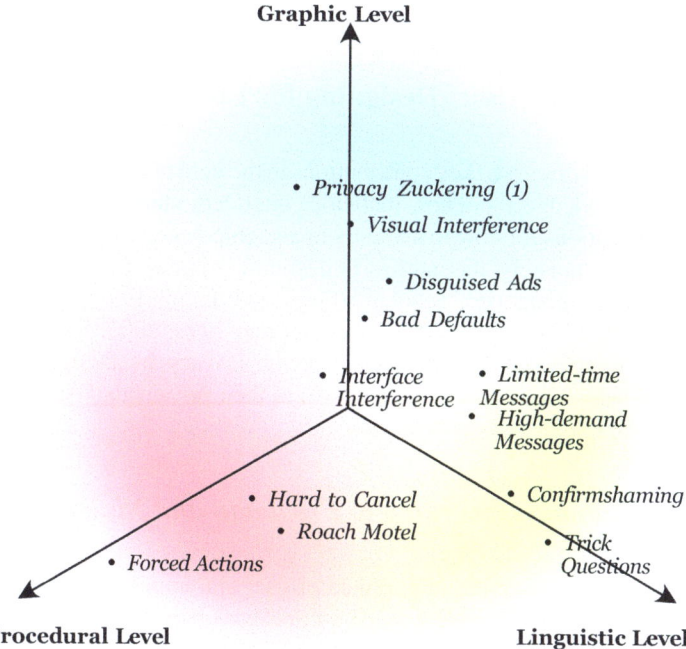

Fig. 3 This graphic presents the discussed dark patterns in the three-dimensional space containing graphic, linguistic, and procedural dimensions. (Source: Own figure)

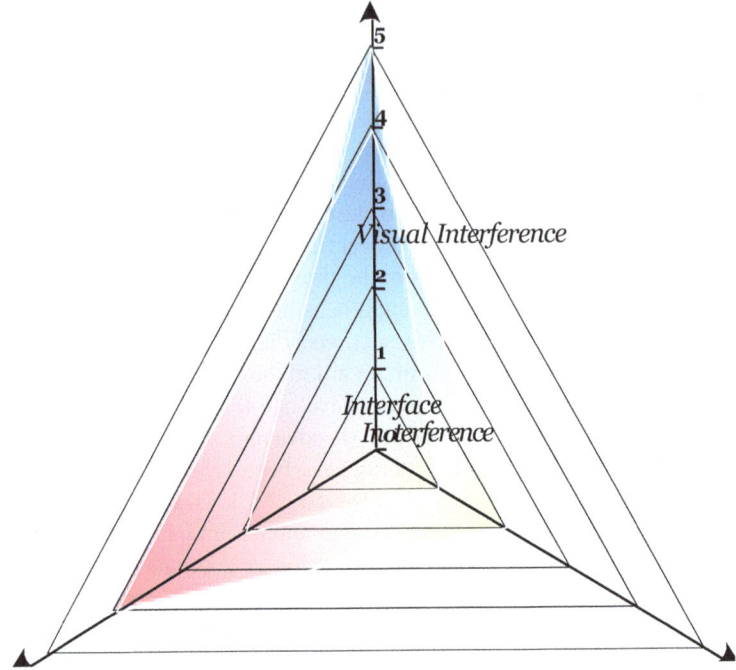

Fig. 4 This radar plot visualizes a comparison between the two dark patterns "Interface Interference" and "Visual Interference" which, although describe similar strategies, utilize the dimensions differently. (Source: Own figure)

6 Empowering the User: Designing for Ethical Interfaces

The previous section discussed key contributions in the field of dark pattern research. Unfortunately, knowledge about how malicious interfaces manifest does not necessarily offer explanations for how to avoid them and empower users to make autonomous decisions. Fortunately, the interest in designing systems that support human values is not new among HCI scholars (Fogg and Tseng 1999; Friedman and Nissenbaum 1996; Millett et al. 2001; Shneiderman 1999, 2000; Suchman 1994; Winograd 2004) and has led to projects like the Privacy by Design guidelines (Hustinx 2010), adopted by Bösch et al. (2016) in their privacy dark strategies.

6.1 User Autonomy According to Friedman and Nissenbaum

With the goal of integrating the importance of user autonomy into the HCI discipline, Friedman et al. (2013) made a decisive contribution by developing their Value Sensitive Design framework. Here, the authors offer certain human values with ethical import as a heuristic for designers when developing systems. While values such as privacy (Friedman and Nissenbaum 1996), trust (Fogg and Tseng 1999), and freedom from bias (Friedman and Nissenbaum 1997; Nass and Gong 2000) each describe important ethical pillars for developing sustainable designs, we want to take a closer look at autonomy, as trends for persuasive technologies limit users' agency, often without their consent. Here, Friedman and Nissenbaum (1997) provide guidance for creating interfaces that communicate their functionalities better, keeping their users in control over their actions. In earlier work, the authors provide five key aspects impacting user autonomy (Friedman and Nissenbaum 1997).

1. *Agent capability* is crucial for enabling users to achieve their goals. Returning to the example of mHealth applications, a fitness tracking app that records various health data but cannot provide an easily comprehensible overview denies users readable access to their own health data. Hence, by missing a specific functionality, such an app limits its capability and, thus, its usefulness for the user.
2. *Agent complexity* describes the need for capable systems to stay within users' expectations without overwhelming them with unnecessary features and options. Especially in setting menus, the task of maintaining individual choices can become a cumbersome exercise. Instead of providing a single option to completely shut off any data forwarding to unwanted parties, many services complicate such intentions by presenting users with too many choices resulting in decision fatigue. Earlier, we outlined this through the "Bad Defaults" and "Privacy Zuckering" dark patterns.
3. *Knowledge about the agent* refers to the importance of transparency and communication of information. A fitness tracking application needs to make information accessible regarding stored information and how it is used. Local storing of health-related data is necessary to track the users' performance allowing them to observe their progression. In case more complex data processes are required to, for instance, make predictions that exceed the computational power available on a mobile device, it would further be understandable if the application would connect to protected servers to carry out necessary but delicate processes.
4. *Misrepresentation* of the agent can lead to uninformed decisions by users. Keeping them in the dark by not communicating important information is one thing, but presenting false or incorrect information cuts even deeper into users' autonomy. This can happen accidentally by not finding the right way to communicate a system's capabilities. Users trying to talk to customer service through text should always be made aware of whom they are talking to—a human or a chatbot. Consequently, a chatbot should never act in such a way that confuses users into thinking they are talking to anything other than a chatbot. As demonstrated by the dark pattern of the same name (Gray et al. 2020), "Misrepresentation" can also be used intentionally to harm users.
5. *Agent fluidity* is required to adopt users' change of mind with regard to their goals. Systems should therefore consider adjustments to users' decisions by keeping a dynamic state and allowing alternative goals. Referring to fitness trackers once more, a user may set out to run five kilometers but may realize that they feel better than expected and want to change their goal to run ten kilometers

Fig. 5 Apps frequently ask users about their usage preferences without providing information on how this data is going to be used. (Source: Own figure)

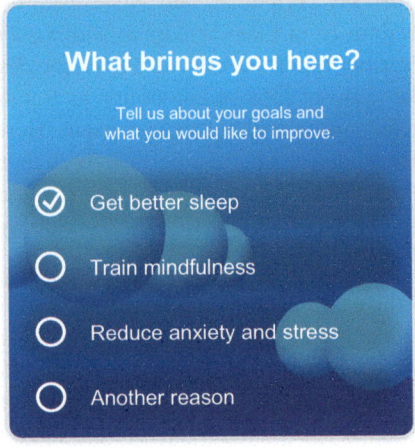

Fig. 6 In the privacy policy, users will learn that their data is, in fact, shared with third parties. (Source: Own figure)

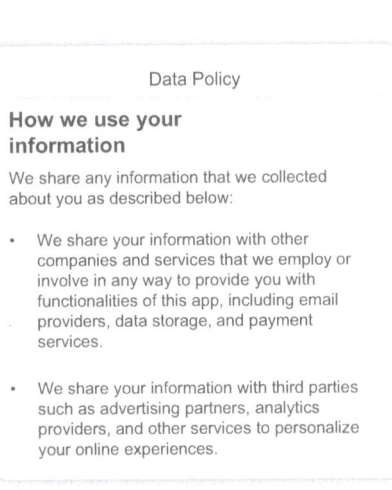

instead. The app needs to be able to allow for this fine-tuning without resetting already accomplished progress.

Together, these five aspects are helpful measures to identify if a system respects users' autonomy. In this regard, limiting users' agency or ability to make informed decisions is detrimental to their experience. As a countermeasure, appropriate testing of new systems with potential user groups is a crucial element in learning about users' expectations and understanding their autonomy to ensure a good user experience. Figs. 5 and 6 illustrate another example of a dark pattern that prevents users from making informed decisions about the usage of their personal data.

6.2 Empowering the User: Data Sovereignty

In addition to ethical design that empowers users of health apps by avoiding dark patterns, users are often data subjects according to the GDPR as they produce personal health data with their behavior. Such health apps are often associated with Big Data practices and extend the data set of Big Data databases. Here, the ethical issues are not initially those of the interface design but concern the self-determination of the users and the authorized use of their data. The German Ethics Council has developed a concept for this, which concerns the ethical design of Big Data practices in the context of health: "Data sovereignty, understood as the responsible shaping of informational freedom, in a manner appropriate to the risks and opportunities presented by Big Data, is the central ethical and legal goal in confronting the challenges and opportunities presented by Big Data" (German Ethics Council 2018). Central principles of data sovereignty, which can undoubtedly be derived from the ethical principle of respect for autonomy, are (1) to maximize the potential of Big Data in healthcare, (2) to promote individual freedom and privacy, (3) to ensure solidarity and equity, and (4) to promote trust by clearly assigning responsibilities for Big Data practices in healthcare and preventing diffusion of responsibility in these contexts. In our view, responsibility is central to practical applicability: Responsibility points to the fact that, on the one hand, the developers and providers of Big Data practices must be clearly identified so they can be held responsible and accountable in case of misuse and other unethical practices. On the other hand, users of health applications linked to Big Data cannot be exempted from all responsibility. Truly autonomous users are, to some extent, responsible for their behavior if they want to achieve autonomy and sovereignty.

7 Conclusion and Future Directions

HCI offers a plethora of strategies and frameworks to develop systems that users will find easy to use. Although certain streams of HCI provide ethical frameworks for systems and interfaces, usability standards do not necessarily cover them. Whether accidentally deployed by failed goodwill or through malicious motivation, interfaces can persuade users in such a way that navigates or dictates their decision-making. Meanwhile, we observe a trend among user experience designers arguing in favor of persuasive design and declaring it a necessity to present users with easy-to-use services (Chivukula et al. 2018; Gray et al. 2018). Suddenly, good design is being defined from a practitioner's point of view with a focus on how easily users achieve their goals, for instance, completing an online purchase. Here, one-click buy options in online shopping sites allow users quick and frictionless purchases but arguably deny them a thorough reflection on their decision.

Yet, there are positive examples of persuasive technologies. From this context, derived principles can be used to support behavior changes that enhance the lives of end users by, for example, helping them to live healthier lives (Asbjørnsen et al. 2020) or motivating the donation of health data (Pilgrim and Bohnet-Joschko 2022) or organs. Similar approaches might also be taken in creating novel online learning opportunities (Alexandrovsky et al. 2021). Importantly, this entails the given consent of the people granting authority to override their autonomy.

As this chapter illustrates, there is no easy answer to whether persuasive designs targeting users' autonomy are good or bad, both in health contexts and outside. Indeed, this assessment appears to be highly context-specific, as seen in the literature surrounding dark patterns. Ultimately, the responsibility to create ethical interfaces resides with the practitioners and legal institutions to regulate otherwise exploitative designs. The traditional ethical frameworks, based on respect for autonomy, cannot provide direct instructions for ethical design. Rather, they should be reflected in ethical frameworks that address user autonomy and the ethical use of health data, including a Big Data perspective. Especially in situations where frameworks for ethical design and legislation are behind schedule due to cultural lags, this chapter demonstrates how easily design can be used to trick people and reminds them about the traditional ethical frameworks that guide sound legislation and design practices.

References

Acar G, Eubank C, Englehardt S et al (2014) The web never forgets. In: Ahn GJ, Yung M, Li N (eds) Proceedings of the 2014 ACM SIGSAC conference on computer and communications security. Scottsdale, 3–7 November 2014, pp 674–689. https://doi.org/10.1145/2660267.2660347

Alexandrovsky D, Friehs MA, Grittner J et al (2021) Serious snacking: a survival analysis of how snacking mechanics affect attrition in a mobile serious game. In: Kitamura Y, Quigley A, Isbister K et al (eds) Proceedings of the 2021 CHI conference on human factors in computing systems. Yokohama, 8–13 May 2021, pp 1–18. https://doi.org/10.1145/3411764.3445689

Andalibi N, Buss J (2020) The human in emotion recognition on social media: attitudes, outcomes, risks. In: Bernhaupt R, Mueller FF, Verweij D et al (eds) Proceedings of the 2020 CHI conference on human factors in computing systems. Yokohama, 8–13 May 2021, pp 1–16. https://doi.org/10.1145/3313831.3376680

Asbjørnsen RA, Wentzel J, Smedsrød ML et al (2020) Identifying persuasive design principles and behavior change techniques supporting end user values and needs in eHealth interventions for long-term weight loss maintenance: qualitative study. J Med Internet Res 22(11):e22598. https://doi.org/10.2196/22598

Beauchamp TL, Childress JF (2019) Principles of biomedical ethics, 8th edn. Oxford University Press, New York and Oxford

Bongard-Blanchy K, Rossi A, Rivas S et al (2021) "I am definitely manipulated, even when I am aware of it. It's ridiculous!"—dark patterns from the end-user perspective. In: Ju W, Oehlberg L, Follmer S et al (eds) Designing interactive systems conference 2021. Yokohama, 8–13 May 2021, pp 763–776. https://doi.org/10.1145/3461778.3462086

Bösch C, Erb B, Kargl F, Kopp H, Pfattheicher S (2016) Tales from the dark side: privacy dark strategies and privacy dark patterns. Proc Priv Enhanc Technol 2016(4):237–254. https://doi.org/10.1515/popets-2016-0038

Brignull H (2010) Deceptive design—formerly darkpatterns.org. https://www.deceptive.design/. Accessed Jul 2023.

Češková E, Šilhán P (2021) From personalized medicine to precision psychiatry? Neuropsychiatr Dis Treat 17:3663–3668. https://doi.org/10.2147/NDT.S337814

Chakravarty K, Antontsev V, Bundey Y et al (2021) Driving success in personalized medicine through AI-enabled computational modeling. Drug Discovery Today 26(6):1459–1465. https://doi.org/10.1016/j.drudis.2021.02.007

Chivukula SS, Brier J, Gray CM (2018) Dark intentions or persuasion? In: Koskinen I, Yk L, Cerratto-Pargman T et al (eds) Proceedings of the 2018 ACM conference companion publication on designing interactive systems. Hong Kong, 9–13 June 2018, pp 87–91. https://doi.org/10.1145/3197391.3205417

Conti G, Sobiesk E (2010) Malicious interface design. In: Rappa M, Jones P, Freire J et al (eds) Proceedings of the 19th international conference on World Wide Web—WWW '10. Raleigh, 26–30. ACM Press, New York, p 271. https://doi.org/10.1145/1772690.1772719

Di Geronimo L, Braz L, Fregnan E et al (2020) UI dark patterns and where to find them. In: Bernhaupt R, Mueller FF, Verweij D et al (eds) Proceedings of the 2020 CHI conference on human factors in computing systems. Honolulu, 25–30 April 2020, pp 1–14. https://doi.org/10.1145/3313831.3376600

Dworkin G (1981) The concept of autonomy. Grazer Philosophische Studien 12:203–213. https://doi.org/10.5840/gps198112/1333

Favaretto M, de Clercq E, Schneble CO et al (2020) What is your definition of big data? Researchers' understanding of the phenomenon of the decade. PLoS One 15(2):e0228987. https://doi.org/10.1371/journal.pone.0228987

Fogg BJ, Tseng H (1999) The elements of computer credibility. In: Williams MG, Altom MW (eds) Proceedings of the SIGCHI conference on human factors in computing systems the CHI is the limit—CHI'99. Pittsburgh, 15–20 May 1999. ACM Press, New York, pp 80–87. https://doi.org/10.1145/302979.303001

Friedman B, Nissenbaum H (1996) Bias in computer systems. ACM Trans Inform Syst 14(3):330–347. https://doi.org/10.1145/230538.230561

Friedman B, Nissenbaum H (1997) Software agents and user autonomy. In: Johnson WL (ed) Proceedings of the first international conference on autonomous agents—AGENTS'97. Marina del Rey, 5–8 February 1997. ACM Press, New York, pp 466–469. https://doi.org/10.1145/267658.267772

Friedman B, Kahn PH, Borning A et al (2013) Value sensitive design and information systems. In: Doorn N, Schuurbiers D, van de Poel I et al (eds) Early engagement and new technologies: opening up the laboratory, philosophy of engineering and technology, vol 16. Springer, Dordrecht, pp 55–95. https://doi.org/10.1007/978-94-007-7844-3

German Ethics Council (2018) Big data and health—data sovereignty as the shaping of informational freedom: opinion executive summary & recommendations: 2017. https://www.ethikrat.org/fileadmin/Publikationen/Stellungnahmen/englisch/opinion-big-data-and-health-summary.pdf. Accessed Jul 2023

Grassl P, Schraffenberger H, Zuiderveen Borgesius F et al (2020) Dark and bright patterns in cookie consent requests. https://doi.org/10.31234/osf.io/gqs5h

Gray CM, Kou Y, Battles B et al (2018) The dark (patterns) side of UX design. In: Mandryk R, Hancock M, Perry M et al (eds) Proceedings of the 2018 CHI conference on human factors in computing systems. Hong Kong, 9–13 June 2018, pp 1–14. https://doi.org/10.1145/3173574.3174108

Gray CM, Chivukula SS, Lee A (2020) What kind of work do asshole designers create? Describing properties of ethical concern on Reddit. In: Wakkary R, Andersen K, Odom W et al (eds) Proceedings of the 2020 ACM designing interactive systems conference. Honolulu, 25–30 April 2020, pp 61–73. https://doi.org/10.1145/3357236.3395486

Greenberg S, Boring S, Vermeulen J et al (2014) Dark patterns in proxemic interactions. In: Wakkary R, Harrison S, Neustaedter C et al (eds) Proceedings of the 2014 conference on designing interactive systems. Vancouver, 21–25 June 2014, pp 523–532. https://doi.org/10.1145/2598510.2598541

Gudivada VN, Baeza-Yates R, Raghavan VV (2015) Big data: promises and problems. Computer 48(3):20–23. https://doi.org/10.1109/MC.2015.62

Heidel A, Hagist C (2020) Potential benefits and risks resulting from the introduction of health apps and wearables into the German statutory health care system: scoping review. JMIR mHealth uHealth 8(9):e16444. https://doi.org/10.2196/16444

Hummel P, Braun M (2020) Just data? Solidarity and justice in data-driven medicine. Sci Soc Policy 16(1):8. https://doi.org/10.1186/s40504-020-00101-7

Hustinx P (2010) Privacy by design: delivering the promises. Ident Infor Soc 3(2):253–255. https://doi.org/10.1007/s12394-010-0061-z

Kupwade Patil H, Seshadri R (2014) Big data security and privacy issues in healthcare. In: Chen P, Jain H (eds) 2014 IEEE international congress on big data. IEEE, Piscataway, NJ, pp 762–765. https://doi.org/10.1109/BigData.Congress.2014.112

Li W, Hong T, Liu W et al (2022) Development of a machine learning-based predictive model for lung metastasis in patients with Ewing sarcoma. Front Med 9(807):382. https://doi.org/10.3389/fmed.2022.807382

Marckmann G (2020) Ethische Fragen von Digital Public Health. Bundesgesundheitsblatt, Gesundheitsforschung, Gesundheitsschutz 63(2):199–205. https://doi.org/10.1007/s00103-019-03091-w

Mathur A, Acar G, Friedman MJ et al (2019) Dark patterns at scale. In: Proceedings of the ACM on human-computer interaction 3(CSCW), pp 1–32. https://doi.org/10.1145/3359183

Mathur A, Kshirsagar M, Mayer J (2021) What makes a dark pattern... dark? In: Kitamura Y, Quigley A, Isbister K et al (eds) Proceedings of the 2021 CHI conference on human factors in computing systems. Yokohama, 8–13 May 2021, pp 1–18. https://doi.org/10.1145/3411764.3445610

Metcalf J, Crawford K (2016) Where are human subjects in big data research? The emerging ethics divide. Big Data Soc 3(1):205395171665,021. https://doi.org/10.1177/2053951716650211

Mildner T, Savino GL (2021) Ethical user interfaces: exploring the effects of dark patterns on Facebook. In: Kitamura Y, Quigley A, Isbister K et al (eds) Extended abstracts of the 2021 CHI conference on human factors in computing systems. Yokohama, 8–13 May 2021, pp 1–7. https://doi.org/10.1145/3411763.3451659

Mildner T, Freye M, Savino GL et al (2023a) Defending against the dark arts: recognising dark patterns in social media. In: Designing interactive systems conference (DIS'23). ACM Press, New York, pp 1–13. https://doi.org/10.1145/3563657.3595964

Mildner T, Savino GL, Doyle PR et al (2023b) About engaging and governing strategies: a thematic analysis of dark patterns in social networking services. In: Proceedings of the SIGCHI conference on Human factors in computing systems—CHI'23. Hamburg, 23–28 April 2023. ACM Press, New York, pp 1–15. https://doi.org/10.1145/3544548.3580695

Millett LI, Friedman B, Felten E (2001) Cookies and web browser design. In: Jacko J, Sears A (eds) Proceedings of the SIGCHI conference on human factors in computing systems—CHI'01. Seattle, March 2001. ACM Press, New York, pp 46–52. https://doi.org/10.1145/365024.365034

Mittelstadt B, Benzler J, Engelmann L et al (2018) Is there a duty to participate in digital epidemiology? Life Sci Soc Policy 14(1):9. https://doi.org/10.1186/s40504-018-0074-1

Molina-Pérez A, Rodríguez-Arias D, Delgado-Rodríguez J, Morgan M, Frunza M, Randhawa G, Reiger-Van de Wijdeven J, Schiks E, Wöhlke S, Schicktanz S (2019) Public knowledge and attitudes towards consent policies for organ donation in Europe. A systematic review. Trans Rev (Orlando, Fla) 33(1):1–8. https://doi.org/10.1016/j.trre.2018.09.001

Munson SA, Krupka E, Richardson C et al (2015) Effects of public commitments and accountability in a technology-supported physical activity intervention. In: Proceedings of the 33rd annual ACM conference on human factors in computing systems. Seoul, 18–23 April 2015. ACM, Seoul, pp 1135–1144. https://doi.org/10.1145/2702123.2702524

Nass C, Gong L (2000) Speech interfaces from an evolutionary perspective. Commun ACM 43(9):36–43. https://doi.org/10.1145/348941.348976

Ngiam KY, Khor IW (2019) Big data and machine learning algorithms for health-care delivery. Lancet Oncol 20(5):e262–e273. https://doi.org/10.1016/S1470-2045(19)30149-4

Norman DA (1990) The design of everyday things, 1st edn. Doubleday/Currency, New York. http://www.loc.gov/catdir/description/random043/89048989.html

Perakslis E, Coravos A (2019) Is health-care data the new blood? Lancet Digit Health 1(1):e8–e9. https://doi.org/10.1016/S2589-7500(19)30001-9

Pilgrim K, Bohnet-Joschko S (2022) Effectiveness of digital forced-choice nudges for voluntary data donation by health self-trackers in Germany: web-based experiment. J Med Internet Res 24(2):e31363. https://doi.org/10.2196/31363

Ryan R, Deci E (2018) Self-determination theory: basic psychological needs in motivation, development, and wellness. Guilford Publications. https://books.google.de/books?id=th5rDwAAQBAJ

Schäfke-Zell W (2022) Revisiting the definition of health data in the age of digitalized health care. Int Data Privacy Law 12(1):33–43. https://doi.org/10.1093/idpl/ipab025

Sharif A, Moorlock G (2018) Influencing relatives to respect donor autonomy: should we nudge families to consent to organ donation? Bioethics 32(3):155–163

Shneiderman B (1999) Universal usability: pushing human-computer interaction research to empower every citizen. ISR Technical Report University of Maryland, College Park, MD

Shneiderman B (2000) Universal usability. Commun ACM 43(5):84–91. https://doi.org/10.1145/332833.332843

Suchman L (1994) Do categories have politics? Comput Supp Cooperat Work 2(3):177–190. https://doi.org/10.1007/BF00749015

Sunstein CR (2017) Misconceptions about nudges. SSRN Electr J. https://doi.org/10.2139/ssrn.3033101

Synofzik M, Vosgerau G, Newen A (2008) Beyond the comparator model: a multifactorial two-step account of agency. Conscious Cogn 17(1):219–239. https://doi.org/10.1016/j.concog.2007.03.010

Tangari G, Ikram M, Ijaz K et al (2021) Mobile health and privacy: cross sectional study. BMJ 373:1248. https://doi.org/10.1136/bmj.n1248

Thaler RH, Sunstein CR (2008) Nudge: Improving decisions about health, wealth, and happiness. New Haven, CT, Yale Univ. Press. http://www.loc.gov/catdir/enhancements/fy0833/2007047528-b.html

Wilbanks JT, Topol EJ (2016) Stop the privatization of health data. Nature 535(7612):345–348. https://doi.org/10.1038/535345a

Winograd T (2004) Categories, disciplines, and social coordination. Comput Supp Cooperat Work 2:191–197

Zagal JP, Bjork S, Lewis C (2013) Dark patterns in the design of games. In: Foundations of digital games conference, FDG 2013, May 14–17, Chania. Greece. http://www.fdg2013.org/program/papers/paper06_zagal_etal.pdf. Accessed Jul 2023

Open Access This chapter is licensed under the terms of the Creative Commons Attribution 4.0 International License (http://creativecommons.org/licenses/by/4.0/), which permits use, sharing, adaptation, distribution and reproduction in any medium or format, as long as you give appropriate credit to the original author(s) and the source, provide a link to the Creative Commons license and indicate if changes were made.

The images or other third party material in this chapter are included in the chapter's Creative Commons license, unless indicated otherwise in a credit line to the material. If material is not included in the chapter's Creative Commons license and your intended use is not permitted by statutory regulation or exceeds the permitted use, you will need to obtain permission directly from the copyright holder.

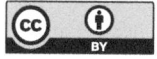

Health Data Pipelines: Moving Away from Excel to Scalable, Sustainable, Insightful, and Future-Proof Infostructure

Martina Cilia and Stefan Buttigieg

Abstract This chapter covers the theme of health data pipelines through the reference of data flow between different health information systems aimed at achieving public health objectives. There is an impending need to move public health and other affiliated healthcare organizations away from data silos to data-driven infostructures. It starts with understanding key concepts, upon which fundamental knowledge of ongoing technological advancements can be further developed. The necessary situational assessments underpinning the definition of goals and objectives intended to direct healthcare organizations away from silos and closer to constructive interaction are critical in the planning of a tailored Data Governance Framework. In this regard, the documentation of a robust and stepwise plan is imperative for sustainable change, which is reinforced through the consolidation of internal resources and/or the acquisition of external ones. Ultimately, each healthcare system and organization must ensure the output is consistent, reliable, and serviceable to all stakeholders. In the context of the European Health Data Space, knowledge is fundamental to successful implementation and communication. Thus, this chapter aims to provide the basics for all healthcare professionals to better comprehend the terms, concepts, and available tools. All this information can dramatically change the public health sector and revolutionize healthcare systems worldwide.

Keywords Data pipelines · Health Information Systems · Infostructure · Health data · Data governance

---

M. Cilia
Mater Dei Hospital, Msida, Malta
e-mail: martina.a.cilia@gov.mt

S. Buttigieg (✉)
Information Management Unit, Ministry for Health and Active Ageing, Pietà, Malta

Faculty of Health Sciences, University of Malta, Msida, Malta

European Public Health Association, Utrecht, Netherlands
e-mail: info@stefanbuttigieg.com

Abbreviations
CRM	Customer Relationship Management
DAL	Database Access Language
DW	Data Warehouse
EDW	Enterprise Data Warehouse
ELT	Extract Load Transform
ERP	Enterprise Resource Planning
ETL	Extract Transform Load
ETLT	Extract Transform Load Transform
PHI	Personal Health Information

1 Data, Databases, and Information Systems

The poorer the quality of the data we produce and work with, the worse the quality of our products, results, and decisions we make in all situations. From board meetings to budget plans, quarterly reports, and their analysis, hiring and firing employees, adjustments in cost and quality-care processes, prescribing medications, and predicting disease onset and severity. The list goes on. The breadth of said list is owed to the fact that data pervades our lives not just in the mathematical, physical, biological, and chemical sense but also in our philosophical and conscientious aspects. Hence, through humanity's mode of daily living, by and through which we create, store, use, and leverage data, it is crucial to point out that data is beyond the simple concept of numbers.

The best way to understand a concept, a word, or an entire subject, is to start from the beginning. Upon skimming through this chapter, the word "data" seems to pop out effortlessly. Yet, as with everything overused, its meaning loses value, becomes overlooked, and consequently loses its elemental explicability. Data is the bedrock of the world we live in. Quite so, it is our brick-and-mortar. Hence, we begin by defining it comprehensively:

1.1 The Basics

1.1.1 Data

To begin with, the etymology of the word "data" originated in the seventeenth century, initially as a term for use in philosophy. It is derived from the singular Latin term "datum." The Latin verb for "datum" is "dare," which means "to give." Accordingly, a datum is a thing given. Nevertheless, the noun "thing" is too abstract for us. Instead, it can be substituted for a premise, predicate, fact, or reference point by which conclusions are drawn from observations or measurements. Data is a recorded truth of an event happening at a particular time. It represents specific objects and phenomena within our reality that can be questioned, compared,

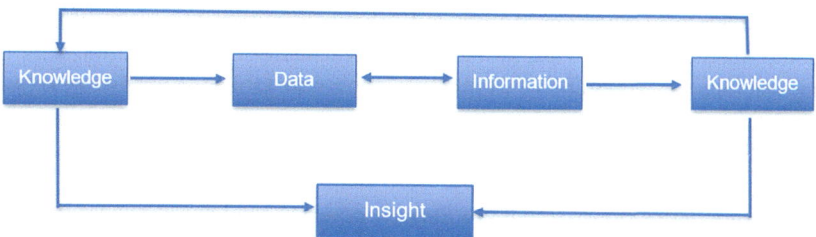

Fig. 1 The creation of data through knowledge and the flow of information that is generated as a result. (Source: Own figure)

explained, understood, and predicted. It is a tool used for decision-making, inference, and interpretation.

In today's technical world, data is stored in digital form. However, storing data requires context. A narrative. Without this, data is meaningless, just a collection of digits. This is even more paramount in the healthcare sector, particularly in an era wherein the four P's (Personalized, Precision, Predictive, Participatory) of healthcare have become more undisputed. Since each patient has their own individual health story and health journey, the context can be divided into three main parts:

- Domain and its subdomain (if present)
- The vocabulary used to represent the data
- The relationships between the data and other related components

As such, these parts are data about data, referred to as "metadata." We can explain metadata by saying it is data that gives us additional information about different aspects of the data in question. It can be viewed as a summary of the distinct components of the data.

Data does not simply exist. It must be created. Data is created through knowledge, which ultimately gives us more knowledge through the information gathered. In the end, the accumulation of knowledge, and the repetitive use of data as an asset, leads to an element of insight that can be harbored by the organization and the people working for it. However, the sequence of such flow is not as linear as expected (Fig. 1).

1.1.2 Data Sets

We have mentioned data in both singular and plural terms. A single observation, essentially a row of information, is called a record. It is regarded as a unit of data entry that, in its multiplicity, makes up a whole. Hence, records numbering in the thousands and billions make up our data. Taking it a step further, each record is divided into portions for storing specific categories of the information in question. These are colloquially known as columns (often referred to as attributes) of data. We have just technically described a data table (colloquially referred to as a table). However, a data table is not synonymous with a data set. Both contain critical distinctions.

A data table is a collection of rows and columns. Conversely, a data set is a collection of data tables. Both are in-memory representations of information with the same structure, i.e., rows and columns. In a single data table, we used to work with only one row at a time. However, by dividing a data set into different data tables, based on the information we aim to group and analyze, we are now capable of working with multiple rows simultaneously.

Thus, data tables organize data to make it easier to read and compare different rows and columns from the data set. Data tables can be regarded as objects that form a data set when grouped and collected (Fig. 2).

A Data Set is known to have data relations between its different components (rows and columns). This is not the case for a Data Table. As a result of these data relations, a data set is governed by rules that ensure data integrity and thereby maintain its relational integrity. These rules are formally called constraints. They are applied to a column, and any related columns, to determine the result when a value in a row, or rows, is updated.

1.1.3 Databases

What Is a Database?

The storage and organization of data in rows and columns is called structured data. A database is an organized collection of structured information (Balusamy et al. 2021). We can say it is a collection of datasets. A database consists of multiple

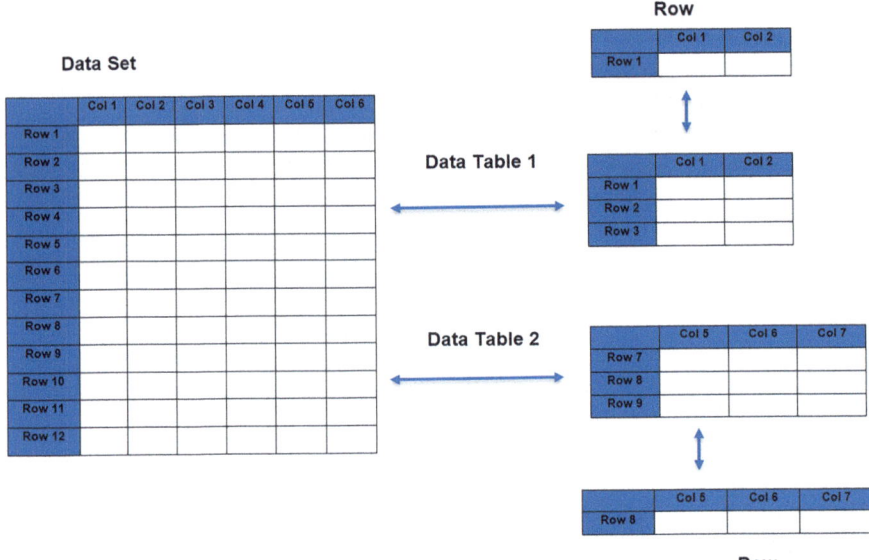

Fig. 2 The hierarchical and inter-relational relationship between a data table and a data set. (Source: Own figure)

Health Data Pipelines: Moving Away from Excel to Scalable, Sustainable, Insightful...

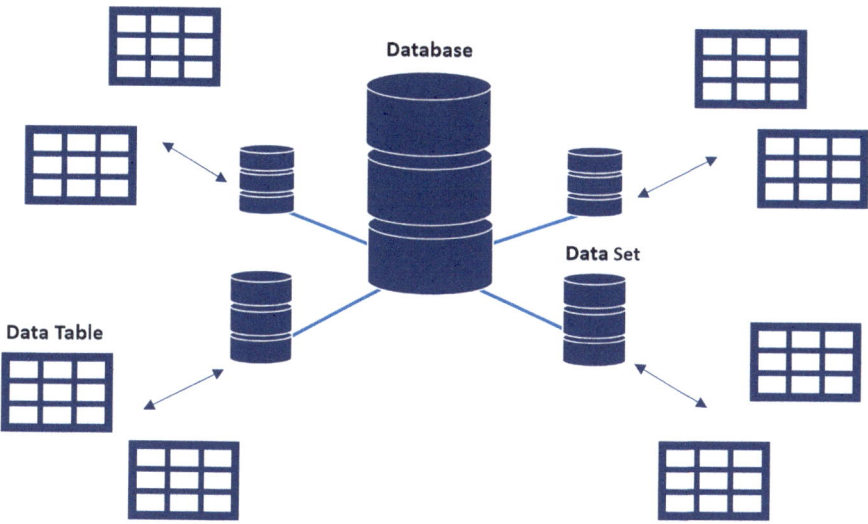

Fig. 3 Database, data sets, and data tables. (Source: Own figure)

records containing interrelated data stored together to serve multiple applications. They are essential for record-keeping and analytical decision-making. One of the most important assets of any organization is its information. In general, databases have two dimensions to store information; rows and columns. It is important to note that a database does not automatically denote a single dataset. A "database" is similar to the concept of an airbase. Wherein airplanes can be safely stored and managed according to a specific operating system. Like a data set, each airplane stores a set amount of equipment and personnel—all of which are units of information that can be grouped according to specific attributes to form data tables (Fig. 3).

What Are the Diverse Types of Databases?

There are distinct types of databases based on their intended purpose and are classified as relational and non-relational (Fig. 4).

A hierarchical database is a relational database management system that represents a collection of databases that are organized in a tree-like form with a parent-child approach to collection, retrieval, and interpretation. The retrieval of data always starts at the "root." Each child record has only one parent (one-to-one relationship), whereas a parent record can have multiple child records (one-to-many relationship). Furthermore, a child record can be a reference parent record for other child records (DAMA International 2017). In the context of a hospital, a hierarchical database will contain healthcare information about various patients, organized in specific levels (Fig. 5).

For example, a patient's health record will be subdivided into Medical Records, Radiological Imaging, and Mental Health Records. Each will have its own level of

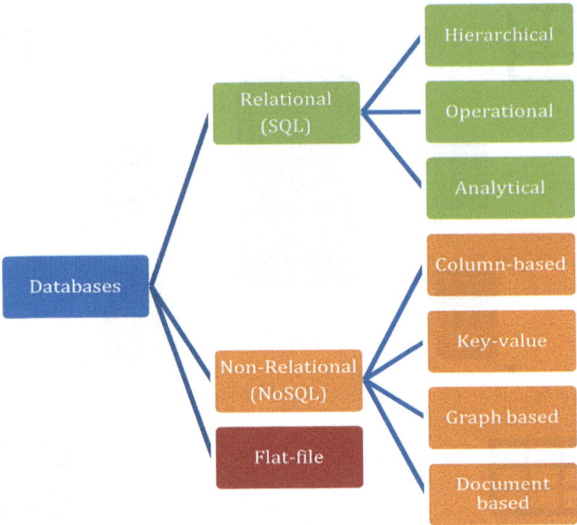

Fig. 4 Different types of databases and their sub-types. (Source: Own figure)

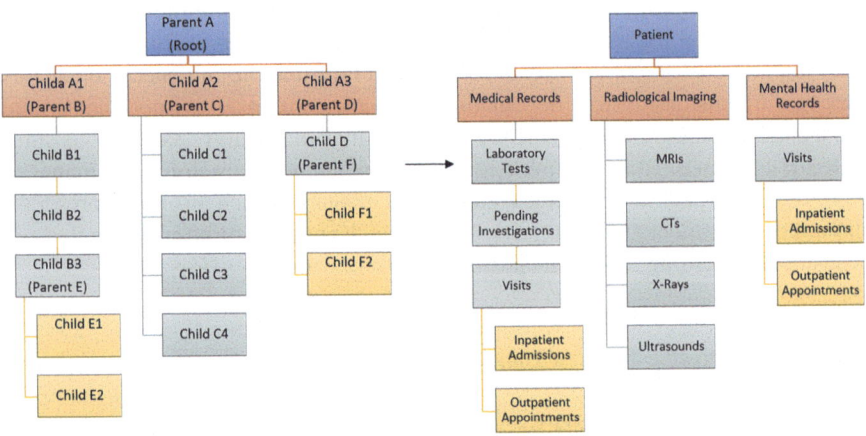

Fig. 5 Parent-child approach in a hierarchical database. (Source: own figure)

information. Medical Records will contain information about past/pending medical visits, laboratory results, pending investigations, medical visits, medical notes written by specialists during outpatient visits or inpatient stays, etc. Each healthcare provider, whether private or governmental, will have established its own hierarchical database management system.

Most often, Hierarchical Databases are supported by Operational Database systems—these work to support operational processes. The main aim is to support the information that is stored. Such databases contain transactional information that can be read, modified (only in specific circumstances), added to, and deleted.

"Transactional information" derives from day-to-day transactions in an organization that any operational database stores and processes. The term "transactional" refers to an exchange between systems and systems, systems and people, and people with people. Some medical-related examples include:

1. A hospital registering a patient at the Emergency Department.
2. An outpatient department or medical clinic booking a patient in for a visit.
3. A patient giving their medical information to a doctor.
4. A health-insurance company paying a patient's hospital bill.
5. A laboratory scientist inputting the blood results of a particular patient into the Laboratory Information System.

These transactions have four fundamental properties supporting operational databases: Atomicity, Consistency, Isolation & Durability. In fact, they are called "ACID transactions." They ensure the integrity and reliability of the data (Databricks 2021). A data storage system that applies these four operational properties is called a transactional system:

- **Atomicity**—each transaction is a single unit, so either it is executed in its entirety or not at all.
- **Consistency**—transactions only make changes to tables in a predefined way (no loss of integrity to tables).
- **Isolation**—when multiple data users read and write from the same table simultaneously, they do not interfere with or affect one another.
- **Durability**—changes to the data done by successful transactions are saved even in the event of a system failure.

The purpose of these operational databases is to "hold" and deliver the requested data at the right time to analyze patient information and operational processes to extract trends, patterns, and inconsistencies in data. Moving from operational data support to in-depth analysis often involves migrating enormous amounts of data from operational to analytical databases (also called decision support databases). Through advanced technological tools, they harness the power to leverage data for comparative insights on specific operational characteristics that allow for informed decision-making about system efficiency and productivity, logistics and supply use.

What Is a Database Management System?

Any system is composed of processes and procedures working together to form a structure of interconnected parts. In general, a management system is simply an operating system, just like Android or iOS, for instance, which is expressly set up to deal with the interaction of distinct parts of the system itself. It ensures the smooth and seamless flow of information aimed at managing a specific service and/or product.

A database management system (DBMS) is a software system, often a set of programs, to create, organize, and manage the database and control the use of the data within it. It provides an interface (environment) between the database and the user to perform operations related to the creation, insertion, deletion, updating, and retrieval of data. Common examples include Microsoft Access, AmazonS3, and Amazon DynamoDB, to name a few.

There are six main components of a Database Management System Environment:

- **Hardware**—a computer and a network of computers.
- **Software**—database management system, operating system, network software, and application programs.
- **Data**—the key component that acts as a bridge between the machines and the human aspect.
- **Database Access Language (DAL)**—a simple and easy-to-use programming language that allows end users to write commands (called queries) to perform specific operations on the data stored in the database in question.
- **Procedures**—instructions and established standard rules, determined by the organization, that need to be followed to design and use a particular database system.
- **People (users)**—application programmers and software developers, end users (clients), and database administrators.
- Database Administrators are an especially important sub-component. They are responsible for:
  – Defining the conceptual schema (framework), the internal and external schemas.
  – Defining security checks.
  – Overseeing data integrity and quality checks.
  – Defining backup and recovery procedures.
  – Liaising with other users and monitoring the performance of the entire system.

These are different from application programmers and software developers. The latter design specific parts of the DBMS that allow other users, including database administrators and other end users, to interact with the DBMS. They do this by using programming languages such as JAVA and C++. The end users then use Database Access Language (DAL) to query the data and perform specific operations according to those queries.

One of the most common DALs used for structured databases is the Structured Query Language (SQL). It is a DAL that allows the selection and modification, through addition, update, and deletion, of the data.

Some popular types of DBMS are DB2 and Informix Dynamic Server by IBM, Oracle, MySQL and RDB by Oracle, SQL Server, and Access by Microsoft. There are many types of DBMS, but one of the most important ones is a relational database management system (RDBMS).

The database created with an RDBMS is a relational database. These relational databases (RDBS) follow the relational model (RM). Most of today's DBMSs follow this model.

1.1.4 The Relational Model and Its Elements

The RM was first described in 1969 by a British computer scientist, Edgar Codd. He described how data can be managed using structure and language consistent with relational algebra. In simpler terms, Codd proposed a method by which data can be modeled in relational databases. In fact, the RM is governed by important terminologies, constraints, and properties.

Within the RM, relational databases store data in tables referred to as relations. So, a table containing data about patients is a relation called Patient (Fig. 5). This is because it often has a relationship with other tables (relations) within the database, such as Medications, Medical History, Address, and so on (Fig. 6).

Each relation has characteristic properties, called attributes, that define and describe the relation. For instance, a related Patient will have attributes such as Patient ID, Patient Name, and Patient Surname. The set of values for a particular attribute is contained within an entire column. Every attribute has a specified domain, which can be considered a pre-defined rule. For example, the attribute patient name can only contain names that are a maximum of twenty characters long with no numbers. Moreover, the patient identification number can only contain numbers between 1 and 6000 with no alphabetical characters. The total number of attributes in a relation is called the "degree of relation." This means that in our patient relation, we have three degrees of relation. Each row of information is called a "tuple," and the number of tuples is referred to as "cardinality" (DAMA International 2017).

The structured combination of the relation with its attributes is called a relation schema, where schema refers to the structured framework and diagrammatic representation of the relation (table).

These relational databases can contain complex data models involving hundreds and thousands of relations (tables). Hence, it was Codd's primary aim to use the relational model as a systematic method that facilitates the organization of relational

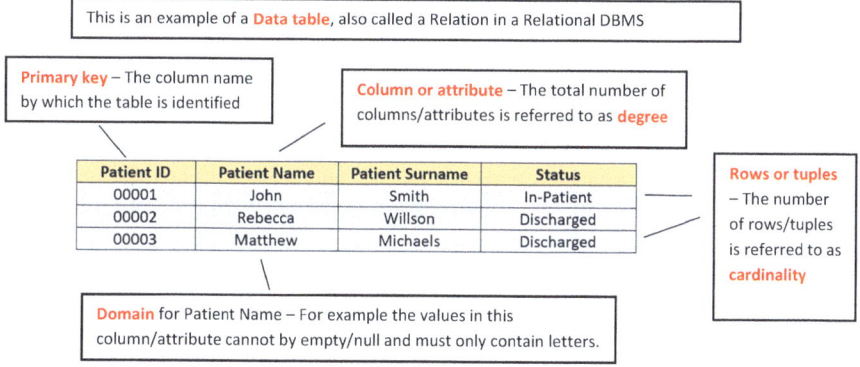

Fig. 6 A relation with its primary key, attributes, and tuples. (Source: Own figure)

databases. The processes and steps in doing this are called "database normalization" (DAMA International 2017).

The normalization process ends up breaking up large tables into many smaller ones. Even though this may seem counterintuitive, it helps ease the retrieval of information from these relational databases, which may contain millions of rows. As data grows exponentially, the need to retrieve the correct data in a timely way has become imperative and can only be ensured with good data modeling.

1.1.5 Data Warehouses

William H. Innmon, an American computer scientist considered the "Father of Data Warehousing," wrote the first book about data warehousing (Inmon 2002). His definition of a data warehouse is still used to this day:

> *A data warehouse is a subject-oriented, integrated, time-variant, and non-volatile collection of data used in the support of management decision-making processes.*

We can clearly see that a data warehouse is a repository of data collected from various sources (internal or external) to make it available for enterprise/organization-wide access, maintenance, and subsequent analysis. As healthcare systems have different data types from various sources, a separate place is needed to converge and analyze it all. Data in a data warehouse is stored in databases referred to as decision support databases.

Innmon's definition of a data warehouse specifically stipulates that it must adhere to four properties:

- **Subject-oriented**—focused on very specific users. For example, some people from the pharmacy department want to see logistical data, or people from the human resources department are interested in employee data.
- **Integrated**—it must have consistent data. For instance, if we want to see the frequency of use for a specific medicine, all the information must be the same. This means standardization of the data, which must be defined as a priority (e.g., micrograms to milligrams). All data is converted to the same convention specified at the beginning to allow the measurement of products. Data type formats are also essential to the standardization process (e.g., prices should be in decimals, not integers (whole numbers).
- **Time-variant**—it gives a historical view of the data, allowing high-level reporting and analysis that organizations can use to make informed decisions.
- **Non-Volatile**—the data is just a copy of the data contained in the operational system, which in turn is just a copy of the data obtained from real life. Keeping the data as it was from the very beginning. Once data is stored in a data warehouse, it must stay the same ad aeternum and cannot be altered. This is the point of having historical data. The only exceptions that require updates are when the hardware/software goes haywire, affecting the operating system (such as default-

ing in inputting data values), and this defective update subsequently translates into the data warehouse.

It is important to note that a data warehouse (DW) is not synonymous with a warehouse of data. The two terms cannot be used interchangeably. A warehouse of data contains data from operational systems, which capture day-to-day processes, and hence are real-time systems. Contrarily, a data warehouse is a system that supports the flow of data from operational systems to decision systems (also called analytical systems). Thus, data from a warehouse of data flows into a data warehouse. Moreover, a data warehouse that serves the entire enterprise, not just a specific department or sector, is called an enterprise data warehouse (EDW).

Some uses of data warehouses in the context of healthcare include the following:

- Segmenting patients into different groups based on their medical history or current treatment plan(s).
- Predicting disease onset and progression using past laboratory test results, imaging results, physiological measurements, medications used and in use, along with past and current lifestyle factors.
- Forecasting which health aspects and disease(s) to focus on primarily.

1.1.6 Data Lakes

Data lakes and data warehouses are widely used to store vast amounts of data (Big Data, a concept we will dive into shortly). It is common for them to be used interchangeably, although they are not the same concepts. The main differing component is the level of processing the data has gone through in each.

A data lake is a central repository that allows the storage of data as-is without having first to structure it (Knight 2022). Thus, it may store any type of data, including images, making all the healthcare data available to allow data employees to analyze it. All data consolidation, processing, cleaning, and profiling come from this single storage of data.

On the other hand, a data warehouse is a repository for structured data, i.e., data that has been processed for a defined purpose.

The use of data lakes took off in the early twenty-first century. They store unstructured data more economically. A database and a data warehouse can handle unstructured data, albeit not in a cost-effective way. As so much of the data produced nowadays is of the unstructured type, this becomes very expensive. Data that goes into databases and data warehouses must be processed before it is stored and used. This can be a long and complicated process, and sometimes not all the collected data is needed. So, data lakes act as these handlers of all types of data in the most cost-efficient way. In fact, there are some key benefits for any organization, including healthcare systems, in investing in the development of a Data Lake (Fig. 7).

A data lake has some specific stages of maturity that are worth mentioning and briefly explaining (Fig. 8):

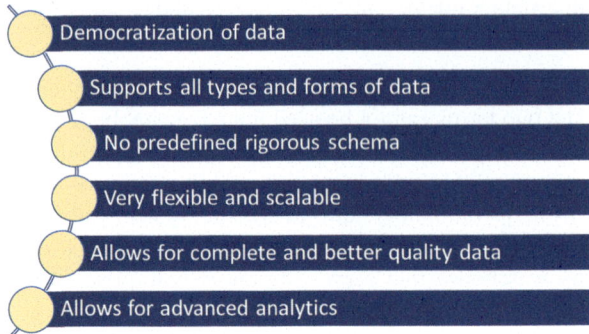

Fig. 7 The benefits of a data lake. (Source: Own figure)

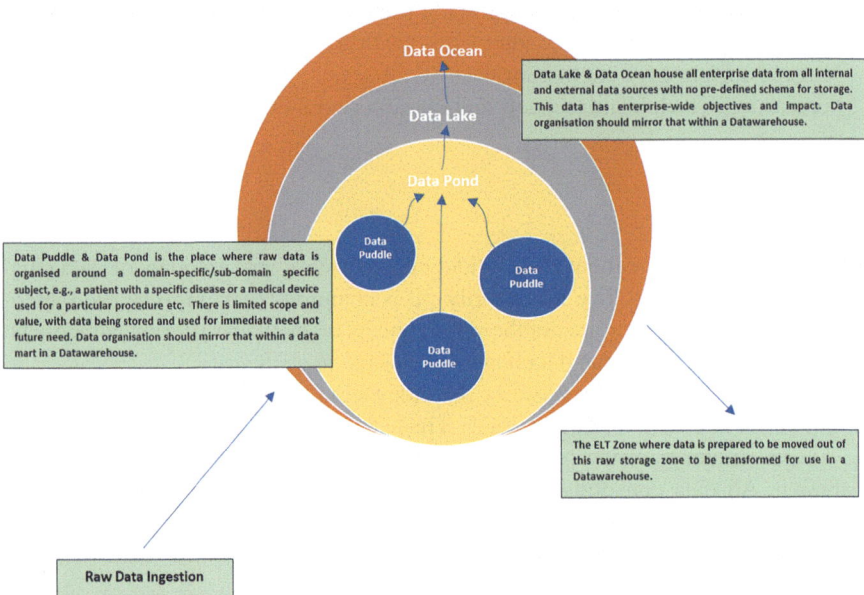

Fig. 8 Stacked Venn diagram showing the logic and maturity of different phases of a data lake. (Source: Own figure)

- **Data puddle**—data that is loaded for a specific project or team.
- **Data pond**—a collection of data puddles. It only contains data for a particular ongoing project, which is only used in a way that the project demands. It still involves a lot of IT-personnel participation and thus is not good in democratizing the access and use of the data within it for business users (self-service).
- **Data lake**—one of its essential aspects is that it supports self-service. Business users can access and use data without relying on IT personnel. In addition, it also

can contain data that business users may want to access and use in the absence of any ongoing project(s). Self-service and democratization are important facets of any data lake.
- **Data ocean**—this expands the democratization, self-service, and data-based decision-making to all enterprise data.

There is an ideal way a data lake architecture is set up and matured. If not, this will lead to a data swamp. A messy storage of any form of raw data that makes it unmanageable. Data that cannot be managed is practically useless, and in today's data-driven world, it automatically translates into the loss of money, resources, and time. In healthcare, this can lead to delayed treatment, undertreatment, over-treatment, or mistreatment, all of which have detrimental effects.

Having a data catalog makes the process of finding the desired data easier within a data lake. A data catalog is an organized digital inventory of an organization's data assets. It is not synonymous with a data dictionary. It is a library or a collection of data assets within the organization. It should be flexible regarding searchability and filtering options that allow users to quickly find relevant data sets for data science, analytics, or data engineering.

The establishment of such a self-service architecture requires crucial prerequisite processes to be cultivated within the development of a data lake (DAMA International 2017). Some ways by which organizations can circumvent this is by working and improving on:

- Metadata and metadata management.
- Data governance (business glossary, data dictionary, and data catalogs) makes the process of finding the desired data easier within a data lake.
- Maintaining all the data's context.

Conclusively, the primary use of a data lake is to 'keep' data stored in its raw state until it can be extracted and loaded into the data warehouse. From here on, it is subjected to specific transformation processes depending on its targeted use (and end users).

1.1.7 Data Lakehouse

As previously mentioned, data lakes are handlers of raw data of any type, and yet they still lack the features of data quality, consistency, and transactional support that data warehouses can provide. Thus, a data lake still loses many benefits that make data warehouses desirable. Data warehouses have been used for analytical decision support and business intelligence for over a decade. However, they are not well suited for dealing with unstructured and semi-structured data on a large scale. This makes them inefficient and costly. With data becoming increasingly complex in terms of variety, faster in terms of production, and bigger in size, another system was developed to address this issue, the data lakehouse (Gorelik 2019).

A data lakehouse is a data architecture solution concept. It converges the data architectural element of a data warehouse and the data management features of a data lake. Merging these two systems into one means that data teams within an organization can work together faster since data does not need to be moved around or accessed from multiple systems. It also ensures that the data teams always have the most complete and updated form of data available (Fig. 9).

The following Table 1 shows some differences and advantages of a data lakehouse (Gorelik 2019).

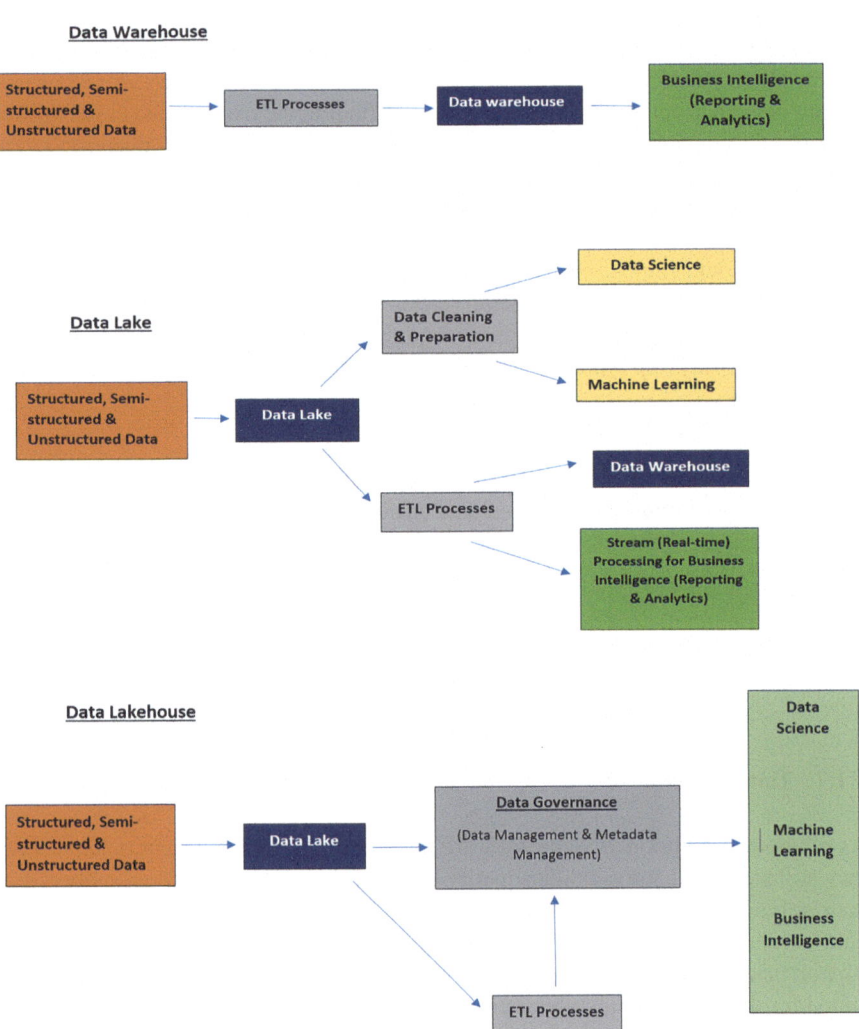

Fig. 9 Comparison of data warehouse, data lake, and data lakehouse system flows. (Source: Own figure)

Table 1 Differences between data warehouses, data lakes & data lakehouses

	Data warehouse	Data lake	Data lakehouse
Use	Traditional architecture	Data storage repository	A blend of data warehouse and data lake
Data	For structured data management, not for complex data types	Supports the storage of large amounts of unstructured, semi-structured and structured data	Collects all data types at a scale and processes any data at scale
Capability	Supports business intelligence	Poor data warehouse capability and business intelligence support	Data lake optimized by adding the ACID transactional layer on top to provide business intelligence support
Storage and Cost	High storage & processing costs	Stores bulk data at low cost	Cost-effective and scalable at low cost
Processing	Limited streaming (real-time) processing abilities but difficult to implement unified processing (batch + streaming)	Difficult to handle stream processing due to large amounts of data	Able to handle large amounts of data for stream processing Includes a unified framework for batch & stream processing workloads in one architecture that improves the efficiency of data transformation
Data Governance	Data catalog	Data quality, security, and compliance are weaknesses that need to be enforced	Open data management architecture
Support System Applications	Does not directly support data science & Machine Learning applications	Does not directly support data science & Machine Learning applications	Data science, Machine Learning & business intelligence reporting & analytics are directly supported. Specifically, data lakehouses provide the ability to pin specific versions of data sets to a Machine Learning model. This makes it easier for other data team members to re-trace and reproduce that same model training for replication and analysis.
Data Quality	Data quality is enforced. Supports ACID transactions	Poor data quality enforcement. Poor performance features for ACID transactions	Ensured data reliability & integrity. Different data warehouse schema support & ACID transactions

Source: Own table

2 Getting Data Ready for the Real World

2.1 The 6 Vs of Data

Big Data is just a blanket term. It refers not only to the large amount of data generated (typically from terabytes upwards) but also its complexity in terms of structure, sources, and the speed by which it is created. There are a few characteristics of Big Data that will help us understand the concept better (Panesar 2021). These are known as the six Vs of Big Data (Fig. 10). Initially, only three were used. However, as data continued growing and became more complex, other characteristics were added to describe it better.

2.1.1 Volume (Data at Rest)

The size of Big Data is always large, although it does not necessarily have to be of a minimal size to be classified as such. In fact, if the data you have stored, and any additional incoming data, is growing so fast that you are finding it difficult to store and manage it with traditional tools, then that is automatically referred to as Big Data. This requires scalable solutions to be able to keep up with it in terms of storage, processing, and analytics (Cavanillas et al, 2016).

2.1.2 Velocity (Data in Motion: Milliseconds to Seconds)

The speed at which data is created in real time. More than 90% of the data in the world has been created in the last two years, and it is calculated that more than three trillion gigabytes of data are created every day. However, velocity is not only referring

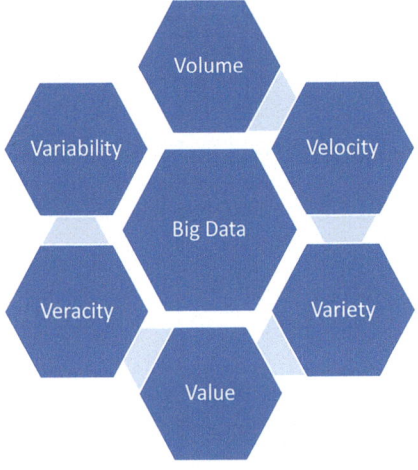

Fig. 10 The six main characteristics of Big Data. (Source: Own figure)

to the speed at which data is created but also to the rate at which it is processed and analyzed. For example, according to Statista, in 2023 there were 5.9 million Google searches every minute, and in 2024 approximately 35 million people updated their Facebook status every minute. This is an analysis of Big Data in real time.

2.1.3 Variety (Data in many Forms)

Variety refers to the diverse types and formats. Generated data arrives in three formats: structured, semi-structured, and unstructured (Table 2). Structured data is organized within a framework of rows and columns and can, therefore, be managed by traditional database management systems. Semi-structured data is an intermediary between both. It exhibits some organization but does not fit the structured data model. Unstructured data, as the name implies, has no definite structure and hence cannot be processed by traditional database management systems.

It is well-established that 80% of data generated worldwide is unstructured, while the remaining 20% is only structured data.

Variety does not only refer to the type of data but also the diverse sources that generate it, such as different internet systems and social media sources.

2.1.4 Veracity (Data in Doubt)

This deals with the following questions: how can an organization or business ensure that the data used is dependable, accountable, and accurate? And to what degree can the organization trust it? These questions refer to data verification and validity, two crucial components of data quality assessment.

Table 2 Distinctive features of the three main types of data

	Structured data	Semi-structured data	Unstructured data
Organization	Well-Organized	Partially Organized	Not Organized
Easy to search	Yes	No	No
Schema	Schema dependent—very rigorous	Has a tolerant schema that allows easier alterations	No schema
Flexibility	Less flexible due to its schema dependency	More flexible but not as much as unstructured data	More flexible since it is not dependent on any schema
Scalable	Difficult to scale	Simpler to scale but not as much as with unstructured data	Easy to scale
Technology	Based on relational database	Based on JSON, XML	Based on characters and binary data
Examples	Databases e.g., financial data	Emails, JSON files	Videos, images, recordings, media posts, HTML documents

Source: Own table

2.1.5 Variability (Data in Discordance)

This refers to the number of inconsistencies in the data, not only in the quality and information provided but also in the speed at which it is created and loaded.

2.1.6 Value (Data as Currency)

This means the usefulness of the data that is gathered for the organization. Large volumes of data do not guarantee usefulness. In fact, if we had to represent all the previous five Vs linearly, they all can be combined to give a degree of value to our data:

$$\text{Volume} + \text{Velocity} + \text{Veracity} + \text{Variability} + \text{Variety} = \text{Value}$$

2.2 Data Types

In computer programming, data can be grouped according to a specific set of characteristics. This is where the concept of different data types emerges. Different data types have distinct attributes that a programming language object can hold (Balusamy et al. 2021).

Most programming languages support a variety of data types (Table 3). Each type of data defines the way its values can be stored, its meaning, how it should be interpreted, and the operations that can be executed on it.

Boolean data refers to how the data language should be interpreted by the machine. A Boolean of 0 represents the logic false, whereas true, which is never a 0, is represented by the Boolean 1.

Table 3 Different data types

Data type	Description	Example	Memory usage
Integer (Int)	Whole number that can be positive, negative, or zero	54,675	2–4 bytes
Float	All the infinite whole numbers (integers) with their fractions and decimals	8.768	4–8 bytes
Character (Char)	Any single alphanumeric character, where the character can be any alphabet, number, or symbol	'M' '£' '7'	1 byte
String	Can hold a list of characters of any length. It can be empty (null), just one character, or many characters. It is always represented using the parenthesis.	'Hello' 'M' 'The cost is $5'	1 byte for each character in the string
Boolean	Can only be either of two values: true or false	True/False	1 byte

Source: Own table

3 Data Pipelines

The data pipeline is divided into five main stages: (1) data sources from which data ingestion occurs (the data ingestion layer), i.e., the data collector layer, (2) the data processing layer, (3) the data storage layer, (4) the data query layer, and (5) the data visualization layer for data reporting and analytics (Balusamy et al. 2021).

3.1 Data Sources

Data sources are data that are available for analysis, coming from all channels. These all point toward the different data origins in terms of differing formats, types, velocities, volume, geographical location, primary or secondary sources, etcetera.

Some examples may include sources such as SQL databases, flat files, semi-structured and unstructured data, social media interactions, website log-ins, mobile application log-ins, IoT devices, search engines, and emails. Figure 11 gives a more detailed and graphical representation of these data sources.

3.1.1 Data Ingestion

This is the first step from which data created from various sources can start its journey in the data pipeline. This data ingestion layer is closely related to the data collector layer. The logic behind this is that as data is ingested, it is prioritized and categorized to facilitate storage, processing, and analysis further down the pipeline.

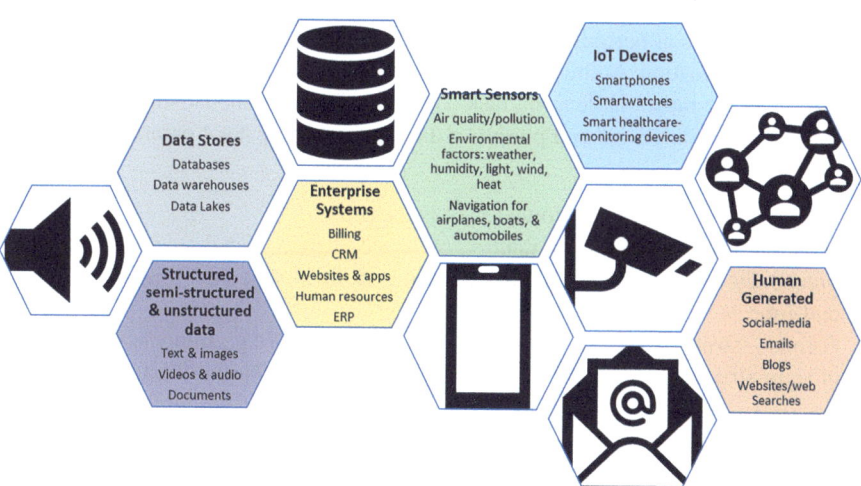

Fig. 11 Different data sources. (Source: Own figure)

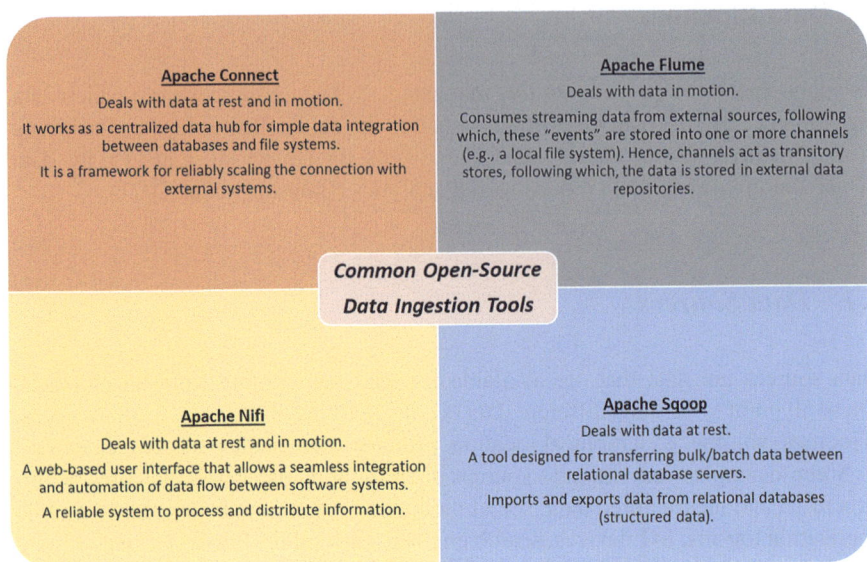

Fig. 12 Common open-source data ingestion tools. (Source: Own figure)

3.1.2 What Exactly Is Data Ingestion?

It is the process of bringing data into the data processing system. Data, especially unstructured data, is moved from where it originated into a system where it can be stored and analyzed. Hence, it is put somewhere where it can be accessed. Data can be streamed in real time or ingested in batches. When it is ingested in real-time, it is ingested nearly as soon as it is created. When data is ingested in batches, data is ingested in chunks at periodic time intervals.

Big Data Ingestion Architecture, the process of building it, and its necessary platforms, is the most challenging task. Data flowing from thousands of sources in various formats is ingested and put into a data center. There are 4 parameters of data ingestion:

- Velocity—the continuous flow at massive speeds.
- Size—enormous volumes of data.
- Frequency—in batch (stored in batches and fixed at some time interval) or real-time.
- Format—structured (e.g., tabular form), unstructured (e.g., images, audio files), or semi-structured (e.g., JSON files (JavaScript Object Notation), CSS files).

Effective data ingestion starts by prioritizing the different data sources, validating the individual files, and routing data items to their correct destination. That is why data should be ingested using the right tools. Various technologies deal with the various steps involved in data ingestion (Fig. 12).

3.2 Data Storage and Retrieval

This layer focuses on how and where to store large amounts of data efficiently. There are two main types of storage: batch and streaming storage. Batch storage is aimed at dealing with large volumes of Big Data. Specialized data stores are needed for streaming and real-time data.

The data storage layer is one of the most important layers as it is where the data lakes occur. Consequently, many Big Data projects often fail due to the inability to focus on and build this layer.

3.2.1 Batch Storage

In Big Data, this is a distributed file-based system. New Big Data tools have been developed to allow organizations to store and analyze large volumes of data effectively. Hadoop is an open-source framework that Yahoo developed with the aim of allowing reliable, scalable, and distributed storage computing. It was developed to bring together storage and computing. It is very well suited to store all forms of Big Data, particularly unstructured and semi-structured. The data stored in Hadoop is then moved into a data warehouse, which distributes the data into data marts where end users can query and analyze the data.

With the introduction of public clouds (as a result of technical evolution), there has been a critical shift in terms of Big Data storage affordability and cost-efficiency for companies. These clouds offer different services for storage and processing.

3.2.2 Streaming Storage

In 2006, Hadoop was designed to address the volume and variety of Big Data. However, as technology continued to develop, the speed at which data started being produced rose exponentially. This then needed to be addressed since there are many instances when data needs to be stored, processed, and analyzed as soon as it is generated. As a result, modern technologies were created to solve this problem.

Open-source technologies include Apache Kafka and Apache Pulsar as distributed streaming technologies. Apache Kafka, created by LinkedIn in 2011, has been more successful in adoption and use by companies. The platform allows high throughput and low latency for real-time streaming analytic data pipelines. Other cloud technologies used for real-time data ingestion and storage include Microsoft Azure Event Hubs, Amazon MSK, and Google Cloud Pub/Sub.

3.3 Data Processing, Preparation, and Model Training

This layer retrieves data from the storage layer and processes it to extract insights. Different transformative techniques are applied to the data that are primarily determined by the dimensions of the data and the type of analytics to be applied to it (Table 4).

Batch and stream processing are important analytical techniques to know about.

Batch processing collects the data in groups (batches) and processes them. This output can be an input for another process. This is suitable for large amounts of data, the processing of which is neither time-sensitive nor critical. Such a process is commonly used in billing, payroll, and data warehouses, where data is collected in batches and analyzed over time. This typically occurs offline since it takes hours to days to finish. This batch data is processed from the batch data store.

Stream processing is the real-time processing of data in a continuous manner as events create it. To further classify real-time processing, the time it takes for such processing is divided into four phases (Balusamy et al. 2021):

- Macro-batch—takes more than 15 min.
- Micro—occurs within 2 to 15 min.
- Near real time—100 ms to 2 min.
- Real time—less than 100 ms.

A few years ago, these processing tasks were done separately. Nowadays, modern tools implement a unified processing approach wherein both batch and stream processing can be dealt with using just one technology. Apache Spark, developed in 2014, is an example and an exceedingly popular one at that.

3.4 Extract, Transform, and Load (ETL)

ETL is the general procedure of copying data from one or many sources into a defined destination system that represents the data differently. The first phase extracts data from databases into what is known as the staging area. The staging area

Table 4 Different types of data dimensions and analytics that determine data processing techniques used

Data dimensions	Type of analytics
Volumes of data (large vs. small)	Artificial Intelligence processing
Latency (high/fast vs. low/slow)	Batch processing
Data in motion vs. data at rest	Stream processing
Offline vs. online	Unified processing (batch and stream)
–	Graph processing
–	SQL processing

Source: Own table

is where the transformation processing occurs, quite like the concept of a physical workbench. These transformations can be done internally by internally set procedures and/or using third-party applications. This transformed data is then loaded into information system databases as loadable tables and file formats.

The extraction process combines all data from several source databases and moves it into the staging area. It is important to note that the extraction process only involves the copying of the data, and it does not in any way alter it. The extraction can be either cross-sectional, a snapshot of the company's data at a particular point in time, or longitudinal, referred to as an incremental extract, whereby changes in the data are detected since the last extraction process.

The transformation process conforms and consolidates the data according to the business user's needs, following which it is loaded into the data warehouse. Such transformation processes are outlined in Table 5.

There exists another process called ELT. The order of execution is different from ETL. Loading of the data occurs before the transformation. This is because ELT is often used in conjunction with data lakes. On moving extracted data, it is stored in its original format in the data lake and then transformed. Hence, with ELT, a staging area is not needed (Gorelik 2019) (Table 5).

In the load process, loadable files and/or tables are moved into the data warehouse in the ETL process or the data lake in an ELT process.

The ETL process is good for maintaining data quality, security, and compliance. However, it lacks flexibility for ingesting unstructured data at high speeds. Contrarily, ELT is faster in ingesting raw data and more flexible in integrating it with other storage solutions and data analytical strategies. However, this occurs at a cost for data security and compliance.

Data warehouses have been evolved and optimized in such a way as to support business intelligence processes for high-level reporting. This is primarily done by transforming data into a relational format prior to loading it into the enterprise data warehouse. Conversely, with ELT, raw data is sent to the data lake, and it is there that transformational processes are applied post-loading. Thus, ELT bypasses the need for a staging area. This removes the option for masking personal health

Table 5 The main procedures followed in the transformation processes

Transformation process	Description
Data Cleaning	• Fixing errors & missing data • Make sure data comply with business rules
Data Conforming	• Provide consistent codes • Standardize any measuring units • Rename and restructure tables so that they make sense to the user • Ensure consistent and correct data labeling for attributes and tables (this is master data management)
Data Delivery	• Redesign data model structures to be used with specific tools by users • Prepare loadable files and database tables to be successfully loaded into the data warehouse

Source: Own table

information (PHI) and personal identifier information (PII), as per the industry's specific compliance requirements, prior to loading. For some organizations, the cost of such a risk is too high. Hence, they either use ETL processes only or use a hybrid approach: the ETLT *(Extract, Transform, Load, Transform)*. The benefit of ETLT is that it speeds up data ingestion while maintaining data security and compliance with the adhered standards. The process is summarized as follows:

1. Extracting raw data from various sources is the first step, and loading it into the staging area.
2. Transformations are made in a pre-load stage that are light, quick, and fast. Particularly removal, or encryption, of PHI, PII, and any other identifiable information. This is done one data source at a time, not simultaneously, each with an independent process.
3. Loading the lightly transformed pre-loaded data into the data warehouse.
4. Transformations are then made post-loading. This step is a complex and multi-source transformation process.

A particular use case for ETLT would be in the case of General Data Protection Regulation (GDPR) standards. The GDPR states that a data controller must pseudonymize data by implementing data masking procedures to any PHI and PII data before loading it. Other confidentiality and privacy acts worth mentioning include HIPAA (Health Insurance Portability & Accountability Act) and the CCPA (California Consumer Privacy Act) in the United States (DAMA International 2017) (Table 6).

Table 6 Comparative benefits of ETL, ELT & ETLT

ETL	ELT	ETLT
Maintenance of data security and compliance.	Rapid data ingestion with no staging area needed. This is good for real-time streaming.	Data security and compliance standards are adhered to.
Greater ability to manage larger datasets since any unnecessary or duplicate information is removed prior to the data being loaded into the data warehouse.	Data that might be needed later is saved and not discarded before loading.	Faster data ingestion of all types of raw data.
The data warehouse processing fees are not more costly than in ELT. Rather, it may appear cheaper with ELT because all the processing is shifted to the data warehouse and is not, in truth, bypassed in any way.	Data is only transformed when needed for specific business use cases. These can be changed, including the data transformation needed to address it.	Greater flexibility in data transformation because different post-load transformations can be done according to the analyses in question.
Data quality is maintained through the standardization and transformation of data in batches.	The transformations are usually done in SQL—a popular coding language. Thus there is no need to find and hire specific people to do this. It is also less costly.	Handles multiple sources and data redundancy.

Source: Own table

3.4.1 Data Serving

Data serving mainly refers to processed data that is ready to be delivered and served to consumer applications. The data in this layer can have many use cases, and each case has its own requirements for representation and accessibility that need to be met.

This data serving is typically conducted through a server platform, that provides services according to other consumer software applications and/or hardware systems.

4 Designing Data Pipelines

A healthcare data pipeline, as the name implies, involves the connection of various technological processes, organized systematically, that reflect and support raw data flow in real life. This permits the movement and transformation of medical data between systems. Further, a high-quality data pipeline allows all healthcare systems and institutions to have timely access to recent, accurate, reliable, and scalable medical data that provides the essence for accurate diagnosis, prognosis, and sustainability in maintaining and upgrading all systems.

Moreover, the unification of all health records gives a broader view of the patient's past, current, and prospective well-being. Healthcare is in an era of preventive and predictive care; thus, data credibility is another important facet of any healthcare data pipeline. Accurate medical data will help drive positive prospective patient results, whereas inaccurate and unreliable medical data can have unintended consequences on patients' health. Having the knowledge, skill, insight, foresight, and vision to develop and sustain high-quality data pipelines is a prerequisite for any healthcare system or institution.

To consolidate and present the best architectural pipeline, all the different steps need to be prepared and presented using appropriate visualizations that represent the entire process. The goal of such an exercise is to gain a graphical perspective that adds value to the concept of what can be done, what cannot, what can be improved, and any bottlenecks that need to be addressed.

Documenting data pipelines lays the foundational groundwork for long-term implementation strategies. Delving deeper into this, we might face situations where a specific data source lacks in-built automation, data connectors, or integrations. There can be an instance wherein the initial step of any project will entail manual intervention, including the extraction of data to a specific location. All these processes and parts need to be identified, automated if possible, and ameliorated.

4.1 Visualizing Data Pipelines

Data pipelines come in different sizes and shapes. Moreover, they act on data asynchronously with long time intervals that are demanded by mechanisms. These may be in the range of weekly reporting or a real-time, large-scale modus operandi, as seen in medical devices that are connected to the Internet of Medical Things (IoMT). Nonetheless, it is essential to mention the three main aspects:

- Origin (Input)
- Data flow (Process)
- Destination (Output)

The data flow component brings together several different aspects that take care of storage, processing steps, workflow, and monitoring. Ensuring coverage of all these different aspects increases your chances of long-term success and sustainability.

4.2 Documentation and Data Engineering Lifecycles

Designing data pipelines can be done on any medium, and multiple tools are available for visualization. The DeMarco Notation (Ghezzi et al. 2002) is an excellent framework to start with. The basic symbols of this notation are: a) arrows (dataflow), circles (process), horizontal line pairs (file) and rectangular box (data source, sink).

After the first step of graphically designing the data pipeline, several complex processes can be outlined. The pipeline diagram needs to be substantiated with additional details that aid quick project implementation. These specific details are brought about by questions such as: must the data be processed in real time? Can it be updated daily? Will it be modeled for use in a dashboard or as input to a Machine-Learning model? These questions shape the various parts of the pipeline, especially in mission-critical organizations such as healthcare and public health (Chonho et al. 2017). Developing this documentation usually lies in the hands of Data Engineers, who in the public health realm most probably would be all-rounders covering different aspects of the data engineering lifecycle. As such, it's critical to mention that as you start developing these pipelines and immerse further into this work you need to also keep in mind the Data Engineering Lifecycle (Generation, Storage, Ingestion, Transformation and Serving Data) and the relevant undercurrents. These undercurrents are now playing a more important role than ever, as they encompass the whole lifecycle and can break or make a data project, such as, security, data management, DataOps, Data Architecture, Orchestration and last but not least, Software Engineering.

5 Conclusion and Takeaway Messages

It has been estimated that in 2024 the world produced 140 zettabytes of information. By the end of 2025, 80% of organizations seeking to scale businesses will fail because they do not take a modern approach to data and analytics governance. This is not only limited to the conventional understanding of a corporate organization but also any governmental and non-profit entity. A consequence of not seeing data from the business perspective will result in a negative return on investment, loss of resources, and increasing costs. By 2026, 20% of high-performing organizations will use connected governance to scale and execute their digital ambitions. The healthcare industry, together with public health, must step up its approach to data to be able to maintain recency, interoperability, accessibility, and usability of health data and healthcare system infrastructure to ensure efficient responses in a health crisis and to further develop innovative treatments. Digital services in the health domain have become an indistinguishable and indispensable component in their functionality and serviceability.

Using the acquired knowledge from this chapter, supplemented with any additional informative resources, public health specialists and other healthcare professionals have the advantage of building, developing, and deploying the necessary assessments, projects, studies, and innovative ideas. This can be done sustainably and effectively in advancing data-driven health-related policies, procedures, recommendations, and legal frameworks.

Data has become a dynamic and ever-growing aspect of our lives. We're now seeing policy making efforts that starting to bear fruit as seem for example from the perspective of the European Union, where an intensive three year legislative process has concluded, resulting in the publication of the European Health Data Space (EHDS) Regulation (European Commission 2025) It is clear to see that Health Data, Data Engineering, Data Science in close association with strong data governance have the potential to dramatically transform the Public Health sector and revolutionize health systems.

References

Balusamy B, Abirami N, Kadry S, Gandomi AH (2021) Big data: concepts, technology, and architecture. Wiley, Hoboken

Cavanillas JM, Curry E, Wahlster W (2016) New horizons for a data-driven economy, 1st edn. Springer, Cham. https://doi.org/10.1007/978-3-319-21569-3

CDC (2023) Improving public health data pipelines | technologies | CDC. https://www.cdc.gov/surveillance/data-modernization/technologies/public-health-data-pipelines.html. Accessed 30 Mar 2023.

Chonho L, Murata S, Ishigaki K, Date S (2017) A data analytics pipeline for smart healthcare applications. https://doi.org/10.1007/978-3-319-66896-3_12

DAMA International (2017) DAMA-DMBOK: data management body of knowledge. Technics Publications, LLC, Denville

Databricks (2021) What are ACID transactions?. https://www.databricks.com/glossary/acid-transactions. Accessed 1 Apr 2023.

DIGITALEUROPE Ecosystem Digital Twins in Healthcare (EDITH). n.d. https://www.edith-csa.eu/. Accessed 30 Mar 2023.

European Commission (2025) European Health Data Space. https://health.ec.europa.eu/ehealth-digital-health-and-care/europeanhealth-data-space_en. Accessed 30 Apr 2025.

Fronza EM, Barochia Rishit G, Sunil G (2022) Building a healthcare data pipeline on AWS with IBM Cloud Pak for Data. https://aws.amazon.com/blogs/architecture/building-a-healthcare-data-pipeline-on-aws-with-ibm-cloud-pak-for-data/. Accessed 30 Mar 2023.

Ghezzi C, Jazayeri M, Mandrioli D (2002) Fundamentals of software engineering. Prentice Hall, Englewood Cliffs

Gorelik A (2019) The enterprise big data lake, 1st edn. O'Reilly Media, Sebastopol

Inmon WH (2002) Building the data warehouse, 1st edn. Wiley, Hoboken

Knight M (2022) What is a data lake?. https://www.dataversity.net/what-is-a-data-lake/. Accessed 30 Mar 2023.

Nelson G (2017) A practical guide to healthcare data: tips, traps and techniques. https://support.sas.com/resources/papers/proceedings17/0831-2017.pdf Accessed 30 Mar 2023.

Panesar A (2021) Machine learning and AI for healthcare—big data for improved health outcomes. Apress, Berkeley

Open Access This chapter is licensed under the terms of the Creative Commons Attribution 4.0 International License (http://creativecommons.org/licenses/by/4.0/), which permits use, sharing, adaptation, distribution and reproduction in any medium or format, as long as you give appropriate credit to the original author(s) and the source, provide a link to the Creative Commons license and indicate if changes were made.

The images or other third party material in this chapter are included in the chapter's Creative Commons license, unless indicated otherwise in a credit line to the material. If material is not included in the chapter's Creative Commons license and your intended use is not permitted by statutory regulation or exceeds the permitted use, you will need to obtain permission directly from the copyright holder.

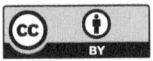

Digital Public Health: An Outlook

Hajo Zeeb, Laura Maaß, Ulrike Haug, Iris Pigeot, Tanja Schultz, and Benjamin Schüz

Abstract This chapter provides a summary overview and an outlook towards different pathways which the future of digital public health may take. We discuss three somewhat distinct potential scenarios, including a dystopian view, a slow transformation scenario and comprehensively digitalized public health landscape, while also summarizing core insights from different chapters of this book.

Keywords Digital public health · Equity, ethics · Empowerment · Future scenarios

The preceding chapters touch upon a broad range of topics in digital public health. They provide ample evidence of the diverse and dynamic, extremely interdisciplinary character of the field, as well as of the fact that many potential developments are still in their infancy. Naturally, this also includes possible consequences of the further digitalization of public health, be it with respect to public health outcomes, interaction and participation, or the digital divide.

In our view, there are three core themes that act as a common thread through the chapters of this handbook: equity aspects (digital divide), ethical aspects (including privacy and data protection), and autonomy/empowerment.

H. Zeeb (✉) · U. Haug · I. Pigeot
Leibniz Institute for Prevention Research and Epidemiology—BIPS, Bremen, Germany
e-mail: zeeb@leibniz-bips.de; haug@leibniz-bips.de; pigeot@leibniz-bips.de

L. Maaß
SOCIUM—Research Center on Inequality and Social Policy, University of Bremen, Bremen, Germany
e-mail: laura.maass@uni-bremen.de

T. Schultz
Cognitive Systems Lab, University of Bremen, Bremen, Germany
e-mail: tanja.schultz@uni-bremen.de

B. Schüz
Institute of Public Health and Nursing Research, University of Bremen, Bremen, Germany
e-mail: benjamin.schuez@uni-bremen.de

Chapter "A Framework to Develop and Evaluate Digital Public Health Interventions" presents a framework for systematically developing digital tools that considers equity aspects. At the same time, chapter "Digital Health Inequality" on the digital divide has illustrated many other issues relevant to social inequalities in the use and benefit of digital tools for public health. However, on a level beyond usability and reach, there are problems created by differential patterns of engagement with digital (public) health tools according to socioeconomic factors. Namely, differential engagement with such tools generates skewed analytic data as well as training data for digital public health tools. Individuals from socioeconomically disadvantaged backgrounds are less likely to volunteer their data for health-related research or engage with (generic and non-tailored) digital health tools; those who do tend to be either particularly interested in health-related matters or personally affected by health problems. This has to be considered in the data interpretation, particularly if the aim is to develop targeted approaches for disadvantaged populations.

The increasing digitalization of public health touches upon the autonomy of individuals and groups, whether it be through functions delivered, medical information sought, or health and social interactions shared. Here, in particular, the autonomy to share or withhold health-related personal data is relevant, but also whether and how digital public health tools allow and cater to individual behavioral decisions—be they health-promoting or not. Many of the great promises of increasing digitalization in public health, such as faster and more reliable monitoring systems, digital infection control systems such as proximity tracking, or individual behavioral recommendations for the prevention of chronic or non-communicable diseases, rely on gathering, processing, and predicting upon large amounts of (personal) data. To which degree individual autonomous decisions to maintain privacy are outweighed by public interest in disease prevention is, in turn, a matter for societal contracts. Differences even between EU countries (with a shared data protection legislation) in their handling of the COVID-19 pandemic provide a stark illustration of these contrasts when considering the type, amount, and usefulness of data available to evaluate, for example, the effectiveness of non-pharmaceutical interventions. To illustrate this point, while Danish data allowed for the estimation of infection risks for vaccinated vs. non-vaccinated family members through data linkage, Germany largely refrained from recording COVID vaccinations within health insurance records and, therefore, will remain unable to conduct similar evaluations in the absence of a vaccination registry.

Privacy and autonomy in the digital space can be threatened by malicious attacks. Cybersecurity—also termed information technology security—is a topic to which we have not devoted a chapter in this handbook partly because this topic would deserve much more space. Even a few chapters would not suffice to adequately provide insights into developments, core issues, regulations, and a plethora of other aspects related to cybersecurity. We also note that cybersecurity is not an issue that specifically impacts digital public health; however, this argument holds for many of the issues discussed in the handbook. Nevertheless, overall developments, discussions, and regulations on cybersecurity will be highly relevant to digital public health.

Digital Public Health: An Outlook

These issues of cybersecurity may well be among the most decisive ones when thinking about possible scenarios in the future development of digital public health. In addition, the discussion on artificial intelligence is rapidly accelerating, and serious risks for public health (and more) have been highlighted. In an attempt to provide a basic structure for discussions regarding the future of digital public health and its fast-changing context, we outline the following scenarios[1] and invite their use and adaptation:

1 Scenario 1: Digital Public Health Dystopia

Mistrust and division have reached unprecedented levels, leading to a substantial disruption of digital communication and the fulfillment of public health functions. This collapse of the digital public health infrastructure exacerbates existing global health challenges and results in dire consequences for individuals and communities worldwide. The rapid spread of misinformation and fragmentation of communication channels, as well as increasing hacker attacks, lead to an erosion of the public health infrastructure. Furthermore, this collapse of trust and communication channels triggers a loss of funding and resources for digital public health development. Without reliable information, marginalized communities face even greater struggles to access accurate health guidance and resources, leading to increased health disparities. Inequities widen, exacerbating existing social and economic divisions.

2 Scenario 2: Slow but Continuous Digital Transformation

The digital transformation advances slower than anticipated by some, as there are many barriers and competing topics, including crises outside the health system. Stakeholders are being engaged in participatory approaches, and the advancement of digital public health is constantly negotiated, with some aspects of current systems where digitalization seems a useful advance changing quickly, whereas others remain largely non-digitalized or transform at a slow pace given that there is limited or no evidence for advantages of digital approaches. Major areas of public health—namely community-based health promotion and public health work with the elderly and marginalized communities—remain strongly analog, using digitalization only

---

[1] In order to illustrate and examine the potential of large language models to discuss public health problems, we asked ChatGPT for a dystopian, an optimistic and a mixed future scenario for the use of digital technology in public health. Somewhat fitting, the dystopian scenario produced corresponded most closely with our own considerations and is therefore reproduced here. The optimistic and mixed future AI-generated scenarios however were much less conscionable with current data and evidence.

on distinct topics and occasions. This slow evolution, however, also leads to sluggish investment and development of public health in general.

3 Scenario 3: Public Health Is Digital

In this scenario, the digital transformation dynamics have increased, and public health functions, in sum, are now mainly fulfilled through digital communication channels and digital tools. Improved and equitable technological access and digital health literacy of individuals, organizations, and systems have become cornerstones of public health advancements, thereby also enhancing trustful exchange and partnerships. Citizens, providers, and other stakeholders communicate mainly digitally, and public health capacity building across all levels includes a major digital skills and services component. The digital divide has been recognized as a core threat, and active countermeasures are taken. Artificial intelligence (AI) is firmly governed by effective regulation and control mechanisms. AI tools are successfully being harnessed as everyday support tailored to public health needs and challenges in local and global circumstances.

These scenarios are certainly not the only ones possible, and there may be good arguments to believe that what we actually expect concerning future digital public health lies somewhere in between. Glimpses of the dystopic scenario No.1 were revealed during the COVID-19 pandemic, where the unholy role of social media, but also the discussions around state actors digitally controlling citizens in the name of public health, came to the forefront. Scenario No. 2 is familiar to many public health stakeholders in both industrialized as well as low- and middle-income countries. However, this scenario can always swerve towards other paths and change speed, for example, in the light of public health crises. Scenario No. 3, as the "positivistic" outlook on digital public health, puts firm belief in an enlightened approach to digitalization in public health, but there are many caveats and learnings necessary to even come close to some of the outlined developments.

In order to turn mainly commercially driven and revenue-oriented development into supporting essential public health services, multinational regulatory approaches are required—which in turn depend on broad societal contracts. Realistic expectations regarding infodemics and mistrust, as well as the huge commercial potential of digital communication that does not always align with public health aims, speak against Scenario No. 3 being an uncontested "winner." Still, the hope and aspiration of public health at large must be that more of this optimistic scenario and less of scenario No. 1 come true.

Strong interdisciplinary cooperation between information and communication technology (ICT), public health, medical, legal, and social science experts (to name a few), as well as a focus on participation and open discussion, will be crucial to advance and develop digital public health in the coming years and decades. There is little doubt that major public health challenges, such as the health and social consequences of climate change, will require intelligent and sustainable use of digital approaches to understand, monitor, and provide solutions to the myriad of problems and factors expected to shape the health of populations in this century and beyond.

The theme of digitalization supporting the achievement of public health aims is also at the heart of the Leibniz Science Campus Digital Public Health Bremen (LSC DiPH), which commences its second phase just after the contributions for this book have been finalized. In this second phase, the campus (represented in this book through many chapter authors) will focus on applying, testing, and expanding the findings and framework reported in this book to address real-world public health problems and sustainably improve population health. As digitization continues to be a core issue in the modernization and adaptation of public health and health systems, there is a need for high-quality, interdisciplinary research to proactively shape this development instead of merely following technological advances.

Key issues remain: improving accessibility and equity of digital public health, developing and applying appropriate methods to produce high-quality evidence to support public health decision-making, and systematically outlining and determining needs and opportunities for digital technology in public health. LSC DiPH is located at the center of these issues and will provide applied research in three major domains: (i) bridging the digital divide through addressing digital literacy needs, developing participatory approaches to digital public health, and supporting the public health workforce in the digital transformation; (ii) making digital technology useful for primary and secondary prevention through generating quality standards, establishing indicators, and systematically support the translation of analog into digital formats where indicated; (iii) guiding public health-related interactions between humans and digital systems through research on dark patterns in digital health tools, developing approaches to combat health-related misinformation in social and other digital media, and improving informed consent procedures to privacy and data protection procedures.

To do this, close interdisciplinary collaboration and the development of new research paradigms is indispensable. We have been fortunate enough to be able to integrate excellent local and international researchers into our campus, and we have been privileged to work with excellent early-career researchers who, through collaborative supervision arrangements, facilitated interdisciplinary work and generated many novel perspectives and questions. We hope that this book and the perspectives developed herein will inspire more research on this critical junction of health sciences, information and communication technology, social sciences and humanities and invite new partners to join us on this research journey. Our door is open for new collaborations, and we look forward to furthering research into this vital topic together.

Open Access This chapter is licensed under the terms of the Creative Commons Attribution 4.0 International License (http://creativecommons.org/licenses/by/4.0/), which permits use, sharing, adaptation, distribution and reproduction in any medium or format, as long as you give appropriate credit to the original author(s) and the source, provide a link to the Creative Commons license and indicate if changes were made.

The images or other third party material in this chapter are included in the chapter's Creative Commons license, unless indicated otherwise in a credit line to the material. If material is not included in the chapter's Creative Commons license and your intended use is not permitted by statutory regulation or exceeds the permitted use, you will need to obtain permission directly from the copyright holder.